MW00562405

PRACTICAL APPROACH TO
Electroencephalography

SECOND EDITION

PRACTICAL APPROACH TO
Electroencephalography

Mark H. Libenson, MD

Director, Clinical Neurophysiology Laboratories
Boston Children's Hospital
Department of Neurology
Harvard Medical School
Boston, Massachusetts
United States

ELSEVIER

Elsevier
1600 John F. Kennedy Blvd.
Ste 1800
Philadelphia, PA 19103-2899

PRACTICAL APPROACH TO ELECTROENCEPHALOGRAPHY, SECOND EDITION   ISBN: 978-0-443-34836-5

Copyright © 2025 by Elsevier, Inc. All rights are reserved, including those for text and data mining, AI training, and similar technologies.

Publisher's note: Elsevier takes a neutral position with respect to territorial disputes or jurisdictional claims in its published content, including in maps and institutional affiliations.

No part of this publication may be reproduced or transmitted in any form or by any means, electronic or mechanical, including photocopying, recording, or any information storage and retrieval system, without permission in writing from the publisher. Details on how to seek permission, further information about the Publisher's permissions policies and our arrangements with organizations such as the Copyright Clearance Center and the Copyright Licensing Agency, can be found at our website: www.elsevier.com/permissions.

This book and the individual contributions contained in it are protected under copyright by the Publisher (other than as may be noted herein).

Notice

Practitioners and researchers must always rely on their own experience and knowledge in evaluating and using any information, methods, compounds or experiments described herein. Because of rapid advances in the medical sciences, in particular, independent verification of diagnoses and drug dosages should be made. To the fullest extent of the law, no responsibility is assumed by Elsevier, authors, editors or contributors for any injury and/or damage to persons or property as a matter of product liability, negligence or otherwise, or from any use or operation of any methods, products, instructions, or ideas contained in the material herein.

Previous edition copyrighted 2010

Content Strategist: Mary Hegeler
Senior Content Development Specialist: Rishabh Gupta
Publishing Services Manager: Shereen Jameel
Project Manager: Gayathri S
Design Direction: Ryan Cook

Printed in India

Last digit is the print number: 9   8   7   6   5   4   3   2   1

Working together
to grow libraries in
developing countries

www.elsevier.com • www.bookaid.org

To Pearl, Lisa, Sara, Andrew, David, and Julia; and to the next generation, Nathan, Isla, Danny, and Vinny, for their love and support

CONTRIBUTORS

Aristides Hadjinicolaou, MD, FRCPC, CSCN (EEG)
Division of Neurology
Department of Pediatrics
Centre Hospitalier Universitaire Sainte-Justine;
Assistant Professor
Department of Neurosciences
Université de Montréal
Montreal, Quebec
Canada

Avantika Singh, MD
Comprehensive Epilepsy Program
Division of Child Neurology
Children's Wisconsin;
Assistant Professor of Neurology
Medical College of Wisconsin
Milwaukee, Wisconsin
United States

ACKNOWLEDGMENTS

Practical Approach to Electroencephalography is based on a personal experience of learning, practicing, and teaching Clinical Neurophysiology and Neurology; as such, many of the ideas presented here reflect concepts shared with me or taught to me by others. No doubt, one of the joys of practicing medicine is the free flow of ideas and culture of teaching among the colleagues and students who work around us and I have benefited immensely from that culture. I consider myself fortunate to have learned the art and science of reading EEGs from a group of extraordinary neurophysiologists, including Drs. Gregory Holmes, Edward Bromfield, and Bruce Ehrenberg, to name a few who provided foundational teaching to me early in my career. I am indebted to many colleagues, past and present, at the Floating Hospital for Children at Tufts Medical Center and at Boston Children's Hospital for what they have taught me. I am also grateful for the expertise of the EEG technologists of those institutions where many of the tracings used in this text were recorded. This is a group of extraordinary professionals who work around the clock and make an invaluable contribution to the care of people with epilepsy and neurologic disorders.

Dr. David Preston has provided invaluable assistance and inspiration at all stages of this project, for both editions of this text, including the initial suggestion that I begin the project. I would also like to thank Jeffrey Marcus, PhD, for his advice and expertise in the fields of electronics and digital signal processing. Dr. Phillip Pearl is a longtime friend and colleague who has provided unwavering support and expert advice in the preparation of this second edition. I would also like to thank the outstanding faculty of the European Stereo EEG Course for sharing their deep knowledge of epilepsy and invasive monitoring.

I wish to thank my editors at Elsevier, including Mary Hegeler, who helped shepherd this project to completion, along with the able development and production staff at Elsevier. I am also grateful for the exceptional expertise of the librarians at the Boston Children's Hospital Library and the Francis Countway Library of Medicine at Harvard Medical School for their wizardry in helping to track down obscure materials with impressive speed.

I would like to thank the many fellows, residents, and students whom I have taught and who have taught me, often by making insightful observations and posing questions that have helped me to think through some of the difficult concepts of Clinical Neurophysiology.

Finally, I would like to thank my wife, Lisa Muto. Without her support—both emotional and editorial—this project would not have been possible.

FOREWORD TO THE SECOND EDITION

From the historical underpinnings of electroencephalography (EEG) to the recent revamping of intensive care monitoring terminology, Mark Libenson has produced the second edition of his renowned text on the fundamentals of understanding and interpreting EEG.

Long considered the primer every neurology resident and aspiring EEGer seeks, this conversational yet concise and highly illustrated book affords the reader the tools needed to understand and interpret EEG. We have used this book year after year in our fellowship program in Epilepsy and Clinical Neurophysiology at Boston Children's Hospital, forming the foundation upon which EEGers understand and use the concepts of montage selection, artifacts, filters, and localization, in addition to a thorough grounding of the normal EEG at all ages. Examples and strategies for the process of EEG localization demystify this process and other aspects of EEG reading, finally providing a truly practical approach to understanding the EEG recording.

There is an exciting, extensive discussion on the age-old question "Where do EEG waves come from?" that includes explanations of ion channels, transmembrane potentials, postsynaptic potentials, and the action potential. The exposition on filters, with detailed discussion on resistor-capacitor (RC) circuits and their role in creating filters of different bandpasses, or frequency ranges, is crucial for a scientific understanding of EEG, one that has eluded many readers.

Following these initial chapters is coverage of EEG background abnormalities, normal variants, epileptiform discharges, and effective EEG report writing. The chapter on the EEG in Epilepsy has been thoroughly updated to conform to the 2017 ILAE terminology that changed the lexicon of seizures and epilepsy. The ACNS 2021 published revisions in ICU EEG terminology are explained in a completely revised chapter on patterns encountered in the intensive care unit. Neonatal and intracranial EEG are covered, both conceptually and in a real-world manner. This is why our fellows, and ourselves, have sought to cover this book for a basic grounding in the principles of EEG used every day in the clinical laboratory. This book is also for the neurology resident, intensive care resident, or other learner to master the art and science of electroencephalography.

As one of multiple metaphors used in Dr. Libenson's warm and clear writing, learning EEG is like driving a car. The classroom sessions are nice, but they cannot replace getting behind the wheel. This marvelous teaching text puts one "behind the wheel," in the EEGer's seat, and gets the reader up to speed so that any record in any situation can be handled with expertise, confidence, and the ability to properly convey the results and meaning of an EEG for clinical care. There could be no better legacy for a teacher of electroencephalography. Kudos on the publication of this edition!

Phillip L. Pearl, MD
Director, Division of Epilepsy and Clinical Neurophysiology
Boston Children's Hospital
William G. Lennox Chair and Professor of Neurology
Harvard Medical School
Boston, Massachusetts

During my neurology training in the 1970s, I learned a great deal from my mentors about how to take care of patients with neurologic disorders. In those pre–computed tomography (CT) and magnetic resonance imaging (MRI) days, we depended a great deal on the history and neurologic examination of a patient, as well as the most valuable ancillary test available: the electroencephalogram (EEG). In addition to helping us determine whether the patient had epilepsy, the EEG provided information regarding the presence or absence of structural lesions, the cause of the metabolic encephalopathy, or the type of encephalitis the patient had. With the advent of CT and MRI, we are now able to image the brain in exquisite detail. The arrival of these neuroimaging techniques led some of my teachers to suggest that the EEG would be relegated to a secondary role in the evaluation of patients with neurologic disorders. While my professors were correct about many things, in this case they were mistaken.

Even as embracing new imaging technologies is warranted, it is now clear that the EEG is becoming more, not less, important in the assessment of individuals with a wide variety of neurologic disorders. Rather than looking at structure at a fixed moment in time, electroencephalography allows one to assess physiological function over time and across sleep and wake states. This ability to assess physiological function second by second over extended periods of time provides data that simply are not matched by those of other technologies.

Although Hans Berger discovered the EEG in the 1920s, it has not remained static; rather, new technology has been added, and the EEG has matured into a time-tested diagnostic test. The digitalization of analogue signals has dramatically increased the information base and flexibility of EEG, greatly expanding the usefulness of the test. Although collecting and displaying this enormously powerful data has become easier, the challenge for physicians is to correctly interpret the findings.

It is therefore timely that Mark Libenson has written *Practical Approach to Electroenchephalography*, a book beautifully designed to teach learners to understand both the physiological and technological basis of the study and to interpret the findings. Although there are other excellent authoritarian textbooks on electroencephalography available, this book fills an important gap by providing a practical approach to how to evaluate the EEG. For the individual new to the field, the book provides an excellent starting point, taking the reader from EEG basic principles to constructing a useful report. Clearly written and beautifully illustrated with more than 450 high-quality figures, the book is a pleasure to read and study.

Although EEG can be useful in the evaluation of patients with a wide gamut of neurologic disorders, it is most widely used in epilepsy. The EEG can provide information on seizure type, epileptic syndrome, and etiology, and is widely used for localization of the seizure onset zone. Understanding the EEG signature of the epileptic syndromes is a critical step in the diagnosis and management of epilepsy. Knowing the importance of epileptic syndromes, Dr. Libenson has devoted an entire chapter to epilepsy, emphasizing the EEG findings of the epilepsy syndromes.

There is little doubt that this book will be widely studied. I plan to recommend it for our neurology residents and clinical neurophysiology fellows. However, this book is not just for trainees; seasoned veterans will learn a lot from Dr. Libenson. I know I did.

Gregory L. Holmes, MD
Chair, Department of Neurology
Professor of Neurology and Pediatrics
Dartmouth Medical School
Dartmouth-Hitchcock Medical Center
Lebanon, New Hampshire

More than a decade has passed since the publication of the first edition of *Practical Approach to Electroencephalography*. A couple of years ago, my editors at Elsevier asked me if I would "freshen up" (but *not* rewrite!) the first edition of this text. At first, I was not sure what there would be to add to what is substantially a "how-to" text—after all, the phase reversal of 2009 is not much different from the phase reversal of 2024. Still, over the course of time, different ways of examining and explaining concepts come to mind. As both a practitioner and teacher of electroencephalography, I have had the opportunity and delight to discuss the topics presented in this book with many outstanding learners who have asked me incisive questions and made me think of the "how-tos" and "whys" of so many things in unexpected, new ways. One of my early mentors told me that, when people give lectures, no one in the room learns more than the lecturers themselves. This idea also extends to the process of writing a textbook. There are so many things that I heard during my training that "everybody knows" about EEG, but when setting them down in a textbook, I had to ask myself whether each of these dictums was true.

What is new in this book? Although the fundamentals of interpreting an EEG have not changed substantially over the past 15 years, there are new classifications and terminologies that have at least partially replaced previous systems. This includes new nomenclature systems for both seizure types and epilepsy syndromes. As for EEG interpretation in the intensive care unit (ICU) setting, an entirely new set of guidelines for making EEG diagnoses in the ICU was put forward in 2021 and is summarized in this text. A new chapter consisting of a brief introduction to invasive EEG recording techniques for patients undergoing epilepsy surgery (an idea proposed by two excellent epileptologists who were trainees at the time and coauthored the chapter with me) has also been added. Finally, the discussion of certain concepts in neurophysiology

has also been expanded, including the electrical behavior of cell membranes and the physiological basis of the EEG.

As mentioned, the goal of this text is not to present an encyclopedic review of the field, but rather to effectively present the ideas of EEG interpretation to new learners (and some of the ideas, I hope, may be useful to more seasoned readers as well). All of us have had the feeling after having spent time mastering a new field of endeavor: if only I could have explained to my previous self the things I finally understand now—it would have saved me so much time! This text therefore, in part, attempts to be a compilation of the variety of morsels of knowledge and explanations that we wish someone had just told us about right at the outset.

When writing a textbook, there is an urge to write in an academic fashion, covering all the bases, considering every facet of the problem, and presenting the information in perhaps too much detail. I am not, however, the first to have this worry in mind when writing an introductory EEG textbook. The original example of this endeavor is *EEG in Clinical Practice* by Dr. John R. Hughes (1982). This was a beautiful little book that approached the task very successfully and which I enjoyed reading when I was an early EEG learner. Interestingly, Dr. Hughes wrote in his preface to that book that his inspiration for the style of his text was Dubin's *Rapid Interpretation of EKG's*, which he said allowed its reader in "less than two hours to arrive at approximately the same level of understanding as a reading of one of the more classical texts that required 10 to 20 hours." Of course, this text will take more than two hours to digest, but it is written with the same philosophy. One of my early mentors described electroencephalography as a "dark science." Indeed, though electroencephalography still holds mysteries for us all, I hope that this book will brighten some of the corners of this fascinating field.

Mark H. Libenson, MD

CONTENTS

Introduction to Electroencephalography

Electroencephalography (EEG) remains one of the principal tools in the practice of clinical neurology. Notwithstanding the development of increasingly sophisticated imaging techniques over the years, including computed tomography (CT) scanning, magnetic resonance imaging (MRI), nuclear medicine imaging, and newer functional MRI techniques, rather than being displaced by these newer techniques, the use of EEG in the assessment of neurological disorders continues to increase. The information learned from EEG testing differs in a number of ways from what is learned from radiological images such as MRI scans. Whereas MRI primarily furnishes anatomical information as a snapshot in time, EEG captures electrical information over time. Just as an x-ray image of the heart does not tell us whether a patient's heart is beating quickly, slowly, or erratically, information easily learned from an electrocardiogram, likewise CT and MRI scans of the brain do not give direct information regarding electrical irritability in the brain or even indicate whether the patient is awake or asleep. Thus, radiological imaging studies and electroencephalography are complementary techniques.

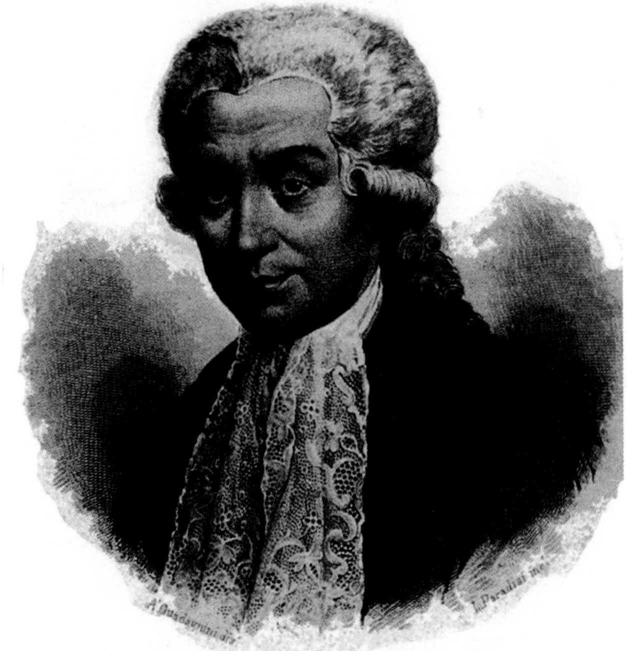

Electroencephalography is used in a variety of clinical situations, but the large majority of EEGs are obtained as a part of the evaluation of seizures or epilepsy. Estimates of the population prevalence of epilepsy range between 0.5% and 1%, suggesting that, for instance, at least 2 million people in North America have epilepsy. EEG is also useful in the evaluation of confusional states and coma, and it can play an important role in separating psychiatric illness from organic disease.

It was not always a given that electricity was an important mediator of biological processes, an idea that we take for granted today. Luigi Galvani, working at the University of Bologna, is credited with making some of the first experimental observations that demonstrated the physiological role of electricity in animal tissues (Figure 1.1). He became interested in the idea when he fortuitously saw the leg muscle of a dead frog twitch when an electrical stimulus was inadvertently applied to its lumbar nerve. He then studied this phenomenon using multiple methods and sources of electricity, including using a Leyden jar, using an electrostatic machine, and placing a copper hook into the frog's spinal cord and attaching it to an iron railing during a lightning storm (Figure 1.2). He theorized that muscle and nerve used an innate form of "animal

Figure 1.1 Luigi Galvani (1737–1798) as a young man. Galvani described the twitch of a frog's leg that was in contact with a pair of scissors during an electrical storm in his notebook in 1786, sparking his interest in the phenomenon of "animal electricity." (From Dibner B. Luigi Galvani: An expanded version of a biography prepared for the forthcoming edition of the Encyclopedia Britannica, San Marino, California, 1971, Burndy Library.)

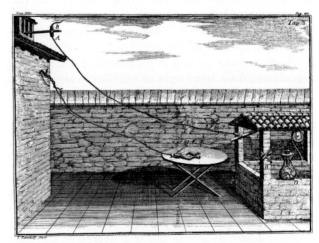

Figure 1.2 An engraving of Galvani's experiment arranged on the terrace of his house, showing that the muscles of frogs respond to atmospheric charges. The exposed, dissected frog is connected by insulated wires that lead from the chimney to the frog, and then from its foot down into the water of a well. A second frog is depicted inside the bottle (labeled 'D') sitting on the edge of the well. This engraving was a part of Galvani's 1791 doctoral dissertation, *De viribus electricitatis in motu musculari commentarius*. (Commentary on the Effects of Electricity on Muscular Motion). Courtesy of Dibner and Galvani, 1971. (From Dall'opera "De viribus electricitatis in motu musculari commentarius" - ampiamente diffusa sul web e dal copyright Scaduto, 1791.)

electricity" to function, in contrast to "natural" electricity (e.g., lightning) or an "artificial" form produced by friction (e.g., the static electricity stored in a Leyden jar). He published his findings in his dissertation, *Commentary on the Effect of Electricity on Muscular Motion*, in 1791 (Galvani, 1791).

Some of Galvani's ideas were initially challenged by the famous physicist Alessandro Volta, who worked to the north at the University of Pavia and who was the inventor of the voltaic pile or first battery, which was the first consistent source of direct current. Eventually, though, Volta came to accept Galvani's ideas and it was Volta who actually coined the term *galvanism* to refer to direct currents in an acknowledgment of Galvani's work. The classic galvanometer—the instrument named for him (and also the immediate progenitor of the more modern EEG-pen recorder), whose needle shifts left or right according to the voltage difference between wires attached to its two poles—was only invented well after Galvani's death. The device was named for him because it was felt that the concept of the twitching motion Galvani first described in the frog muscle was, in a way, the first galvanometer (Dibner, 1971).

Electroencephalography is a relatively young science. One hundred years ago, it was not yet a settled fact that there was electrical activity in the human brain. In 1875, Richard Caton was the first to report an observation of electrical activity from the brains of monkeys and rabbits, though techniques available at the time did not allow him to record these waveforms for posterity (Figure 1.3). Caton made his observations using a device called *Thomson's mirror galvanometer* (Caton, 1877). This device, invented by William Thomson (who was later elevated to the House of Lords as Lord Kelvin, and for whom the absolute temperature scale is also named), included a mirror mounted on a vertical swivel that rotated (rather than sweeping left and right) according to the voltages attached to its terminals (Figure 1.4). Caton projected the oscillations of light that bounced off the swiveling mirror affixed to the galvanometer onto the wall of his laboratory. He described "a graduated scale, some eight or nine feet in length, being placed on one of the walls of the theatre, a beam of light from an oxyhydrogen lamp was thrown on to the mirror of the galvanometer, and thence reflected to the scale" (see Figure 1.4). His report that "feeble currents of varying direction pass through the multiplier when the electrodes are placed on two points of the external surface, or one electrode on the grey matter, and one on the surface of the skull" is considered the first description of an EEG wave (Caton, 1875). This is also a nice description of a hunt for a good reference electrode, a process described later in this text. Thereafter, successful recordings were made by Caton and others from the brains of dogs, monkeys, rabbits, and cats, although some still claimed that the recorded waves were related to the pulsations of cerebral blood vessels rather than to brain electrical activity. Of course, because Caton's demonstrations of EEG waveforms consisted of a light oscillating on his laboratory wall, no actual recordings exist, only written descriptions. In an interesting change of career trajectory, Caton was elected Lord Mayor of Liverpool at the end of his tenure at its university.

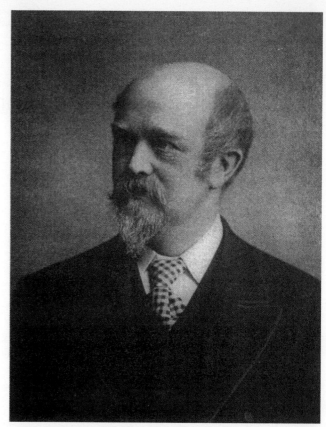

Figure 1.3 Richard Caton (1842–1926), credited with observing the first electroencephalogram from the brains of a variety of animals, first reported in 1875, using Thomson's mirror galvanometer. (From Cohen of Birkenhead, 1959)

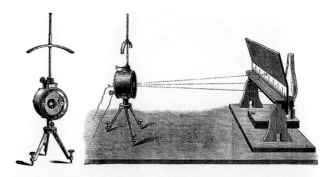

Figure 1.4 This drawing shows the setup of a Thomson galvanometer similar to the type that Richard Caton used to observe the first EEG in a variety of animals. The device stands on three leveling screws. The two electrode inputs can be seen attached to the back of the galvanometer. The rotation of the mirror attached to the vertical swivel allowed a moving light to be projected onto the scale on the right side of the figure. (Enhanced image Courtesy of the Brainclinics Foundation, Nijmegen, Netherlands, https://brainclinics.com/pioneers-of-the-eeg/)

Hans Berger, considered the father of modern electroencephalography, was the first to record EEG in humans (Figure 1.5) while working as a professor of Psychiatry at the University of Jena in Germany. His previous work included precise measurements of cerebral pulsations in both animals and humans and, later, the measurement of brain temperature

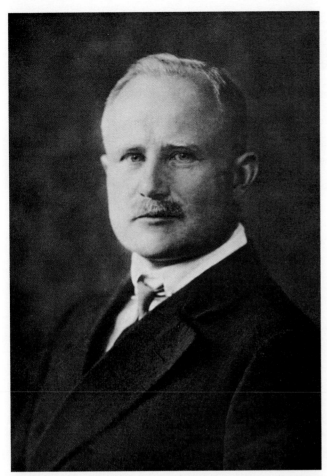

Figure 1.5 Hans Berger at age 52 (1925), one year after he began his work on the human electroencephalogram. (Courtesy Mrs. Ursula Berger. With permission, from Berger H, Gloor P. On the electroencephalogram of man; the fourteen original reports on the human electroencephalogram [Gloor P, translator and editor], Amsterdam and New York, Elsevier, 1969.)

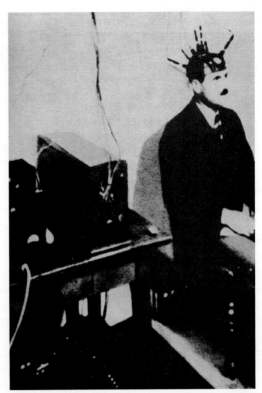

Figure 1.6 This photograph shows one of the first attempts at recording the electroencephalogram in humans. The patient had undergone a left-sided trepanation. The recording attempt was made with silver electrodes secured to the scalp with adhesive tape but was unsuccessful. This patient was recorded sitting up; later patients were studied lying on a couch with glass legs for electrical isolation. (With permission, from Berger H, Gloor P. On the electroencephalogram of man; the fourteen original reports on the human electroencephalogram [Gloor P, translator and editor], Amsterdam and New York, Elsevier, 1969.)

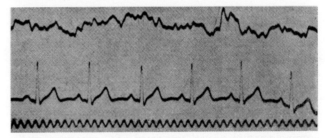

Figure 1.7 The first published recording of an electroencephalogram in a human. The top trace shows an electroencephalographic signal recorded from two needle electrodes in the area of a large bone defect. The middle trace shows the electrocardiogram and the bottom trace shows a 10 Hz calibration signal. (With permission, from Berger H, Gloor P. On the electroencephalogram of man; the fourteen original reports on the human electroencephalogram [Gloor P, translator and editor], Amsterdam and New York, Elsevier, 1969.)

variations in animals to determine whether temperature fluctuated in different behavioral states. His first attempts at recording brain waves in 1924 were carried out using a string galvanometer designed to record electrocardiograms. The first attempts at recordings were made in subjects with areas of missing cranial bone, either from palliative trepanations (creation of a window in the skull bone) for relief of increased intracranial pressure from brain tumors or from skull defects related to injuries sustained during the First World War. Because of these patients' skull defects, he was able to place his needle electrodes only a few millimeters away from the brain surface (Figure 1.6).

In his first report, titled "On the Electroencephalogram of Man" and published in 1929, Berger outlines the path toward his first successful observation of the EEG of man (which he did not, at the time, have the equipment to make a permanent recording). The observation was made in 1924 in a 17-year-old boy who had undergone palliative trepanation over the left cerebral hemisphere for a brain tumor. The first published recorded rhythm, shown in Figure 1.7, was obtained in a 40-year-old man who had had a large bone flap removed to relieve pressure from a brain tumor. The recording was made with needle electrodes placed subcutaneously which, in this patient, represented the epidural space. The patient died from his tumor a few weeks later.

Berger's initial work was met with considerable skepticism, in part because the action potential of single nerves was

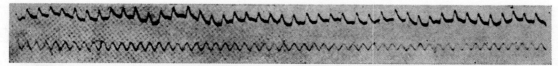

Figure 1.8 The first successful recordings of the EEG in man recorded from a patient with an intact skull were made in Hans Berger's son, Klaus, using needle electrodes. This particular example was obtained when Klaus was 16 years old. The top trace of this figure shows an EEG signal derived from a pair of electrodes "in the midline of the skull anteriorly within the hair line of the forehead and posteriorly two finger breadths above the external occipital protuberance." The bottom channel shows a 10 Hz calibration signal. (With permission, from Berger H, Gloor P. On the electroencephalogram of man; the fourteen original reports on the human electroencephalogram [Gloor P, translator and editor], Amsterdam and New York, Elsevier, 1969.)

just then under study. It was difficult to reconcile the short duration of the action potential, approximately 1 millisecond, with the much longer duration of the waves that comprised the "Berger Rhythm," the wavelengths of which were closer to 100 milliseconds or longer.

Berger also attempted recordings in subjects with intact skulls, starting as early as 1920 with unsuccessful attempts in a bald medical student "who put himself most obligingly" at Berger's disposal. The first series of successful recordings made in a subject with an intact skull were obtained from Berger's son, Klaus, when he was aged between 15 and 17 years (Figure 1.8). Berger continued to publish a series of papers, each entitled "Über das Elektrenkephalogramm des Menschen" ("On the Electroencephalogram of Man") on a yearly basis or more from 1929 until 1938 when retirement from the university was forced upon him related to disagreements with the Nazi authorities.

PLAN OF THE TEXT

The chapters in this text are ordered so that they can be read sequentially, although individual chapters may be referenced out of turn as necessary. Chapter 2, "Visual Analysis of the Electroencephalogram," begins with a general introduction to the appearance of the normal EEG during wakefulness, drowsiness, and sleep. A number of general EEG terms are also introduced in this chapter, essential information for all beginning EEG readers. After these basic concepts and visual features of the normal EEG are described, a discussion of general EEG terminology follows. The vocabulary of EEG is intertwined with certain EEG concepts; this review of EEG terminology and several associated EEG concepts are discussed together in Chapter 3, "Introduction to Commonly Used Terms in Electroencephalography."

Chapter 4, "Electroencephalographic Localization," is the most important chapter in this text. Without excellent localization skills, it is impossible to become an excellent electroencephalographer. EEG localization techniques tell us much more than the location from which a wave originates. Localization techniques allow us to translate a group of waves on an EEG page into a three-dimensional map of charge on the scalp surface and to understand how the shapes on that map vary over time. No less important, localization is also the key skill necessary to master a surprisingly vexing problem in EEG interpretation: how to distinguish true brain waves in the recording from electrical artifacts that arise from other sources.

The ordering of the display of EEG channels generated from a specific electrode set and how those electrodes are paired is called the *EEG montage*. Montages are discussed in detail in Chapter 5, "EEG Electrodes, Channels, and Montages and How They Are Chosen." Different montage strategies and electrode placements help the electroencephalographer to understand the distribution and polarity of different types of discharges. Visualizing these three-dimensional maps is not simply an academic exercise. The ability to classify specific EEG waveforms as to whether they are normal or associated with disease depends significantly on the topography suggested by their polarities and localizations. The topography of an EEG event indicates whether it was generated in a specific part of the brain, or whether it originated from the brain at all. This latter possibility, that a wave on the EEG page has not come from the brain at all, brings us to a major topic in electroencephalography: the identification of EEG artifacts.

One of the main attractions of learning EEG interpretation is the prospect of understanding more about the phenomenology of the wave patterns that the brain generates. It may come as a surprise to the new student of electroencephalography how much time is spent analyzing and identifying waves in the EEG that are caused by stray electrical activity or the patient tossing and turning or blinking the eyes: so-called EEG artifacts, which is the topic of Chapter 6, "Electroencephalographic Artifacts." The considerable problem of identifying artifacts in the EEG is related to the high amplifier gains necessary to record the microvolt-level EEG signals that are the object of our interest. A by-product of the high levels of amplification necessary to produce the beautiful EEG traces that EEG technologists produce and to which we have become accustomed is that everything electrical on the scalp surface gets amplified, including noncerebral electrical events. Experienced electroencephalographers will often be heard to say that "half of EEG is correctly identifying the artifacts." Although many artifactual waves are easy to identify as not being of cerebral origin, some may closely mimic true brain wave activity. Artifact recognition involves both pattern recognition and careful localization and topographic understanding of the wave in question, a skill that is absolutely essential in EEG interpretation.

All EEG signals are passed through a set of filters before being displayed. As discussed in Chapter 7, "Filters in the Electroencephalogram," filters may have a significant impact on the appearance of EEG waves, with the potential to enhance, suppress, or even distort EEG information.

Although knowledge of filter circuit design is not required for fundamental EEG interpretation, the electrical and digital strategies used to create simple high- and low-frequency filters are covered in this chapter. Learning how filters behave in terms of how they change the appearance of EEG waves may not be the first skill you will need to acquire when learning to read EEGs, but it is a subject you will eventually want to master. It would not be unreasonable to defer the review of this chapter until EEG reading skills are already crystallizing. The design and behavior of the circuits used to create these filters, discussed at the end of this chapter, will be of interest only to a subset of readers because these technical topics are not necessary for daily EEG interpretation.

Often the only representation to the outside world of the time and thought that the electroencephalographer has put into the interpretation of the EEG is the written EEG report. The EEG report must include a distillation of the technique used to record the EEG, what the EEG tracing looked like and, most importantly, the EEG findings and their clinical implications. Strategies for producing useful EEG reports are discussed in Chapter 8, "The Structure and Philosophy of the EEG Report."

Before the advent of modern neuroimaging, EEG was an important tool for localizing anatomical lesions such as brain tumors and strokes in addition to its role in diagnosing seizure disorders. Although EEG abnormalities can still be divided into epilepsy- and nonepilepsy-related groups (albeit with considerable overlap), the evaluation of possible seizure disorders has become the most common reason for EEG testing. Chapter 9, "The Abnormal Electroencephalogram," discusses both epileptic and nonepileptic EEG abnormalities in the EEG and describes the types of clinical disorders associated with each.

Chapter 10, "The Electroencephalogram in Epilepsy," examines these associations from the opposite point of view, reviewing selected epilepsy syndromes and describing the EEG findings expected to be associated with each. The chapter begins with a review of the classification of seizure types and seizure syndromes, the foundation for how we think about seizure disorders. The most recent seizure and epilepsy classifications at the time of this writing are also reviewed.

Over the past 90 years, a variety of EEG findings that were initially felt to be abnormal, either because of their resemblance to epileptiform activity or because of their rarity in the normal population, have been classified as "normal variants." The clinical significance of some of these variants is still under debate. This interesting group of EEG findings is discussed in Chapter 11, "Normal Variants in the Electroencephalogram."

EEG is an important tool for assessing neurological prognosis in coma. Although EEG is not used as a sole or required criterion for the determination of brain death, it is sometimes used as a confirmatory study in patients in whom brain death is suspected. Chapter 12, "Electroencephalogram Patterns in Stupor and Coma," discusses how the EEG can be used to evaluate patients in coma and the technical requirements for performing recordings in the setting of suspected brain death. The newer and fairly complex terminology system introduced by the American Clinical Neurophysiology Society (ACNS)

in 2021 for classifying EEG diagnoses in ICU-based EEGs is also introduced along with their definitions and how they relate to older terms still in use.

The EEG begins to attain adult patterns in patients as young as 2 months of age. Before that point, however, the form of the EEG in babies is remarkably unlike that of older patients. Different and unique EEG patterns evolve with surprising rapidity from the earliest clinical recordings obtained in extreme prematures at 22, 23, and 24 weeks post-conceptional age, to recordings performed in newborns at term (40 weeks postconceptional age), and after term when early adult-type patterns finally appear. Chapter 13, "The Electroencephalogram of the Newborn," provides an introduction to this distinctive and unique progression of EEG patterns seen in premature and mature newborns.

Chapter 14, "A Brief Introduction to Invasive EEG Monitoring," is a new addition to this edition of this text. The purpose of this chapter is to provide a first glimpse into some of the invasive recording techniques used to define a patient's seizure focus in preparation for epilepsy surgery. These techniques include placing specially designed EEG electrodes either on the surface of the brain or directly within the substance of the brain. Another new addition to this edition of the text is found in Appendix A: "Where do EEG waves come from?" This appendix includes a description of the behavior of ion channels, an introduction to how voltages across nerve cell membranes are maintained and behave, and how these behaviors contribute to the appearance of the EEG waves we see on the display screen. This discussion of basic neurophysiological principles is not a prerequisite for EEG interpretation and, therefore, may be deferred for later review depending on the individual reader's interests.

Much like driving a car, electroencephalography cannot be learned just by reading a textbook. While reading this text, the reader is encouraged to interpret as many EEG records as possible. Many students start to learn EEG record review by reading "over the shoulder" of a more experienced EEG reader. The real work of learning electroencephalography is done by "getting behind the wheel" and reading records alone, forming an opinion of the EEG's findings uninfluenced by the opinion of others, and then comparing your results to those of a more experienced reader.

REFERENCES

Caton R: The electric currents of the brain [abstract], *BMJ* 2:278, 1875.

Caton R: Interim report on investigation of the electric currents of the human brain, *BMJ* (Suppl), May 5, 1877.

Cohen of Birkenhead: Richard Caton (1842–1926) pioneer electrophysiologist, *Proc R Soc Med* 52(8):645–651, 1959.

Dibner B: *Luigi Galvani: An expanded version of a biography prepared for the forthcoming edition of the Encyclopedia Britannica*, San Marino, California, 1971, Burndy Library.

Galvani L: *Commentary on the effect of Electricity on muscular motion. De viribus electricitatis in motu musculari commentarius*, Doctoral Dissertation, 1791.

SUGGESTED READINGS

Berger H, Gloor P: In Gloor P, editor: *On the electroencephalogram of man; the fourteen original reports on the human electroencephalogram*, Amsterdam and New York, 1969, Elsevier.

Brazier MAB: *A history of neurophysiology in the 17th and 18th centuries: from concept to experiment*, New York, 1984, Raven Press.

Brazier MAB: *A history of neurophysiology in the 19th century*, New York, 1988, Raven Press.

Brainclinics Foundation, Nijmegen, Netherlands, https://brainclinics.com/pioneers-of-the-eeg/

2

Visual Analysis of the EEG: Wakefulness, Drowsiness, and Sleep

An orderly approach to visual analysis of the EEG is important, especially for those who are beginning to hone their EEG reading skills. Although not all EEG records necessarily lend themselves to a single reading approach, it is useful to start the process of record interpretation with a preplanned analysis strategy that is based on the findings of a typical EEG, such as the EEG of a normal adult or child. The approach can be modified from this starting point when more atypical tracings are encountered.

There are two fundamental strategies for EEG analysis, and a good approach to reading includes a combination of both strategies. The first strategy consists of making a mental list of the EEG elements that one would expect to see in the EEG given the patient's age and sleep state and identifying and analyzing each of these elements in turn. The second strategy consists of examining the array of waveforms present on the page, identifying each, and classifying each as a normal element, an abnormal element, or an artifact. In summary, the first strategy consists of making a list of "what do I expect to see?" and attempting to find each element in the list of expected items in the EEG record. The second step is to survey the landscape of the EEG page and to identify each waveform that one sees. Of course, the two strategies are complementary and can be carried out in either order; combining the two strategies ensures that the reader will consider everything that does appear on the EEG page but will also notice what is absent from the EEG record but should be there. This chapter discusses each of the two strategies in turn.

The purpose of this chapter is to give a brief overview of a normal EEG tracing, including transitions from wakefulness to sleep, and then back to wakefulness. Next, the elements involved in these transitions are examined more closely. The figure captions include additional detail regarding the features of each stage.

QUICK TOUR: TRANSITION OF THE EEG FROM WAKEFULNESS TO DROWSINESS, SLEEP, AND AROUSAL FROM SLEEP

Wakefulness

Figure 2.1 shows the typical appearance of the EEG in a patient who is awake with eyes closed. The basic setup of the EEG page is summarized in the figure's caption, which is worth reviewing in detail if you are new to EEG. The most prominent rhythm on the page is denoted by the solid black arrows and is called the posterior rhythm. Note that this waveform is highly rhythmic and sinusoidal (i.e., shaped like a sine wave). It is of highest voltage in the posterior or occipital channels (black arrows) and becomes much less prominent in the anterior channels. The posterior rhythm is best seen when the patient is awake with eyes closed. In fact, you can prove to yourself that a waveform is the posterior rhythm by ascertaining that it has three main features: it is seen best **posteriorly**, it is only seen when the patient is **awake**, and it *disappears* when the patient **opens the eyes** and visually fixes on something in the environment.

Another typical feature of wakefulness is the presence of an anteroposterior gradient of voltage and frequency. This term may sound complicated but is merely a shorthand term to summarize where waves of different frequencies and voltages are most prominent in the awake EEG. Anteriorly, waves are generally of lower voltage and higher frequency. Posteriorly, waves are of higher voltage and lower frequency.

Summary of Transition from Wakefulness to Sleep in the Routine EEG	
Awake	Eyes closed: posterior rhythm present Eyes open: low-voltage, nondescript pattern seen posteriorly, posterior rhythm absent, eyeblink artifacts
Drowsy	Mild slowing of the posterior rhythm in some Slow roving lateral eye movements appear Disappearance of posterior rhythm in the occipital areas, replaced by low-voltage theta activity Diffuse increase in theta range activity, particularly at the vertex
Stage I Sleep	Vertex waves of sleep
Stage II Sleep	Sleep spindles appear, vertex waves continue K-complexes
Arousal	High-voltage hypersynchronous (rhythmic) slowing in some Return of posterior rhythm and typical waking patterns

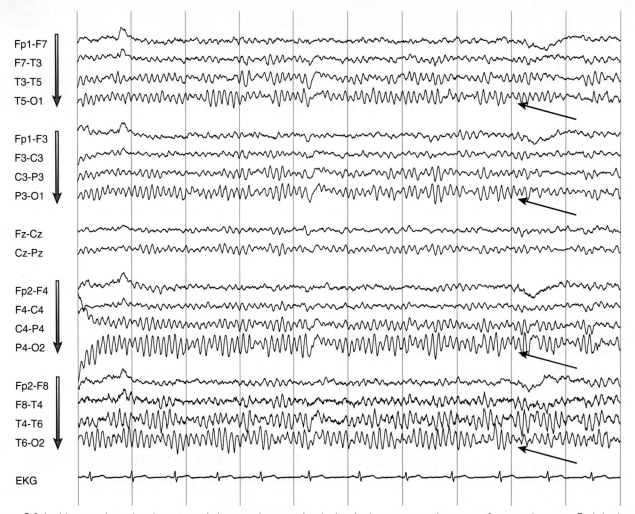

Figure 2.1 In this normal, awake electroencephalogram, the posterior rhythm is the most prominent waveform on the page. Each horizontal EEG wave is generated by recording from the pair of electrodes denoted in the left margin. Each vertical division represents one second. Odd-numbered electrodes are placed on the left side of the scalp and even-numbered electrodes are on the right; those with z-subscripts (for "zero") are in the midline. The initial letters of the electrode names represent different brain regions: (Fp) frontopolar, (F) frontal, (T) temporal, (P) parietal, (C) central, and (O) occipital.

Each of the four major chains of electrodes can be examined from the anterior to posterior direction, as indicated by the four shaded vertical arrows on the left side of the page. These arrows signify that the sweep from the front to the back of the head in each of these chains corresponds to scanning each chain from top to bottom (e.g., from the Fp1-F7 channel to the T5-O1 for the first chain of four). The posterior rhythm, a well-formed sinusoidal rhythm, becomes more prominent as each chain is scanned from the front of the head to the back of the head, and is best defined in the channels that include the occipital electrodes, O1 and O2 (solid arrows). In this patient, as in most, the posterior rhythm is of slightly higher voltage over the right occipital area (bottom two solid arrows) compared with the left (top two solid arrows).

The normal awake EEG tracing often manifests two types of voltage and frequency transitions seen between anterior and posterior head regions, termed the anteroposterior gradient of the EEG: going from the front of the head to the back, the amplitude (or height) of waves generally increases and the frequency of waves decreases, paralleling the shading of the arrows on the left. Note that anteriorly in the brain (the top channels of each set of four), voltages are low, and more fast activity is seen. Posteriorly (bottom channels of each set of four, indicated by solid arrows), voltages are higher and waves are slower. In this example, posterior waves are higher because of the presence of the posterior rhythm, approximately 10 Hz in this sample.

Comparing the first line and the fourth line of this figure bears out these relationships. The top channel is relatively flat and has a lower voltage, higher frequency (faster) waveform. The fourth line has a higher voltage, lower frequency (slower) waveform. This is what is meant by the antero-posterior gradient: in normal, awake patients, waves in the front of the head tend to be of lower voltage and have faster activity, while waves toward the back of the head tend to be of higher voltage and show somewhat slower activity. Additional examples of the anteroposterior gradient are given later in this chapter.

As seen in Figure 2.2, the posterior rhythm suppresses or disappears completely with eye opening and fixation of gaze. When the eyes are closed, the posterior rhythm returns. In summary, the posterior rhythm is a rhythm of wakefulness that is present when the eyes are closed. During wakefulness

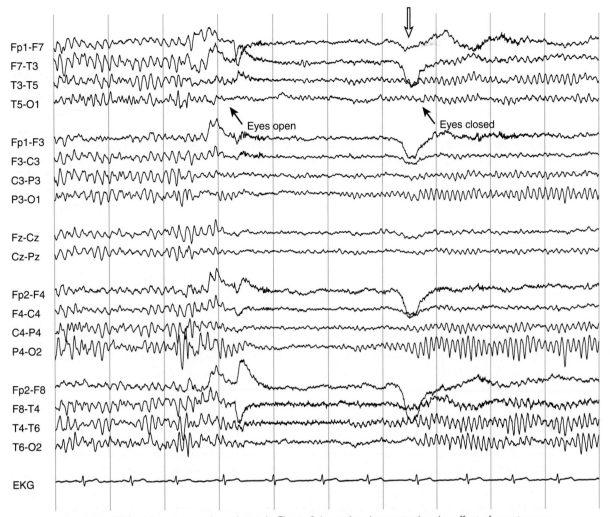

Figure 2.2 EEG of the same patient shown in Figure 2.1, awake, demonstrating the effect of spontaneous eye opening and closure on the posterior rhythm. The posterior rhythm suppresses dramatically with eye opening. Note also that the posterior rhythm actually begins to return 1.5 seconds before the eyes close, suggesting a brief period of relative visual inattention just before eye closure. The exact moment of eye closure is marked by the eye-closure artifact seen in the frontal leads (hollow arrow).

with the eyes open, the EEG shows a lower voltage, nondescript pattern in the occipital region, as is seen in Figure 2.2, between eye opening and closure. Typically, eyeblink artifacts are also seen in the EEG during wakefulness when the patient's eyes are open.

Drowsiness

It is easy to tell from the EEG when drowsiness starts in normal individuals. One of the first EEG changes seen in drowsiness is a subtle slowing of the posterior rhythm. In Figure 2.3, the posterior rhythm is seen to slow over the course of the page from 10 Hz (waves per second) in the first second of the page to 8 Hz in the seventh second, an early indication of drowsiness in this patient. However, this brief period of posterior rhythm slowing is not always identifiable; often the posterior rhythm simply "drops out"

without an observable period of slowing. Another more subtle finding is that of slow roving lateral eye movements of drowsiness, which are indicated by the shaded rectangles (see figure caption for further explanation). Such slow roving eye movements are commonly detected by the EEG because eye movements create electrical artifacts in the EEG tracing. In fact, most are surprised to learn that our eyes rove left and right when we are drowsy, a fact hidden to casual observation by closed eyelids. Although the appearance of slow roving eye movements in the EEG technically represents an artifact (because they are not actual brain waves), they still provide useful information to the reader regarding onset of drowsiness. The EEG appearance of slow roving eye movements is discussed in more detail in Chapter 6, "Electroencephalographic Artifacts." Thus, the signs of early drowsiness are possible slowing of the

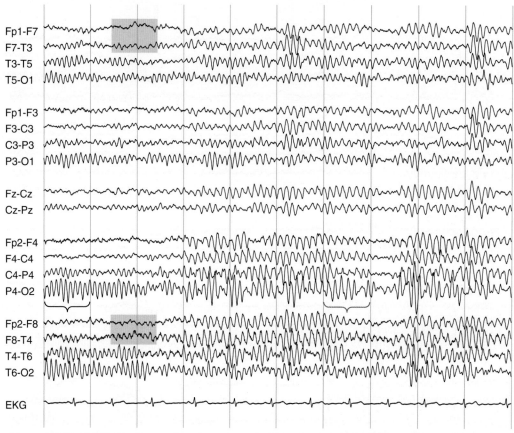

Figure 2.3 The initial transition to drowsiness is marked here by a slowing of the posterior rhythm. A frequency of 10 Hz can be counted over the black brace in the first second of this page. The frequency falls to approximately 8 Hz by the seventh second over the gray brace. Artifact from slow roving eye movements can also be seen: note the subtle spreading apart of the waveforms of the two channels that include F7 (top red rectangle) compared with a relative narrowing together of the two channels that include F8 (bottom red rectangle). The appearance of this artifact is caused by a slow roving movement of the eyes to the left, a sign of early drowsiness, and why these eye movements appear in the EEG as they do is described in more detail in Chapter 6.

posterior rhythm, dropout of the posterior rhythm with replacement by low voltage irregular and slower activity, and the appearance of slow-roving lateral eye movements.

The next EEG page (Figure 2.4) in this example shows two additional important changes that mark advancing drowsiness: first, the posterior rhythm has dropped out nearly completely. Second, there is an increase in theta-range (slow) activity throughout the tracing. Characteristically, theta activity appears first at the vertex, particularly in the midline central (Cz) electrode (arrow), although it may be seen in other locations as well.

On the following EEG page (Figure 2.5), the first true vertex waves of sleep are seen, marking deeper drowsiness. These midline sharp waves are a marker of Stage I sleep and may occur in dramatic bursts. After they are established, assuming no subsequent arousals, vertex-wave bursts continue in a periodic fashion through Stage II sleep.

Stage II Sleep

The onset of Stage II sleep is defined by the appearance of sleep spindles. The sleep spindles that occur early in Stage II sleep are usually of maximum voltage in the central electrodes (C3 and C4) and at the central vertex (Cz), as is seen in this example. They consist of lower voltage, regular 14 Hz waves lasting from one to a few seconds. As it happens, sleep spindles are most lengthy in infants and of shorter duration in adults. In deeper Stage II sleep, the field of sleep spindles may include both the frontal and central areas. Figure 2.6 shows the appearance of the first, bicentral sleep spindles in this patient, intermixed with vertex waves. By the next page, the sleep spindles become more sharply defined (Figure 2.7) and continue to be intermixed with repetitive vertex waves. The combination of repetitive vertex waves and spindles marks well-established Stage II sleep. An example of the fields of spindles and vertex waves is shown in Figures 2.8 and 2.9, and schematically in Figures 2.10 and 2.11.

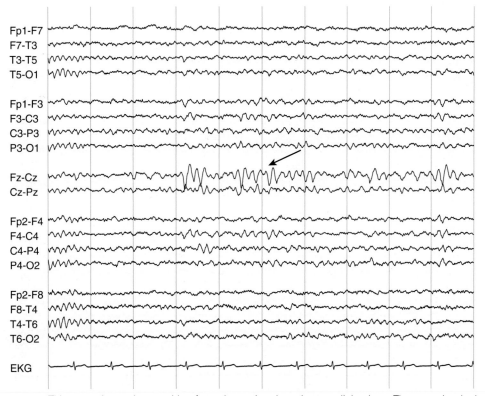

Figure 2.4 This page shows the transition from deepening drowsiness to light sleep. The posterior rhythm completely disappears after the first second and vertex activity increases (black arrow) in the form of theta waves. More low voltage theta range (slow) activity is seen in other brain areas as well.

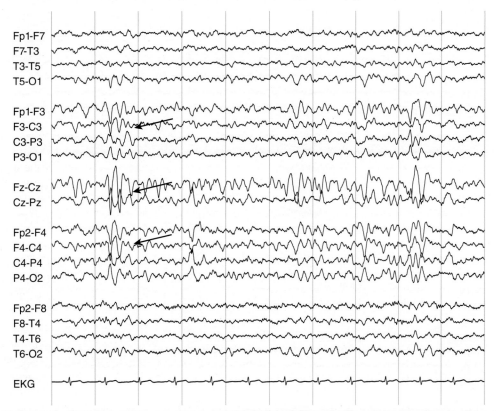

Figure 2.5 In this figure, vertex waves become well established. Note that the vertex wave voltage is highest in the C3, Cz, and C4 electrodes (as evidenced by phase reversals in those locations—see black arrows). A second set of vertex waves is seen near the end of the page. Rhythmic vertex theta can be seen between these two larger vertex-wave bursts. The appearance of vertex waves marks the onset of deeper drowsiness.

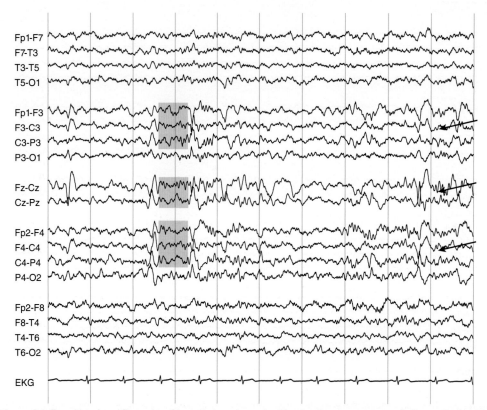

Figure 2.6 Transition from Stage I to Stage II sleep is marked by the first appearance of sleep spindles. The sleep spindles are the lower voltage, sinusoidal 14 Hz waves that are following close on the heels of the vertex waves (a portion of the spindles is highlighted by the red rectangles). Sleep spindles are also seen surrounding the later vertex wave on the right side of the page (arrows). The spindles become better defined in the next examples.

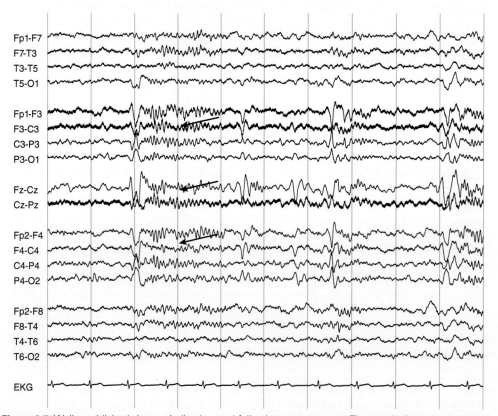

Figure 2.7 Well-established sleep spindles (arrows) following a vertex wave. These spindles are maximum in the frontocentral regions and in the midline. Repetitive vertex waves continue. Note that spindles often follow vertex waves, although the link between the two is not always consistent.

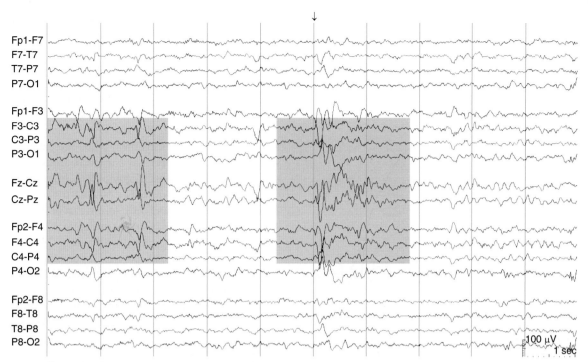

Figure 2.8 The red rectangles highlight the brain areas in which vertex waves and spindles are seen most prominently, here displayed in a bipolar montage. Note that the temporal chains, represented by the four-channel groupings at the top and bottom of the page not included in the red rectangles, are relatively uninvolved with the vertex wave and spindle waveforms.

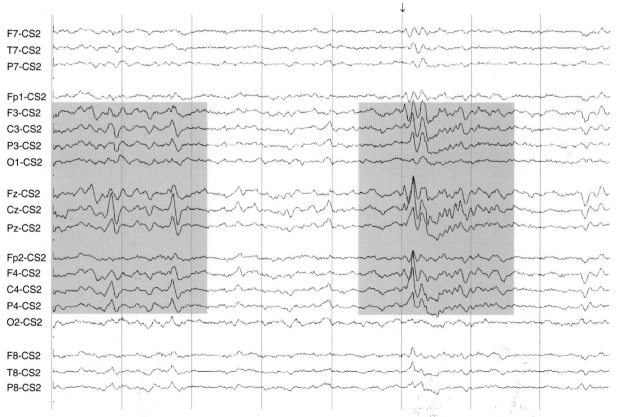

Figure 2.9 The same vertex waves and spindles displayed in a referential montage. Because referential montages dedicate one channel to each active electrode (compared to a pair of active electrodes per channel in bipolar montages), the individual electrodes that pick up the spindle and vertex-wave discharges are easier to discern. The red rectangles highlight the field of these waves, which primarily include the central, frontal, and midline regions. Note that the phase (up or down direction) of these waveforms changes between the bipolar montage and the referential montage. You will become an expert on why this happens as you proceed through this text.

The final hallmark finding of Stage II sleep is the *K-complex*. These bursts of high voltage waves occurring across nearly all channels may be seen sporadically in sleep. These normal discharges can be dramatic and, because of

their bursting quality, are sometimes mistaken for spike-wave discharges, an epileptiform abnormality, which would be considered abnormal. K-complexes may be triggered by stimuli (such as a noise) in the environment of the sleeping patient that cause a mild subarousal (an increase in the level of arousal or a lightening of the sleep state that is not strong enough to awaken the patient fully). In fact, EEG technologists often demonstrate K-complexes in the EEG by tapping a pencil on the EEG instrument while the patient is in light sleep. The tapping sound may elicit a subarousal and an associated K-complex. Most K-complexes, however, appear to occur spontaneously without an obvious trigger. The field of a K-complex is diffuse, and differs from that of sleep spindles or sleep vertex waves and is shown in Figure 2.12. K-complexes may or may not be intermixed with a sleep spindle, as occurs in the example shown in Figure 2.13. Therefore, the hallmark findings of Stage II sleep are repetitive vertex waves, the first and repetitive appearance of sleep spindles, and the sporadic appearance of K-complexes. By definition, the onset of Stage II sleep is marked by the first appearance of sleep spindles.

Arousal from Sleep

Arousal from sleep may occur uneventfully with a simple return of the posterior rhythm and other patterns of wakefulness described earlier. At other times, arousal from sleep may be marked by a dramatic run of diffuse, high-voltage rhythmic waves called an arousal hypersynchrony. Figure 2.14 shows a fairly simple arousal with a brief increase in rhythmic

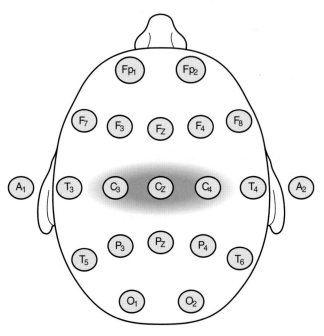

Figure 2.10 A schematic of the approximate field of vertex waves of sleep is shown. The maximum activity of vertex waves is at the Cz electrode with lesser voltages measured at the adjacent C3 and C4 electrodes.

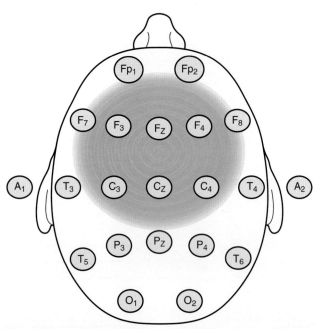

Figure 2.11 Classically, spindles are centered over the central areas, particularly the C3 and C4 electrodes. In many examples such as the EEG traces shown in Figures 2.8 and 2.9, spindles are also seen to spread frontally (F3 and F4 electrodes). The field of spindles only occasionally spreads laterally to the midtemporal electrodes where they should be of lower voltage compared with the central electrodes or not seen at all.

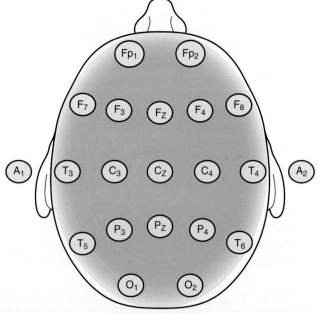

Figure 2.12 The field of a K-complex is diffuse and may include all brain areas. This helps differentiate it from simple spindles, which are maximum frontocentrally and concentrated in the midline and parasagittal areas as described in Figure 2.11. A sleep waveform of an intensity just as strong in the temporal areas as in the midline is not likely to represent a sleep spindle or vertex wave but may represent a K-complex.

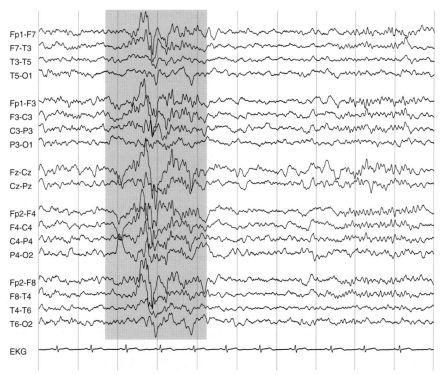

Figure 2.13 A K-complex is seen during Stage II sleep (red rectangle). At first glance, the K-complex resembles a vertex wave followed by a sleep spindle. Note, however, that the high-voltage waves preceding the spindles in this example do not have the typical distribution of a vertex wave of sleep. Although vertex waves are maximum in C3, Cz, and C4, the example of this particular wave shows frontal voltages that are just as high in the temporal chains (Fp1-F7, F7-T3, Fp2-F8, F8-T4) as in the parasagittal chains. The broad field extending to the temporal chains of the high-voltage wave that precedes the spindles is the tip-off that this complex is not simply a combination of a vertex wave and sleep spindles but a K-complex.

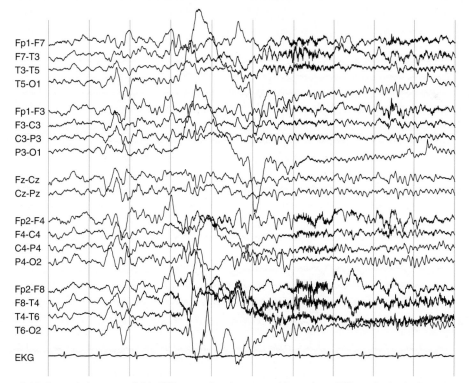

Figure 2.14 Several elements of this EEG page signal an arousal from sleep. Diffuse rhythmic slow waves, as seen in the second second of this tracing, are typical of arousal and sometimes much more dramatic than in this example. The very high-voltage deflections that cross into neighboring channels are large motion artifacts, often seen at the time of arousal from sleep, which is typically associated with body movements. The very fast waves that turn some channels dark black, most prominent in the temporal chains at the top and bottom of the page, represent muscle artifact associated with movements related to arousal. Note the reappearance of the posterior rhythm in the second half of the page following the high-voltage motion artifact.

slowing followed by high-voltage motion artifact generated from the patient stirring in bed. This is followed by a return of the posterior rhythm.

The sequence of wakefulness to drowsiness to sleep is shown in a second patient in Figures 2.15 through 2.20, with fewer figure markings to help the reader practice identification of normal sleep waveforms.

Natural Sleep

The foregoing example represents a quick tour through wakefulness, drowsiness, into light sleep, but any drowsiness-related by an arousal and return to wakefulness. The reader may ask why this sequence does not include examples of deeper sleep such as sleep Stages III and IV and rapid eye movement (REM) sleep. In practice, these deeper sleep stages are not typically encountered during the recording of routine EEGs in the outpatient laboratory. The amount of sleep recorded during a routine EEG study is usually less than 20 to 30 minutes and sometimes just a few minutes of sleep is recorded if much time has been spent getting the patient to fall asleep for the test. During routine EEG testing, few patients enter Stage III, IV, or REM sleep because these stages typically only appear after more prolonged sleep, longer than is practicable during the recording of routine outpatient

EEGs. Examples of these patterns are seen in Figures 2.21 through 2.23.

During natural sleep, normal individuals sequentially cycle through Stages I through IV and then back up to Stage I, after which they may enter a brief REM stage after 1 to 2 hours. The first third of the night's sleep is dominated by slow-wave sleep, whereas REM sleep is most plentiful during the early morning hours before awakening, at which time the portions of the cycle devoted to REM sleep are lengthier. An example of normal sleep cycling is illustrated in the hypnogram shown Figure 2.24.

VISUAL ANALYSIS OF THE EEG: IDENTIFICATION OF EXPECTED ELEMENTS

Wakefulness

The Posterior Rhythm

A good first step in the interpretation of the awake EEG is identification of the posterior rhythm, often the most distinctive and easily identifiable feature of the waking EEG. The posterior rhythm is, as the name implies, best seen in the posterior head regions, although how far the field of the posterior rhythm spreads forward varies among patients. In some patients, the

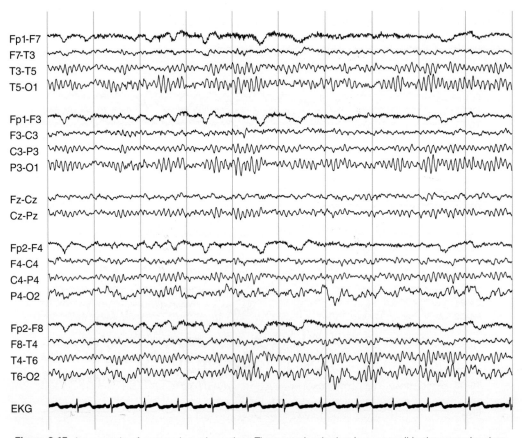

Figure 2.15 An example of a normal, awake patient. The posterior rhythm is seen well in the posterior channels: T5-O1, P3-O1, Cz-Pz, P4-O2, and T6-O2. The frontal channels in each chain of four—Fp1-F7, Fp1-F3, Fp2-F4, and Fp2-F8—are darker than others because of artifact from the frontalis muscle. Bobbing waves seen in those channels represent artifact related to vertical eye movements made under closed eyelids (the eyes are known to be closed based on the presence of the posterior rhythm).

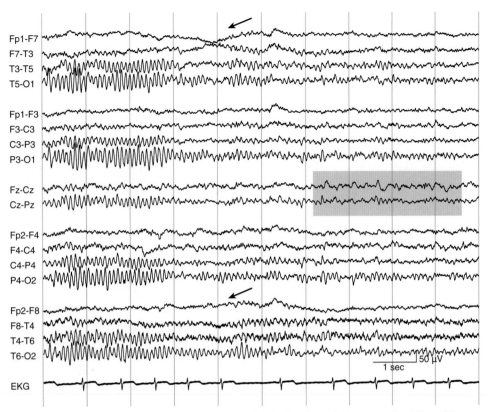

Figure 2.16 During the course of this page, the posterior rhythm drops in frequency by 1 Hz and becomes less prominent (seen best in T5-O1, P3-O1, P4-O2, and T6-O2). Slow roving lateral eye movements are seen as evidenced by approximation of the Fp1-F7 and F7-T3 channels at the same time as a mild "bulging apart" of the Fp2-F8 and F8-T4 channels (arrows). The reason that lateral eye movements create this appearance is explained in more detail in Chapter 6. An increase in theta activity, another sign of drowsiness, is seen at the vertex in the seventh and eighth seconds in the Fz-Cz channel (red rectangle).

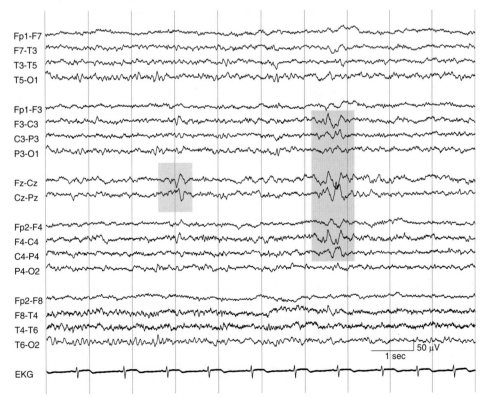

Figure 2.17 The first vertex wave appears at the beginning of the fourth second exclusively in Cz, visible in the Fz-Cz and Cz-Pz channels (small red rectangle). The second vertex wave appears in the seventh second and now includes both Cz and the central electrodes, seen in the channels that include C3 and C4 (large red rectangle).

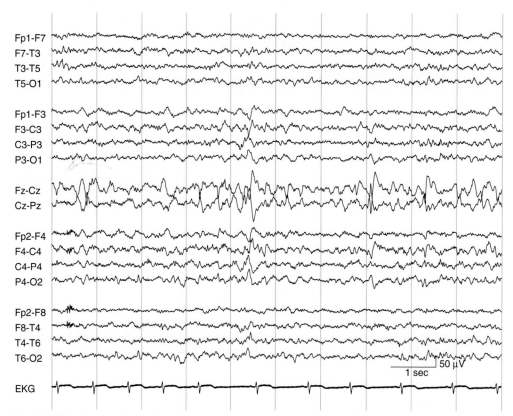

Figure 2.18 Cascades of vertex waves of sleep are seen regularly in the midline channels (Fz-Cz and Cz-Pz) as stage I sleep becomes well established in deeper drowsiness. Overall, the background shows an increased number of low-voltage slow waves.

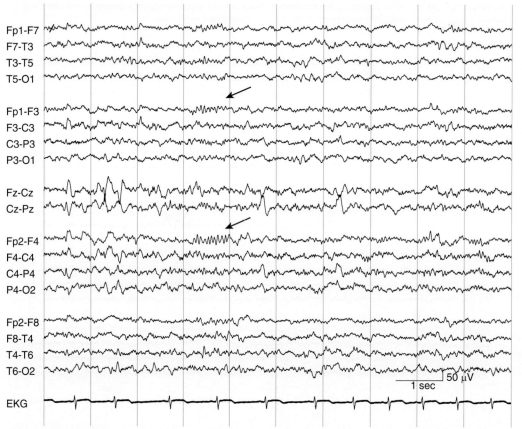

Figure 2.19 Vertex waves continue, and sleep spindles now make their appearance (arrows), marking the onset of Stage II sleep.

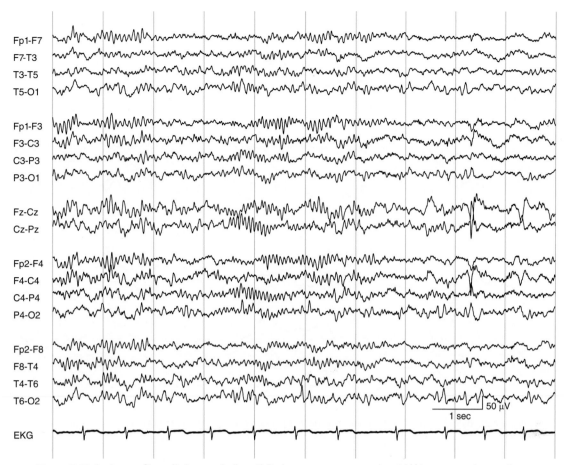

Figure 2.20 In deeper Stage II sleep, spindle activity becomes more prominent. Vertex waves also continue, seen in the last 2 seconds of the page.

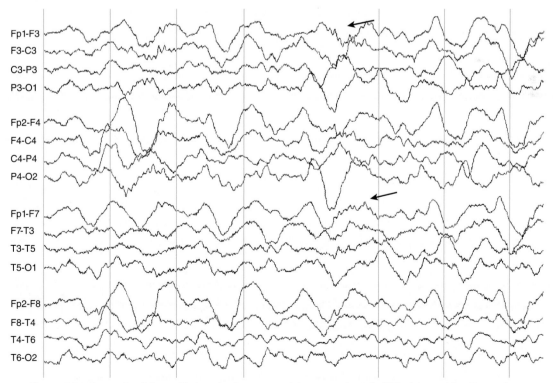

Figure 2.21 A sample of Stage III sleep is shown containing approximately 50% delta activity. Some sleep spindle activity persists (arrows) but is more difficult to appreciate against the backdrop of the slow wave activity.

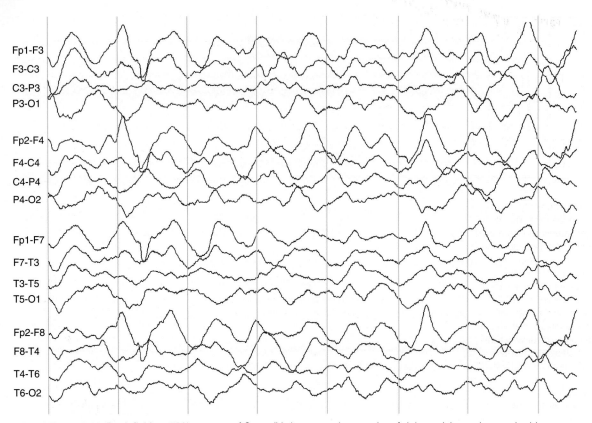

Figure 2.22 By definition, 50% or more of Stage IV sleep samples consist of delta activity, as is seen in this sample.

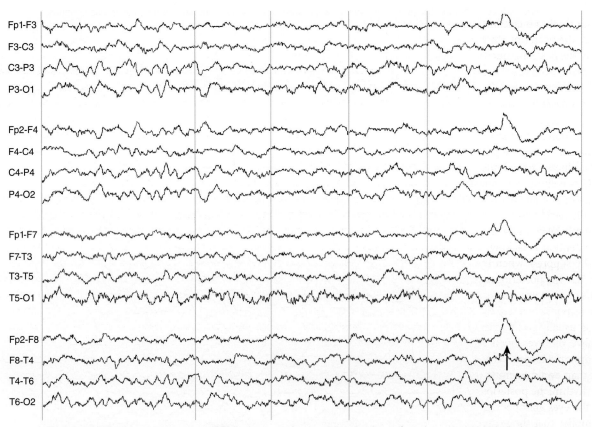

Figure 2.23 Rapid eye movement (REM) sleep, or dream sleep, is also referred to as paradoxical sleep because of the overall decrease in voltages that somewhat resembles an awake pattern. REMs are best seen in specialized channels designed to pick up eye movements but may also be detected in the frontal electrodes that are near the eyes, such as the large deflection seen in the four frontal channels in this example (arrow).

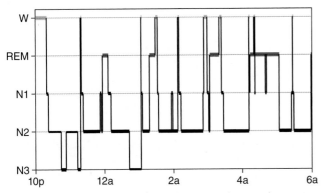

Figure 2.24 Sleep polysomnography has many elements in common with EEG recordings. This hypnogram was generated from an overnight sleep study and represents a graphical representation of the time spent in different sleep stages through the night. Note that this patient falls asleep soon after 10 p.m. and progresses immediately to Stage I (N1), and then to Stage II sleep (N2). After a longer period of time, the patient enters deeper sleep, Stages III and IV (N3). REM periods are shaded red and the first REM period does not occur for several hours and is relatively brief. REM periods then become more frequent and longer in the early morning hours. Looking at this pattern, it becomes clear why REM sleep, and even the deeper stages of slow wave sleep, are not typically recorded during the relatively brief routine EEG recordings of normal subjects obtained in the outpatient laboratory. (W = Wakefulness, REM = REM sleep, N1 = Stage 1 sleep, N2 = Stage II sleep, and N3 includes both Stages III and IV sleep. The AASM 'N' nomenclature used in this figure is summarized later in this chapter under the paragraph "Sleep Stages used for Sleep Scoring.") Hypnogram courtesy of Dr. Jonathan Lipton.

posterior rhythm is confined to the occipital areas, but in many subjects, the posterior rhythm spreads forward to include the whole of the posterior quadrants (see Figure 2.15), and at times the field may even reach the superior frontal electrodes (F3 and F4), as was seen in Figure 2.1. The posterior rhythm should not be visible in the frontopolar electrodes—any rhythm that spreads this far forward is likely some other rhythm.

In addition to its location on the head, two other distinctive qualities define the posterior rhythm. First, it is a rhythm of wakefulness. Indeed, the posterior rhythm is the hallmark of EEG wakefulness in those patients who manifest such a rhythm—it is a fair bet that a patient in whom the posterior rhythm is seen is awake. Second, the posterior rhythm is predominantly seen when the subject's eyes are closed or when visual attention is lacking. The posterior rhythm should dramatically suppress when the eyes are opened, as was seen in Figure 2.2. The posterior rhythm suppresses equally well when patients open their eyes spontaneously as when they open their eyes in response to a request. Although visual attention and eye opening usually go together, during certain intervals a patient may have the eyes open but may not be attending visually (fixating) on a target. Because it is specifically visual attention rather than eyelid opening that causes suppression of the posterior rhythm, the posterior rhythm is sometimes seen at times when the eyes are open but the subject is visually inattentive. This implies that the posterior rhythm can be considered an "idling rhythm" of the occipital (visual) cortex. Though it may seem counterintuitive, when visual cortex is busy processing

visual information, the posterior rhythm wave disappears. When visual cortex is idle, the wave reappears.

Although the posterior rhythm can be identified in the great majority of patients, in a small number of normal individuals no posterior rhythm is seen on scalp-recorded EEG. Absence of the posterior rhythm as an isolated finding is not necessarily considered an abnormality because a small minority of normal individuals do not have a scalp-recordable posterior rhythm.

Most often, the shape of the posterior rhythm is sinusoidal, which is to say that the peaks and troughs of the waveform are similarly rounded and regular. In a minority of individuals, the posterior rhythm waveform is sharpened on one side (often the bottoms of the waves in bipolar montages) and rounded on the other. This is referred to as spiky alpha variant and is considered a normal variant (Figure 2.25). The spiky shape of the posterior rhythm in these patients should not imply an epileptiform abnormality.

A Note on the Term "Alpha Rhythm"

Because in adults and older children the posterior rhythm's frequency is normally in the alpha range (8–13 Hz), the posterior rhythm is sometimes referred to casually as the *posterior alpha rhythm* or simply the *alpha rhythm*. This terminology is not preferred for several reasons, in particular because the posterior rhythm may have a frequency below the alpha range in many clinical situations. A posterior rhythm below the alpha range is seen frequently in children, especially in the first few years of life, an age at which a posterior rhythm under 8 Hz is expected (and therefore in the theta rather than the alpha range). Adults may also manifest a slowing of the posterior rhythm below 8 Hz, most often marking a pathological state or occasionally a pharmacological effect. Finally, rhythms in the alpha range (between 8 and 13 Hz) may be found elsewhere in the EEG and in different brain areas. These, too, could correctly be called *alpha rhythms*, which could lead to some confusion. Use of the term posterior rhythm or *posterior dominant rhythm* rather than alpha rhythm avoids the awkwardness of referring to an "alpha rhythm" that may, in fact, be in the theta range.

Amplitude Asymmetry of the Posterior Rhythm

The amplitude of the posterior rhythm usually differs between the two hemispheres. Most often, the posterior rhythm is of higher voltage over the right hemisphere (the non-dominant hemisphere) compared with the left hemisphere. Although some amount of asymmetry of posterior rhythm amplitude is normal and, indeed, expected, a large asymmetry of the posterior rhythm may reflect an abnormality of one of the hemispheres; the posterior rhythm amplitude may be lower on one side because that hemisphere has been damaged or is abnormal in some way. Usually, the difference in the posterior rhythm amplitude between the two sides does not exceed 20%. Because the posterior rhythm is typically asymmetric in normal patients, but *too much* asymmetry might be a sign that one hemisphere is abnormal, it is useful to set a threshold for posterior rhythm asymmetry beyond which an amplitude difference is called abnormal.

The following rule for determining when an asymmetry of the posterior rhythm is abnormal is somewhat arbitrary and

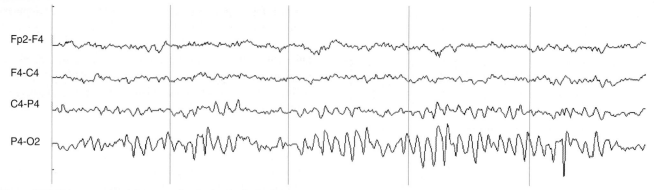

Figure 2.25 This example of the posterior rhythm is distinctive because portions are not sinusoidal (i.e., rounded on both the tops and bottoms) but rather have a "spiky" appearance at the bottom of the waves. It is important not to mistake this pattern for true spikes in the EEG. The clue that these spiky waveforms do not represent spikes is that they clearly fit into the posterior rhythm; true spikes would appear to interrupt the rhythm.

is also fairly conservative (i.e., designed so that not too many patients are labeled abnormal). Start by remembering that the dominant hemisphere is usually the left hemisphere. In the majority of patients, the left hemisphere usually has the lower voltage posterior rhythm. If, in a given patient, the posterior rhythm is unexpectedly seen to be of higher voltage on the left, it is still accepted as normal if it is up to twice the voltage of the right side. In the more typical situation in which the posterior rhythm is of higher voltage on the right side because it is already expected to be higher on that side, up to a three-fold asymmetry of voltage is considered acceptable.

Stated more formally, when the posterior rhythm is of higher voltage over the nondominant hemisphere (the usual case), if it is more than threefold higher than that of the dominant hemisphere, it is considered abnormal. When the posterior rhythm is of higher voltage over the dominant hemisphere (the less common case), if its amplitude is more than twofold greater than that of the nondominant side, it is considered abnormal.

One theory that has attempted to explain why the posterior rhythm is of higher voltage over the nondominant hemisphere is based on the observation that in several settings, EEG waves are of higher voltage at times when a brain area is not busy with mental processing. A simple example of this phenomenon is the posterior rhythm itself: as mentioned above, when the occipital lobes are involved in visual processing, the posterior rhythm disappears and low voltages are seen in the occipital areas. When the occipital lobes are idle during periods of eye closure or visual inattention, occipital voltage increases in the form of the posterior rhythm. There is an analogous idling rhythm of the motor cortex called the central mu rhythm (see Chapter 11), which classically disappears when a motor movement is made or contemplated in the contralateral upper extremity and reappears when the limb is at rest.

The analogy of higher voltages during idle states can even be extended to sleep. Sleep waves are generally of higher amplitude than waking rhythms and presumably represent the higher voltage electrical activity of a more sleepy and therefore more "idle" brain compared with the lower voltage waves of the waking EEG. Returning to the phenomenon of the posterior rhythm being of lower voltage over the left hemisphere compared with the right, the theory holds that

the dominant hemisphere tends to be more occupied with neural processing because of the nature of the tasks it handles (sometimes humorously referred to as the "smarter" hemisphere), processing language and mathematical calculations. In comparison, the nondominant (usually right) hemisphere is considered to be more "idle" and therefore would be expected to generate a higher amplitude posterior rhythm (the "not-as-smart" hemisphere). Although this theory may be useful in helping the electroencephalographer remember the side of the brain on which the posterior rhythm usually manifests higher voltage, the idea is unproven, and its greatest value may be as a mnemonic memory device.

Symmetry of Frequency of the Posterior Rhythm

The frequency of the posterior rhythm should be the same over each hemisphere. Although a mismatch in the frequency of the posterior rhythm between hemispheres should be considered an abnormality, true differences in the fundamental frequency of the posterior rhythm between hemispheres is very uncommon. Most examples of apparent mismatches of the posterior rhythm frequency are actually caused by an intermixing of slow-wave activity into the posterior rhythm on one side. In these cases, the fundamental posterior rhythm frequency may be the same on both sides, but on one side the rhythm may be partly obliterated by a slow wave (e.g., a theta wave), creating the illusion of different posterior rhythm frequencies over each hemisphere when counted out.

The Posterior Rhythm in Infancy and Childhood

The posterior rhythm can be first recognized as early as 3 to 4 months of age in infants born at term, although in infancy, reactivity to eye closure is more difficult to demonstrate. At 3 to 4 months, a posterior rhythm frequency of 3 to 4 Hz is expected. Through the first decade, the posterior rhythm's frequency increases and reaches the adult range, which is between 8 and 13 Hz. Because a posterior rhythm below 8 Hz is considered abnormal after age 8 years, the rule of "eight by eight" can be applied, meaning that by 8 years of age a posterior rhythm frequency of 8 Hz must be reached to be considered normal. Realistically, 8 years can be considered the outer age limit by which the posterior rhythm is expected to reach 8 Hz. In practice, some normal children will attain a posterior rhythm frequency of 8 Hz by as early as 2 years of age. This illustrates the distinction between knowing the typical as opposed to the limit of normal posterior rhythm frequencies at different ages. The limit of normal of the posterior rhythm for a particular age dictates the cutoff used between normal and abnormal (an interpretation of abnormal implying an increased probability that a pathological state is present). By contrast, typical ranges for the posterior rhythm represent what the reader will commonly encounter during the interpretation of a large number of EEGs in different age groups. These typical values are generally higher than the cutoff values used for determining normal versus abnormal. The figures that represent the lower limit of normal are, perhaps, the most important to commit to memory because these numbers will determine which tracings the reader will label normal or abnormal (Table 2.1).

Beta (Fast) Activity

EEG fast activity is usually low-voltage activity. Because of its low amplitude, it is easy for fast activity to escape notice on first review unless the reader makes a point of looking for it. These lower voltage fast waves generally range from 13 to 30 Hz and sometimes look like nothing more than low-voltage "noise" or fuzziness that rides on the larger, slower waves (Figure 2.26). Indeed, fast activity arising from the brain can appear fairly similar to the artifact from the electrical activity that muscles generate ("muscle artifact" or electromyogram artifact, usually called "EMG artifact"). Because electroencephalographers train themselves to filter out muscle artifact mentally to "see" the cerebral activity, it can be easy for fast activity's features to be missed during this visual filtering process. For this reason, fast activity in the EEG should be deliberately analyzed separately.

Although there is no official upper limit to the frequency of what can be called beta activity in the EEG, there are practical

TABLE 2.1 Typical Frequencies of the Posterior Rhythm and Lower Limits of Normal by Age

Age	Typical Posterior Rhythm (Hz)	Limit of Normal (Hz)
4 months	3–4	*
5 months	5	*
1 year	6	5
2 years	7	
3 years	8	6
6 years	9	7
8 years		8
13 years	≥10	

*Because a posterior rhythm may be difficult to discern in these age ranges, a lower limit of normal is not given.

limits to what can be seen on the EEG recording. Because it is known that the majority of very fast activity in routine EEG recordings represents electrical noise rather than brain wave activity, the filter settings routinely used for most recordings are designed to screen out any very fast activity that might present, be it from the brain or from an artifact source. Other technical constraints of the recording instrument also limit the amount of very fast activity that can be seen. These constraints include the specific design of amplifier circuits and, in the case of digital EEG machines, the sampling rate at which EEG data is acquired, in addition to limitations of the display. In fact, the analysis of very fast activity (so-called "fast ripples" or "high frequency oscillations") has become an important area of ongoing research interest, but it does not yet play a part in the interpretation of routine EEGs.

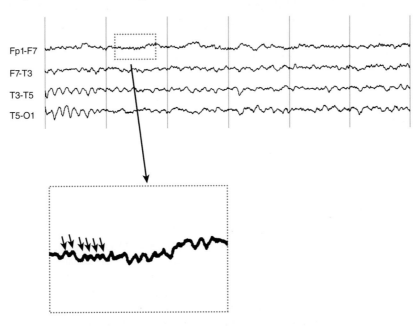

Figure 2.26 This figure shows a close-up of the beta activity present in the top channel of a bipolar montage. The small arrows indicate each beta wave. Note that in the unmagnified version, it would be easy to skip past this low-voltage fast activity without noticing it.

The Anteroposterior Gradient

The concept of the anteroposterior gradient of the EEG is meant to describe the pattern of distribution of two features of the background waves in the normal waking EEG: where the fast activity is most plentiful and where the higher voltage waves are most plentiful. Fast activity is usually most prominent in the anterior brain regions and becomes less conspicuous in the posterior regions. At the same time, the overall voltage of all waves in the EEG during wakefulness generally increases going from the anterior to the posterior head regions. This gradual decrease of fast activity and gradual increase in amplitude going from front to back head regions during wakefulness is referred to as the *anteroposterior gradient* of the waking EEG. This gradient is shown in a referential montage that uses the nose as the reference electrode (the comparison point) in Figure 2.27 and also in a bipolar montage in Figure 2.28. You should typically be able to see this anteroposterior gradient in the waking EEG of a normal person, but whether absence of this usual gradient represents an abnormality is dependent on the specific clinical context.

Fast activity may appear to be absent from the EEG for technical reasons related to EEG instrument settings. When a particular EEG tracing has intrinsically high background voltage, amplifier gains are usually set lower so that high-amplitude channels do not cross other channels and obstruct each other. Because fast activity is usually low-voltage activity (and when the amplitude of slow wave background activity is increased the fast activity is not necessarily increased with it), the low amplifier gains used to display high-voltage EEGs disadvantage the display of any fast activity, which may become visually lost. When this occurs, high-voltage slow waves attain a "smooth" appearance. Resetting the amplifiers to more standard settings allows the lower voltage fast activity to reappear, although the remainder of the tracing may be rendered more difficult to interpret (Figure 2.29). When a tracing appears to be devoid of fast activity, the possibility that amplifier gains are set low to "tame" a high voltage background should be considered. Alternatively, use of more aggressive low-filter settings is a more advanced technique that can be used to display fast activity in a high-voltage record, discussed in Chapter 7.

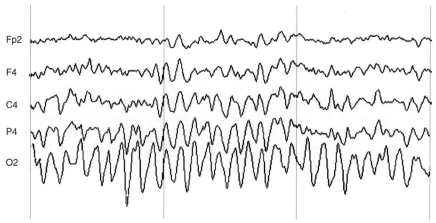

Figure 2.27 This referential recording of an awake patient shows the anteroposterior gradient of fast activity diminishing from front to back, and an opposite gradient of slower activity. Low-voltage fast activity is most prominent in Fp2 and diminishes in the posterior channels. Slower activity, in the form of the posterior rhythm, diminishes in amplitude in the more anterior leads.

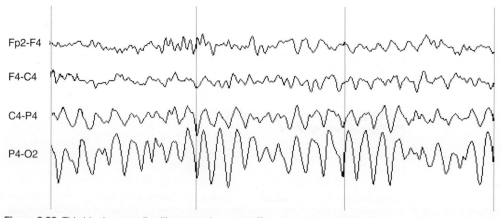

Figure 2.28 This bipolar recording illustrates the same effect as was seen in the previous example, with more plentiful faster rhythms seen frontally and higher voltage slower rhythms seen posteriorly.

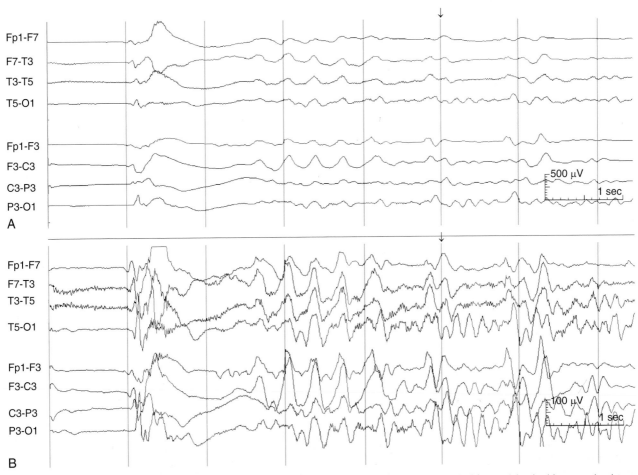

Figure 2.29 (A) The tracing shown in this portion of the figure appears "smooth" and relatively devoid of fast activity. In this example, the apparent lack of fast activity is, however, a consequence of the low amplifier gains used (note the calibration bar in the lower right-hand corner). Because some of the waves are of 400 to 500 µV, amplifier gains were set low, which has resulted in the lower voltage fast activity being lost to the eye. (B) The exact same tracing is shown here with amplifier gains at settings that are fivefold higher. Plentiful fast activity can now be appreciated. When a tracing appears to lack fast activity, the possibility that amplifier gains are set low should be considered.

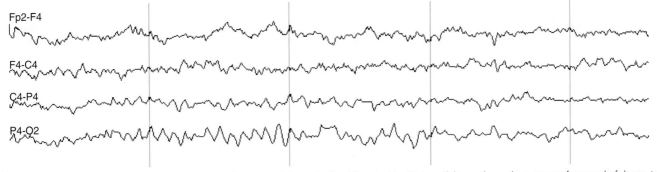

Figure 2.30 The posterior rhythm, seen in the P4-O2 channel, is gradually obliterated by theta activity as the patient passes from wakefulness to drowsiness. Theta waves are seen in other channels as well. The persistence of theta waves in the location previously occupied by the posterior rhythm is confirmation of a transition to drowsiness (see Figure 2.36 for comparison).

DROWSINESS
Theta Activity

Theta activity refers to activity between 4 and 8 Hz. Waves in the theta range are generally considered abnormal in the adult EEG during wakefulness; however, the appearance of theta waves is one of the hallmarks of the onset of normal drowsiness. Theta waves are usually of low voltage and can appear in any brain area; in some patients, theta waves are most prominent occipitally in early drowsiness (Figure 2.30). Theta waves may also be seen in the temporal regions during drowsiness and, in others, they may be seen diffusely. Occasionally, theta waves (or slower delta waves) can be seen at onset of drowsiness in rhythmic, hypersynchronous runs (Figures 2.31 and 2.32). These rhythmic slow-wave runs seen on falling asleep, referred to as hypnagogic hypersynchronies, can be quite

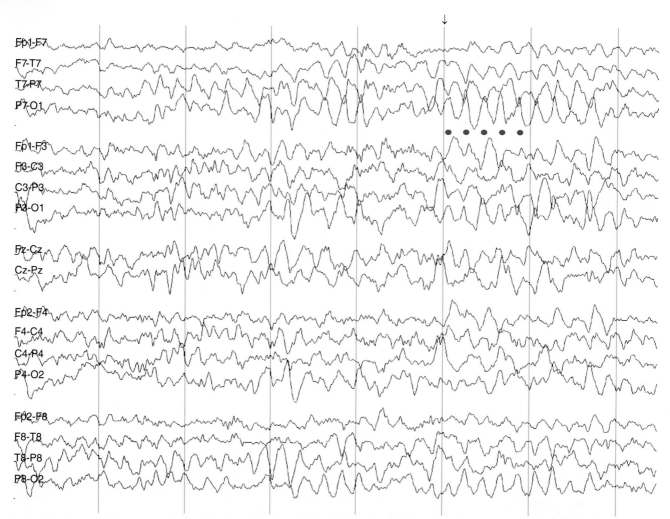

Figure 2.31 Hypersynchronous slowing with drowsiness. As this patient transitions from wakefulness to drowsiness, a fairly dramatic 5Hz rhythmic slow wave is seen in multiple locations on the page, but most prominently in the posterior regions in this patient. A few of the hypersynchronous waves from the left occipital area are highlighted by the red dots. This pattern may be seen during evolution to Stage II sleep.

dramatic at times (hypnagogic = falling asleep). Similar runs can also be seen on arousal, so-called hypnopompic hypersynchronies, which can also be quite dramatic and lengthy (hypnopompic = arousal to wakefulness) (Figures 2.33 and 2.34). Occasionally, these types of sleep-related hypersynchronies may be mistaken for seizure activity, which can also express as a high-voltage, rhythmic discharge. Usually, hypnagogic and hypnopompic hypersynchronies are not difficult to distinguish from epileptic seizure activity in that the hypersynchronies maintain a consistent frequency throughout their duration (rather than speeding up or slowing down as electrographic seizures typically do), and they lack clear sharp components. Although not a change in brain wave activity *per se*, onset of drowsiness is also marked by a reduction and disappearance of muscle, motion, and eyeblink artifact on the EEG, which causes the tracing to appear to "clean up." This, of course, correlates with the muscle relaxation and decrease in spontaneous body movements that come with falling asleep.

Fast Activity

Although fast activity is detectable in most waking EEGs, a relatively sudden, diffuse increase in beta activity can mark

onset of early drowsiness (Figure 2.35). In some, this increase persists into light sleep, but any drowsiness-related increased beta activity usually becomes less noticeable in Stage II sleep and beyond. This type of increase in beta activity with drowsiness is not seen, however, in all patients.

Posterior Rhythm

One of the earliest signs of drowsiness is a subtle decrease in the frequency of the posterior rhythm, although this slowdown is usually seen only briefly before the posterior rhythm disappears entirely. In general, the posterior rhythm frequency only slows by approximately 1 to 2 Hz before it disappears, and such a deceleration is not seen in all patients. Before it finally disappears, theta activity may intermix with the posterior rhythm. When the posterior rhythm disappears completely, low-voltage, irregular theta activity can be seen in its place.

Consider then that, when the posterior rhythm disappears, there are two main possible explanations: either the patient's eyes have opened or the patient has become drowsy. These two possibilities can be distinguished by close assessment of the EEG. When the posterior rhythm suppresses because of eye opening, it is usually replaced by a flat, nondescript tracing as

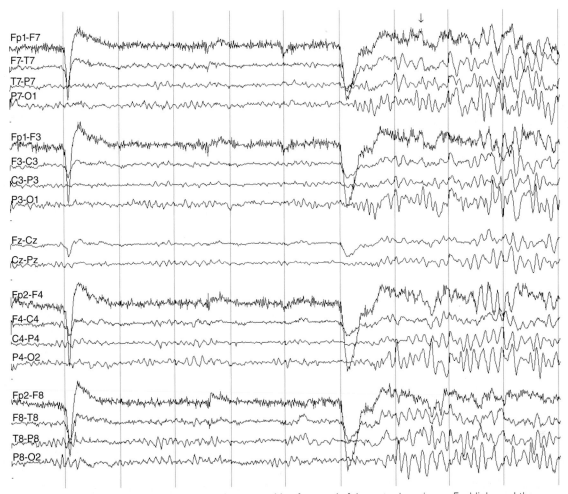

Figure 2.32 This figure shows a more abrupt transition from wakefulness to drowsiness. Eyeblinks and the posterior rhythm are visible on the first half of the page, followed by diffuse, rhythmic theta heralding the drowsy state during the last 3 seconds.

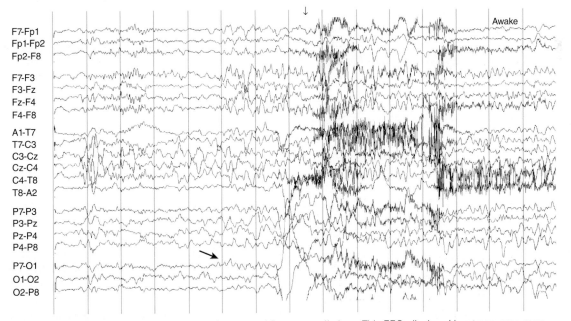

Figure 2.33 A typical appearance of an arousal from stage II sleep. This EEG, displayed in a transverse montage, shows a vertex wave and spindles in the first 3 seconds, followed by 4 seconds of rhythmic, hypersynchronous activity that represents a hypnopompic (arousal) hypersynchrony. The appearance of the posterior rhythm (arrow) and muscle artifact herald wakefulness.

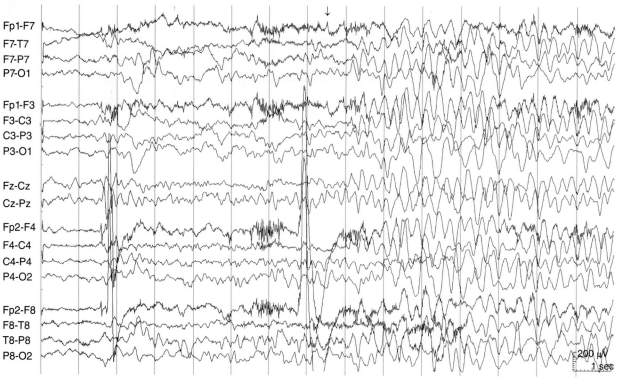

Figure 2.34 High-voltage rhythmic waves dominate the second half of this page and represent an arousal hypersynchrony. The darkened channels and high-voltage deflections seen particularly on the first half of the page represent muscle and motion artifact related to the arousal. Note that this hypnopompic hypersynchrony maintains its 4Hz frequency throughout.

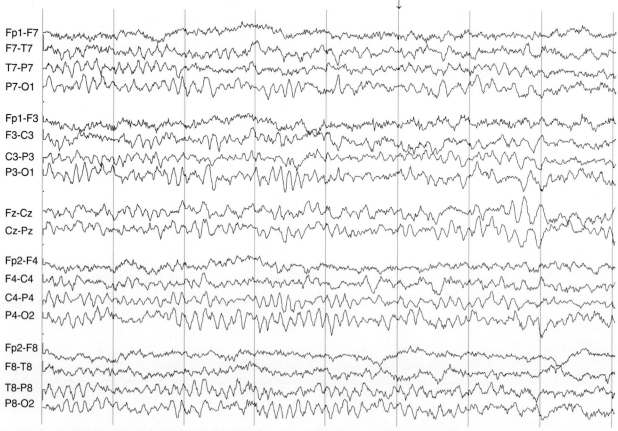

Figure 2.35 Increased fast activity associated with onset of drowsiness. Note the increased amount of very low-voltage fast activity riding the larger waves in nearly every channel. Although most obvious in the frontal channels, the increased fast activity can even be seen superimposed on the posterior rhythm. Increased fast activity is not necessarily seen at the onset of drowsiness in all patients.

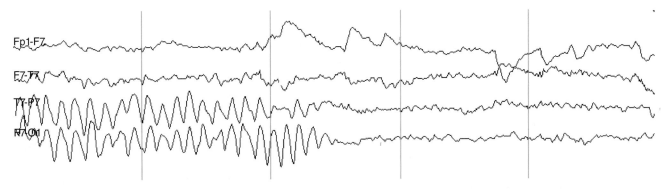

Figure 2.36 In contrast to Figure 2.30, in this example the posterior rhythm transitions to a nearly flat pattern in the bottom two channels suggesting suppression of the posterior rhythm from visual attention or eye opening rather than from onset of drowsiness. This idea is backed up by the presence of the jagged eye movement artifact seen in the top channel (Fp1-F7), caused by quick lateral eye movements, which also suggests that the patient is awake and alert.

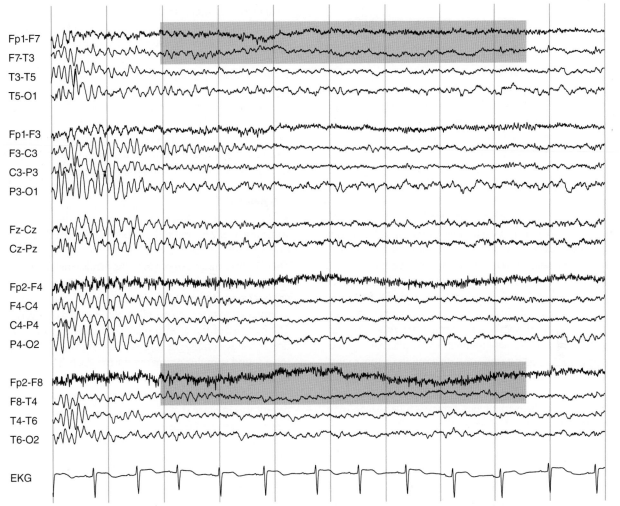

Figure 2.37 Slow roving eye movements are noted in the anterior temporal channels in the form of slow, phase-reversing waves, marking drowsiness. Note that the channels that include the F7 electrode (top red rectangle) become closer to each other at the same time that the channels that include the F8 electrode (bottom red rectangle) become farther apart. This distinctive pattern is consistent with lateral eye movement artifact. The reason that lateral eye movement artifact has this appearance is discussed in more detail in Chapter 6.

in Figure 2.36. Also, continued eyeblinks may be seen, indicating that the eyes remain open. When the posterior rhythm drops out because of drowsiness, it is usually replaced by mixed theta frequencies as was seen in Figure 2.30. If disappearance of the posterior rhythm is related to drowsiness, the EEG record may show other evidence of drowsiness, such as slow roving

eye movements (discussed next), an increase in beta activity, or increased theta activity in other locations.

Slow Roving Eye Movements of Drowsiness

Eye movement artifacts seen in the EEG do not represent electrocerebral activity, but they may provide valuable information to the electroencephalographer regarding sleep state. In drowsiness, after the patient's eyes are closed, slow lateral eye movements can be appreciated by virtue of the artifacts they produce in the anterior leads of the EEG (Figure 2.37). Although not all patients manifest such eye movements, they occasionally represent the only identifiable sign of drowsiness.

Knowing whether a patient is drowsy can be important in a variety of reading situations. For instance, if theta waves are present in the tracing of an alert adult patient, their presence could constitute an abnormality. If, however, the electroencephalographer notes that slow roving eye movements accompany the theta waves, then it can be surmised that the segment in question represents early drowsiness, and the theta waves could be considered normal "drowsy waves."

IDENTIFICATION OF EXPECTED ELEMENTS: SLEEP

Vertex Sharp Waves of Sleep

Vertex sharp wave transients appear in Stage I sleep and continue into Stage II sleep. These waves are often of high amplitude, especially in children, and have a voltage maximum in the central electrodes, in particular at the central vertex, electrode, Cz, and its flanking electrodes, C3, and C4, as was seen in Figure 2.5. These waves can be multiphasic, meaning that each wave may include more than one up-and-down deflection. In some patients, they are blunted in appearance, but in others they can be quite sharp. The polarity of vertex sharp waves of sleep may be either positive or negative, but they are more often negative (wave polarity is discussed in more detail in Chapter 4, "Localization"). When light sleep is well established, vertex waves appear every several seconds in a more or less rhythmic or semiperiodic fashion. Indeed, when the semiperiodic appearance of vertex waves is established and then is interrupted, this is often a clue that rather than continuing into deeper sleep, there has been a subarousal, perhaps caused by a noise in the environment or an internal stimulus. Sleep apnea may also be a cause of such arousals or subarousals. Occasionally, a tracing may show vertex waves that are sporadically asymmetric (seen better over one central area compared to the other) as a normal variant, but if there is a persistent asymmetry, this may reflect an abnormality.

Sleep Spindles

By definition, the appearance of sleep spindles marks the onset of Stage II sleep. The term spindle refers to the fusiform, or sausage-shape, of the spindle waveform as it evolves over one to several seconds, resembling the shape that thread winds onto a wooden spindle. Despite their name, spindles often do not manifest a spindle shape; many spindles maintain a relatively constant amplitude throughout their evolution (as was seen in Figure 2.7). Spindles are easily recognized by their characteristic frequency and location. The most typical spindle frequency is 14 Hz, although slower spindle frequencies at the bottom of the 12 to 14 Hz range are occasionally seen. Likewise, the most typical spindle location is at the vertex and adjacent central areas bilaterally (Cz, C3, and C4 electrodes), similar to the field of vertex waves as described in

the previous paragraph. Especially in children, spindles may appear to migrate anteriorly with deepening Stage II sleep, at which time they may become most prominent in the frontal regions. Especially when they appear more frontally, spindle frequencies may fall as low as 12 Hz (Figure 2.38).

Spindle duration varies to some extent according to age, with longer spindles seen in infancy and early childhood. In infants, spindles of 3 to 4 seconds and even longer are common, whereas in adults, spindles of 1 to 2 seconds are more typical. Spindle interhemispheric synchrony (the tendency for spindles to occur on both sides of the brain at the same time) also occurs as a function of age. Particularly in infants aged under 18 months, the initial spindles seen at onset of Stage II sleep are often asynchronous, occurring first on one side of the brain and then on the other (Figure 2.39). As Stage II sleep deepens, even in infants, there is a tendency for spindles to become more synchronous. After 24 months of age, spindles are expected to occur bisynchronously, even at the onset of Stage II sleep.

Asynchrony of sleep spindles should be distinguished from asymmetry of sleep spindles. In the case of asynchrony, spindles may occur over one hemisphere, then over the opposite hemisphere; but over time there should be a tendency for the number of spindles to "even out" right compared to left. When spindles show a persistent asymmetry, either in their amplitude or in the number that appear over each hemisphere, an abnormality should be suspected.

K-Complexes

K-complexes are complex, polymorphic (meaning that they contain waves with multiple shapes), and often dramatic bursts that occur during sleep, sometimes with sharpened components. There is some disagreement as to the precise meaning of the term K-complex. Some have used the term synonymously with vertex waves of sleep. Others have used the term K-complex to refer to a combination of a sleep spindle superimposed on a vertex wave. The best use of the term probably remains the original definition of the K-complex: a complex of waveforms generated during a sound stimulus occurring during sleep. These waves were recognized as the burst of activity seen when a noise occurred, planned or unplanned, in the recording environment while the patient was in Stage II sleep. Although such complexes often do contain a mixture of spindles and vertex-wave activity, it is not required that these elements be identifiable within a K-complex. The broader definition is important because K-complexes elicited by sound often manifest an electrical field that is much more widespread than those of spindles and vertex waves. Unlike spindles and vertex waves, which are particularly concentrated in the central areas (Cz, C3, and C4) and much less-so in the temporal areas, K-complexes often involve all brain areas at once. The difference in the field distribution of sleep spindles and K-complexes can be seen when comparing Figure 2.6 and Figure 2.13 and is schematized in Figures 2.11 and 2.12.

Because some K-complexes can bear some resemblance to spike-wave discharges, it is important to be able to distinguish between this normal sleep finding and abnormal epileptiform activity. Although K-complexes may occur with auditory stimuli, for several reasons it is not necessary to prove that a sound has elicited the waveform to identify a K-complex.

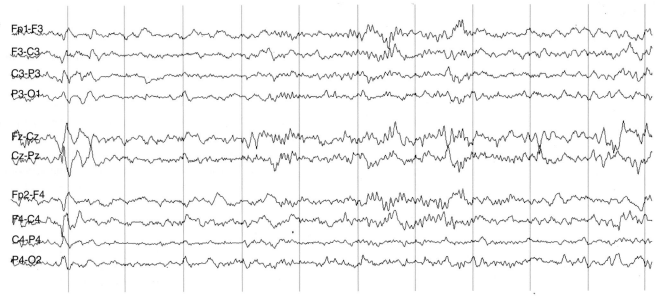

Figure 2.38 In some subjects, especially in deeper Stage II sleep, the sleep spindle field becomes more anterior (frontal and central) rather than purely central. Note that in this example, the spindles are most visible in the Fp1-F3, F3-C3, Fz-Cz, Cz-Pz, Fp2-F4, and F4-C4 channels.

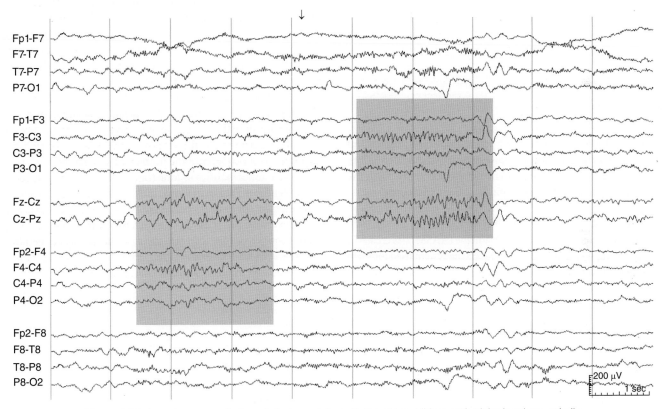

Figure 2.39 Asynchronous spindle activity in an infant. Unlike older children and adults in whom spindle activity generally occurs synchronously over both hemispheres, in infants spindles may alternate over the hemispheres in early Stage II sleep. In deeper Stage II sleep, even in infants, spindles often become bilaterally synchronous.

First, one may not know whether a sound has occurred in the patient's environment because this fact is not always noted on the EEG or audible if sound is being recorded. Second, K-complexes may be associated with subarousals, which may also be caused by nonauditory stimuli, even internal stimuli, which could be impossible for an outside observer to identify.

Slow Wave Activity: Theta and Delta Activity

Theta activity (4-8 Hz activity), and especially delta activity (activity below 4 Hz), are hallmarks of slow wave sleep. In addition to the appearance of K-complexes, vertex waves, and sleep spindles, Stage II sleep may contain up to 20% delta activity. By definition, Stage III sleep epochs contain 20% to 50%

Summary of Stages of Wakefulness and Sleep

Sleep Stage	Sleep Depth	Findings
Wakefulness	Awake	Posterior rhythm identifiable when eyes closed, anteroposterior gradient
Stage I	Early Drowsiness Deeper Drowsiness	Possible slowing of posterior rhythm, followed by complete dropout of posterior rhythm and replacement by low voltage theta waves Appearance of vertex waves of sleep
Stage II	Light Sleep	Sleep spindles, vertex waves, and K-complexes
Stage III	Deep Sleep	Delta activity (20%–50%), some sleep spindles, some K-complexes
Stage IV	Very Deep Sleep	Delta activity (>50%), some K-complexes
REM	REM/Dream Sleep	Lower voltages, faster frequencies (resembles wakefulness), REMS, frontal sawtooth waves

delta activity. Sleep spindles may persist into Stage III sleep and are seen intermixed with the slow-wave activity. By definition, Stage IV sleep contains more than 50% delta activity. With the appearance of Stage IV sleep, spindles all but disappear.

Sleep Stages Used for Sleep Scoring

The American Academy of Sleep Medicine (AASM) has created a sleep scoring system that closely parallels the system used for sleep staging in EEG interpretation. In the AASM system, Wakefulness corresponds to **W**, Stage 1 corresponds to **N1**, Stage II corresponds to **N2**, and Stages III and IV are collapsed into a single stage, **N3**. REM sleep is scored as **R**. The N-terminology was used so that it would always be clear which sleep staging/scoring system was being used, the EEG system or the AASM system.

Identification of Expected Elements: Arousal

Although in some cases arousal from sleep is marked by an unceremonious transition from a sleep pattern to an awake pattern, in many a hypersynchronous run of slowing accompanies the transition. In addition, because most patients stir somewhat during an arousal, it is typical to see a combination of muscle and motion artifact when patients awaken (see Figure 2.33).

VISUAL ANALYSIS OF THE EEG: IDENTIFICATION OF ABNORMAL ELEMENTS

The second step of the process of visual analysis is identification of abnormal findings in the EEG. Although it may be useful to ask the question, "do I see spikes here?" epileptiform activity will often come to the EEG reader's notice without the need to go through a formal inventory of possible abnormalities. Other types of abnormalities, such as voltage asymmetries, are more subtle and it is worthwhile to run through a list of the various frequency bands one-by-one during visual analysis as such asymmetries may not be immediately obvious to the eye without specifically searching for them. Voltage asymmetries are best consciously inventoried according to frequency band, sequentially asking whether delta, theta, alpha, and beta activity are similar on both sides of the brain. Asymmetries of specific elements may also be seen, such as asymmetric sleep spindles or asymmetry of the posterior rhythm.

Other abnormalities to look for include the broad category of epileptiform abnormalities, including spikes, sharp waves, spike-wave complexes, polyspike-wave complexes, and certain repetitive patterns. Continuous slow waves and intermittent slow waves may also represent abnormalities, depending on the context. These and other types of EEG abnormalities are discussed in more detail in Chapter 9.

REVIEW QUESTIONS

1. The posterior rhythm.
   a. may be seen while the patient is either awake or asleep.
   b. disappears when the eyes open and the patient looks at something.
   c. is a sign of coma.
   d. can be seen in the frontopolar electrodes.

2. Which of the following is not a sign of drowsiness?
   a. Acceleration of the posterior rhythm.
   b. Disappearance of the posterior rhythm.
   c. Slow roving eye movements.
   d. Diffuse high voltage slow waves.

3. Which is true?
   a. The terms "alpha rhythm" and "posterior rhythm" are essentially synonymous.
   b. Sleep spindles are a sign of early drowsiness.
   c. The field of vertex waves of sleep is similar to the field of sleep spindles.
   d. K-complexes are a fairly reliable sign of epilepsy.

4. Regarding the posterior rhythm,
   a. if an adult has no observable posterior rhythm, the EEG should be considered abnormal.
   b. suppression of the posterior rhythm is more related to paying visual attention than to eyelid opening.

c. in most patients the posterior rhythm is of higher voltage on the left side.

d. despite good health, the posterior rhythm tends to disappear with old age.

5. Regarding hypersynchronies (rhythmic slow waves) in sleep transitions,
   a. it is normal to see hypersynchronies both at onset of drowsiness and on arousal.
   b. hypersynchronies typically change frequency throughout their course.
   c. it is common for hypersynchronies to be asymmetrical.
   d. hypersynchronies are a sign of epilepsy.

6. REM sleep is not usually recorded in the EEG lab because
   a. patients are usually too nervous when having a test get into dream sleep.
   b. special polysomnographic electrodes are necessary to demonstrate REM sleep.
   c. routine EEG recordings done in the EEG lab are usually not long enough for a patient to have REM sleep.
   d. REM sleep cannot be recorded after childhood.

7. Regarding sleep staging,
   a. vertex waves are not seen in Stage II sleep.
   b. K-complexes are characteristic of Stage II sleep.
   c. stage IV sleep is defined by >20% delta (slow waves).
   d. copious delta activity is characteristic of REM sleep.

8. Which is true?
   a. Sleep spindles are expected to occur synchronously on both sides of the head in any age group.
   b. By 8 years of age, the posterior rhythm should have reached at least 8 Hz.
   c. Slow roving eye movements come from patient anxiety regarding who is in the room during testing.
   d. When falling asleep, once spindles are seen, vertex waves are expected to appear soon after.

ANSWERS

1. ANSWER: **B**. The posterior rhythm is defined as a rhythm that is maximum in the posterior area of the head, present during wakefulness, and disappears with eye opening and fixation. The posterior rhythm is not present during sleep, nor would it be seen in comatose states. The posterior rhythm may have a field that spreads well forward of the occipital areas, but it should never reach the frontopolar electrodes.

2. ANSWER: **A**. Signs of drowsiness include a slow-down (never an acceleration) of the posterior rhythm, followed by drop-out (disappearance). Slow roving eye movements are a useful sign of drowsiness in the EEG and create a distinctive artifact. Diffuse, high-voltage slow waves (hypersynchronies) occur in some patients with drowsiness.

3. ANSWER: **C**. The terms "alpha rhythm" and "posterior rhythm" should not be used interchangeably. Although (especially in adults) the posterior rhythm is often in the alpha range, in abnormal adult subjects and in normal younger children, the posterior rhythm may be below the alpha range. The term "alpha rhythm" can correctly be applied to any rhythm (in any location) between 8 and 13 Hz. Sleep spindles are not seen in early drowsiness, but do appear at onset of Stage II sleep. Vertex waves and sleep spindles are often maximum in approximately the same electrodes: C3, Cz, and C4. K-complexes are a normal feature of Stage II sleep and should not be mistaken for an epileptiform discharge.

4. ANSWER: **B**. In a minority of normal adults, a posterior rhythm cannot be recorded at the scalp. Therefore, absence of the posterior as an isolated finding should not be considered an abnormality. Suppression of the posterior rhythm comes from paying visual attention rather than the position of the eyelids; subjects whose eyes are open but who are not actively paying visual attention may manifest a posterior rhythm. In the majority of the population, the posterior rhythm is of higher voltage on the right side of the brain. The posterior rhythm continues to be present in normal elderly subjects.

5. ANSWER: **A**. Hypersynchronous slow, while not seen in all patients, is a characteristic sign of both the advent of drowsiness and arousal from sleep in many individuals. Drowsy and arousal hypersynchronies maintain the same frequency throughout, which helps distinguish them from other types of epileptiform activity. For instance, the frequency of seizure discharges usually changes throughout their course. In normal patients, such hypersynchronies are expected to be more or less symmetrical.

6. ANSWER: **C**. Although patient anxiety may hinder a patient's falling asleep, if sleep is of sufficient duration, dream sleep should eventually occur. Although special PSG leads can be helpful in detecting REMS, they are not necessary to identify this sleep state, which is characterized by a dramatic decrease in voltage from slow-wave sleep patterns. Also, artifacts caused by REMS are often visible in the anterior temporal leads in the standard EEG electrode set, aiding identification of REM sleep. REM sleep is not often recorded in routine EEG recordings because it does not appear until much later in sleep, and routine EEGs are often not of sufficient duration for the patient to enter a REM cycle. REM sleep (and its equivalent, even in the case of newborns) can be recorded in all ages.

7. ANSWER: **B**. Although vertex waves first appear in Stage I sleep, they continue during Stage II sleep (along with appearance of sleep spindles). K-complexes first appear in stage II sleep. Stage IV sleep is defined by >50% delta activity. In REM sleep, rather than copious delta activity (which is characteristic of stage IV sleep), a low voltage, faster pattern is seen, more similar to waking patterns.

8. ANSWER: **B**. Although it is true that sleep spindles occur synchronously over each hemisphere after 2 years of age, asynchronous sleep spindles are common and considered

normal before age 2 years. The posterior rhythm is expected to reach 8 Hz by 8 years of age ("8 by 8" rule) to be considered normal, though it often reaches 8 Hz well before 8 years of age. Slow groving eye movements are a useful sign of drowsiness and are not related to visual behaviors as the subjects eyes are closed when they occur. After falling asleep, vertex waves typically appear first (Stage I sleep) followed by the appearance of sleep spindles (Stage II sleep).

SUGGESTED READINGS

A manual of standardized terminology, techniques and scoring system for sleep stages of human subjects edited by Allan Rechtschaffen and Anthony Kales, National Institutes of Health, Publication no. 204, Neurological Information Network, 1968.

Beniczky S, Schomer DL: Electroencephalography: basic biophysical and technological aspects important for clinical applications, *Epileptic Disorders* 22(6):697–715, 2020 Dec 1.

Berry RB, Brooks R, Gamaldo C, et al. AASM Scoring Manual Updates for 2017 (Version 2.4).

Loomis AL, Harvey EN, Hobart G: Brain potentials during hypnosis, *Science* 83:239–241, 1936.

3

Introduction to Commonly Used Terms in Electroencephalography

In this chapter, we review the basic terms used in electroencephalography and strategies for communicating EEG findings to others. The creation of a concise description of an EEG tracing is a key part of the art and science of EEG interpretation. The ideal EEG description allows its reader, on the basis of reading report alone, to visualize the appearance of the EEG even in the absence of the tracing. The report also includes a section that describes the technique used to record the EEG and a separate clinical interpretation of the results that discusses the potential implications that the findings might have for the patient. The specifics of EEG reporting are discussed in more detail in Chapter 8, "The Structure and Philosophy of the EEG Report." The main purpose of this chapter is to review the terminology used in describing the EEG.

Careful use and understanding of EEG terminology brings specific advantages to both the writers and readers of EEG reports. The most obvious benefit is that strict use of EEG terminology facilitates unambiguous communication of EEG findings to others. The use of idiosyncratic terms or a personal EEG vocabulary should be avoided because they may not be fully understandable to others. In some instances, certain unique terminology is well understood by the group of neurophysiologists working in a particular lab, but may not be well understood if a report is circulated more widely. Standard definitions for EEG terms were published in 1974, 1999, and more recently in 2017 (see "Suggested Readings"). Another reason for using a common vocabulary is to aid in the matching of EEG findings (e.g., "spikes" or "intermittent rhythmic delta activity") to the clinical syndromes that may be associated with those findings. This is important in both clinical diagnosis and the conduct of research involving EEG. Finally, using the most precise term possible in a description helps discipline the EEG reader during both the interpretation phase and the report preparation process.

DESCRIPTION OF EEG WAVES

As mentioned, an ideal description of an EEG waveform would allow the reader to visualize or perhaps even produce an accurate drawing of the wave on the basis of the written description alone. If a wave can be drawn two or more fundamentally different ways based on a particular written description, the ambiguity in the description provides a clue as to how it could be improved. In general, a complete

TABLE 3.1 Some Wave Parameters with Specific Descriptive Examples of Each	
Descriptive Parameter	**Examples**
frequency	given in cycles per second (cps) or Hertz (Hz) or by frequency range: delta, theta, alpha, or beta
location	occipital, frontopolar, generalized, multifocal
morphology	spike, sinusoidal waveform
rhythmicity	rhythmic delta, irregular theta, semirhythmic slow waves
amplitude	high voltage slowing, a 75 μV sharp wave
continuity	continuous slowing, intermittent theta, periodic sharp wave

description of an EEG wave or event includes the following features: location, voltage (amplitude), shape (morphology), frequency, rhythmicity, continuity, and the amount of the wave seen and in which particular clinical states (awake, drowsy, asleep) it occurs in the record (Table 3.1). For instance, a left temporal theta wave could be described as follows: "Occasional examples of intermittent, medium voltage, sinusoidal 6–7 Hz waves are seen in the left temporal area during drowsiness."

FREQUENCY

Frequencies are quoted either in cycles per second (cps) or in Hertz (Hz). The terms *cps* and *Hz* are synonymous. For historical reasons, each frequency band in the EEG is named using one of four Greek letters. By convention, the names of the letters are written out: delta, theta, alpha, and beta; the symbols for these Greek letters are not used in this context. The terms delta, theta, alpha, and beta are used as a shorthand to refer to rhythms in specific frequency bands and are defined as follows:

delta	0 to < 4 Hz
theta	4 to < 8 Hz
alpha	8 to 13 Hz
beta	> 13 Hz

These frequency ranges are straightforward, but a few observations are worth noting. Note that according to the formal definition, the alpha range is the only "all-inclusive" range, and includes both boundary frequencies (8 and 13 Hz). The other frequency ranges include the boundary frequency on only one side of the range. For example, the theta range, for which the boundary frequencies are 4 and 8 Hz, includes 4 Hz but does not formally include 8 Hz (which belongs to the alpha range), although it does include 7.9 Hz.

Very Fast and Very Slow Activity

Although the list above implies that beta-range frequencies are unbounded on the high side, in reality EEG activity recorded at the scalp with routine EEG instruments rarely exceeds 30 to 40 Hz. High-frequency filtering and other inherent equipment limitations make it difficult to see faster frequencies in routine recordings, even should they be there to record. The assumption behind using high filters (filters that remove higher frequency activity) is that little or no cerebral activity exceeds 30 to 40 Hz so that any signals above this range likely represent electrical noise or "artifact" from muscle, electrical interference, or other sources—hence, the strategy to filter out most activity above this range. In the early days of EEG, frequencies above 30 Hz were said to be in the gamma range, but the term (and the concept) was later discouraged. More recently, there has been renewed interest in "gamma activity" or so-called *high-frequency oscillations*. Although such very fast activity has yet to establish its place in the mainstream of conventional EEG interpretation, it is currently an area of active research, especially with invasive recordings, and may prove useful in identifying abnormal areas of cortex.

Similarly, although the lower bound of the delta frequency range is "zero Hz," it was initially felt that there was little cerebral activity below 0.5 Hz. Newer techniques have successfully recorded very slow activity, which are termed *DC potentials* because they resemble shifts of the baseline (direct currents) rather than oscillations. Again, because standard recording techniques usually exclude most such very slow activity, frequencies much below 0.5 Hz are usually not reliably observed in conventional EEG recordings. Despite the possible existence of some very slow potentials in the EEG, in most situations, the great majority of activity below 0.5 Hz usually represents motion or electrical artifact rather than electrocerebral activity. Conventional filtering techniques attempt to remove these large baseline shifts from the recording because they usually represent artifact related to movement and other sources and may render the EEG tracing unreadable (see Chapter 7, "Filters").

The term *slow activity* refers to any waves for which the frequency falls below the alpha range (i.e., delta and theta activity—activity between "zero" and 8 Hz). Likewise, the term fast activity refers to all activity above the alpha range (e.g., beta activity—activity above 13 Hz).

Frequency, Wavelength, and the Relationship of Frequency to Wavelength

The simplest way to assess the frequency of a wave is to count how many times it cycles within 1 second. If a wave cycles four times (i.e., manifests four "peaks" and four "troughs") in 1 second, then it is said to be a 4 cps or 4 Hz wave. At times, however, a wave cannot be counted for a full second because it lasts less than 1 second. Luckily, it is possible to determine the frequency of a wave not just by counting how many times it cycles within a second, but simply by measuring its duration or wavelength (measured from peak to peak or from trough to trough). The result of a straightforward calculation shows that if a wave cycles five times per second then each wave's duration must be one fifth of a second or 0.2 seconds. Similarly, if a wave cycles eight times per second, each wave will last one eighth of a second or 0.125 seconds. This yields the easy to remember relationship below, where λ gives the wavelength and f is the wave's frequency:

$$\lambda = \frac{1}{f}$$

The rearrangement of the above relationship is also useful and allows estimation of a wave's frequency by measuring its duration (wavelength) on the page, even if only a single wave is available for analysis:

$$f = \frac{1}{\lambda}$$

Both of these simple relationships always hold true. This allows the EEG reader to measure the duration (or wavelength) of any particular wave seen in the EEG (in seconds) and by taking the reciprocal, to determine its frequency (in cps or Hz). Because standard EEG recordings show pages with vertical divisions of 1 second, the wavelength of a given wave can usually be easily measured or visually estimated by determining what fraction of a second it occupies. Such measurements can also be made with the digital time cursor provided by the EEG software. To measure a complete wave cycle, measure the wave from wave peak-to-peak or trough-to-trough (for rhythmic spike-wave complexes, it may be easiest to measure from spike-to-spike). The reciprocal of the wavelength measurement is calculated, yielding the frequency.

A Note on Units

The foregoing examples assume that wavelengths are stated in seconds, but it is common practice to quote wave durations in milliseconds (msec). Rather than stating that a wave lasts 0.2 seconds, it is often said that the wavelength is 200 msec. Using milliseconds is perfectly satisfactory, except when it comes to using the formula cited above to calculate frequency. The reciprocal of 200 (i.e., 1/200) is 0.005, which clearly is not the correct frequency of a wave of 200 msec duration. This is because inserting a wavelength measurement in milliseconds into the formula would yield the result in the undesirable unit of "cycles per millisecond." To yield the frequency in cycles per second, or Hertz, the wavelength measurement used in the formula must be given in seconds (1 cycle/0.2 sec = 5 cps). Examples of how the frequency of alpha, delta, theta, and beta activity are assessed are shown in Figures 3.1 through 3.4.

Waves of Mixed Frequency and the Fourier Theorem

The preceding discussion deals with descriptions of simple waves of a single frequency. However, after a brief look at actual EEG recordings, it is clear that few, if any, of the waveforms seen on the EEG page resemble the pure sine waves seen in math textbooks. Indeed, as a rule, EEG waves represent a mixture of waves of different frequencies and amplitudes. Part of the reason for this mixture of frequencies is that the waveform recorded at the scalp often consists of a mixture of the products of different wave generators from various locations in the brain. In addition, wave-generating circuits in the brain may produce complex, nonsinusoidal waveforms.

One important skill in EEG interpretation is the ability to "deconstruct" EEG waves visually into their component frequencies. The idea that a repetitive complex wave can always be broken down into simpler, fundamental waves was proved by Joseph Fourier in a mathematical theorem now called the

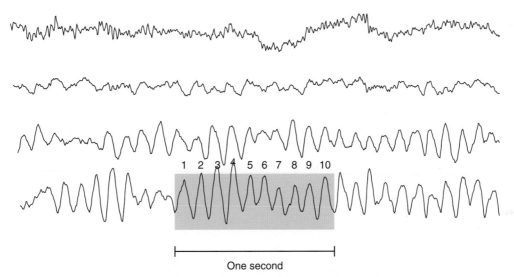

One second

Figure 3.1 The frequency of the wave in the red rectangle is most easily determined by counting the number of wave peaks or troughs seen in 1 second. These waves are rhythmic, fairly sinusoidal in shape, and vary in amplitude. In this example, 10 wave peaks are counted in a 1-second time period, indicating that this is an example of fairly regular 10 Hz alpha activity. This method works best for sustained waves that last a full second. This particular tracing represents an example of the posterior rhythm of a 7-year-old boy.

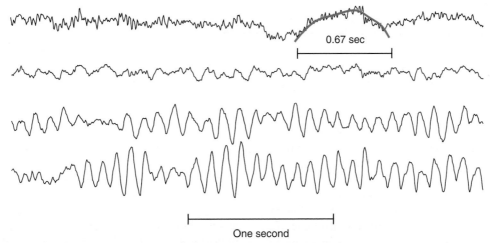

One second

Figure 3.2 The frequency of the nonrepeating slow wave denoted by the penstroke in the top channel is most accurately assessed by measuring its wavelength. The wave in this example is 0.67 seconds in duration, measured from wave trough to wave trough. The simple relationship of wavelength to frequency described in the text in which frequency is the reciprocal of wavelength (1 cycle / 0.67 seconds = 1.5 cycles per second) tells us that this is a single 1.5 Hz delta wave. Note that the wave's frequency can be determined even though it stands alone and does not repeat, and also that the shape of this slow wave can be seen despite the superimposed fast activity. If a wave of this size did repeat, it can be visually estimated that 1.5 such waves would fit into 1 second.

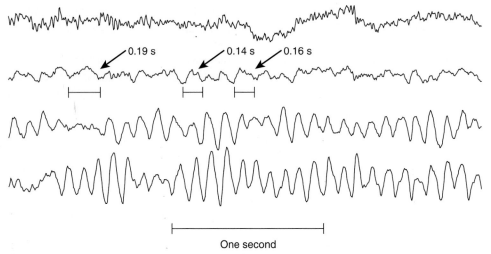

One second

Figure 3.3 The frequency of irregular (nonrepeating) theta waves can be assessed using the same technique of measuring wavelength that was used for the previous figure. In the second channel of this figure, several semirhythmic theta waves can be seen with the durations shown in the figure. Although the waves indicated by the arrows do suggest some rhythmicity, each varies to some extent in wavelength and cadence. By calculating their reciprocals, the measured wavelengths of 0.19, 0.14, and 0.16 seconds correspond to frequencies of 5.3, 7.1, and 6.3 Hz, respectively, all of which are in the theta range (4–8 Hz).

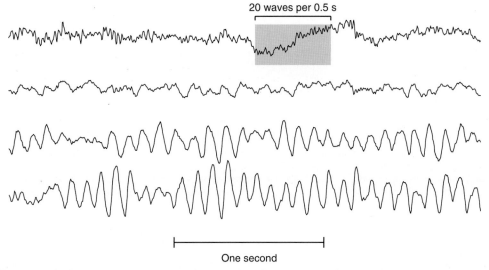

One second

Figure 3.4 The fast activity seen in the shaded area of the first trace is too fast to make an accurate measurement of wavelength and would be cumbersome to count for a full second. Here, in the half-second interval denoted by the shaded rectangle, 20 waves are counted, implying a frequency of 40 Hz.

Fourier theorem. This theorem states, in simplified terms, that any waveform, no matter how simple or complex, can be exactly described by the summation of a sufficient number of simple sine waves. Although a comprehensive discussion of the Fourier theorem is beyond the scope of this text and not necessary to EEG interpretation, this theorem reminds us that even the most complex EEG waves may be thought of as the sum of some number of fundamental sine waves. For example, the apparent complex wave shown in Figure 3.5 actually represents the combination of a 2 Hz wave, an 11 Hz wave, and a 34 Hz wave, of various amplitudes. It is not necessarily the electroencephalographer's goal to identify all of the component parts of any particular EEG wave, but it is useful to be able to identify the fundamental wave and the main superimposed waves of an EEG signal. Figures 3.6 through 3.8

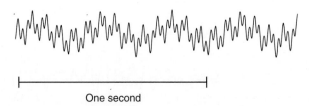

One second

Figure 3.5 The complex waveform shown in this figure represents the summation of three separate sine waves of different amplitudes with frequencies of 2 Hz, 11 Hz, and 34 Hz wave. The three individual contributing components of the wave are shown in the following figures. A 1-second scale is shown.

illustrate the component waves that make up the complex wave of this example.

For those interested in the basic mathematics that describe these waves, a review of the formula for a simple sine wave

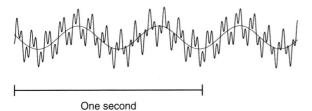

One second

Figure 3.6 The original 2 Hz component of the mixed wave is seen in red superimposed on it. Some of the gradual "up and down" or rollercoaster shape of the complex wave is seen to be explained by this underlying 2 Hz slow-wave component.

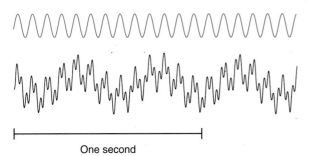

One second

Figure 3.7 The same wave as Figure 3.6 with the 11 Hz component isolated and shown above the original wave. The 11 Hz component of the complex wave can be seen without too much trouble, riding the "rollercoaster" of the 2 Hz wave (look for waves in the original wave that are the exact width of the 11 Hz wave drawn at the top of the figure).

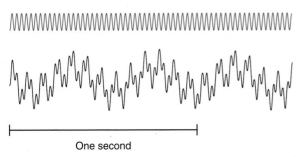

One second

Figure 3.8 The 34 Hz component of the initial wave is probably the easiest to identify. It is seen to "ride" atop the lower frequency waves.

function helps us to recall some of the features of a wave that can be described, thus:

$$f(x) = A*sin(bx + \phi).$$

final wave shape

amplitude

frequency

phase shift

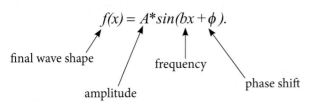

In this formula, varying the coefficient A higher or lower will change the height or amplitude of the resulting sine wave. Varying b will change the frequency of the wave (which is the same as saying that it will make the individual waves wider or narrower). Finally, changing the value of ϕ will shift the wave to the left or right on the x-axis, which is also referred to as shifting the phase of the wave. It is not necessary to know this formula to interpret EEGs, but some may find it helpful to keep the general concepts of this formula and its coefficients in mind when learning to visually separate out and describe the features and component parts of wave mixtures (Figure 3.9A–D).

Although addition of one sine wave to another can be described with mathematical formulas, it is more useful to become accustomed to the appearance of how sine waves add *visually* as opposed to mathematically.

Figure 3.10 shows the result of superimposing or adding a lower voltage 10 Hz wave onto a higher voltage 1 Hz wave. Note that the lower voltage fast activity appears to "ride" the hills and valleys of the slower wave. The key is that both individual waves can still be visually appreciated even though they are mixed together.

When two waves are mixed and one has a frequency that is a multiple of the other, the higher frequency multiple is called a *harmonic*, and the lower frequency wave may be called the *fundamental frequency*. (Occasionally, the lower frequency wave may be called the *subharmonic* if the higher frequency wave seems to be the main frequency.) For instance, if a brainwave has a 5 Hz fundamental frequency, in some cases there may also be a superimposed 10 Hz harmonic. When a wave is mixed together with its harmonic, the resulting wave often has a particular appearance of regular notching.

Figure 3.11 shows an example of adding a 2 Hz wave to its 4 Hz harmonic. Note how the shoulder of the slower wave is regularly notched by the faster wave in this idealized example. The notching may appear on the upslope, downslope, peak, or trough of the slower wave, depending on how the phase of one wave is lined up with the phase of the other when the two are added together. This pattern is important to recognize because the notching patterns created by these harmonics can occasionally be mistaken for spike-wave discharges.

Figure 3.12 shows how the appearance of the superimposition of the same 2 Hz and 4 Hz waveforms can differ depending on how the phase of one is shifted to the right or left in comparison to the other.

Figure 3.13 shows the result of adding a fundamental 2 Hz wave (top trace) to a 7 Hz wave of slightly varying amplitude (middle trace). In reality, the important skill is not necessarily to be able to predict what the result will be of adding two particular waves together but, rather, the reverse process: to be able to look at the bottom trace in Figure 3.13 and to be able to visually "deconstruct" and identify the distinct 2 Hz and 7 Hz rhythms contained within the more complex waveform. Although the examples shown in these figures are of idealized sine waves, the same visual skills apply to the deconstruction of actual EEG waveforms. Of course, the idealized waves seen

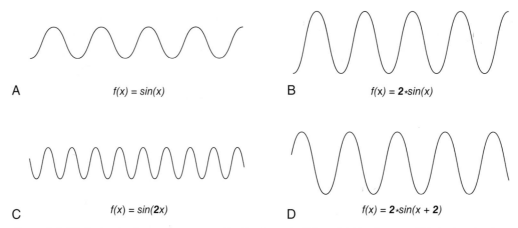

A $f(x) = sin(x)$

B $f(x) = \mathbf{2}*sin(x)$

C $f(x) = sin(\mathbf{2}x)$

D $f(x) = \mathbf{2}*sin(x + \mathbf{2})$

Figure 3.9 (A) A simple sine wave generated by the formula $f(x) = sin(x)$ is shown, which is the simplest form of the general equation $f(x) = A*sin(bx + \phi)$ equation mentioned in the text (where A = 1, b = 1, and $(\phi = 0)$. **(B)** The sine wave formed by $f(x) = 2\ sin(x)$ is equivalent to setting the 'A' coefficient to 2. Note that the height of the wave is doubled, but all other aspects stay the same. **(C)** The sine wave formed by $f(x) = sin(2x)$, equivalent to setting the 'b' coefficient to 2, doubles the frequency of the wave, but it remains the same height. **(D)** The sine wave formed by $f(x) = 2\ sin\ (x + \phi)$ looks just like the wave formed by $f(x) = 2\ sin(x)$ seen just above it in panel B (same height and same frequency), but the resulting wave is shifted horizontally by a certain amount.

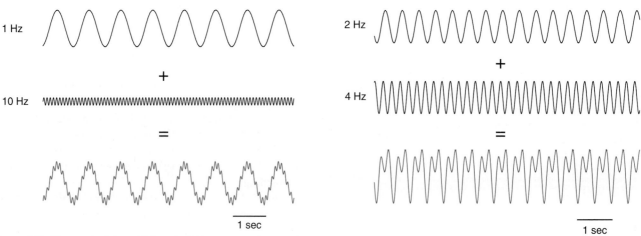

1 Hz

+

10 Hz

=

1 sec

2 Hz

+

4 Hz

=

1 sec

Figure 3.10 The result of the addition of a 1 Hz wave to a lower voltage 10 Hz wave is shown. The top trace shows a 1 Hz sine wave at an amplitude of 100 µV, and the middle trace shows a 10 Hz wave at 20 µV. When the 1 Hz and 10 Hz waves are added together, the bottom wave results, showing the 10 Hz wave "riding" on the fundamental 1 Hz frequency.

Figure 3.11 This figure illustrates the addition of a fundamental wave to its harmonic. The top trace shows the fundamental 2 Hz wave at 25 µV, and the middle trace shows a 4 Hz sine wave of the same amplitude. When a wave is added to another wave that is a multiple of the first wave's frequency (i.e., a harmonic frequency, 2 Hz compared to 4 Hz), the distinctive tracing seen in the bottom trace results. Note the regular "notching" pattern of the smaller wavelet riding on the upslopes of the larger wave. Because the two waves partially reinforce, the summation wave has an amplitude of 40 µV in this example. The degree to which the two waves reinforce and the particular shape that results is partly a function of how the two waves are shifted in the left–right axis with regard to one another (phase shift).

in these examples do not occur in such pure forms in biological systems such as the brain, which are complex and subject to considerable variation.

Figures 3.14 and 3.15 show examples of other ways that pure sine waves can vary, such as in frequency and amplitude, and represent somewhat more realistic approximations of real-life EEG waves.

Figure 3.16 shows a close-up of a recorded EEG wave that contains mixed frequencies.

LOCATION

The location of an EEG event is usually best described in terms of the electrode(s) it involves. The proper placement of the EEG electrodes is the job of the EEG technologist who

produces the recordings. The schema used for electrode naming and placement is called the *International 10-20 system*, formalized by Jasper in 1958. Two 10-20 electrode systems are in use today, the system using the original electrode nomenclature and a modified 10-20 system in which some of the electrode positions have been renamed. Luckily, the great majority of the electrodes have the same name in both systems. Unfortunately, to date, neither system has established primacy over the other, and use of both systems is still widespread. At the risk of some confusion, examples of both

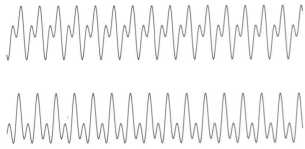

Figure 3.12 The two waves shown here represent the summation of the exact same two component waves (top and middle waves) from the previous figure, except that the phase of the second wave is shifted to the left or right a slightly different amount compared with the first wave before the two are added together. Such combinations of fundamental waves with their harmonics do occur in cortical circuits and should not be mistaken for spike-wave discharges.

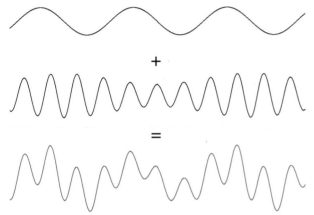

Figure 3.13 The top trace shows a 2 Hz wave of constant amplitude, and the middle trace shows a 7 Hz wave of slightly varying amplitude. The bottom wave shows the result of adding the top wave to the middle wave. In this example, the 7 Hz activity is most readily appreciated in the combined wave, whereas the 2 Hz component is less obvious, although it makes a definite contribution to the final wave's shape. Looking only at the bottom wave, could you sense that there is a slow (2 Hz) component added into the fundamental 7 Hz component?

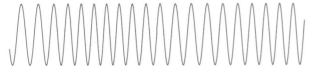

Figure 3.14 The sine wave shown has a constant amplitude (height) but a 15% variation in frequency. Note that the width of each wave increases and decreases perceptibly. Such slight variations in frequency are common in physiologic EEG waves.

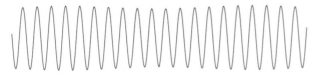

Figure 3.15 This sine wave has the same average frequency as the previous wave, but in this example, the frequency is held constant, and there is a 10% variation in the wave's amplitude.

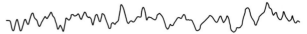

Figure 3.16 An EEG signal acquired from a patient shows a complex, "real-world" mixture of delta, theta, and faster rhythms. Although some sinusoidal elements can be appreciated, many of the waveforms are irregular.

systems are used in this text so that readers will gain some familiarity with each. Some feel the newer system is more logical, whereas others do not feel it offers enough advantages to overturn decades of tradition in the original nomenclature. Because no single electrode name is used to indicate different positions in the two systems, the two conventions can coexist unambiguously side by side. Although it may be tempting for new electroencephalographers to memorize only the newer system because it may seem to represent the "wave of the future," it is probably best first to memorize the system in use in one's own laboratory but to have at least a passing acquaintance with the other nomenclature if called on to read records or reports that come from other laboratories.

The term *10-20* is based on the general strategy of measuring the distance between two fixed anatomical points, such as the nasion (the point where the bridge of the nose meets the forehead) and the inion (the prominent bony point on the occiput), and then placing electrodes at 10% or 20% intervals along that line. This 10-20 system represented an improvement over previous electrode placement systems, some of which relied on absolute measurements (instead of percentages) but failed miserably when heads of different sizes were studied—imagine the effect of using the same system of absolute measurements on the heads of adults or patients with hydrocephalus and the smaller heads of newborns or even premature infants. The general plan for the placement of the 21 primary electrodes of the original 10-20 system is shown in Figure 3.17. The electrode nomenclature for the modified 10-20 system is shown in Figure 3.18. The four electrode positions for which names have changed are shown shaded.

As a note of historical interest, it is not always immediately obvious what part of the brain any particular location on the scalp overlies. When the initial 10-20 electrode system was proposed by Jasper and colleagues, a subcommittee was assigned to determine the relationship between each 10-20 electrode position as placed on the scalp and the underlying surface anatomy of the brain. Jasper's report described that,

after these electrode positions were agreed upon, anatomical studies were carried out with the help of Dr. Penfield, Dr. McRae, and Dr. Caveness to determine the cortical areas over which each position would lie in the average brain. Two methods were employed: (1) metal clips placed along the Central and Sylvian fissures at operation were then used to identify these fissures in x-ray studies of the skull after the EEG electrodes had been applied, and (2) electrode positions were carefully marked in the head of cadavers, drill holes placed through the skull and the cortex marked with India ink in each position before removing the brain for examination.

The result of these studies is shown in Figure 3.19 from the 1958 Report. It is important to remember that an electrode may record from a larger area of cortex (or deeper area of cortex) than the specific anatomical location that it overlies.

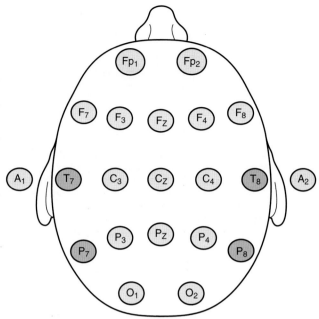

Figure 3.18 Primary electrode names for the newer "modified" 10-20 electrode system are shown. Note that the majority of electrode names are unchanged; the more darkly shaded electrodes represent the name modifications proposed by this new system. In addition to those electrodes shown, this system also establishes names for electrodes in additional intermediate positions that are not routinely used in standard EEG recordings (see Figure 3.22). This modified 10-20 system has not yet been universally adopted, however.

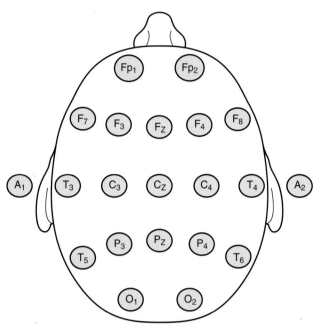

Figure 3.17 The electrode nomenclature for the original 10-20 electrode system is shown. This original naming system is still in use in many EEG laboratories.

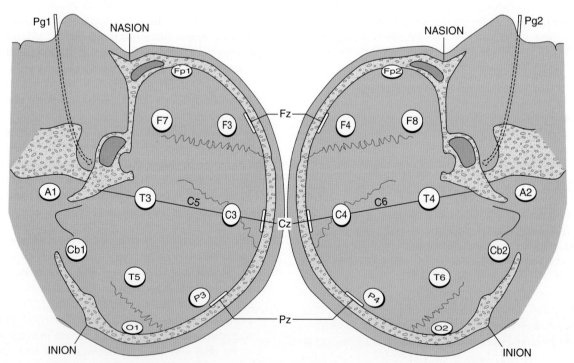

Figure 3.19 These lateral views of the head were based on lateral skull x-rays that Jasper and his colleagues obtained to determine the relationship between the 10-20 electrode positions and the principal fissures of the brain, which are sketched into the figures. (With permission from Jasper 1958, Report on the Committee on Methods of Clinical Examination in Electroencephalography. Electroencephalography and Clinical Neurophysiology, 10, 370-375. https://doi.org/10.1016/0013-4694(58)90053-1.)

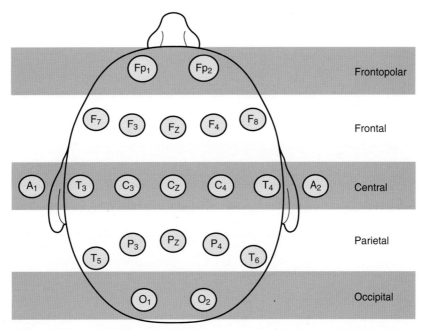

Figure 3.20 The international 10-20 systems group electrodes into five primary transverse planes as shown. One of the goals of the modified 10-20 system was to increase consistency of electrode names in these planes by allowing all of the positions in the parietal plane to begin with the letter 'P' (see Figure 3.18).

Comparison of the Original and Modified 10-20 Systems

The electrode nomenclature used in the original International 10-20 system has different strengths and weaknesses. Most of the electrodes are named using a letter to denote the area of the brain they overlie: F for frontal, Fp for frontopolar, T for temporal, C for central, P for parietal, and O for occipital. The earlobe electrode is denoted by an A. Electrodes over the left hemisphere are subscripted with odd numbers and those over the right hemisphere are subscripted with even numbers. Electrodes in the midline are denoted with a z-subscript, standing for "zero." The electrode nomenclature is generally based on longitudinal and transverse arrays (see Figures 3.20 and 3.21). Although electrode names may be written with subscript nomenclature such as F_7, many EEG instruments (as well as this text) use an unsubscripted format ("F7") to increase readability.

Certain idiosyncrasies common to both systems should be noted. Although the F7 and F8 electrodes are, indeed, placed over a portion of the frontal lobes as their names imply, these electrodes best reflect activity from the anterior temporal lobes and, for this reason, activity recorded from F7 and F8 is often described as anterior temporal lobe activity, despite the fact that they carry an F in their names. The C3 and C4 electrodes are referred to as the central electrodes even though there is no central lobe of the brain. These electrodes derive their names from the central sulcus which divides the adjacent precentral and postcentral gyri, the primary motor and sensory areas.

Certain features of the old system that were deemed undesirable have been addressed by the new system. In general, it was considered preferable that the electrodes running in each sagittal chain (the chains that run from front to back) use the same numeric designations when possible. For instance, in the original 10-20 system, the electrode names for the chain

that runs along the temporal lobe (F7, T3, and T5) each have a different numeric designation, and there was an urge to correct this by replacing the subscripts with '7's. Second, in the original system, some of the letter designations appear in more than one of the transverse rows, such as T3 and T5, which appear both in the transverse chain that links the earlobes but also in the transverse chain just posterior to that.

The modified system of EEG electrode placement proposed by the American Electroencephalographic Society addressed these problems making only minimal modifications (see Figure 3.18). In the modified system, all of the electrodes in the sagittal temporal chains carry a label that includes the number 7 or 8 (e.g., F7, T7, and P7), thus conforming to the idea of using as few numbers as possible in each sagittal plane. Individual letter designations now appear in only one coronal plane (the rule that electrode names T3 and T5 broke in the original system). T5 and T6 were renamed P7 and P8 so that all of the electrode names in that row start with 'P.'

Finally, new, intermediate electrode positions are given standardized names—there are now 75 electrode positions, which include electrode placements lying in between the standard positions described by the original International 10-20 system. These include electrode names such as F5 (for the position between F3 and F7), FC3 for the position between F3 and C3, and so on. This more comprehensive system of electrode naming is also called the *10-10 system* or *10-10 terminology* (Figure 3.22). The many additional electrodes designated by the 10-10 system are not typically used in routine recordings but may be used when special circumstances require them. Because this system modification required the renaming of 4 of the 21 standard electrode positions, many laboratories felt the introduction of the new system would be confusing and have not elected to adopt the modifications,

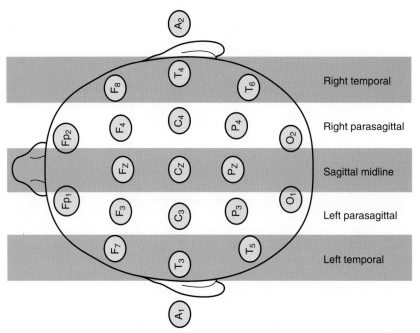

Figure 3.21 The numbering systems for the international 10-20 systems is based on five primary sagittal planes as shown. One goal of the modified 10-20 system was to increase the consistency of the electrode names' number subscripts, allowing the names of all the electrodes in the lateral (temporal) chains to end in 7 or 8 (see Figure 3.18).

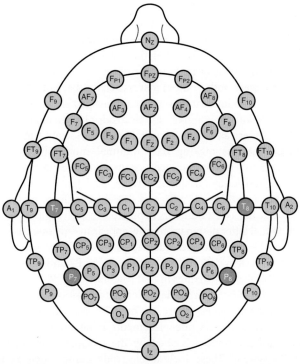

Figure 3.22 The full 10-10 combinatorial system is shown. Note that intermediate electrode positions are given official names and measured positions. Only the electrode positions shown with darker backgrounds have had their names changed in this modified version of the basic 10-20 system. (*From American Clinical Neurophysiology Society Guideline 5: Guidelines for Standard Electrode Position Nomenclature.* J Clin Neurophysiol *2:107–110, 2006.*)

preferring to remain with traditional system instead. The English names for the different electrode positions are given in Table 3.2. These terms are important to know by memory;

TABLE 3.2 Frequently Used Names for Each Electrode Position

Electrode	Common Name
Fp1 and Fp2	frontopolar or frontal polar
F7 and F8	anterior temporal
F3 and F4	superior frontal
Fz	frontal midline
T7 and T8 (T3 and T4)	midtemporal
C3 and C4	central
Cz	vertex or central midline
P7 and P8 (T5 and T6)	posterior temporal
P3 and P4	parietal
Pz	parietal midline
O1 and O2	occipital

Although there is some variation in the common English names given to the different electrode positions, the table above gives names that are most frequently used for each electrode position. The original 10-20 nomenclature appears in parentheses when the electrode name differs.

even though the formal 10-20 electrode name is used in the Description section of EEG reports (e.g., "a spike was seen in F4"), the English name is used in the Interpretation and Clinical Correlation sections of the report (e.g., "a spike was seen in the right superior frontal electrode") to assist nonelectroencephalographers in reading reports.

Focal, Lateralized, Multifocal, and Generalized

These localization terms are essentially self-explanatory. A focal discharge or wave is confined to a single brain area, usually to a tightly clustered group of electrodes but occasionally to a single electrode. A lateralized event is localized to a single hemisphere, and most or all of the hemisphere is involved with the activity in question. A multifocal phenomenon involves three or more brain areas independently; for example, a patient with spikes occurring at different times in Fp1, O2, and T7 can be said to have multifocal spikes. It is generally held that not all of the locations should be in the same hemisphere. A generalized discharge involves all scalp areas or almost all scalp areas in a synchronous fashion, as in the example of generalized spike-wave discharges. Generalized waveforms may still have an area of maximal involvement.

VOLTAGE

Because the EEG waves recorded in any given channel essentially consist of continuous voltage readouts between two given points, the voltage of an EEG wave is simply reflected by its amplitude or height on the page. Indeed, measuring the voltage of a wave is as simple as measuring its height, as long as the extent to which it has been amplified is factored in. Therefore, even though a wave may appear to be large on the tracing, it is not necessarily a high-voltage wave; it may simply be that the amplifier gain has been turned up. Likewise, waves that appear small on the EEG page may actually be of much higher voltage than the visual impression they make if the amplifier gain has been turned down. In fact, without knowing how the amplifier gain has been set, it is impossible to know a wave's true voltage, whether or not it looks big or small on the page. EEG wave voltage is measured from the top of the wave to the bottom of the wave, i.e., from peak to trough.

Gain Versus Sensitivity

The job of the amplifier is to create readable pen deflections from what are, in absolute terms, very low voltage electrical events on the scalp (measured on the microvolt scale). One reasonable way to describe the strength (or gain) of an EEG amplifier would be to quote how many millimeters it can make an EEG pen deflect for each microvolt of input it receives from the scalp. Amplifier gain can, therefore, be described in millimeters per microvolt (mm/μV)—the stronger the amplifier, the more millimeters it can make the pen deflect for a microvolt of input. Looked at in this way, as the amplifier gain increases, the resulting wave looks bigger and bigger on the page, which makes good intuitive sense. As it happens, however, EEG amplifier settings are *not* traditionally described in gain, but in sensitivity.

Amplifier Sensitivity

When the question "how sensitive is this amplifier?" is asked, this is similar to asking "how many microvolts of input are necessary to make this amplifier deflect a standard of one millimeter?" If the amplifier setting is "strong," then only a few microvolts would be required to generate the 1 mm deflection. If the amplifier is weak, it takes a larger input in microvolts to generate the 1 mm deflection. It follows that the unit of sensitivity is microvolts per millimeter (μV/mm)—this is

the standard way in which amplifier strength is described in clinical electroencephalography. Because of the situation in which a stronger amplifier setting requires fewer microvolts to deflect a millimeter, the stronger the amplifier gain, the lower the number to describe the sensitivity. Given the same EEG scalp activity, the display would show waves of greater heights with settings of 2 μV/mm and waves of much lower heights when the setting is 20 μV/mm (by a factor of 10). Because the unit of sensitivity (μV/mm) is the reciprocal of the unit of gain (mm/μV), this leads to a somewhat nonintuitive situation that can take some getting used to: as an amplifier's strength or gain increases (i.e., it make the waves on the page look bigger) the corresponding sensitivity number goes down:

$$\text{gain} = \frac{\text{millimeters}}{\text{microvolt}} \left(= \frac{\text{mm}}{\mu V} \right)$$

whereas

$$\text{sensitivity} = \frac{\text{microvolts}}{\text{millimeter}} \left(= \frac{\mu V}{\text{mm}} \right)$$

The units for amplifier *gain* are discussed here only for explanatory purposes. It is the sensitivity expression that is used in clinical electroencephalography. When a sensitivity of 10 μV/mm is used, it can be useful to understand this sensitivity with the mental construct: "It takes 10 μV of scalp EEG activity to make every millimeter of wave." If the sensitivity is then changed to 5 μV/mm, the thought would be: "Now it only takes 5 μV of scalp activity to make a millimeter of wave—the amplifier setting is now stronger, and the displayed waves should look bigger."

If an EEG is printed on standard EEG paper, figuring the actual voltage of an EEG wave is easy after the sensitivity is known. This is accomplished by simply measuring the height of the wave in millimeters and multiplying by the sensitivity. The product is the wave voltage. For instance, a wave that measures 5 mm in height when the amplifier sensitivity is 7 μV/mm is a 35 μV wave. This follows mathematically because the millimeter unit cancels out in the expression:

$$5\,\text{mm} \times \frac{7\,\mu V}{\text{mm}} = 35\,\mu V$$

This was the simple system for measuring wave heights with a millimeter ruler when EEGs were written with pen and ink on paper: the height in millimeters was simply multiplied by the sensitivity setting of the amplifier. However, few of us are reading EEGs on paper printouts any longer. Instead, our EEG pages are displayed on computer display screens. With the advent of digital EEG, EEG software designers were then confronted with the challenge of not knowing just how big the display screen might be that the reader is using. In fact, if an EEG is displayed on a giant screen in a large lecture hall, it is easy to see how quickly the concept of 5 µV per millimeter loses its meaning. As something of a holdover from the old days of being able to measure EEG waves with a physical ruler, most EEG software will still allow you to measure your screen size and input the measurement so that the microvolt per millimeter sensitivities figures are converted to be physically correct. Doing so would still allow you to hold a ruler up to the screen and multiply the measurement in millimeters by the screen-calibrated sensitivity figure to ascertain the voltage of a wave. However, few readers today calibrate their displays and use a physical ruler to measure voltages. Instead, EEG software provides two simple ways of assessing voltage. The first is an available digital calibration marker that can be displayed on the page (as in Figures 3.23 and 3.24) and compared to a given wave. The second is the use of digital calipers that can be placed on a wave to measure its voltage. Thus, the "mm" term in "µV/mm" is really obsolete and a vestige of the days

when all EEGs were printed on paper—it persists because no better practical term has been found to replace it. Also, retaining this (somewhat false) unit has allowed a specific advantage. Because the proportions of the old paper EEG pages are *similar* to the proportions of pages displayed on computer screens, wave heights that were printed at 5 µV/mm on paper still appear proportional and quite similar to wave heights displayed on a computer screen at the same sensitivity.

How high should the EEG amplifiers be set at any given time? The technologist should choose amplifier settings in real time in such a way as to create a readable EEG tracing "as recorded." The amplifier sensitivity can be further adjusted by the reader at the time of interpretation to bring out different features in the tracing. In general, the amplifier should be set so that EEG waves are large enough to appreciate detail, but not so large that they become distorted or overlap with the channel above or below. The amplifier sensitivities used can have

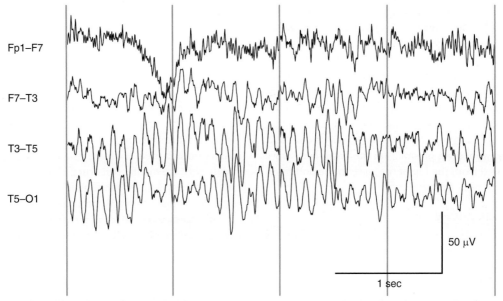

Figure 3.23 Several seconds of wakefulness are recorded. The posterior rhythm is best seen in the bottom two channels, T3–T5 and T5–O1. The amplifier sensitivity is set at 10 µV/mm. Wave morphology is easy to appreciate at these settings, although some of the channels do occasionally cross over into others.

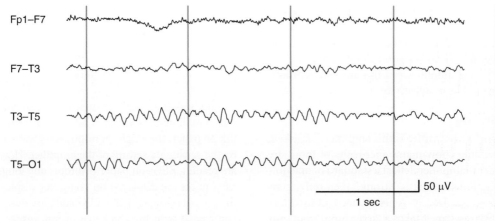

Figure 3.24 The same EEG segment is shown as in the previous example, but this time displayed at 50 µV/mm. The posterior rhythm is still easy to identify and count, but there is a considerable loss of detail in the lower voltage, fast activity.

striking and sometimes unexpected effects on the apparent shape of EEG waves. Figure 3.23 shows a typical EEG tracing during wakefulness recorded at a reasonable sensitivity. In Figure 3.24, the sensitivity is high, and some wave detail is lost. In Figure 3.25, the sensitivity is set too low, resulting in channels crossing each other, and the general impression that all of the waves are spiky in appearance. This same phenomenon is evident again in Figure 3.26 in which the very same posterior rhythm segment is displayed at three sensitivities, giving three different appearances. A similar effect is noted in

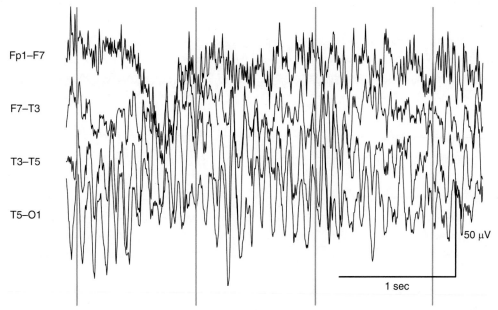

Figure 3.25 The same EEG segment shown in the previous two figures is displayed at a sensitivity of 5 µV/mm. Channels cross frequently making it difficult to discern some of the waves. The posterior rhythm takes on a spiky appearance (compare to the sinusoidal appearance of the posterior rhythm in the previous figure). If only the display of this EEG segment were considered, the reader might question whether the waves of the bottom two channels represent a succession of rapid spikes rather than the posterior rhythm.

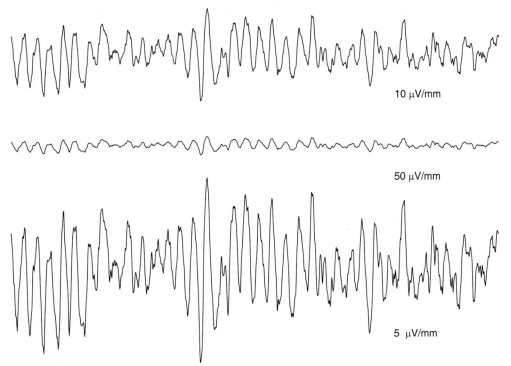

Figure 3.26 A highlight of the posterior rhythm from the previous examples is shown. Note that the peaks and troughs of the posterior rhythm become sharpened when high amplifier settings are used. Although there is little question that this is an "innocent" and typical sinusoidal posterior rhythm when displayed at 10 and 50 µV/mm, the appearance at 5 µV/mm might suggest the possibility of epileptiform activity to some if the low amplifier sensitivity were not noted. Keeping in mind that all three sweeps are representations of the exact same brain wave activity, the importance of the choice of display settings is clear.

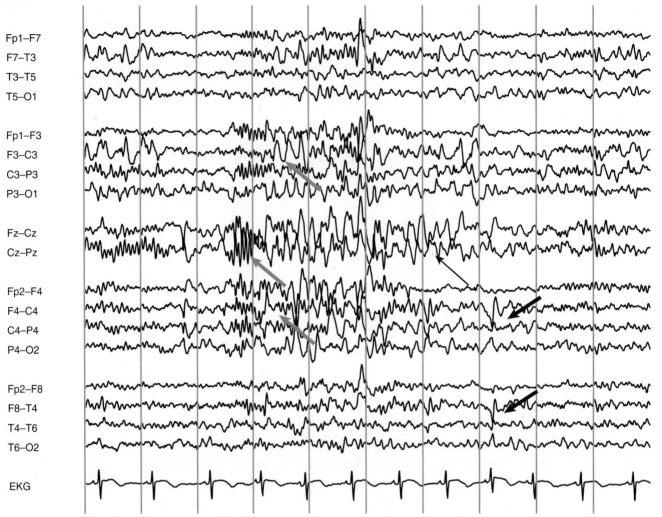

Figure 3.27 A 10-second segment of Stage II sleep is displayed at 20 μV/mm. Sleep spindles are seen at the vertex and in each central area (three red arrows). A cascade of vertex waves of sleep is seen at the vertex (thin black arrow). Compare the appearance of these and other waves to the following two figures. This patient also happens to have right centrotemporal sharp waves (two heavy black arrows).

the examples of a Stage II sleep recording shown in Figures 3.27 through 3.29. The lesson of these figures is that the reader must always be alert to the amplifier settings and whether those settings bias toward underemphasis or overemphasis of the sharpness of waves.

High, Medium, and Low-Voltage Waves

It should come as no surprise that there is no uniform definition for what constitutes a high, medium, or low-voltage wave in conventional EEG. This is partly because different waveforms in the EEG typically appear at different voltages. For instance, a sleep spindle that appears to be of relatively high voltage (for a sleep spindle) may be of lower voltage than a low-voltage spike-wave discharge. Guidelines for high, medium, or low-voltage examples for specific waveforms in specific situations such as ICU recordings have been proposed (see Chapter 12, "EEG Patterns in Stupor and Coma."). However, defining ranges for these terms for all types of EEG waves would be cumbersome, and would also suffer from the disadvantage of requiring both the reader and writer of the report either to have committed all of the ranges to memory

(an unlikely proposition), or to have a table at hand to decode the meaning of these modifiers. Therefore, a certain amount of leeway is usually granted in the use of these terms. Stating that the posterior rhythm is of low voltage implies that it is of lower voltage than most other posterior rhythms you are used to seeing. When you feel it is desirable to communicate the actual voltage of an EEG phenomenon, it is simplest to state the voltage of the wave (e.g., "200 μV delta waves were seen in the frontal regions"), a reporting strategy that will be understood by all.

Synchrony and Desynchronization

At first glance, one would expect that higher voltage EEG waves imply more neuronal activity under the recording electrode and that flatter EEG waves imply less activity. However, the opposite is often the case. EEG waves will only achieve a significant voltage when the neurons below the measuring electrode are acting in unison. Rather than measuring the activity of a single neuron, a scalp EEG electrode measures the summation of the activity of millions of neurons below its location on the scalp. When the neurons under a single

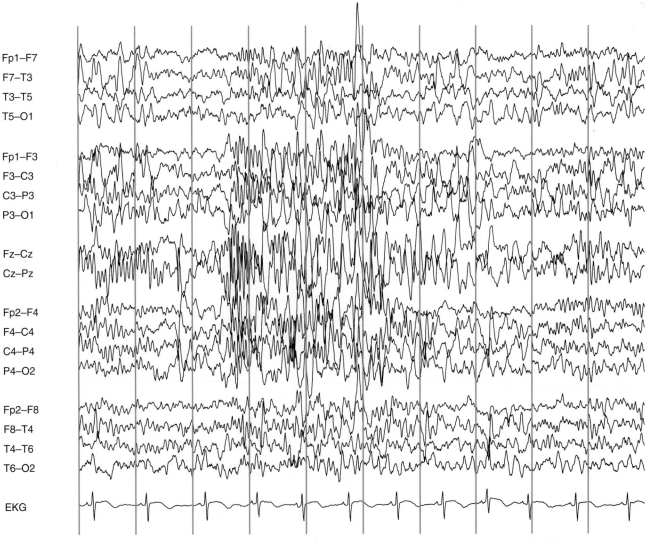

Figure 3.28 The same 10-second segment of Stage II sleep from the previous figure is displayed at 10 µV/mm. The sleep spindles, which are generally of low voltage, take on a misleading, dramatic appearance. The shapes of the vertex waves become difficult to discern, the spindles appear sharp, and the right centrotemporal sharp waves are harder to pick out from the surrounding rhythms, making a 10 µV/mm sensitivity for display of this segment a poor choice.

electrode are manifesting the same type of charge shift at the same time (e.g., from negative to positive), the measuring electrode will "see" a net voltage change toward positive. However, if half of the neurons below the electrode make a net shift to positive at the same time as the other half make a net shift to negative, even though all this charge-shifting reflects that the neurons below the electrode are "hard at work," the positive-shifting population and negative-shifting population will average out to zero. When averaged, no net change will be "seen" by the scalp electrode.

Thus, it follows that EEG waves are of highest voltage when the neurons in the measured area are acting in unison, or in synchrony with one another. This is to say, if all of the neurons under the electrode are manifesting the same charge shift, a large wave will be created. In contrast, another group of neurons under a similar electrode may be shifting charge just as actively, but if each is behaving in a fashion different from that of its neighbor the summed activity will

be cancelled out, and the measuring EEG electrode detects little net change in voltage when averaging the activity of all of the neurons in its recording area. This phenomenon of EEG flattening when neurons in an area do not shift charge in unison is called *desynchronization*. Figure 3.30 shows a schematic of synchronized neurons under a measuring electrode producing an EEG wave. In Figure 3.31, the neurons are equally active in terms of changing charge but are not doing so in unison. The result of this lack of synchrony is a flattening or "desynchronization" of the recorded EEG wave. In electroencephalography, saying that a tracing has become desynchronized is synonymous with saying that it has flattened.

As described above, flattening of the EEG in a particular brain region does not necessarily indicate that that brain area is less active or "resting." Indeed, the opposite is often the case. Several types of biological EEG waveforms manifest lower voltage waves when the area is carrying out a more complex

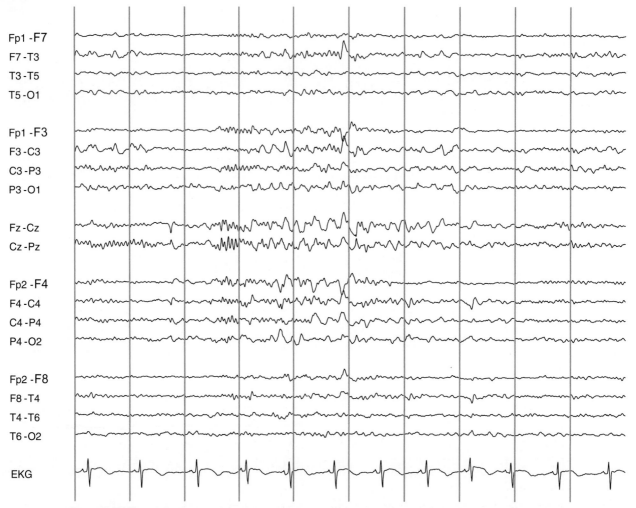

Figure 3.29 The same 10-second segment as shown in the previous two figures is displayed at 50 μV/mm. Although the vertex waves and spindles can still be appreciated, the detail of the fast activity is lost to a great extent, giving the tracing a "smoother" appearance. The right centrotemporal sharp waves have lost some of their sharp character and could be missed with these display settings.

task but show larger waves when comparatively idle. The posterior rhythm is a good example of this phenomenon. The occipital region is primarily responsible for interpreting visual information. The posterior rhythm is a well-formed sinusoidal rhythm appearing in posterior areas when the subject is awake but with eyes closed. When the subject's eyes open and visual activities begin to take place in the occipital lobes, the posterior rhythm desynchronizes, or flattens. During visual processing, it can be imagined that each neuron gets a different task to carry out. When the occipital lobes are idle (eyes closed), it can be imagined that individual occipital neurons do not each have a separate task and that they can be more easily "influenced by others," for example, by neural generators from deeper centers. Thus it is theorized that pacemakers from deeper centers can more easily recruit *idle* neurons to become synchronized to form a discernible wave. When the occipital lobes are occupied with visual processing, each occipital neuron gets a different task to do as part of its job of visual interpretation. The neurons shift charge in a nonsynchronous fashion, the activity of some groups cancels out the activity of other groups and, when averaged by the recording

electrode, the posterior rhythm flattens. Similarly, in normal subjects, the EEG attains its highest voltage during sleep, in particular, during slow-wave sleep, a period of relatively decreased cognitive activity. Of course, EEG flatness does not always reflect the activities of a busy brain. In the examples of large strokes or deep coma, EEG flatness may also represent a simple absence of neuronal activity. The distinction between the two is usually easily made from the context of the clinical recording.

Note that the word *synchrony* can appear in different contexts with different meanings. In this section, *synchrony* refers to the synchronous behavior of nearby neurons. Below, in the section on synchrony and independence, the synchrony of waves between different hemispheres is discussed, and the same word is used to refer to a different phenomenon.

RHYTHMICITY AND CONTINUITY

In reality, most EEG waves recorded in clinical practice do not really resemble the perfect sine waves shown in some of the figures in this chapter, many of which would be more at

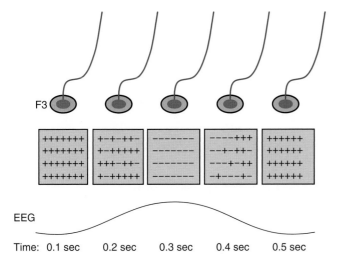

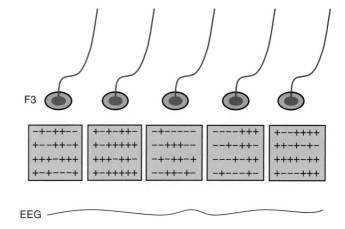

Figure 3.30 This schematic "imagines" a single electrode's view of 28 separate neurons whose polarities shift between positive and negative over time. At the beginning of the time period (first square), all of the neurons have positive polarity. By the middle of the time period, the successive squares show the population of neurons has shifted toward all negative (middle square), and by the end they have returned to all positive (final square). The recording electrode senses the "net" or "averaged" change in polarity of the population. Because, on average, the neurons are changing in unison (in a synchronized fashion), the recording electrode registers a net change in charge and generates the EEG oscillation shown.

Figure 3.31 Although the individual neurons in this figure shift charge between positive and negative more often than in the previous figure, the changes are not occurring in synchrony. The "net" or "averaged" change in charge under the recording electrode is small between each square. Each neuron's behavior is not synchronized to that of its neighbor, and despite the fact there is more overall neuronal activity in this example (more examples of '+'s changing to '−'s and vice versa per second), because the activity does not occur in unison, a relatively flatter, desynchronized EEG trace results.

home on the pages of a mathematics textbook than on the pages of an electroencephalogram. But in what ways do typical EEG waves tend to differ from idealized sine waves? We have already discussed variations in amplitude and frequency that can occur over time, in addition to the fact that many EEG waves consist of a mixture of different sine waves. Beyond voltage and frequency parameters, EEG waves may also vary according to their rhythmicity and continuity.

Rhythmicity

A wave's rhythmicity is a reflection of its regularity and, therefore, its predictability. If an EEG wave is highly rhythmic, it should be easy to predict when the next wave in a series will appear. A continuous sine wave is an example of an ideally rhythmic wave. If you see four peaks of a sine wave in a row, you will know exactly where the fifth peak will fall. Actual EEG waves never manifest this level of perfect rhythmicity, although some highly rhythmic waves come close, such as those shown in Figure 3.32. In some cases, a wave is less regular, but there is still some predictability to its pattern. Such a wave can be described as semirhythmic (Figure 3.33). Finally, a wave may appear with no predictability of cadence at all, in which case it can be described as irregular as in Figure 3.34. A less commonly seen pattern is a periodic pattern. A periodic pattern consists of a wave or complex of waves that appears more or less rhythmically. The older definition of a periodic discharge referred to a waveform occurring every 1 or more seconds with some rhythmicity, therefore applying to slower rhythmic or semirhythmic patterns (typically below 1 Hz). A newer definition for a periodic discharge is for waveforms that occur with some rhythmicity but with background

activity between each complex. Although they seem different at first glance, the two definitions have considerable overlap because the large majority of waveforms that appear less frequently than once per second are bound to have intervening background activity. A periodic pattern following a seizure is shown in Figure 3.35. In general, rhythmic delta activity (RDA) can be visually distinguished from periodic patterns: RDA appears more "oscillatory" (like a hand tremor) and indeed, rhythmic, without intervening background activity between the individual delta waves. Periodic patterns are usually repetitive complexes, with intervening and unrelated EEG activity seen between them, like a hand tapping out a very slow beat on a tabletop, but remaining motionless between each tap.

Continuity

A background pattern may appear continuously or discontinuously (in an on-and-off pattern). In the case of slow waves, continuous slowing in an area may have a different clinical implication than intermittent (discontinuous) slowing. For instance, a patient may have a persistent theta wave in the left temporal area (continuous theta)—the theta wave is almost always there, or at least there for significant periods of time, when you look for it. Alternatively, a pattern may be seen in which a brief run of theta waves or even single theta waves appear every now and then (intermittent theta). A schematic of a frankly discontinuous waveform is shown in Figure 3.36 in which periods of relative flatness interrupt the higher voltage activity.

In the case of neonatal EEG, the concept of continuity is of central importance. In the newborn, different stages of wakefulness and sleep are distinguished in part by the continuity or discontinuity of EEG background activity according to gestational age. In general, after the neonatal period almost all normal EEG background activity is continuous, which is

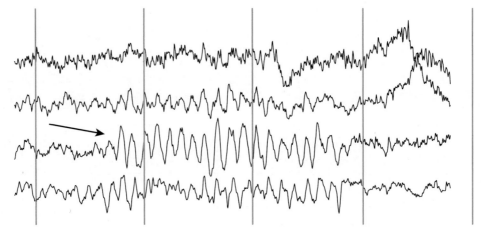

Figure 3.32 The waves in the third channel (arrow) represent an example of the posterior rhythm. Over the 2 seconds followed by the arrow, the peaks and troughs of the waves appear in a predictable fashion and can be described as highly rhythmic.

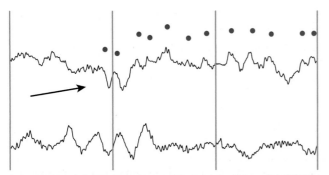

Figure 3.33 The theta waves shown in this example do not appear in a strictly rhythmic pattern, but there is still some predictability to the cadence of their appearance, which could be described as semirhythmic. The red dots are placed above the wave peaks to highlight the fact that the wave's rhythm is far from random.

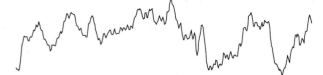

Figure 3.34 This wave is a mixture of irregular frequencies. Looking at any particular portion of the wave, it would be difficult to predict what comes next.

to say that start-and-stop or on-and-off background patterns are not expected. In contrast, in newborn EEGs, many normal background patterns manifest discontinuous patterns. Figure 3.37 shows a normal discontinuous pattern in a newborn at 35 weeks gestational age. Figure 3.38 shows the same baby's EEG pattern while awake showing continuous activity. These newborn patterns are discussed in further detail in Chapter 13, "The Electroencephalgram of the Newborn." Discontinuous patterns are also important in certain patterns seen in coma, such as the burst-suppression pattern.

Synchrony Versus Independence

The term *synchrony* can be used to describe the timing of how electrical events occur in different brain areas relative to one another. (This use of the term is not related to the concepts of neuronal synchronization and desynchronization discussed earlier.) For instance, if we are told that a young woman has sharp waves in both the left and the right central areas, this does not tell the whole story. Do these bilateral central sharp waves appear at the same time (i.e, synchronously), or do they occur at some times on one side and at other times on the other side (i.e., independently or asynchronously)? When an event occurs at the same time on both sides, it can be said

to be interhemispherically or bilaterally synchronous. The term *bisynchronous* can be used as shorthand for bilaterally synchronous to describe activity that occurs synchronously between the two hemispheres. The example of the newborn EEG shown in Figure 3.37 shows examples of both a bisynchronous burst and independent bursts.

PAPER SPEED

Not that long ago, almost all EEG studies were directly recorded onto paper for review. Today the majority of laboratories have adopted digital EEG equipment. In digital EEG laboratories, almost all studies are viewed on a computer monitor and are rarely printed on paper. Even though paper is a thing of the past for most laboratories, the issue of "paper speed" is still an important consideration in EEG interpretation. On paper systems, the display of an EEG wave could either be "pulled apart" or "squeezed together" like an accordion by varying the speed at which the paper was pulled by a motor under the writing pens. The standard paper speed was 30 mm/sec. The correlate to paper speed on digital systems is the number of seconds displayed on each page (essentially, on each screen) at a time, referred to as the timebase. Displaying many seconds on a screen compresses the appearance of the waves and is similar to a slow paper speed. Displaying only a few seconds on the monitor screen has the same impact as a fast paper speed. On many digital instruments, despite the complete absence of paper in the recording process, the term *paper speed* is still used and described in millimeters per second. The *millimeter* term in

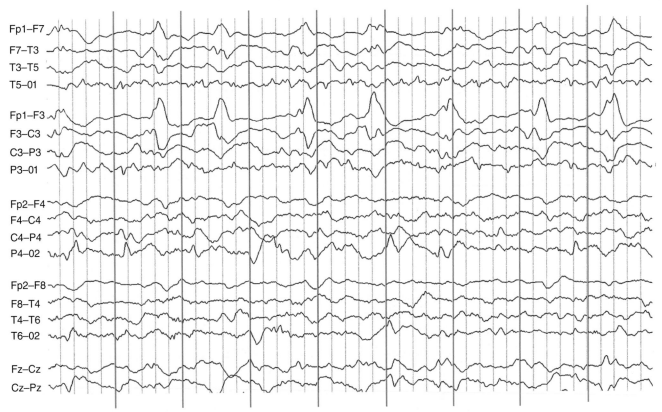

Figure 3.35 Wave complexes that appear only once every 1 or more seconds may be termed periodic. Here, a periodic waveform is seen in the left frontal area firing at a rate of just less than one per second following a seizure. Note that these periodic discharges also conform to the newer definition of periodic waveforms because each is separated by background activity.

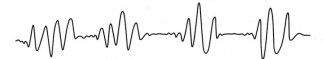

Figure 3.36 This schematic of a discontinuous waveform shows an on-and-off pattern of EEG wave activity separated by brief periods of relative quiet.

this expression is technically obsolete for the same reasons the *microvolt per millimeter* term is obsolete for sensitivity as discussed in the earlier paragraph on amplifier sensitivity—the millimeter term loses its meaning when the EEG software does not know the size of the screen you are using. Some instruments use the related units of seconds per page to avoid this problem.

The paper speed chosen for the display (or seconds of EEG displayed per screen) actually has a large impact on the shape and appearance of EEG waves. The apparent sharpness of a wave is strongly affected by how the software is asked to "stretch out" or "squeeze together" a waveform according to the paper speed chosen. Slower paper speeds (i.e., higher numbers of seconds per page) can sharpen the appearance of any waveform considerably. Figures 3.39 and 3.40 show how wave shapes can dramatically change according to the paper speeds at which they are displayed. The same spike-wave complexes are shown displayed at three paper speeds in Figure 3.41.

The standard paper speed used for recording routine EEGs is 30 mm/sec, which was a rock solid standard when EEGs were printed on paper. Today, we keep in mind that the terms 30 mm/sec or 7 µV/mm have lost their literal meaning, which becomes obvious when an EEG is displayed on a big screen in an auditorium as compared to a smartphone. For this reason, on digital equipment it is good to use the mm/sec expression as a general benchmark, but it is best to make use of the major vertical divisions on the page (each of which equals 1 second) or the calibration bar to understand wave durations. If the 1-second vertical divisions look close together on the page display, then you are reading at a slow paper speed and waves will tend to look sharper. Compare the appearance of the wider vertical divisions in Figure 3.35 to the narrower spacing of the vertical divisions in the neonatal recordings shown in Figures 3.37 and 3.38, reflecting the fact that newborn EEGs are traditionally recorded at the slower paper speed of 15 mm/sec.

Epileptiform Activity

The term *epileptiform activity* refers to EEG events or waves that stand out from the underlying rhythm and usually have a peaked or sharp appearance. The presence of epileptiform discharges does not guarantee a diagnosis of epilepsy. Rather, the presence of epileptiform activity suggests an increased risk for seizures from that area but does not definitely establish whether the patient has had or will ever have epileptic seizures.

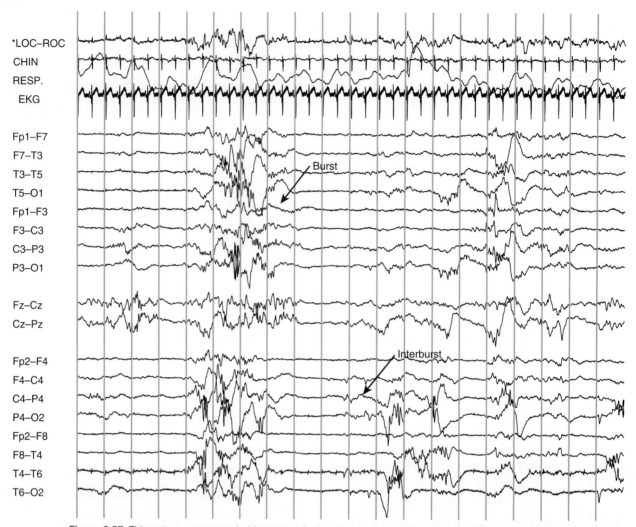

Figure 3.37 This pattern was recorded in a normal, sleeping newborn of 35 weeks gestational age and is discontinuous. There are bursts of EEG activity lasting 3 to 4 seconds, surrounded by much quieter/flatter periods (interbursts). The EEG appears to "turn on" and "turn off" for several seconds at a time. Compare this discontinuous pattern to what is seen in the next figure, which was acquired in the same baby during wakefulness. Note that the periods of discontinuity in this figure differ somewhat between hemispheres. The first burst is essentially bisynchronous (appearing in both hemispheres at about the same time). The next burst occurs first over the right hemisphere and then over the left hemisphere (asynchronously or independently).

A careful distinction is made between ictal activity (seizure activity) and interictal activity (activity recorded between seizures). Strictly speaking, the term *epileptiform activity* should not be used for ictal activity; rather the expression *epileptiform activity* is reserved specifically for interictal activity.

It is fortuitous that the EEGs of seizure patients manifest abnormal discharges *between* seizures. If it were only possible to make the diagnosis of seizures by having the luck of recording actual seizure activity in the EEG laboratory, then EEG would only occasionally be a useful diagnostic tool in epilepsy. Except in the small minority of patients who have very frequent seizures, it is relatively uncommon to record an actual seizure during a standard EEG recording. It is these interictal "footprints" that make the EEG such an effective tool in the diagnosis of seizures. Epileptiform activity is felt to represent increased cortical excitability or irritability. Apart

from epileptiform activity, the EEG may also provide indirect clues that may aid in the diagnosis of epilepsy, such as regions of abnormal slow-wave activity or other findings.

The difference between interictal activity and electrographic seizure activity is usually straightforward. For example, the sporadic individual anterior temporal spikes seen in patients with temporal lobe epilepsy would not be mistaken for actual seizure activity. The patient looks and feels perfectly well while these spikes are firing. It is important to communicate this distinction to patients and their families (and also to referring physicians) who may incorrectly assume that epileptiform activity in the EEG implies that the patient is experiencing ongoing seizure activity that had not been recognized. The patient should be informed that the abnormal discharges seen are a sign of electrical irritability in a particular location and increase the *chances* that a seizure will arise from that

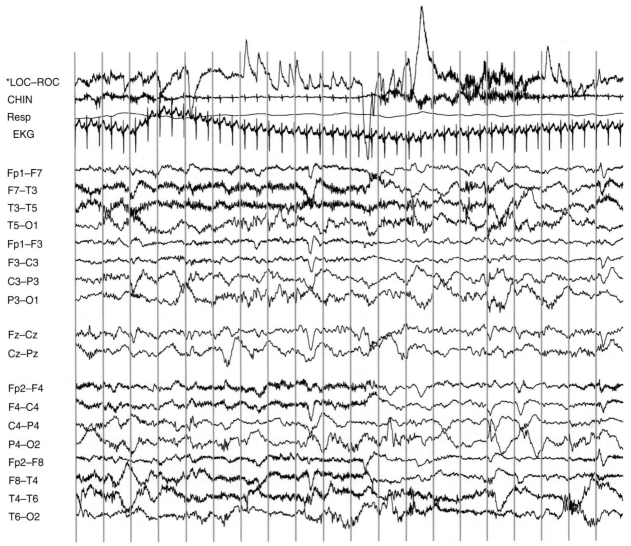

Figure 3.38 This recording was obtained in the same baby while awake. Note that the EEG activity is fairly irregular, but it is continuous. There is no sense of an "on-and-off" pattern as was seen in the previous figure. Some of the channels appear "dark" with muscle and motion artifact as a consequence of the baby's movements.

area, but they do not mean that a seizure has or is occurring in that area, nor do they guarantee that a seizure will occur in that area in the future.

A Note on Clinical Seizures, Electrographic Seizures, and Interictal Epileptiform Activity

A clinical epileptic seizure can be defined as a change in neurologic function associated with and caused by an abnormal, hypersynchronous discharge in the brain (Figure 3.42). Usually, but not always, that discharge can be recorded by routine EEG techniques using scalp electrodes. Even if not recordable at the scalp, this definition implies that during true epileptic seizures, there would always exist some theoretical electrode placement (perhaps even deep within the substance of the brain itself) that could record the abnormal discharge.

An *electrographic* seizure refers to a seizure discharge seen in the EEG in the absence of any associated demonstrable clinical change in the patient. The change in neurologic function experienced during a clinical seizure can range from complete loss of consciousness with dramatic motor symptoms (such as a generalized convulsion) to more subtle changes such as confusional states, psychic symptoms, or visual or sensory phenomena. The definition of an epileptic seizure implies that a change in function, potentially evident to an outside observer or reportable by the patients themselves, has occurred during the episode. In some cases, however, an electrical seizure pattern is recorded on the EEG without any evidence of clinical change. For such "subclinical" electrical events, the terms *electrographic seizure* or *electrographic seizure pattern* are used. These terms are best used when there has been no clinical change associated with the discharge or when the electroencephalographer does not or cannot know whether there has been a clinical or neurologic change. Whether such electrographic seizures should be treated in the same way as electroclinical seizures is an important question in epileptology that has not yet been resolved and is probably situation-dependent.

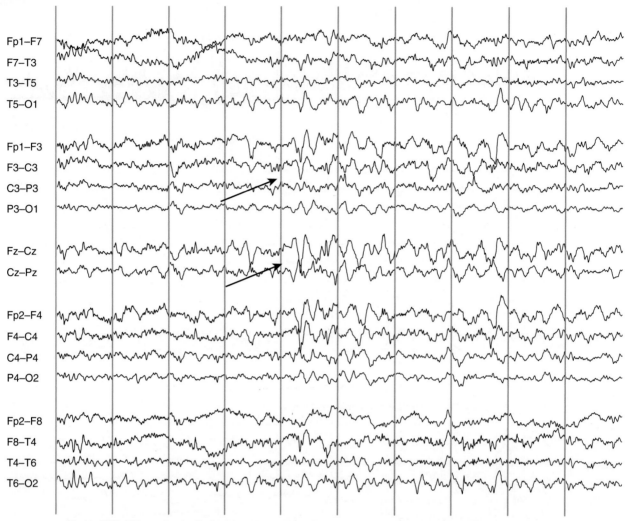

Figure 3.39 This tracing is displayed at 10 seconds per page. The arrows show theta waves (vertex waves) with slightly rounded peaks.

Types of Epileptiform Activity

The most common epileptiform discharges in the EEG are spikes, sharp waves, polyspikes, and spike and slow-wave complexes (also referred to as spike-wave complexes in this text). Spike is a descriptive term for an EEG wave that stands out from the background, has a sharp peak, and whose duration (base) is 70 msec or less (Figure 3.43). Sharp waves are EEG waves with a sharp peak that also stand out from the background whose duration (base) is between 70 and 200 msec (Figure 3.44). Although this definition seems precise, the duration cutoff between a spike discharge and a sharp-wave discharge is somewhat arbitrary and in most cases is not clinically important. In fact, in some patients the same discharge may vary during a recording so that some examples would be considered spikes and others sharp waves, even though they all clearly represent the same electrical phenomenon. There are few situations in which deciding whether a discharge of borderline duration is a spike as opposed to a sharp wave changes the clinical implications of the wave. Nevertheless, the terms are descriptively useful in that each conveys a specific image

to the reader and certain clinical EEG phenomena do tend to manifest either as spikes or as sharp waves.

Sharpness

The sharpness of a wave is difficult to quantify and is somewhat subjective. Interestingly, the quantitative difference between sharp waves and spikes described above is based on the base of the wave rather than the sharpness of the peak. Furthermore, as examples in this chapter have shown, waves can appear sharper visually when displayed at higher amplitudes or slower paper speeds. The difficulty of defining sharpness is reflected by some of the amusing ways it has been defined: "if you touch it, it will feel sharp" or "if you sat on it, it would hurt!"

The term spike-wave complex refers to a pattern in which a spike is immediately followed by a slow wave (Figure 3.45). Occasionally the initial sharp component of the complex is more than 70 msec in duration (i.e., a sharp wave), and the term sharp-and-slow-wave complex can be used. Even in the case of discharges that have been

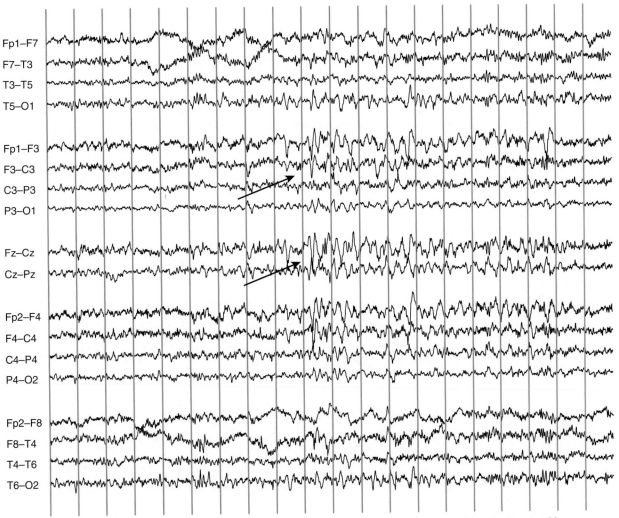

Figure 3.40 The figure shows the same theta waves from the previous figure (arrows) but displayed at 20 seconds per page. Note that the apparent sharpness of the waves is significantly accentuated at this display setting. Slower paper speeds compress the horizontal aspect of the display and increase apparent sharpness.

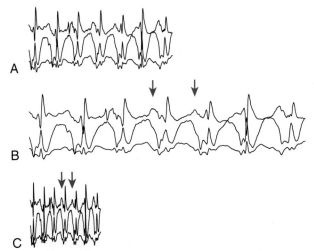

Figure 3.41 The paper speed chosen for display can have a large impact on the appearance of wave shape. Here, the same spike-wave complexes are displayed at three paper speeds: (A) a typical paper speed, (B) a fast paper speed, and (C) a slow paper speed. Note that the same spikes that appear quite sharp in panel A acquire a more rounded appearance in panel B. In panel C, even the aftercoming slow waves begin to acquire a sharpened appearance: compare the large and round appearance of the aftercoming slow waves displayed with fast paper speed in panel B to the same slow waves, now sharp-appearing, recorded at slow paper speed in panel C (arrows).

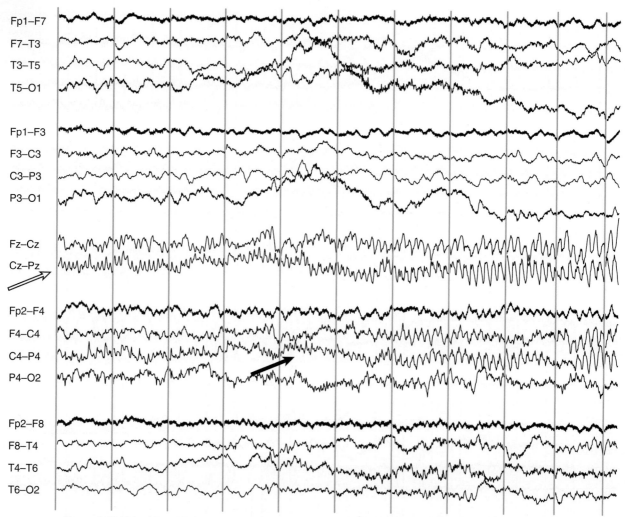

Figure 3.42 This seizure discharge is seen active at the vertex electrode (Cz) at the beginning of the segment (hollow arrow) and spreads to involve the right central area several seconds later (solid arrow).

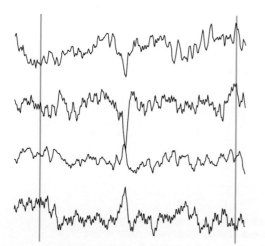

Figure 3.43 The appearance of a spike across a bipolar chain. Each vertical division represents 1 second (or 1,000 msec). Because the bases of these waves are of less than 70 msec in duration, they are classified as spikes rather than as sharp waves.

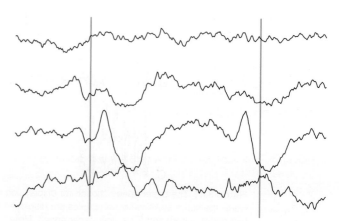

Figure 3.44 Two sharp waves are seen in the third channel. Each vertical division represents 1 second (or 1,000 msec). Because the bases of these waves are of approximately 150 milliseconds in duration, they are classified as sharp waves rather than spikes.

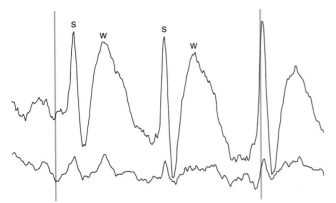

Figure 3.45 Three spike-wave discharges demonstrating classic spike-wave morphology are shown, somewhat enlarged for the purposes of the illustration. Each vertical division represents 1 second. An "s" denotes the spike component, and the "w" denotes the aftercoming slow wave.

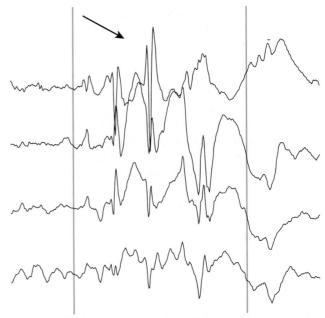

Figure 3.46 Polyspike-wave discharges are displayed in a bipolar chain. Each vertical division represents 1 second. The discharge is classified as a polyspike and slow wave because the initial spike component has multiple (up and down) phases (arrow) before the following slow wave.

called *simple spikes* or *sharp waves*, careful examination can reveal a sometimes subtle aftercoming slow-wave component. Polyspike or polyspike-and-slow-wave discharges are similar to spike-wave complexes except that there are multiple phases (up-and-down sweeps) to the spike component (Figure 3.46).

With only a few exceptions, the use of the terms spike and sharp *wave* connotes abnormal EEG activity. One common exception is vertex sharp waves of sleep, which are normal sleep phenomena. When spikes or sharps are known to be benign from their context, the electroencephalographer has the option of using the essentially synonymous but more neutral-sounding terms *transient* or *sharp transient* to avoid the connotation of abnormality that the terms *sharp* and *spike* suggest to some. The term *transient* is a generic engineering term that refers to any very fast (short duration) electrical event, and such very fast electrical events because they are so narrow, almost always look sharp or spiky. Therefore, most spikes and sharp waves can also be considered transients and there is a large overlap between the terms. In something of an unwritten rule, it is customary to reserve the term *transient* for sharp activity that the reader suspects is benign, such as positive occipital sharp transients of sleep (POSTS) and various normal sharp activity seen in the newborn EEG (e.g., frontal sharp transients). Likewise, one might write "transients seen in F8 likely represent electrode artifact" to avoid using the term *spike*, which may sound more ominous when it is not meant to be.

REVIEW QUESTIONS

1. The preferred method to describe the rate at which a repetitive EEG wave appears is to state
   a. how often it appears in cycles per second (cps).
   b. how often it appears per page of EEG.
   c. whether the wave's frequency is faster or slower than the background frequency.
   d. how often it appears in Hertz (Hz).
   e. a and d

2. The term *slow wave* refers to waves in which range(s)?
   a. Delta
   b. Theta
   c. Alpha
   d. Beta
   e. a and b

3. The term *fast activity* refers to waves in which range(s)?
   a. Delta
   b. Theta
   c. Alpha
   d. Beta
   e. c and d

4. EEG filters attempt to remove activity above 30 to 40 Hz because in scalp-recorded EEGs?
   a. most such activity is artifact (i.e., it comes from some source beside the brain, such as the scalp muscles).
   b. much of this fast activity does come from the brain, but it is not believed to aid in clinical decision-making for the patient.

c. conventional EEG machines cannot record very high frequency activity.

d. EEG filters are not designed to remove activity above 30 to 40 Hz.

5. Regarding the relationship between a wave's frequency and its wavelength, which statement is true?
   a. There is an exact relationship between frequency and wavelength that always obeys a simple formula.
   b. Wavelength can only be used to estimate a wave's frequency if the wave repeats for 1 second or longer.
   c. The relationship between frequency and wavelength only holds well for faster waves and is less accurate for slower waves.
   d. A wave's wavelength and frequency are not strictly related to one another.

6. Regarding complex waveforms, which statement is true?
   a. A good electroencephalographer separates out the different component waves by applying the mathematical principles of the Fourier theorem.
   b. During routine EEG interpretation, electroencephalographers do not use mathematical formulas to divide up complex waves into their component frequencies, rather it is all done visually.
   c. In a complex waveform, the highest voltage component is the most clinically important component.
   d. The human brain cannot be expected to visually sort out the different frequencies in complex waveforms, and this must be done with EEG software.

7. When amplifier sensitivity is adjusted, this will most likely cause a change in
   a. the number of times the waveform repeats on the page/screen.
   b. the apparent height of the wave on the screen.
   c. the left-right position of the wave on the screen.
   d. the shape of the waves on the screen.
   e. b and d

8. Which statement is NOT true?
   a. Changing the amplifier setting increases the voltage of the displayed wave.
   b. Changing the "paper speed" will change the number of times a rhythmic wave will appear on a page/screen.
   c. As amplifier sensitivity goes down, wave heights go up.
   d. As amplifier gains go up, wave heights go up.

9. EEG desynchronization
   a. refers to a situation where the waves in the left hemisphere have a different behavior from the waves in the right hemisphere.
   b. increases the voltage of the wave in the desynchronized area.
   c. often occurs when the recorded part of the brain is idle.
   d. occurs because, when an area of brain is active, the neuronal activity under the recording electrode cancels out through averaging and the EEG wave from that area flattens.

10. Which of the following is not an example of epileptiform activity?
    a. A single spike
    b. A train of spike-wave complexes
    c. Sharp waves
    d. Electrographic seizure discharge

11. Which of the following is true?
    a. A spike is always a transient.
    b. A transient is always a spike.
    c. A spike has a duration of 70 to 200 msec.
    d. A strict definition of sharpness is used in order not to confuse sharp waves with nonepileptiform activity.

ANSWERS

1. ANSWER: **E.** How often a repetitive wave appears is equivalent to stating its frequency. Wave frequencies are stated in cycles per second (cps) or Hertz (Hz), which are synonymous. The number of times a wave occurs on an EEG page is not a reliable measure of frequency because the duration or time-width of an EEG page is not a fixed figure, and can be changed by the EEG software.

2. ANSWER: **E.** The slow wave range encompasses both the delta (0–4 Hz) and theta (4 to <8 Hz) bands, which is to say that any wave with frequency under 8 Hz is considered a slow wave.

3. ANSWER: **D.** Fast activity is defined as waves with a frequency above 13 Hz, which therefore includes the beta range, but not the alpha range (8–13 Hz) or slow wave (delta and theta) ranges.

4. ANSWER: **A.** Although newer research suggests that very fast frequencies may contain potentially valuable information, conventional EEG machines are not well-designed to record this activity, especially from the scalp, and interpretation of very fast activity is not currently a part of routine EEG interpretation. In fact, most activity recorded on conventional EEG above 30–40 Hz does not arise from the brain and much of it represents muscle artifact. For that reason, it is desirable to reduce its representation in scalp-recorded EEG with the use of filters. Although high-frequency filters do, indeed, decrease the amount of high

frequency activity in the EEG display, the reduction is not absolute, but gradual and partial (see Chapter 7, "Filters in the Electroencephalogram").

5. ANSWER: **A**. Wavelength and frequency are reliably related, with one the reciprocal of the other. The simple formulas $f = 1/\lambda$ and $\lambda = 1/f$ where f is the frequency in cps or Hz and λ is the wavelength in seconds show this reciprocal relationship. For example, a wave with a frequency of 8 Hz will have a wavelength of 1/8 or 0.125 seconds. The formula can be used to estimate a wave's frequency, even if it only appears once and does not occur repetitively (e.g., for longer than a second) by measuring the wave's wavelength (λ) from trough to trough or peak to peak and plugging the value into the formula above.

6. ANSWER: **B**. Although the concept of the Fourier theorem is used in this text to introduce the strategy behind separating a complex waveform into its different frequencies, the electroencephalographer does this visually rather than mathematically. Though some EEG software does have the ability to use related mathematical concepts (Fourier transform) to measure the contribution of each frequency to a complex waveform, this is not done as a part of routine EEG interpretation.

7. ANSWER: **E**. Decreasing the amplifier sensitivity (i.e., increasing its gain) will make the displayed waves taller, but it will not change the number of times the wave cycles per page of EEG. Stretching the height of EEG waves by decreasing amplifier sensitivity will also change the shape of the waves, and can make some waves look more spiky. In general, amplifier changes should not shift a waveform discernibly left or right.

8. ANSWER: **A**. Changing an amplifier setting will change the display height (amplitude) of a given wave, but it does not change the wave's voltage. The wave measured from the brain has a predetermined voltage at the scalp (e.g., 50 μV), and the amplifier and other machine settings simply change the manner in which that 50 μV-wave is displayed, causing it to appear taller or shorter, or narrower or wider, but the voltage is already determined by the measurement on the scalp. Paper speed changes will affect how many of a repetitive waveform will appear on the screen, much like pulling apart or pushing together the ends of an accordion. Decreasing amplifier sensitivity (measured in μV/mm) or increasing amplifier gain (measured in mm/μV, though this latter term is not commonly used in EEG practice), which are synonymous, increases the amplitude of the displayed wave.

9. ANSWER: **D**. The term *EEG desynchronization* refers to the apparent flattening of EEG activity that occurs when a functional area of brain becomes involved in a processing task. The most frequently observed example of this phenomenon is the posterior rhythm seen over the occipital lobes (visual areas), which flattens out (desynchronizes) with visual attention and reappears with visual inattention. When waves behave differently between the left and right hemispheres, this is an example of interhemispheric asynchrony.

10. ANSWER: **D**. Spikes, sharp waves, and spike-wave complexes are the most common forms of epileptiform activity. The term *epileptiform* is not meant to be used for actual seizure discharges, however.

11. ANSWER: **A**. The term *transient* refers to any waveform that is very fast (i.e., very brief). Because spikes have, by definition, a duration of 70 msec or less, all spikes are transients. Many transients that occur in the EEG are not spikes, however, because many represent artifacts arising from muscle electrical activity, patient motion, or surrounding electrical interference, to name a few. Sharp waves (rather than spikes) have a defined duration of 70 to 200 msec. Unfortunately, it has not been possible to establish a strict definition of visual "sharpness" in EEG interpretation, but this skill develops through experience as EEG interpretation is learned.

SUGGESTED READINGS

A glossary of terms most commonly used by clinical electroencephalographers. *Electroencephalogr Clin Neurophysiol* 37: 538–548, 1974.

Guideline 5: Guidelines for standard electrode position nomenclature, *J Clin Neurophysiol* 23:107–110, 2006.

Guideline 7: Guidelines for writing EEG reports, *J Clin Neurophysiol* 23(2):118–121, 2006.

Jasper HH: The ten-twenty electrode system of the international federation, *Electroencephalogr Clin Neurophysiol* 10: 371–373, 1958.

Jasper H: Report of the Committee on Methods of Clinical Examination in Electroencephalography, *Electroencephalogr Clin Neurophysiol* 10:370–375, 1958. https://doi.org/10.1016/0013-4694(58)90053-1

Kane N, Acharya J, Benickzy S, Caboclo L, Finnigan S, Kaplan PW, Shibasaki H, Pressler R, van Putten MJAM: A revised glossary of terms most commonly used by clinical electroencephalographers and updated proposal for the report format of the EEG findings. Revision 2017, *Clin Neurophysiol Pract* 2:170–185, 2017.

Noachtar S, Binnie C, Ebersole J, et al: A glossary of terms most commonly used by clinical electroencephalographers and proposal for the report form for the EEG findings, *Electroencephlaogr Clin Neurophysiol* Suppl 52: 21–41, 1999.

4

Electroencephalographic Localization

It is easy to underestimate the importance of learning the skills of precise EEG localization compared with the bigger picture of EEG interpretation. On the face of it, the purpose of localization is to identify the location in the brain at which a recorded EEG event has occurred. Indeed, if this were the only benefit of learning accurate localization, it would still be a key skill in EEG interpretation. However, as we shall see in this chapter and elsewhere in this text, localization can help answer not only where an EEG event has occurred but also *what an EEG event is* and whether it really arises from the brain. Some may be surprised to learn that understanding the topography and polarity of a discharge is the first step in deciding whether an EEG event is truly of cerebral origin or is instead an electrical artifact. Consider for a moment the potential negative impact on patient care of reporting an electrical artifact as an abnormal cerebral discharge. Some electrical artifacts can resemble epileptic spikes, and this type of reading error could culminate in a normal EEG being called *abnormal*, leading to a patient being given the diagnosis of epilepsy and started on seizure medication in error. In fact, mistaking artifact for brain electrical activity (and vice versa) is probably the most frequent significant reading error in EEG. As we shall see, the shape or distribution of certain EEG discharges can be ascertained as being inconsistent with cerebral activity because the localization does not make either topographical or biological sense. In addition, certain discharge topographies can suggest a specific category of discharge and the clinical syndrome to which the discharge might belong, a major aid in clinical diagnosis.

Complete localization of an event includes pinning down both the event's location and its polarity. For instance, an accurate localization would include not only the fact that an event occurs in the left anterior temporal electrode (location) but also whether it is negative or positive at the scalp surface (polarity). Almost all types of EEG events can be localized, whether they be spikes, sharp waves, slow waves, or even voltage asymmetries. In the following discussion, the examples used are spike-like discharges, partly because they are easy to visualize, although the principles discussed here apply equally well to almost all types of EEG events (e.g., sharp waves, slow waves, etc.).

Of all the topics in this book, the skills discussed in this chapter are perhaps the most important for forming a solid foundation in EEG interpretation. Readers who have not mastered the concepts of this chapter will be prone to making significant interpretation errors going forward. A good understanding of the examples in this chapter is a good first step toward becoming an expert electroencephalographer.

FOCAL EVENTS, ELECTRIC FIELDS, AND GENERALIZED EVENTS

Focal Events

A focal EEG event is one that occurs on a limited part of the brain surface rather than over the whole brain surface. Occasionally, an event may be so focal that it occurs in only one electrode. The large majority of discharges from the brain, in addition to appearing most prominently in the electrodes where they are maximal, will also be detectable, though perhaps more weakly, in adjacent electrodes. The electrode position that picks up the highest voltage, be it positive or negative, is referred to as the discharge's *maximum*. Although the discharge may be best seen at its point of maximum, adjacent electrodes often pick up varying amounts of the discharge as well. The schematic of the hypothetical discharge shown in Figure 4.1 shows a discharge maximum in the right parietal electrode (P4) with a field that includes the right posterior temporal electrode (T6) and, to a lesser extent, the right occipital electrode (O2). A focal discharge having a broader field, such as the one shown in Figure 4.2, can have a maximum at one electrode (C4 in this example) but involve a substantial part of one hemisphere.

Rarely, an EEG event may occur so focally that its activity is only recorded in a single electrode, such as the example of the highly focal right parietal discharge shown in Figure 4.3. According to the schematic, the discharge would only be detected by the single electrode (P4), and adjacent electrodes would be electrically quiet. In practice, such highly focal discharges are uncommon and represent the exception rather than the rule (although this phenomenon of highly focal discharges is more commonly seen in newborns). The first two examples given above in which a discharge is detected by a group of electrodes is the more commonly encountered situation. The pattern of how strongly the discharge is picked up in various electrodes helps define the shape of the discharge's electric field as discussed next.

Electric Fields

Several analogies have been used to describe the shape of the electric field of a typical discharge on the scalp surface and how its intensity drops off with distance from the maximum. The analogy of a pebble dropped into a quiet pool of water

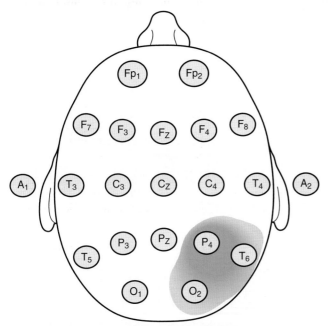

Figure 4.1 This is a depiction of a negative discharge in the right posterior quadrant of the scalp. This depiction can be imagined as a "puddle of negativity" as viewed from above. The darker areas indicate where there is increased intensity of the discharge. In this case, this is a focal discharge with a clear maximum in P4, but the electric field of the discharge extends to include T6 and O2. Rather than seeing a discharge occur at a single electrode position, this is the more common situation in which the maximum of a focal discharge is picked up in one location (P4 in this example) but the discharge can be detected to a lesser extent in adjacent electrodes (T6 and O2). In this case, the discharge can be said to be maximum in P4 with a field that extends to T6 and O2. Note that, if you were standing above the head and observing this spike's "puddle of negativity" in real time, you would see the puddle appear and disappear in less than a tenth of a second.

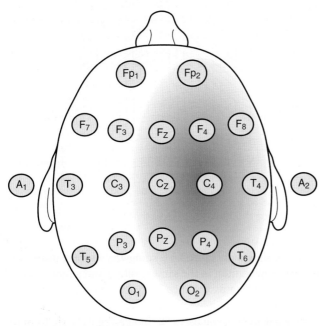

Figure 4.2 In this case of a lateralized discharge, the field of the discharge is maximum at C4 but involves either a whole or nearly a whole hemisphere. In this example, the discharge can be said to be lateralized to the right hemisphere.

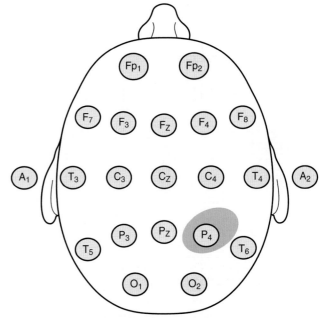

Figure 4.3 The discharge depicted here is highly focal and is only detected by a single electrode (P4). The adjacent electrodes are electrically "quiet." This highly focal pattern is relatively uncommon for brain discharges; most focal discharges affect multiple electrodes at once, at least to some extent. When an electrical event on the scalp is limited to a single electrode, the possibility of an electrode artifact (rather than true brain wave activity) should be considered.

can be used to describe the way a simple field's strength dissipates as it becomes more distant from the point of highest intensity (the splash where the pebble first hit the water). The wave formed from the pebble is strongest at the point of impact but diminishes with increasing distance from that central maximum. This example is useful because many electric fields measured on the scalp do show this radially symmetric (circular) shape but, in practice, many electric fields dissipate from the point of maximum with varying shapes.

Rather than showing a smooth and steady decrease in voltage in every direction from the central maximum point, it is possible for fields to dissipate gently in one direction and more abruptly in another. A better analogy for the shape of some electric fields is the visualization of mountain peaks and ranges. Mountain peaks give a more realistic picture of the variability in shape of EEG fields because they need not be so perfectly symmetrical in shape as the circular waves caused by a pebble hitting water. Imagining the terrain around a 5,000 foot mountain peak, we might expect that the height of land surrounding the peak will fall off with varying steepness in each direction. Likewise, electric fields may manifest a steeper slope of voltage decrease in one direction and a more gentle slope in another direction. An abrupt and immediate falloff in voltage from a central point in all directions as shown in Figure 4.4 would correspond to a thin needle of land (resembling the Empire State Building) 5,000 feet high with nothing surrounding it, an uncommon finding both in geography and in electroencephalography but similar in concept to the discharge depicted in Figure 4.3.

The mountain peak analogy reminds us that an electric field can be visualized as a surface in three dimensions. Just

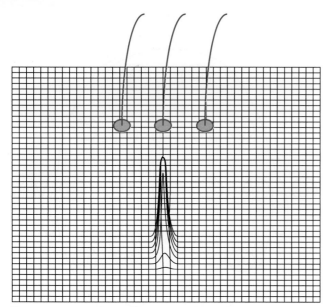

Figure 4.4 This schematic illustrates three imaginary electrodes recording over a highly focal discharge. Note that because of the pin-point location of the discharge, only the middle electrode detects the discharge.

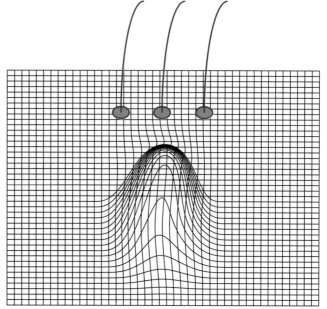

Figure 4.5 The discharge depicted here has a more broadly sloping electric field and, although the middle electrode picks up the biggest voltage change, adjacent electrodes pick up lower voltage changes on the "shoulders" of the field. This scenario is a more realistic depiction of how adjacent electrodes usually pick up brain wave activity.

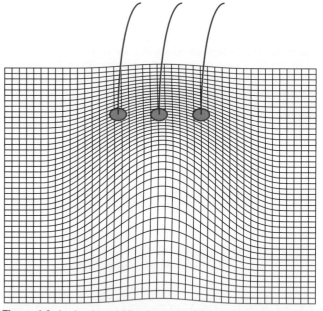

Figure 4.6 Again, the middle electrode picks up the maximum voltage, but the adjacent electrodes also pick up a significant portion of the discharge on the slopes of its electric field.

as slope refers to the steepness of a curve imagined in two dimensions at a given point, the steepness of a surface imagined in three dimensions at a given point is referred to as the gradient at that point. (The slope of a curve at a given point is the slope of a line tangent to that curve at a given point. Similarly, the gradient of a surface at a given point is defined by the slope of an imaginary plane tangent to the surface at that given point.) The rate at which the terrain that surrounds the summit of a mountain falls off is the steepness of the terrain. Unless the mountain is fairly circular in shape, the steepness of the descent may be different if you descend the mountain toward the north, for instance, compared to descending toward the west. The rate at which an electric field changes intensity at a particular point on a surface is called the *electrical gradient* and it, too, depends on the direction in which the field is explored; the two properties are analogous. The exercise of visualizing the shapes of electric fields is similar to visualizing the contours and steepness of a region of mountain terrain. Just as we would never confuse the area of *maximum altitude* of a mountain with the point of *maximum steepness* of a mountain (which may or may not be in the same vicinity), so we will take care not to confuse the point of maximum voltage of an EEG event with the point of the maximum gradient (or change in voltage) of the field surrounding the maximum.

The illustration in Figure 4.4 depicts a highly focal discharge, similar to that shown in Figure 4.3. The plane of the rectangular grid is a representation of the voltages measured on the scalp surface. In this figure, areas fairly close to the discharge's peak are not involved, and relatively nearby electrodes would not "perceive" any change in voltage. Such highly restricted or "punched-out" discharges, if generated by the brain, are relatively uncommon, just as 5,000 foot mountains in the shape of a thin, conical needle are uncommon.

The field shown in Figure 4.5 is somewhat more realistic, with a peak or maximum in the same position, but a more gradual falloff in voltage as distance increases from the maximum point. In this example, adjacent electrodes would pick up somewhat weaker voltages with increasing distance from the point of maximum. Figure 4.6 shows a discharge with a broad field and, although the middle electrode would pick up the highest voltage, the adjacent electrodes would detect a voltage

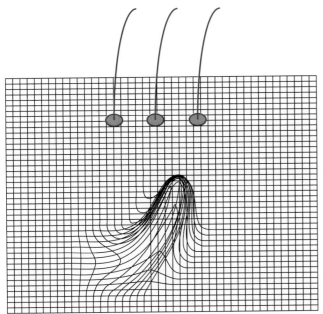

Figure 4.7 The intensity of the field of this focal discharge slopes off more steeply to the right and more gradually to the left. Such asymmetric gradients are common.

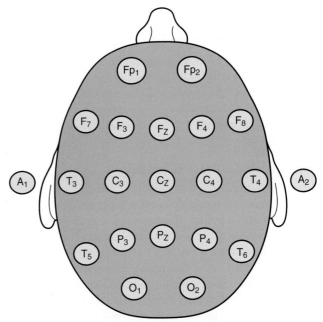

Figure 4.8 This is a depiction of an idealized generalized discharge. The shading of this figure implies that the event is distributed in a perfectly even fashion, although in actual recordings, some amount of unevenness is usually seen even in the fields of generalized discharges.

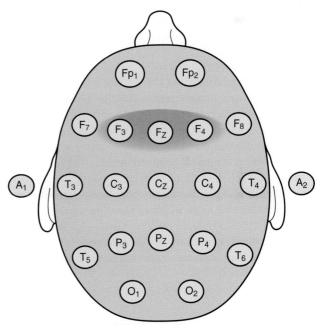

Figure 4.9 This generalized discharge has a clear maximum in the superior frontal and midline frontal electrodes, F3, F4, and Fz. This is a common localization pattern for the "classic" generalized spike-wave discharge, as will be discussed later in this text.

intensity of more than half that detected by the middle electrode. Figure 4.7 reminds us that, quite often, the electric field can slope off asymmetrically from its peak. In clinical electroencephalography, discharges are seen that resemble all of the basic shapes in the preceding figures (in addition to an endless variety of possible shapes). Our task will be to imagine how EEG events of varying shapes display on the EEG page, and also how different discharge patterns on the EEG page correspond to electric fields of different shapes. If we see a discharge that resembles the Empire State Building that involves only a single electrode, we will suspect that this may represent an electrical artifact rather than a signal generated by the brain. Signals generated by the brain are more analogous to a pebble splashing in a pool, creating a big disturbance at the point of maximum but smaller disturbances in surrounding territory.

Generalized Events

In contrast to the focal events described earlier, some events occur in all brain areas at once and are said to occur in a *generalized* distribution. Figure 4.8 depicts a discharge with a perfectly even electric field. With cerebral discharges, even in the case of generalized discharges, there is almost always some unevenness to the field, and an area of maximum intensity can almost always be identified. In Figure 4.9, the discharge affects all brain areas and is, therefore, generalized, but the intensity is highest in the F3, Fz, and F4 electrodes.

The purpose of this chapter is to help the reader become adept at translating the patterns of pen deflections recorded on the EEG page into the particular localizations, polarities, and the shapes of the gradients that those patterns imply. In short, we examine the patterns that EEG pens will draw when they encounter electrical fields of various shapes, including the types depicted in the figures discussed earlier. Ideally, after analyzing an EEG discharge on an EEG page, the reader will be able to imagine a "mountain range" configuration that accurately depicts the shape and the gradients of the discharge's electric field.

EEG WAVES AND EEG POLARITY

What Makes the Pen Go Up versus Down?

An understanding of what causes the EEG instrument's pen to go up or down is the foundational concept of EEG localization and is one of the central skills to master in this chapter. Luckily, the convention is easy to understand. The challenge is to remember to apply it consistently when analyzing EEG patterns.

EEG Channels Are Fancy Voltmeters

A voltmeter measures the potential difference or "voltage drop" between two points. Because voltages are always *differences*, whenever a voltage measurement is made, the reader should be aware which two identifiable points are being compared. Even when we speak as if the voltage at a single point is being described, it is implicit that the point is being compared with some other standard location that is serving as a presumed "neutral" point. Likewise, even though there may be a temptation to think of the output of an EEG channel as representing the activity at some single point on the scalp, every channel deflection we see on the EEG is, in reality, a comparison of two different points on the body (or occasionally a combination of more than two points, as we shall see in later chapters). Any wave seen on the EEG is, therefore, a comparison of the electrical potential between two locations rather than an absolute measurement made at a single location. The waves that we are analyzing are, indeed, the outputs of constantly fluctuating voltmeter readouts comparing two inputs (Figure 4.10).

Inherent to the concept of the voltmeter is, therefore, the idea of differences, or subtraction. Another term for voltage is *potential difference*. If one probe of a voltmeter contacts a point at an idealized voltage of 105 µV and the second probe contacts a point that is at 100 µV, the voltmeter will read out 5 µV. Likewise, if the pair of points recorded is −112 and −117, or even 3 and −2, the voltmeter will read out the same result: the difference of 5 µV. The result of 5 µV that the voltmeter yields gives no clue as to which of these pairings generated it: 105 and 100, −112 and −117, or 3 and −2. The fact that an EEG channel only shows us the difference between two points rather than absolute values has both advantages and limitations. Because each wave displayed on the EEG is a continuous voltmeter output, the reader should always have in mind the following question: which two points are being used to make this channel look this way?

Regarding the question posed at the beginning of this section, the reader may be wondering which would be more logical, for the pen to go up or for the pen to go down in the example in the preceding paragraph in which the difference between Electrode 1 and Electrode 2 is positive 5 µV. The answer to this question is not something that one could derive using mathematical or physical principles. Rather, it is simply an arbitrary convention that was decided by EEG machine manufacturers in the early days of EEG—and one that we have to memorize. The answer for the earlier question is that, if Electrode 1 is more positive than Electrode 2, the pen goes down. The convention assumes that there are two input terminals to the voltmeter/amplifier, Grid 1 and Grid 2, which can also be called *INPUT1* and *INPUT2*. The convention is:

> "INPUT1 more negative: pen goes up. INPUT1 more positive: pen goes down."

This convention is stated first in terms of INPUT1 being more negative (pen goes up!) because it happens that interesting events recorded in EEG are more often negative than positive.

From the amplifier's point of view, INPUT1 is no more important than INPUT2 and its job is merely to subtract one input from the other and amplify the result. However, in the world of EEG, very often the electrode attached to INPUT1 is the "electrode of interest" and INPUT2 is merely a comparison point (this is particularly the case with referential montages, discussed later). Especially if focusing on INPUT1, some may find this convention counterintuitive because in most areas of mathematics and science, values are graphed above the x-axis when they are positive and below the x-axis when they are negative. Alas, in electroencephalography, the opposite is true; this "upside-down" convention is here to stay and can take some getting used to. It may be helpful to use the counterintuitive nature of the convention to help remember it.

Here is how the convention works in more detail: as noted, every EEG amplifier has two principle inputs, which we will refer to as INPUT1 and INPUT2. The EEG technologist essentially decides which electrodes are plugged into INPUT1 and INPUT2 for every channel by choosing a specific EEG montage, which could start with an electrode pair such as Fp1-F7 (meaning Fp1 is attached to INPUT1 and F7 is attached to INPUT2 for the first channel). The situation of INPUT1 being more negative than INPUT2 can be stated in a number of ways, such as: "the difference between INPUT 1 and INPUT 2 is negative" or "INPUT1 is more negative than INPUT2," or as the mathematical expression: "INPUT1 − INPUT2 < 0." In such cases the amplifier's pen deflects upward. Of course, the opposite holds true for the reverse situation: when INPUT1 is more positive than INPUT2, the pen deflects downward as in the example below (Figure 4.11).

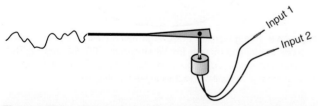

Figure 4.10 An EEG channel can be thought of as a pen attached to the end of a continuously recording voltmeter with the two inputs specified by the recording montage in use. In fact, the EEG channel screen outputs produced by today's digital EEG machines are designed to mimic the pen outputs of older paper EEG machines. These machines recorded literally by placing a pen at the tip of a swinging voltmeter arm as shown in this figure and pulling paper underneath the pen to create an EEG trace.

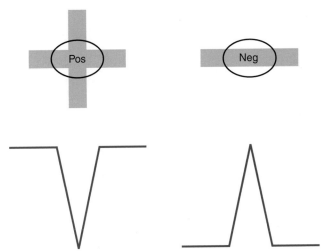

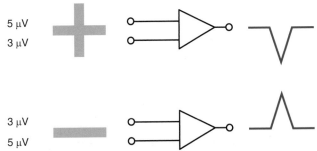

Figure 4.11 The convention for pen movement is best memorized relative to what's going on at the INPUT1 electrode or "Electrode 1." When Electrode 1 is more positive than Electrode 2, the pen goes down. When Electrode 1 is more negative than Electrode 2, the pen goes up. For this reason, in referential montages in which the electrode of interest is attached to INPUT1 and a "neutral" reference electrode is attached to INPUT2, negative events on the scalp appear as upgoing deflections.

When INPUT1 is **more positive** *than INPUT2, the pen goes* **down**.

When INPUT1 is **more negative** *than INPUT2, the pen goes* **up**.

Of all the ways to state this rule, the subtraction expression "if INPUT1 − INPUT2 > 0..." is most correct because it deals with all the possible combinations of each of the two inputs being some combination of positive, negative, or zero. One could quibble with the idea of saying that −3 is "more positive" than −5 because neither is positive. In this text, we use this simpler shorthand, stating that one electrode is "more positive" or "more negative" than another without regard to the sign of the electrodes' absolute voltages for simplicity's sake. Figure 4.12 shows another representation of this convention.

EEG Amplifiers

To understand the meaning of pen deflections, it is useful to consider the nature of the amplifiers used in the electroencephalograph. Perhaps the simplest conceivable amplifier design would be the single-end input amplifier. This type of amplifier would take a single signal as its input and furnish an amplified version of that signal as its output (Figures 4.13 and 4.14). This is not, however, the type of amplifier used in EEG machines, and for good reason. A single-end amplifier is essentially using the building's electrical ground as the comparison input; however, such grounds are usually much too electrically contaminated or "dirty" to be useful for this purpose.

Actual EEG amplifiers, like the voltmeters described earlier, use two inputs (Figure 4.15). The signal from INPUT2 is subtracted from the INPUT1 signal; the result is then amplified and serves as the output. This type of amplifier is also called

Figure 4.12 When the common mode rejection amplifiers used in EEG recording encounter a more positive voltage in INPUT1 compared with INPUT2, the pen goes down as is seen in the top panel. Likewise, when the voltage in INPUT1 is more negative compared with INPUT2, the pen goes up, as is seen in the bottom panel. The top panel shows a 5 µV wave presented to INPUT1 and a 3 µV wave presented to INPUT2. The difference is positive and, by convention, the pen goes down. The bottom example shows the result of switching the input voltages. Now INPUT1 is sensed as more negative and the pen goes up.

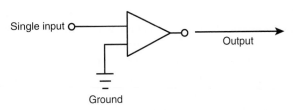

Figure 4.13 A single-end amplifier takes a single active input and compares it to electrical ground, theoretically an electrically neutral position, and amplifies the difference. In practice, building grounds available to us are often contaminated with significant amounts of electrical noise from other devices attached to the ground at other locations in the building. When compared with and subtracted from the weak EEG signals in the single active input, the noisiness of the ground could swamp the low-voltage brain wave signal. For this reason, this simple type of amplifier is not used in electroencephalograph circuits.

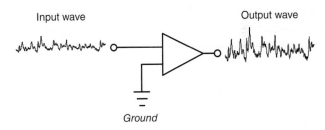

Figure 4.14 This idealized single-end amplifier takes a single signal as input and outputs an amplified version of the same signal. This is not the type of amplifier setup used in EEG machines for a variety of reasons.

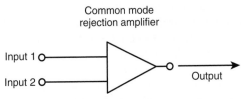

Figure 4.15 The common mode rejection amplifier accepts two inputs, each usually from a single electrode, subtracts one from the other, and yields a single amplified output.

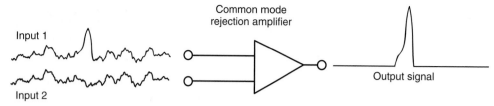

Figure 4.16 An idealized view of a CMR amplifier processing two signals. Note that there is a single difference between the INPUT1 and INPUT2 signals, a single upward deflection seen in INPUT1. The complex underlying waveform that is common to both inputs cancels out or is "rejected." The "difference signal," INPUT1-INPUT2, consisting of the upward deflection, is amplified and becomes the channel output. In this example, one can imagine that the waveform recorded from INPUT2 is obtained from a location such as the earlobe and consists solely of electrical noise found all over the head. The signal recorded from INPUT1, which has been placed on the nearby scalp, is contaminated by the same electrical noise as the earlobe but also contains a single "brain wave," the upward deflection. The result of the CMR amplifier's action is to subtract out the common noise signal which looks the same in both electrodes, and display an amplified brainwave.

a *common mode rejection* (CMR) *amplifier*. As we shall see, the strategy of subtracting one input signal from the other has several important advantages. Figure 4.16 shows how a CMR amplifier behaves with two sample electrical inputs. Note that the component of each signal that is common to both inputs is cancelled out, or "rejected." Only the difference between the two signals appears in the output, and that difference is amplified. Why would eliminating the part of the signal that is common to both electrodes be an advantage? This technique of amplification is especially useful in the field of electroencephalography in which the signals of interest—brain waves—are of very low voltage compared with the electrical noise from external sources that runs through the patient's body. Because the pattern of this external noise signal tends to be nearly the same in the various scalp electrodes, CMR amplifiers cancel out much or all of the external noise component of the signal, ideally leaving only the cerebral component for amplification and interpretation.

Event Localization Using a Bipolar Montage

The examples that follow consider a theoretical spike discharge on the scalp and how it would appear on the EEG record. The first example we examine is a hypothetical spike in the left central region of the brain (the area under the C3 electrode). A spike is, by definition, a quick event, and in this example it will have a negative polarity (the scalp region where the spike occurs becomes momentarily negative while the surrounding scalp remains neutral). The electrode set we use to record the spike is a single chain of standard electrodes that goes along the scalp from front to back just to the left of the midline: Fp1, F3, C3, P3, and O1 (the left frontopolar, superior frontal, central, parietal, and occipital electrodes, respectively). The technique used for the following examples is the typical strategy for creating a bipolar chain with these electrodes by looking at a succession of pairings of adjacent electrodes from front to back: Fp1 to F3, then F3 to C3, C3 to P3, and P3 to O1. The output from each electrode pair (the line of EEG we eventually read) is a subtraction of one electrode in the pair from the other. The term bipolar is used because each EEG channel generated represents a comparison of two cerebral locations. Each of the two electrodes in the pair can be said to be "of interest" because both reflect brain activity, and it is possible that a clinically important event could arise from under any of

the five electrodes. (In the contrasting situation of referential montages described in more detail later, INPUT1 is connected to an electrode over the brain, and INPUT2 is connected to some other reference point that is presumably not "of interest" but is used for the purpose of subtracting noise. One might expect the opposite of the bipolar technique, the referential technique, to be "monopolar" or "unipolar," but that is not at all the case—even in referential montages, each output channel represents the comparison of two or more points and is therefore technically no less "bipolar.") Note that there are five electrodes in this chain but there are necessarily only four possible sequential pairings. Thus, a chain of five consecutive electrodes will produce four channels of EEG in a bipolar chain.

The "Negative Phase Reversal"

Figure 4.17 depicts the field of a –50 µV spike occurring at C3 with no activity at all in the surrounding electrodes. On the right, the four channels representing the output of the bipolar chain are depicted. It is worthwhile to go through each line of the output to understand exactly why the voltage measurements shown on the left side of the figure are associated with the EEG trace on the right side of the figure. The example of a surface-*negative* spike is given first because they are more common than surface-positive spikes, though both occur. While this process of going through EEG channels line-by-line and predicting the direction of pen deflection is somewhat tedious, you will not need to be doing this routinely when reading EEGs. Understanding these step-by-step fundamentals now will allow you to recognize the different patterns going forward and quickly understand what they represent.

Channel 1: The first channel, Fp1-F3, is measuring the difference between 0 µV at Fp1 and 0 µV at F3. Because there is no difference, the Fp1-F3 channel remains flat.

Channel 2: The second channel, F3-C3, is comparing 0 µV in INPUT1 (F3) and –50 µV in INPUT2 (C3). Because the convention is that if the first electrode is "more positive" than the second, the pen goes down, and a downward pen deflection is produced.

Channel 3: The third channel, C3-P3, compares –50 µV in INPUT1 to 0 µV in INPUT2. Now Electrode 1 is more negative than Electrode 2 (the opposite of what occurred in Channel 2), so the convention tells us that the pen goes up.

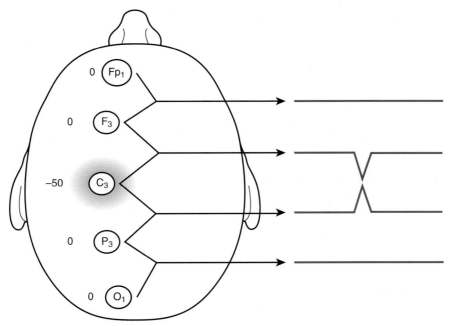

Figure 4.17 EEG channels 1, 2, 3, and 4 on the right side of the figure depict a negative phase reversal corresponding to a focal negatively-charged spike that is confined to the C3 electrode—none of the negativity of the spike is detected by adjacent electrodes. The numerical voltages that each electrode detects are shown to the left of the electrodes. The dark shading denotes the region of the scalp that becomes negatively charged during the spike. The resultant EEG trace seen in a bipolar chain (channels 1 to 4 corresponding to Fp1-F3, F3-C3, C3-P3, and P3-O1 in this example) is shown to the right and the reasons for each specific pen deflection are described step-by-step in the text.

Channel 4: Finally, in the fourth channel, there is no voltage difference measured between P3 and O1 (both 0 µV), so the channel remains flat.

The resulting trace shows one of the classic patterns of EEG waves, the phase reversal, a concept that is expanded on below. For the time being, note that in this example where the pen deflection reversed direction, or phase (in this case from going down in the second channel to going up in the third channel), the electrode in common to the channels where the phase reversed from down to up (C3 since the phase reversed between F3-C3 and C3-P3) points to the location of the discharge's maximum.

As discussed earlier, focal EEG events on the brain surface rarely occur solely in an isolated pinpoint area of the scalp as in the example in Figure 4.17. Instead, there is typically a point of voltage maximum around which lower voltages can be detected. The example shown in Figure 4.18 is more similar to real-world events that arise from the brain. Although the C3 electrode is the point of maximum intensity of this event, the adjacent areas measured by F3 and P3 are also affected, but not as strongly. This gradual drop-off in intensity of voltage shows that the event has a somewhat broader field, even though we are still dealing with a −50 µV spike in C3. A good description of this spike would be that the spike has *a maximum negativity at C3 but a field that also includes F3 and P3*.

Now let's return to Figure 4.18, which shows a more realistic gradient around a spike focus at C3. The resulting EEG trace is similar to the one we saw earlier but with some notable differences:

Channel 1: Fp1-F3 is measuring the difference between 0 and −30 µV. Because Electrode 1 is "more positive" than

Electrode 2, the pen deflects downward an amount corresponding to the difference of 30 µV.

Channel 2: F3-C3 compares −30 µV in Electrode 1 (F3) and −50 µV in Electrode 2 (C3). Because the first electrode is still "more positive" than the second, a downward pen deflection is produced in this channel as well, but of lower amplitude compared to the previous channel, corresponding to the smaller difference of 20 µV.

Channel 3: C3-P3 compares −50 µV in Electrode 1 to −30 µV in Electrode 2. For the first time as we travel down this chain, Electrode 1 is more negative than Electrode 2 (the opposite of the case in the second channel), so the convention tells us that the pen now goes up.

Channel 4: Finally, in the fourth channel, Electrode 1 measures −30 µV, and Electrode 2 measures 0 µV. The pen again deflects upward, corresponding to the fact that Electrode 1 is more negative than Electrode 2 by a 30 µV difference.

Comparing the pattern of EEG waves in Figure 4.18 to the previous figure, we see that there are now deflections in all four channels. This reflects the fact that the field of this spike involves both adjacent electrodes, F3 and P3, and that the gradient of the field stretches out more broadly from the center than in the first example. Stated another way, there is now an electrical gradient (difference) between all four channel pairs. The fact that there is a deflection in each channel reflects the fact that no two adjacent electrodes measure the exact same voltage and that there was an increase or decrease in voltage in every comparison. Because in channels 1 and 2 the pen goes down and in channels 3 and 4 the pen goes up, we say there is a phase reversal occurring between channels 2 and 3. A phase reversal is the point along a bipolar electrode chain at which the

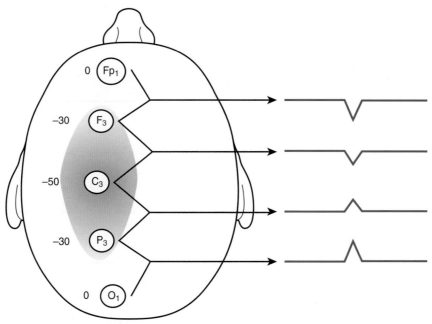

Figure 4.18 A −50 µV spike in C3 with a field extending to include F3 and P3 viewed in a bipolar montage. The F3-C3 and C3-P3 channel deflections reflect the 20 µV difference between those electrode pairs. The larger deflections seen in the top and bottom channels, Fp1-F3 and P3-O1, reflect the 30 µV gradient between those electrode pairs.

direction of the pen deflections changes (from down to up or from up to down). Because in this example C3 is the electrode common to channels 2 and 3, the two channels between which the phase "reversed" is the point of the discharge's maximum.

A second interesting observation can be made about this recording: the point of this spike's maximum voltage (C3) does not correspond to where the spike appears tallest on the EEG page. Even though the biggest pen deflections can be seen in channels 1 and 4, the actual maximum of the discharge lies between Channels 2 and 3. This apparently paradoxical result occurs because, in this example, the electrical gradient was steeper at some distance from the maximum (nearer the forehead and occiput), similar to the example of a mountain peak in which the terrain could be steeper around the base of the mountain, where you begin your hike, and less steep as you get near its summit. Still, the "peak" is at C3, even though the deflections in Fp1-F3 and P3-O1 are larger. Clearly, in bipolar montages the maximum of a discharge cannot be located simply by finding the biggest waves—a pitfall to be avoided. This is because the measuring stick used to determine wave heights in bipolar montage tracings is the differences between pairs of points rather than the absolute value of the voltage at any given point. In bipolar montages, rather than using wave heights, the maximum is located by finding the phase reversal.

Each EEG channel in a bipolar chain passing from front to back along the head is, in reality, answering the question in its march along the brain: "Is the next electrode getting more negative or more positive compared to the one I'm at right now?" The following analogy illustrates this process in another way, and is similar to what it would be like to walk down the scalp from front to back with a voltmeter, measuring voltages.

A farmer has a large field and would like to build his house at the highest point in the field to have the best view of his crops

from the house. The farmer does not have a standard instrument to measure height (such as an altimeter), and he does not trust himself to find the highest point visually (perhaps it's foggy that day). Rather, his only tool to locate the highest point in the field is a crude instrument that reports the difference in height of his current position (where he is standing) compared to the location 10 feet in front of him. The instrument only has a single readout, a pen that points downward if the point 10 feet in front of him is higher than his current position, or upward if the point 10 feet in front of him is lower than his current position. The bigger the change in height, the bigger the deflection of the pen up or down. He will use this instrument to take pen readings as he follows a straight path across the field (Figure 4.19). Taking readings as he walks every 10 feet forward, he can create a "chain" of comparisons: first location to second location, second location to third location, and so on. As he walks forward through his field, it is easy to imagine a strategy he can use to locate the highest point along any track he walks, looking only at the instrument's pen direction.

Imagine that the farmer turns on the instrument, which senses his starting position, and at the same time senses the relative height of the field 10 feet directly ahead. At his starting point, the instrument, comparing the starting position to the position 10 feet ahead, reports "it's getting higher" (the pen goes down). Now walking forward those 10 feet so he is standing on the previous comparison point, it reports that "it's getting higher" again (the pen goes down again). After walking forward the next 10 feet, it reports "it's getting lower" (the pen now goes up). For the final 10 feet, the instrument again reports "it's getting lower" (the pen continues to point up). Looking back at his measurements jotted on a piece of paper, which only consist of four pen deflections (down, down, then up, up) he notes the location at which the pen direction flipped

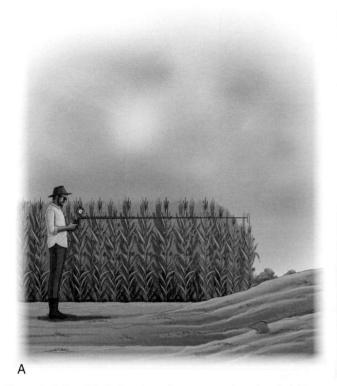
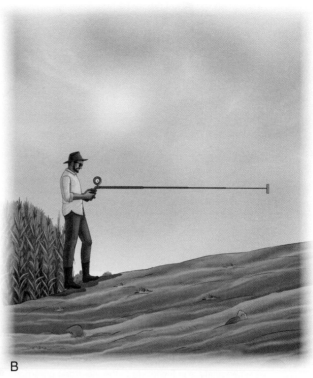

Figure 4.19 Panel A: An imaginary farmer can only make a height-map of his field by using an instrument that is 10 feet long and compares the height of the field where he is standing to the height of the field 10 feet along the path ahead of him. The information comes to him on a display meter in the form of an upgoing or downgoing arrow (the bigger the arrow deflection up or down, the bigger the difference in heights between the two points). The arrow is pointing down, indicating that the next location is higher than the current location. Panel B: The farmer walks 10 feet ahead and now uses the instrument to record a new comparison measurement between the two new locations. He plans to continue on as such in a straight line across his field, paying careful attention to when the wave indicator flips from "down" to "up," as this will indicate that he has just passed a point of maximum height in his field. Of course, translating this example to the world of electroencephalography, the field is the scalp, the height of the field is (negative) voltage, and the farmer is you!

from down to up, which he considers the point of "pen direction reversal" or "phase reversal." We can see what it means if the farmer is making repeated measurements that show the pen pointing down, and then past a certain point the pen flips and now continuously points up. There is only one possible explanation: at the point the pen flipped, the farmer passed a peak of height in his field. To make it even simpler, as long as he is walking forward and the pen points down, he is climbing. As long as he is walking forward and the pen points up, he is descending. If he is walking along a straight line and the pen, which had been pointing down, suddenly switches to up, he must have just passed a point of maximum height in his field.

If you have found the technique that the farmer in the field used to locate the highest point in his field easy to understand, then you will be pleased to hear that the strategy of comparing adjacent points in a bipolar EEG chain is exactly equivalent. However, it may require looking at the bipolar chains on an EEG page in a slightly different way than you may have become accustomed to. You have likely already guessed that the farmer's crude instrument is analogous to a voltmeter, and that downward pen deflections on his instrument that were indicating increasing height in his field are analogous to downward pen deflections on our EEG machines denoting increasing negative voltage as we proceed from Electrode 1 to Electrode 2. Walking past the highest point, which also marks

the transition from climbing to descending is, indeed, the equivalent of a phase reversal in a bipolar chain on the EEG.

As we explore the head from front to back with EEG electrodes and note downward pen deflections, this indicates increasingly negative voltage from point to point. Once we take a further step forward along the head and the pen finally flips upward for the first time, this suggests the next sampled position in the chain is now more positive, and we know we have just passed the point of peak negative voltage. Thus, as we look down a bipolar chain of channels, *downward deflections tell us that voltage is getting increasingly negative*. At the point of the phase reversal (pens newly pointing upward), voltage is now getting less negative (more positive) and the common electrode at the point of phase reversal is the point of maximum negative voltage. What is new about the way we are looking at the set of pen deflections shown in Figure 4.18? Many of us are used to zeroing in on the point of phase reversal to identify the location of maximum voltage, which continues to be a valid strategy. However, considering this bipolar chain as the pen readings from a farmer walking across a field (or an EEG reader walking down the head), note that the direction and height of each wave tell us the contour or steepness in the shape of the electric field the chain is exploring (Figure 4.20).

To complete the farmer's quest of finding the highest point in the field, before making a final decision on where to build

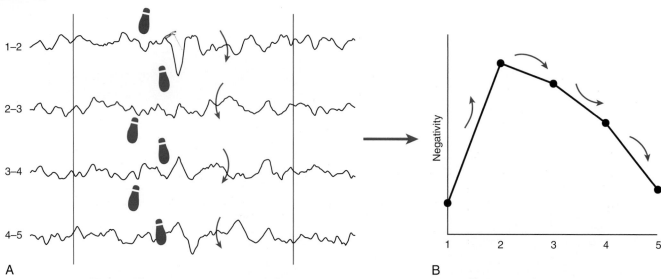

Figure 4.20 When the eye scans a bipolar chain from top to bottom, the voltage contour implied by the upward and downward deflections is visualized in a way similar to the technique of the farmer walking across his field. In this EEG segment, the voltage contour suggested by the upgoing and downgoing sharp waves is depicted on the right side of the figure, which is a graph of negativity. The first wave in the series is large and downgoing, suggesting a sharp rise in negativity (remembering that a downgoing wave means "it is getting more negative" when scanning in the top to bottom direction). The next three waves are upgoing, but by smaller amounts, suggesting that "it is getting more positive" but by smaller increments. Note that the change in the direction of the waves (phase reversal) between channels 1-2 and 2-3 indicate that the peak negativity is in Electrode 2, the electrode common to both channels.

his house he will want to make a topographic map of the whole field by making the same top-to-bottom walk along the field in several parallel lines. Assuming there are four original tracks running from north to south, each of his tracks may have a phase reversal indicating the greatest height along each of those those tracks, but to be even more complete, he might repeat the measurements walking on parallel tracks from west to east (at right angles to the original paths). Using this strategy and recording the amount his pen deflects on every measurement, he would eventually be able to draw a relative topographic map of the whole field, something like the grid shown in Figure 4.6.

Figure 4.21 shows the farmer attacking the same problem in a bigger area, mapping the contours of a mountain range near his farm. Of course, the plan is to convert geography to electricity—the mountain range in this figure is an analogy to an electric field. It is easy to imagine that if the farmer explores the range with his instrument from south to north along the black paths, and then explores the same range from west to east along the red paths, the results won't look the same. Recording the wave deflection on his instrument at every stop and drawing them in a vertical column would create something that looks like a readout of a bipolar EEG chain of height (voltage) information. Mapping the mountain heights first with a set of south-to-north paths, then with a set of west-to-east paths, would be the equivalent of mapping the field of a spike on the scalp surface first with an anteroposterior (front of the head to back of the head) bipolar montage and then mapping the same spike with a transverse bipolar montage. Integrating the information from both bipolar chains could give a pretty good picture of the contours of the

mountain range (or the shape of the electric field of the spike). In the case of this mountain range, the pen deflections will be much higher when recorded along the south-to-north paths because those paths have much larger altitude changes between readings, but there will be a phase reversal when he passes the top of the ridge. When traveling the west-to-east routes, there will still be a phase reversal when he passes the highest point along each path, but each pen deflection will be of much lower amplitude. This is one of the reasons that it is good practice to scan an EEG with both longitudinal bipolar and transverse bipolar montages. In the occasional cases where the electric field of an event is more oblong like in Figures 4.18 and 4.21, the event will be more obvious when scanning in one direction (anteroposterior versus transverse) compared to the other.

In these examples, greater altitude in the farmer's field is analogous to EEG voltage becoming more negative. This suggests a different way to visually interpret a bipolar montage, looking at the set of four chains from top to bottom. Scanning down an EEG page, the EEG reader can imagine "walking down" or scanning a bipolar chain along the scalp, such as from Fp1 all the way to O1 and monitoring pen deflections. This is akin to the farmer, sensing, as the pens go down as he walks, that "it's getting more negative"; and then, as the pens finally reverse direction, that "it's getting more positive" (see Figure 4.20). When there is a larger deflection, it has gotten a lot more negative (or positive). When there is only a small deflection, there has been little change in the voltage between the two positions compared in the channel. When the pen switches direction, this implies that the point of maximum voltage was passed, identifying the position of the voltage maximum of the spike. Figure 4.22 shows the deflections

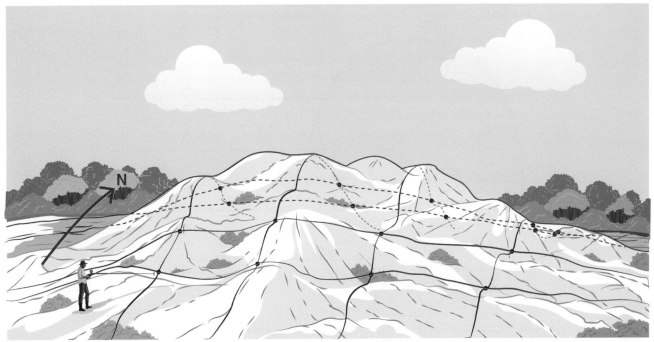

Figure 4.21 The farmer now intends a more ambitious project: to make an altitude-map of the mountain range next to his farm using the same instrument. He starts by walking across the ridge toward the north along the first black path shown on the left, recording the readout of the display meter with every comparison. He then returns to the original side of the mountain range and walks across the ridge on the next black path, parallel to the first, getting a new set of readings, and so on, until he has obtained readings for all four of the parallel black paths that cross the range from south to north. The next step is to make similar comparison readings, but now going from west to east (left to right), along the red paths. Note that the south-to-north gradients can be joined with the west-to-east gradient information (black paths now linked together with the red paths) to get an accurate picture of the contours of the mountain range. The readings from two perpendicular sets of paths in this example would be similar to the EEG process of first examining an AP (anteroposterior or front-to-back) bipolar montage and then joining that information to a transverse (left-to-right) bipolar montage to get an idea of the three-dimensional voltage gradient of an EEG wave. Finally, note that the very same altitude maximum will be easier to see from the south-to-north (e.g., AP bipolar) readings, which will show bigger deflections, than it will be from the shallower west-to-east (transverse bipolar) readings, though each technique is measuring a peak of the same height.

that the farmer's instrument might generate while walking along a single path as he walks across a hill, or likewise what an EEG machine might detect when exploring the left parasagittal chain when there is a spike maximum at C3. Note that the thought process of these examples involves first imagining a surface or an electric field and guessing what kind of EEG pattern the contours would generate. During EEG interpretation, the process is reversed: we examine the channel outputs and ascertain the shape of the underlying field.

The "Positive Phase Reversal"

Next, consider the situation of a positive spike occurring on the scalp, again at C3, as shown in Figures 4.23 and 4.24:

Channel 1, Fp1-F3, reflects the difference between 0 and 20 µV. Because Electrode 1 is "more negative" than Electrode 2, the pen deflects upward an amount corresponding to 20 µV.

Channel 2, F3-C3, compares 20 µV in Electrode 1 (F3) and 50 µV in Electrode 2 (C3). Because the first electrode is again "more negative" than the second, another upward pen deflection is produced, this time corresponding to the difference of 30 µV, so it's a bit bigger than the previous pen deflection.

Channel 3, C3-P3, compares 50 µV in Electrode 1 to 20 µV in Electrode 2. Now Electrode 1 is more positive than Electrode 2 (the opposite of the case in the second channel), so the convention tells us that the pen goes down. As you can see, this is

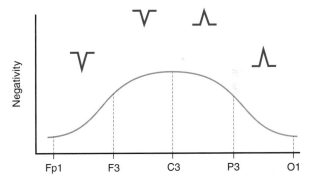

Figure 4.22 This figure shows the sequential readouts from an imaginary "walk" down a bipolar chain extending from the frontopolar area (Fp1) to the occipital area (O1). (Note that the y-axis shows degree of negativity so that more negative voltages cause the curve to go up.) The red curve represents the intensity of the negativity on a path along the electrodes from Fp1 to O1 and shows a maximum negativity at the C3 electrode. The pen deflections at the top of the figure show that as. As the curve goes up, the successive measurements (Fp1 to F3, F3 to C3) show progressively increasing negativity causing downward pen deflections (the pen deflections are placed between electrode positions since they represent comparisons of electrode pairs). After the comparisons have passed over the "voltage hump" of the C3 electrode (C3 to P3 and P3 to O1), the first electrode in the comparison pair is newly more negative than the second electrode, and the pen begins to point up. When the maximum point (C3) is passed, the pen direction reverses phase (from down to up), and this phase reversal marks the maximum.

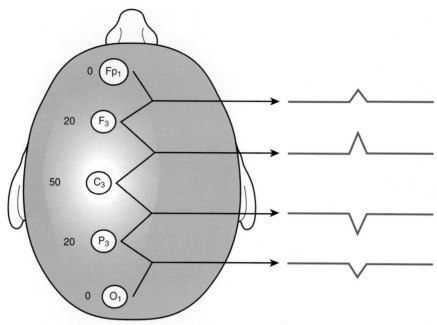

Figure 4.23 The diagram shows an example of a positive phase reversal with pens pointing away from each other and, therefore, a maximum positivity in C3. As in previous diagrams, dark areas are more negative than light areas so that, in this example, the light area around C3 depicts a maximum positivity of 50 μV in the C3 electrode. The strength (field) of the positivity drops off with increasing distance from the maximum point. The upgoing deflections in the first two channels indicate that the field is becoming more strongly positive traveling from Fp1 toward C3. The downgoing deflections in the third and fourth channels indicate that the field becomes more negative (less positive) after traveling past C3. This combination of events marks C3, the point of phase reversal, as the point of maximum positivity in this bipolar chain.

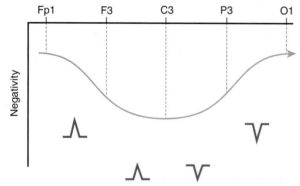

Figure 4.24 This figure shows a two-dimensional representation of a positive event with a maximum at C3 (compare to Figure 4.22). The upward deflection of the pens in the first two channels reflects the fact that, in the first two comparisons of Electrode 1 to Electrode 2 (Fp1 to F3 and F3 to C3), Electrode 2 is more positive than Electrode 1 (recalling that Electrode 1 being more negative causes the pen to go up). In the third and fourth channels, the comparison shows that Electrode 1 is more positive than Electrode 2, and so the pens go down. The phase reversal with pens pointing away from each other between F3-C3 and C3-P3 marks C3 as the point of maximum *positivity*.

the moment of the phase reversal (i.e., the pen direction has changed).

Channel 4, Electrode 1 measures 20 μV and Electrode 2 measures 0 μV. The pen again deflects downward,

corresponding to the fact that Electrode 1 is more positive than Electrode 2 by 20 μV.

In contrast to the type of phase reversals illustrated in Figures 4.17 and 4.18, Figures 4.23 and 4.24 show an example of a second type of phase reversal, the positive phase reversal. This type differs from the first in that the first represented a transition of pens going down to pens going up as the eye proceeds down the page. At the point of phase reversal, the pen deflections face toward each other. In this second type of phase reversal, there is a transition of pens going up to pens going down, or pen deflections facing away from one another at the point of phase reversal. The phase reversal with the pens-down-to-pens-up transition marks an area of maximum negativity, and the second type of phase reversal with the pens-up-to-pens-down transition marks an area of maximum positivity. As shorthand, the first type of phase reversal with the pens pointing toward each other can be called a negative phase reversal, and the second type with the pens pointing away from each other a positive phase reversal (see Figure 4.25). It will be important for the reader to successfully work through the above two examples of the two major types of phase reversals and to be convinced that it is always the case that, in a bipolar montage:

When the phase-reversing waves point toward each other, the point of maximum intensity is a point of maximum negativity.

When the phase-reversing waves point away from each other, the point of maximum intensity is a point of maximum positivity.

This generalization always holds true because of the basic convention of direction of pen deflection and polarity. In the case of the negative phase reversal, the transition from pens going down to pens going up is the same as passing from "getting more negative" to "getting more positive" comparisons. The opposite story holds true for the positive phase reversal with deflections that face away from each other. As you scan downward through a bipolar chain with upgoing waves, the upgoing pens imply that the field is getting progressively more positive. After the waves flip to downward, the opposite is true: the field is now becoming progressively more negative, implying that a point of peak positivity has been passed. Returning to the famer's field analogy, when the farmer sees his instrument shifting from downward-pointing waves to upward pointing waves, he knows he's just walked over a relative peak in his field. If he starts out on his path with upward-pointing readings and then they switch to downward-pointing, he knows he's just crossed the trough of a valley and he is now climbing up. Once you have convinced yourself that the above examples of the concepts behind the two types of phase reversals (and that the diagram in Figure 4.25 always hold true), you will no longer need to step through all of these pen-up/pen-down comparisons for a given discharge to tell if a recorded event has negative or positive polarity.

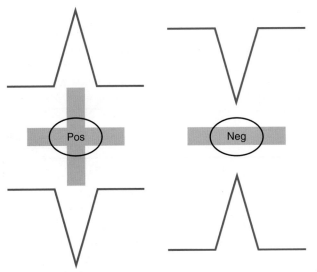

Figure 4.25 This diagram serves as a reminder that in bipolar montages, in the case of a phase reversal in which the pens point away from each other, there is an area of maximum positivity at the common electrode. Conversely, when the pens point toward each other, the phase reversal denotes the location of maximum negativity. The fact that there is only enough space to fit a minus sign between the points tips of the negative phase reversal but that there is enough space to fit a plus sign between the points tips of a positive phase reversal can serve as a memory device to recall which pattern corresponds to which polarity.

The "Isoelectric Phase Reversal"

So far, we have examined examples of a discharge's maximum intensity when that maximum occurs at the very point at which an electrode has been placed. Sometimes, however, a voltage maximum may occur *between* two electrode positions, and it is worthwhile to consider how this can change the appearance of a phase reversal. Figure 4.26 shows just such an example. The maximum negativity of −50 occurs by chance *between* the F3 and C3 electrodes. At the F3 and C3 electrodes, voltages of −40 are measured. In the resulting bipolar recording, the expected negative phase reversal is seen, this time between the first and third channels, with the spikes pointing toward each other since this is an example of a maximum negativity, as expected. This time, however, because F3 and C3 have the same voltage, the second, intervening channel is flat. This occurs because F3 and C3 are isoelectric with respect to one another (they have the same voltage), and because a comparison of two electrodes with the same voltage would generate no pen deflection, it is no surprise that this intervening channel is flat. This example illustrates the general concept that a phase reversal is still "valid" even with an intervening flat channel.

In such examples of an isoelectric phase reversal with an intervening isoelectric (flat) channel, it is tempting to conclude that the maximum always lies in between the two electrodes of the isoelectric channel, as depicted in Figure 4.27A. Although this is often the case, other field topographies are possible. For instance, given these pen deflections, it could be that 40 μV is, indeed, the maximum and is shared by F3 and C3—the field may be "flat" between these two points as shown in Figure 4.27 B. In the case of this isoelectric type of phase reversal, as long as the two electrodes in question are fairly close to one another (such as F3 and C3), we generally assume that the true maximum is somewhere between F3 and C3, inclusive. In reality, we cannot know the true contour of the field between F3 and C3 based on the tracing at hand; if it were necessary to know more, we would need to place additional intervening electrodes. An example of an isoelectric phase reversal recorded from the brain in an actual EEG is shown in Figure 4.28 and its companion Figure 4.29.

Event Localization Using a Referential Montage

In referential montages, each channel shows a comparison of an electrode placed over a brain "area of interest" to a reference point elsewhere on the head or body that is chosen with the hope that it will be electrically quiet (but perhaps share the noise signal present in the "electrode of interest"). The "electrode of interest" is almost always over a brain region and may also be referred to as the active electrode (again, reflecting the hope that the reference electrode will be inactive). The reference electrode, attached to INPUT2 of the amplifier, is located at some other point (or points) on the body, sometimes near the brain but sometimes at a distance from the brain. Examples of points chosen for the reference electrode include the earlobes (A1 and A2), the skin over the mastoid processes (M1 and M2, the bony promontory

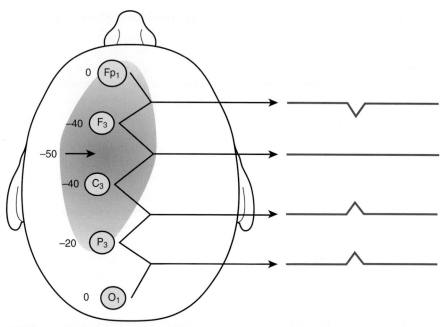

Figure 4.26 An isoelectric phase reversal is shown. In this example, the point of the measured maximum negativity of –40 µV is shared by the F3 and C3 electrodes. The diagram for this example implies that the true maximum negativity of –50 µV lies between the F3 and C3 electrodes and is not directly measured since there is no intervening electrode between F3 and C3. The resulting trace on the right side of the figure shows an example of an "isoelectric phase reversal." Here, the location of the maximum is actually marked by a flat line in the second channel (F3-C3) because those two electrodes are measuring the same voltage (–40 µV) and are said to be isoelectric (of equal voltage). Still, this can be considered a true phase reversal since the pen (or the "farmer in the field's" instrument indicator) is flipping or "reversing" from down, then to neutral, then to up through channels 1, 2, and 3.

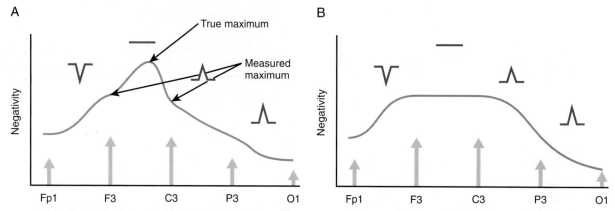

Figure 4.27 Two of the many possible shapes of a voltage gradient are shown that could account for the type of isoelectric phase reversal shown on the right side of Figure 4.26. Panel A shows a gradient in which the true voltage maximum is actually located in between the isoelectric electrodes (F3 and C3), similar to the situation shown in Figure 4.26. Panel B shows another possibility: that there is a plateau of maximum voltage between the two electrodes. If it were necessary to distinguish between these and other possibilities, additional electrodes would have to be placed between F3 and C3.

just behind the ears), the nose, the chin, the Cz electrode, and the base of the neck (CS2). Another strategy for creating a reference electrode is to use the mathematical average of some or all of the brain or other electrodes as a virtual reference electrode. The comparative advantages and disadvantages of different reference electrode strategies is discussed in detail in the chapter on montages.

The active electrode is customarily attached to INPUT1 of the amplifier, and the reference electrode is attached to INPUT2. The strategy of this type of montage, in the best of all possible worlds, is to find an electrode pair in which the INPUT1 electrode contains the brain activity of interest (plus the unavoidable contaminating electrical noise), and INPUT2 contains *only* the contaminating electrical noise of INPUT1, but none of its

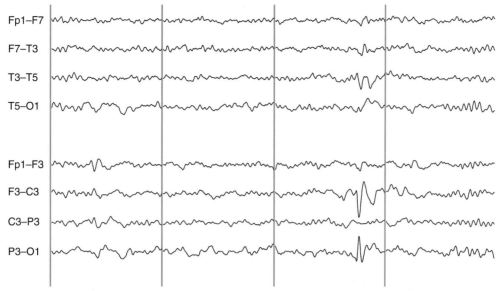

Figure 4.28 A nearly isoelectric phase reversal is seen surrounding the C3-P3 channel, which is nearly flat. This nearly flat channel tells us that the C3 and P3 must be of nearly the same voltage. The downward deflection in F3-C3 indicates that C3 is more negative than F3. The upward deflection in P3-O1 indicates that P3 is more negative than O1. All of these relationships can be confirmed when examining Figure 4.29, which shows the same spike displayed in a referential montage.

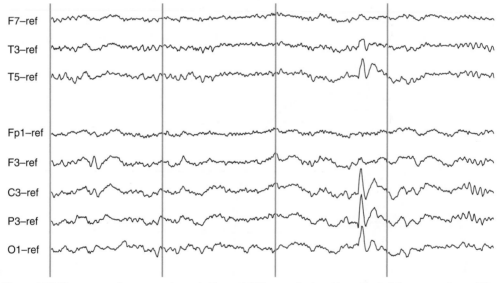

Figure 4.29 The same spike as was shown in Figure 4.28 is now displayed in a referential montage. As could be predicted by its appearance in the bipolar montage, C3 and P3 are the areas of maximum negativity, but they are also of the same voltage (C3-ref and P3-ref are of the same height). Fp1 and F3 are neutral and the field of the discharge's negativity spreads a smaller amount to O1. Whenever we see two adjacent channels in a referential montage that look identical, we can predict that the comparison of those channels in a bipolar montage will look flat.

brain activity. With this type of ideal pairing, the result of subtracting INPUT2 from INPUT1 would be a cancellation of the electrical noise, leaving a pure trace of the brain activity picked up under the active electrode that is attached to INPUT1. This is an example of the ideal active electrode/reference electrode pair that is strived for in a good-quality referential recording. For the purposes of the idealized schematic examples in this chapter, we have assumed ideal, noise-free active and reference electrodes that yield electrically noise-free recordings.

In some ways, the setup of referential montages makes them easier to interpret. Despite their many advantages, however, referential montages are often not the easiest montages

to read. It is useful to compare the relative advantages and disadvantages of the referential technique to its cousin bipolar technique as we discuss them.

We now reconsider some of the same examples used earlier, starting with the simplest case of the highly focal negative spike in C3. Figure 4.30 shows the result of comparing each electrode in the parasagittal chain to an ideal reference electrode: Fp1-ref, F3-ref, C3-ref, P3-ref, and O1-ref. In these examples, the "ref" electrode is a hypothetical neutral reference electrode with a voltage of zero. Because in this example the spike's field does not extend to the adjacent electrodes, there is no voltage difference between those electrodes

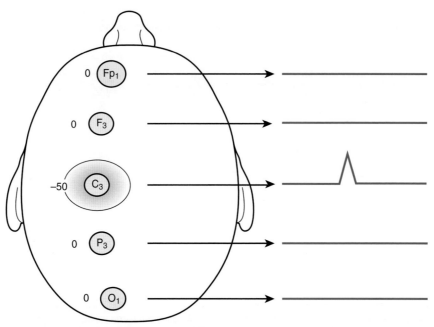

Figure 4.30 A highly focal –50 µV spike limited to the C3 electrode is displayed with a referential montage. The five channels correspond to Fp1-ref, F3-ref, C3-ref, P3-ref, and O1-ref, where "ref" represents an idealized, electrically neutral reference electrode. Because C3 is more negative than the neutral reference electrode, the pen deflects upward. The other pens are silent because the surrounding electrodes are neutral. This type of situation where an electrical event is only seen in a single electrode and all the surrounding electrodes are electrically quiet is uncommon for events that arise from the brain. This pattern, if encountered on an actual EEG, would therefore be suspicious for electrode artifact in C3 rather than true electrocerebral activity.

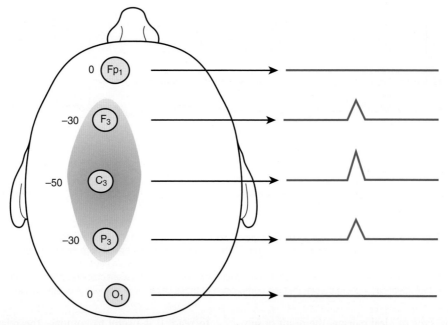

Figure 4.31 A –50 µV spike in C3 with a field extending to F3 and P3 viewed in a referential montage. The C3-ref channel deflects an amount corresponding to –50 µV, just as it did in Figure 4.30. Because the field of this discharge now also involves F3 and P3 in this example, deflections corresponding to –30 µV are seen in F3-ref and P3-ref. Note that the spike amplitude in these channels is only 60% that of the C3-ref channel, reflecting the diminishing field in F3 and P3.

surrounding C3 (Fp1, F3, P3, and O1) and the reference (all are zero). C3, in contrast, is more negative than the reference, causing the pen to deflect upward (first electrode more negative—pen up!). This results in an EEG with four flat lines representing the four surrounding neutral electrodes and one visible spike generated by the C3-ref channel. There is a

convenient simplicity to the result displayed in a referential montage: the pen only moves in a channel that corresponds to an electrically active electrode. This is different from the same example we saw in the bipolar chain illustrated in Figure 4.17 in which a single electrode's activity caused the pens to move in two channels.

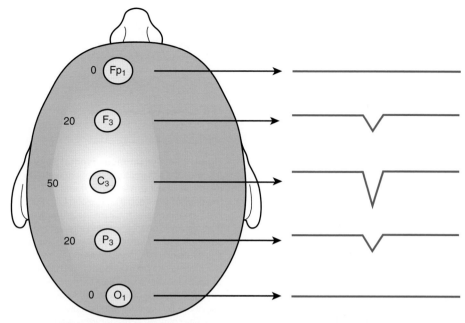

Figure 4.32 A 50 μV "positive spike" in C3 with field extending to F3 and P3 (the white area is meant to depict positivity). Because the active scalp electrodes are more positive than the neutral reference, the pens go down. The biggest pen deflection marks the maximum positivity of the spike's field at C3.

Next we examine a −50 μV spike in C3 that has a lower voltage field in the adjacent electrodes, F3 and P3. Figure 4.31 shows the output of a referential montage for a spike with the same field as was illustrated in Figure 4.18 in a bipolar montage. Once again, the output seems relatively simple, with a −50 μV deflection seen in the C3-ref channel and lower amplitude deflections seen in the flanking channels, F3-ref and P3-ref, reflecting the fact that the spike's field also involves those electrodes, although to a lesser extent. All of the deflections are upgoing because all of the active electrodes are negative when compared with the neutral reference. The height of the deflection is proportional to the strength of the field in microvolts at each point.

Finally, we look at the example of a 50 μV "positive spike" in C3 with a field that includes F3 and P3. Figure 4.32 shows the EEG corresponding to such a spike using a referential montage. The main difference between this example and the previous ones is that the pens go down because the active electrodes are now more positive than the neutral reference electrode. Again, the relative heights of the spike in each channel correspond to the relative voltages at each electrode in the example. In a referential montage, knowing the height of a wave in millimeters and the sensitivity setting of the amplifier makes measurement of a wave's absolute voltage a matter of simple multiplication (Figure 4.33). Alternatively, the height of each wave can be measured directly with the digital calipers provided by your EEG software. Note that you don't even have to think about phase reversals when reading referential montages—with a clean reference the highest wave marks the location of the highest voltage. If it is assumed that the reference is neutral, polarity is easy to assess by whether the pen goes up (negative) or down (positive).

Comparison of the Bipolar and Referential Recording Techniques

According to the descriptions given earlier, the technique of the referential montage has multiple advantages over the bipolar montage technique: each channel includes only one "electrode of interest" or active electrode. Compare this to the more complex situation with bipolar montages in which a deflection in the Fp1-F3 channel could indicate an event involving only Fp1, only F3, or both Fp1 and F3, but to different extents. The voltage of the event in a referential channel is directly proportional to the height of the wave, which has the major advantage of simplicity. This is not necessarily true in bipolar montages, in which the point of maximum voltage can even be a flat channel, as we have seen in the example of the isoelectric phase reversal shown in Figure 4.26. Worse yet, in certain situations where there is synchronous activity in nearby electrodes, that activity will display realistically in the referential montage, but the activity may cancel out almost completely in a bipolar montage because of the technique of subtractions used. An example of this phenomenon is shown in Figure 4.34.

Why, then, does it often seem easier to read bipolar montages? The answer is partly related to the unpredictability of the assumption of the "clean" reference used in these examples. Ideally, we would like the reference to include only the exact same noise that is present in the active electrode and nothing else. In this idealized situation, where Fp1 would have brain waves plus noise and the reference electrode only contains the *very same* noise and nothing else, running the channel pair Fp1-ref through the CMR amplifier will give a beautiful representation of the pure brain wave signal at Fp1 with all of the noise "subtracted out," much as was seen in Figure 4.16. In practice, references often have noise of their own, sometimes to the point that they obliterate important signal information in the active electrode, at times rendering the recording unreadable. This is not to say that, sometimes, a near-ideal reference cannot be found. With different patients during different parts of a given EEG recording, depending on the patient's behavior and other factors, the ability to make a clean referential recording varies greatly. In a given patient, different reference electrode locations

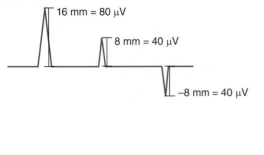

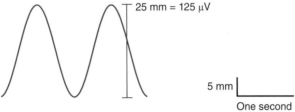

Sensitivity = 5 microvolts/mm

Figure 4.33 When reading an EEG with a calibrated screen (where you have told your EEG software your screen size), the first step in ascertaining the voltage of a wave in an EEG trace is knowing the recording sensitivity used, stated in microvolts per millimeter. The sensitivity tells the reader how many microvolts of voltage each millimeter of pen deflection represents. In this example, the sensitivity is 5 μV/mm. In the top trace, the measured heights from the baseline of the spikes are 16 mm, 8 mm, and 8 mm, respectively. The relationship of millimeters to voltage is found by a simple multiplication: 16 mm × (5 μV/mm) = 80 μV (note that the mm unit cancels out in this multiplication leaving the result in the expected unit of μV). Voltage measurements of sinusoidal waves as shown in the lower trace are made by measuring the peak-to-trough height of the waves, as shown. Because of variations of screen size, reading is often done on uncalibrated monitors (the EEG software does not necessarily know the size of the screen you are viewing the EEG on). In this more common situation, amplitude measurements can also be made either with digital measuring calipers provided by the software or by comparison to a scaled voltage/time bar as seen in the corner of this figure.

can yield large differences in the quality and readability of the tracing. Each recording technique has its own advantages and disadvantages, which are summarized in Table 4.1.

A Return to the Question of "What Makes the Pen Go Up?" and "The Right Wrong Answer"

Now that we have some expertise in how bipolar montages work, let's return to the basic question: what makes the EEG pen go up or down? Imagine that you are asked a very simple question: what does it mean in an EEG channel if the pen goes down (imagining a single downgoing spike)? When new electroencephalographers answer this question, the most common response is "it is positive." This is the "right wrong answer," as we shall see. So why is "it is negative" if the pen goes up or "it's positive" if the pen goes down the "right wrong answer?" Counterexamples are easy to find. Imagine you are reading and come upon a *downward* deflection in Fp1-F3.

Fp1-F3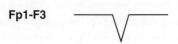

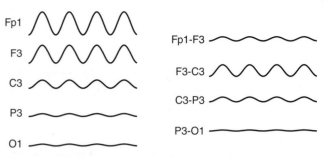

Figure 4.34 Synchronous Frontal Slow in Two Montages. This figure shows a schematic of a patient with a large frontal slow wave that expresses itself similarly in Fp1 and Fp3, and then fades away toward the back of the head (C3, P3, and O1). Panel A shows the slow wave in an idealized referential montage using a good, indifferent reference that displays the location and intensity of this slow wave perfectly—essentially the "truth" about what's happening on the scalp. When this situation is displayed in a bipolar montage (Panel B), however, the waveforms can be misleading. Even though we know this slow wave to be of maximum voltage in the Fp1 and F3 electrodes, when the Fp1-F3 channel is displayed in the bipolar montage, the highly similar activity in Fp1 and F3 almost completely cancels itself out leaving a near-flat channel. A reader who would only inspect the bipolar montage might think that the slow wave is excluded from the very front of the head and that it is only present a bit more posteriorly, a conclusion that would be erroneous.

Considering this deflection alone, if you answer "it is positive" the first question you would be asked is "what is positive?" You might then reply, "Fp1!" This answer would be correct… sometimes. Yes, Fp1 could be positive in this scenario, but it is equally possible that Fp1 is neutral and that F3 is negative, as well as other combinations. Therefore, a more complete answer to this downgoing deflection question would be that Fp1 could be more positive *or* F3 could be more negative. Indeed, both situations are easy to imagine using real-life examples (see below).

Real-life example #1 on the left side of the figure is eyeblink artifact. In the case of eyeblink artifact, Fp1 is more positive than F3 and, indeed, the pen goes down in the Fp1-F3 channel when there is eyeblink artifact. This is explained by the presence of a positivity in Fp1 that comes from the positive charge on the cornea that bobs upward toward Fp1 during an eyeblink. We are used to seeing downward pen deflections in Fp1-F3 with eyeblink artifacts. So with the example of eyeblink artifact on the left side of the figure below, it was correct to say that when the pen goes down in Fp1-F3, it was *because Fp1 is positive*.

For real-life example #2 on the right side of the figure, if there is a negative spike in C3, the pen in the Fp1-F3 channel may still go down exactly as it did with the eyeblink artifact example, but for the opposite reason. The successive channels on the right side of the figure below tell the rest of the story. The phase reversal in C3 tells us that the pen went down in Fp1-F3 *because F3 was negative*. (It is negative because it is near C3, the location of a negative phase reversal, and therefore a maximum negativity in the chain.) These are two nice physiological examples of the same downward pen deflection in Fp1-F3 reflecting *either* a positivity in INPUT 1 (as in eyeblink artifact) *or* a negativity in INPUT 2 (as with a negative spike in C3 with a field that extends to F3).

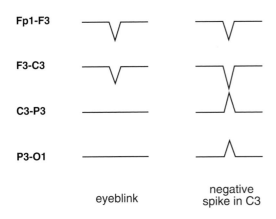

Fp1-F3

F3-C3

C3-P3

P3-O1

eyeblink

negative
spike in C3

Note that the top two lines of each of these events, the eyeblink and the negative spike in C3, can look almost identical. Once your eye scans down the remainder of the page, you learn the rest of the story, which is revealed by the bottom two channels. It becomes clear that the pair of nearly identical pen deflections in the top two rows can represent very different scenarios: an anterior positivity (eyeblink artifact) or a more posterior negativity (C3 negative spike). It is clear from these two examples that the simple response "it is positive" to describe the deflection in Fp1-F3 does not correctly describe what is going on in all circumstances. In particular, it does not describe what is going on in a circumstance like what is happening in the right half of this figure that represents a negative central spike—a situation where there is nothing accurately described by saying, "It is positive!"

The reason that "it's positive" is a *right* wrong answer is that it still remains true in many cases. When an electrode

of interest (e.g., Fp1) is attached to INPUT1 and a relatively quiet reference (e.g., the nose) is attached to INPUT2 creating an Fp1-nose channel, a downgoing deflection does suggest a positive event in Fp1. And yes, there is also a small chance that it could also represent a negative event in the nose!

PREDICTING THE APPEARANCE OF THE BIPOLAR MONTAGE ON THE BASIS OF THE REFERENTIAL MONTAGE

The following section consists of a set of exercises designed to aid the reader in visualizing how various EEG waves might appear differently depending on whether they are displayed in a bipolar or a referential montage. The ability to complete these exercises correctly implies an excellent understanding of the differences between the two montage types and how each type works. The reader may choose to solve the 14 montage problems, each shown on the following odd-numbered pages. The solutions are shown on the overleaf of each page.

We will start by looking at events in a referential montage and determine what their appearance would be in a bipolar montage. The examples used focus on a single chain of five electrodes, extending from the left frontopolar region to the left occipital region: Fp1, F3, C3, P3, and O1. This chain of electrodes is referred to as the left parasagittal chain. Again, to keep things simple, a single spike is used for these examples. In reality, the same line of reasoning applied to this spike can also be applied to any type of wave, such as sharp waves or slow waves. You may wish to look at the figures whose

TABLE 4.1 · The Comparative Advantages and Disadvantages of Bipolar and Referential Recording Techniques

	Bipolar Montages	Referential Montage
Locating the electrical maximum	Maximum point is found by determining the point of phase reversal—the electrode in common between the two phase reversing channels is the point of maximum.	Maximum point is found by locating the channel with the largest deflection (tallest wave). The active electrode in that channel is the point of maximum. Phase reversal has no specific meaning.
Measuring wave voltage	True absolute voltage cannot be accurately determined by measuring wave amplitudes; only relative voltages between electrodes can be determined.	Absolute voltage of a wave can be determined by measuring the wave's height, assuming a neutral reference.
Number of channels in EEG output	There is one fewer channel than the number of electrodes in a chain since they are presented in pairs.	There is the same number of channels as the number of electrodes in a chain.
Appearance of negative and positive polarities	Negativity is marked by phase reversal with deflections pointing toward each other. Positivity is marked by phase reversal with deflections pointing away from each other.	Assuming a neutral reference, negativity is marked by an upgoing deflection. Positivity is marked by a downgoing deflection.
Drawbacks of technique	Absolute voltages are difficult to ascertain. Highest deflections do not necessarily mark point of maximum voltage. Similar activity in adjacent electrodes can cancel out and be lost or understated.	A noisy reference adds noise to all channels. It can be difficult to find an "ideal" reference.

captions start with "Question" first (starting with Figure 4.35) to attempt to solve the conversion problems before reading the narrative that follows that includes an explanation of the answers.

Figure 4.35 shows a simple event localized to a single electrode, C3. The appearance of this event in the bipolar montage can be predicted by imagining a series of subtractions. First, it should be noted that in a five-electrode chain, the referential montage displays five channels (Fp1-ref, F3-ref, C3-ref, P3-ref, O1-ref), but the bipolar montage solution will only include four channels, each channel representing a pairing of electrodes (Fp1-F3, F3-C3, C3-P3, P3-O1). For the purpose of solving these problems, the height of each wave can be measured in any unit (inches, millimeters, etc.)—the graphical answers are independent of the unit of measure used.

To determine what the appearance of the discharge in Figure 4.35 will look like in a bipolar montage, the value of the first bipolar channel is determined by finding the difference between the magnitudes of the discharge in Fp1 and F3. Because the value of each is zero, the difference between the two channels is also zero, and the resulting Fp1-F3 channel is flat (Figure 4.38). The situation is different when determining the appearance of the F3-C3 channel. In this example, on the basis of an examination of the referential montage, F3 is zero, but C3 is upgoing by 5 units (implying that C3 is negative by 5 units). Because in the F3-C3 channel Electrode 1 is zero and Electrode 2 is negative, the pen goes down. Why is this? Because, as discussed earlier, according to the convention, when the first input (F3) is "more positive" than the second input in the pair (C3), the pen goes down. The most succinct way of stating this relationship is "F3 is 'more positive' than C3, so the pen goes down." The words "more positive" are in quotes because F3 is not, strictly speaking, positive , just "more positive" than C3.

Moving to the next electrode pair, C3-P3, now the pertinent comparison is a negative voltage in C3 minus a potential of zero in P3. C3 is more negative than P3, so the pen deflects upward. The final comparison is between P3 and O1, both of

which have a zero value, so the comparison yields a flat line, reflecting a difference of zero. This succession of comparisons yields the appearance of Figure 4.38, the solution to the problem. This figure shows a typical-appearing phase reversal for a localized, negative surface event.

The next example, shown in Figure 4.36, shows a discharge that resembles the previous example, a negative event with maximum in C3, but this time there is a field surrounding the C3 electrode. Examination of the figure reveals that the intensity of the field in C3 is exactly twice the intensity measured in the F3 and P3 electrodes. As a result, when going down

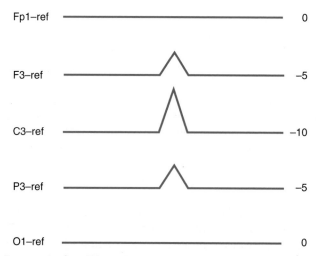

Figure 4.36 Question 2. Predict how this discharge, displayed in a referential montage, will appear in a bipolar montage. Like the previous example, this tracing shows a focal spike in C3, but this time with a larger field surrounding C3 as evidenced by the smaller upward deflections in F3 and P3. Note that the field dissipates in an even fashion with distance from C3. Absolute voltage measurements are given on the right side of the figure.

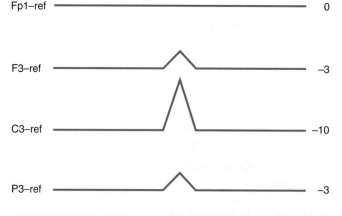

Figure 4.37 Question 3. Predict how this discharge displayed in a referential montage will appear in a bipolar montage. This discharge is similar to the previous example except for the fact that voltage falls off more abruptly between C3 and its adjacent electrodes, F3 and P3. This steep gradient around C3 should be reflected in the appearance of the corresponding bipolar recording (shown on the next page).

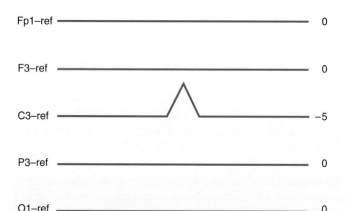

Figure 4.35 Question 1. Predict how this discharge, displayed in a referential montage, will appear in a bipolar montage (answers to all questions appear on the overleaf page). The discharge consists of a simple, highly focal spike with a pure negativity in C3. The adjacent electrodes are inactive, implying that there is no gradient or gradual "falloff" in voltage in the surrounding electrodes.

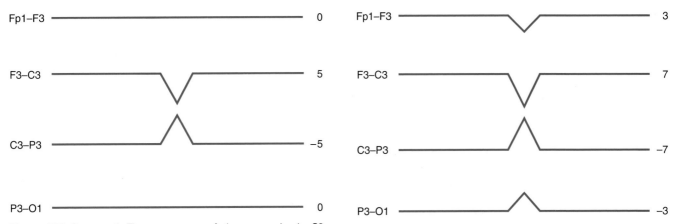

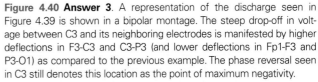

Figure 4.38 **Answer 1**. The appearance of the same simple C3 spike shown on the previous page displayed in a bipolar montage. The flat lines in Fp1-F3 and P3-O1 reflect the fact that there is no electrical gradient between the outermost channels (Fp1 and F3, P3 and O1), which is to say that this electrical event in C3 has no surrounding field. Although such highly focal discharges involving only a single electrode may, indeed, be of cerebral origin, when an electrical event only involves a single electrode, an electrode artifact should be suspected.

Figure 4.40 **Answer 3**. A representation of the discharge seen in Figure 4.39 is shown in a bipolar montage. The steep drop-off in voltage between C3 and its neighboring electrodes is manifested by higher deflections in F3-C3 and C3-P3 (and lower deflections in Fp1-F3 and P3-O1) as compared to the previous example. The phase reversal seen in C3 still denotes this location as the point of maximum negativity.

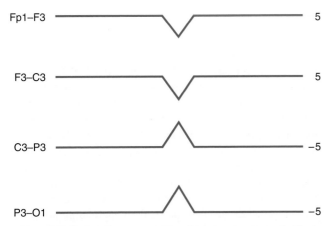

Figure 4.39 **Answer 2**. In the referential montage shown in Figure 4.37 the height of the wave at C3 is evidence that the maximum negativity is located in that electrode. In the bipolar montage, the indication that C3 is the point of maximum negativity is the phase reversal at C3 as seen in this figure. The similar deflections seen in the outer channels, Fp1-F3 and P3-O1, reflect the fact that there is a gentle and steady gradient of decreasing negativity with increasing distance from the C3 electrode. This is one of the most common configurations seen for focal negative events arising from the brain. Deflections in all four channels in this figure confirm the presence of a field extending away from the discharge's maximum.

identical downward deflections, the height of which is exactly the same as the difference between the adjacent electrodes' voltage. The third bipolar channel, the C3-P3 comparison, has the same magnitude of difference as the previous comparison, but now because C3 is more negative than P3, the pen goes up but by the same number of units. This flipping of the pen direction (phase reversal) now that the voltage trend has changed (from successive electrodes becoming more negative to successive electrodes becoming more positive) defines the point of maximum negative voltage. This change in voltage trend causing the wave to flip its phase is the essence of the phase reversal. The phase "reverses" because, as the parasagittal chain is explored from front to back, the trend of successive voltage comparisons is no longer one of increasingly negative measurements but instead becomes one of increasingly positive measurements. Finally, the last two channels, P3 and O1, have the same 5-unit difference with P3 more negative than O1, yielding the final 5-unit upgoing deflection. Figure 4.39 shows the expected phase reversal at C3.

The discharge shown in Figure 4.37 is quite similar to the preceding example, with a negative discharge seen in C3 and a diminishing field seen in F3 and P3, but with a subtle difference. The example differs from the previous one in that the intensity of the discharge drops off more abruptly from C3 to F3 and P3 (the gradient is steeper between C3 and F3 and between C3 and P3). When this type of field is shown in the bipolar montage, the location of the phase reversal at C3 has not changed (Figure 4.40). The fact that the heights of the discharge in second and third channels (F3-C3 and C3-P3) of Figure 4.40 are much higher than those in the outer channels (Fp1-F3 and P3-O1) reflects the fact that the gradient of the voltage drop-off immediately around C3 is steeper in this example compared to the previous example. This is analogous to the example of a mountain peak that is quite steep near its summit and but less steep farther out along its base.

Figure 4.41 shows an interesting discharge in the referential montage that has a result that may be unexpected in the bipolar

through the electrode pairs, if F3 and P3 measure 5 units in height and C3 measures 10 units in height, the Fp1-F3 channel will reflect a 5-unit difference (and display a wave that is 5 units in height going downward because Electrode 1 is more positive than Electrode 2). Likewise, F3-C3 will deflect the exact same amount in the same direction because the difference between that electrode pair is the same, again with the first electrode being "more positive" than the second. For that reason, the first two channels of the bipolar solution are

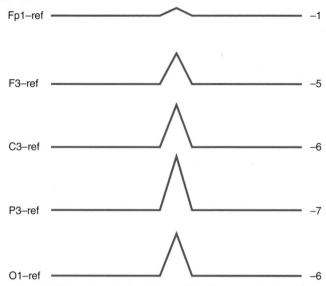

Fp1–ref ——————————⌒—————————— –1

F3–ref ——————————⌒—————————— –5

C3–ref ——————————⌒—————————— –6

P3–ref ——————————⌒—————————— –7

O1–ref ——————————⌒—————————— –6

Figure 4.41 Question 4. Predict how this discharge, displayed in a referential montage, will appear in a bipolar montage. This interesting discharge has a clear maximum at P3, but its field is wide and spreads almost, but not quite, to the frontal pole where it quickly dissipates.

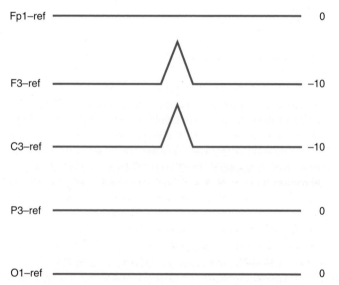

Fp1–ref ——————————————————— 0

F3–ref ——————————⌒—————————— –10

C3–ref ——————————⌒—————————— –10

P3–ref ——————————————————— 0

O1–ref ——————————————————— 0

Figure 4.42 Question 5. Predict how this discharge, displayed in a referential montage, of equal voltage in F3 and C3 but with surrounding electrodes quiet, will appear in a bipolar montage.

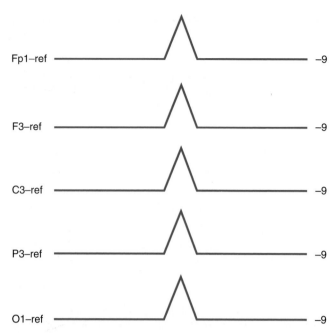

Fp1–ref ——————————⌒—————————— –9

F3–ref ——————————⌒—————————— –9

C3–ref ——————————⌒—————————— –9

P3–ref ——————————⌒—————————— –9

O1–ref ——————————⌒—————————— –9

Figure 4.43 Question 6. Predict how this discharge, a negatively charged event that is spread evenly across the whole electrode chain, will appear in a bipolar montage.

montage. There is a negative discharge centered near the back of the head that has a rather large field and a maximum voltage at P3. Note that the field only dissipates slightly in P3's adjacent electrodes, C3 and O1 and even reaches F3 with considerable strength. Finally, by Fp1, there has been a considerable drop-off in voltage. This example provides an excellent demonstration of one of the relative weaknesses of the bipolar recording technique. Note the misleading, but correct, representation of this discharge in the bipolar montage shown in Figure 4.44. For those new to EEG, the eye could be drawn immediately to the large deflection in Fp1-F3 and this pattern could be erroneously interpreted as an anterior discharge, which it is not. Why

does this occur? As we have learned, the correct interpretation of the bipolar representation shown in Figure 4.44 is properly based on the appearance of the diminutive but definite phase reversal shared by C3-P3 and P3-O1, correctly indicating that the discharge's maximum is in P3. As the reader well understands by now, the height of a wave in the bipolar montage does not represent the absolute voltage in that location, but rather the rate of falloff of the voltage or the voltage gradient of the electric field between the two compared electrodes. In bipolar montages, the point of maximum is always marked by the position of the phase reversal, even if the deflections of the phase reversal do not have particularly high amplitudes. This observation helps emphasize the concept that, in bipolar montages, independent of voltage, phase reversals mark the point of maximum, whereas in referential montages, it is the greatest wave height that marks the point of maximum.

Figure 4.42 shows a discharge with a maximum shared between the F3 and C3 electrodes. Note that, on the basis of this configuration, it is possible that the discharge is "flat" in the region between the two electrodes or, alternatively, there may be an even higher maximum point somewhere between the F3 and C3 electrodes (a schematic of these possibilities was shown in Figure 4.27). The two possibilities cannot necessarily be distinguished from the information provided by the tracing, and it is not necessary to know which of the two possibilities is the case to solve this problem. A discharge with equal maximum points appears as a particular type of phase reversal in a bipolar montage, as is shown in Figure 4.45. This pattern may be called an isoelectric phase reversal because the phases reverse around a flat, or isoelectric channel (F3-C3). Here again, the interpreter of the bipolar montage pattern must be aware that, despite the fact that this channel is

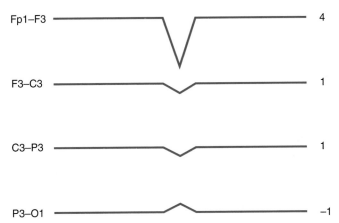

Fp1–F3 ————————⌄———————— 4

F3–C3 ————————⌄———————— 1

C3–P3 ————————⌄———————— 1

P3–O1 ————————⌃———————— −1

Figure 4.44 Answer 4. This solution may come as a surprise since the electrical "action" is clearly centered in the back of the head based on the information in the referential recording, but the biggest deflection in this bipolar representation is in the front of the head. As described in the text, this occurs because the fall-off in voltage is most abrupt between Fp1 and F3, but the area of maximum negativity is still reliably localized to P3, marked by the relatively subtle phase reversal seen in the bottom two channels.

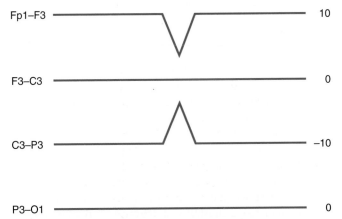

Fp1–F3 ————————⌄———————— 10

F3–C3 ———————————————— 0

C3–P3 ————————⌃———————— −10

P3–O1 ———————————————— 0

Figure 4.45 Answer 5. The discharge shown on the previous page manifests as an isoelectric phase reversal when displayed here in a bipolar montage. A flat channel is seen between the two phase-reversing channels. Because there is no voltage difference between the F3 and C3 electrodes (which share the maximum), there is an apparently paradoxical appearance where the point of maximum voltage is marked by a flat channel in the bipolar representation.

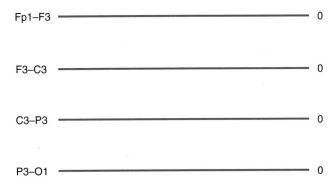

Fp1–F3 ———————————————— 0

F3–C3 ———————————————— 0

C3–P3 ———————————————— 0

P3–O1 ———————————————— 0

Figure 4.46 Answer 6. Because there is no gradient (difference) across any of the electrodes in this chain, all channels are flat in the bipolar montage. Although this result may appear to represent a loss of information (after all, a spike did seem to be present in all the channels of the referential montage), when scalp events occur at nearly the exact same voltage across wide areas of the head, they often represent electrical noise from a distant source. Electrical activity of cerebral origin usually manifests with a gradient (varying voltages) across the scalp. Thus the cancellation of such external noise activity is one of the main advantages of bipolar recording techniques.

be of similar voltage across a wide region of the head, a discharge that arises from the brain with exactly equal voltage across all scalp electrodes is rarely, if ever, encountered. The most common explanation for this type of pattern is electrical noise from an external source. Because of the noise's external origin, it is possible for the noise signal to be of equal voltage all across the scalp. By contrast, discharges of cerebral origin almost always vary in voltage across the scalp and, therefore, are almost always discernible on bipolar montages.

Although the solution of four flat lines shown in Figure 4.46 may seem uninspiring, it represents the triumph of the bipolar montage technique. This tendency to cancel out common noisy activity is what gives bipolar montages their "cleaner" appearance and can make them easier to read. The efficiency with which bipolar montages can cancel out external noise is one of the major advantages of the bipolar recording technique. Less commonly, this type of cancellation of electrical events that are widely represented across the head can be a disadvantage. Occasionally, genuine cerebral activity (e.g., sharp waves or slow waves) can have a wide, synchronous field across the scalp. Displaying such waves in a bipolar montage can result in a large amount of cancellation of such potentials, leading the reader to underestimate the voltage of the events. More often, however, the reader is happy that external noise sources are cancelled with the bipolar technique because this renders the underlying true electrocerebral activity easier to appreciate.

Figure 4.47 shows a downgoing spike, implying that the spike has positive rather than negative polarity. There is a surrounding field consisting of smaller positivities in F3 and C3. The appearance in the bipolar montage seen in Figure 4.50 is that of the classic "positive phase reversal" in which the phase-reversing waves point away from each other. Although epileptiform discharges more commonly show a negative polarity at the scalp (as explained in Chapter 2), occasionally they will

flat, because the phase of the discharges reverses in the surrounding channels, this flat line marks the region of maximum voltage.

The wave pattern illustrated in Figure 4.43 represents a commonly encountered type of electrical event seen in referential montages. This example consists of an apparent sharp wave with the exact same intensity across the whole parasagittal electrode chain (and perhaps across the whole scalp). Because there is no potential difference between any of the electrodes in this chain, the resulting bipolar tracing (Figure 4.46) shows flat lines in all of its four channels—the apparent sharp wave cancels out completely in each of the four comparisons. Although it is not impossible for a discharge to

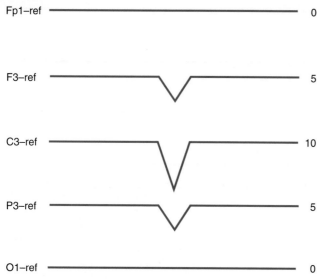

Figure 4.47 Question 7. Predict how this discharge, displayed in a referential montage, will appear in a bipolar montage. The figure shows a positive spike with maximum at C3 and with smoothly diminishing voltages at F3 and P3.

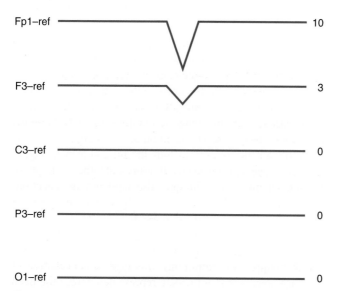

Figure 4.48 Question 8. This pattern, displayed in a referential montage, suggests a strong positivity in Fp1 with diminishing strength in F3 and no field in C3, P3, and O1. Predict its appearance in the bipolar montage. What physiological phenomenon does this pattern resemble?

show positive polarity, as in this example. Many nonepileptiform EEG waves may also manifest positive polarity, such as vertex waves of sleep, which can have both positive and negative components.

Figure 4.48 shows another frequently encountered waveform. In this example, there is a strong positivity in Fp1. The field of the positivity stretches into F3, but with less intensity. The remaining three electrodes (C3, P3, and O1) do not detect the discharge. The corresponding tracing in the bipolar montage shows one of the most commonly seen deflections in the EEG of awake individuals. The Fp1-F3 channel goes

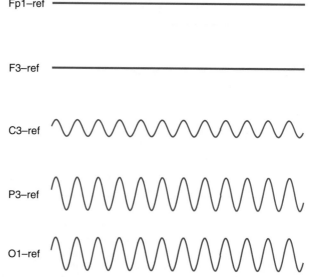

Figure 4.49 Question 9. Predict how this pattern, displayed in a referential montage, will appear in a bipolar montage. Sinusoidal waves are present in this recording, most prominently in the posterior two electrodes, and at half the voltage in the C3 electrode. This pattern is similar to what might be seen as the posterior (occipital) rhythm in some patients. In this example, the P3 and O1 signals are perfectly in phase, which is not always the case in actual patient recordings.

down, reflecting the fact that Fp1 is "more positive" than F3. Likewise, F3-C3 shows a downgoing wave because F3 is more positive than C3, although the difference is not as great. The final two channels (C3-P3 and P3-O1) are flat because C3, P3, and O1 are all neutral.

The wave illustrated in this figure is a representation of an eyeblink artifact, which is common in the awake EEG (described in more detail in Chapter 6, "Electroencephalographic artifacts"). Its appearance in the bipolar montage is illustrated in Figure 4.51. Because there is a net positive charge on the front of the globe of the eye, when the eyes are closed, the eyes bob upward (the so-called *Bell's phenomenon*), causing a momentary positivity in the most anterior electrodes. Working through this problem yields the explanation for a surprising feature of eyeblink artifacts in EEG—they look similar in referential montages and bipolar montages, with big anterior downward deflections seen in both!

The pattern seen in Figure 4.49 suggests the familiar appearance of the posterior rhythm seen in the occipital lobes, but with a twist. The visual subtraction of sinusoidal curves such as those seen in this example is somewhat more challenging than subtracting the simple spikes we have been looking at so far, but the principles are the same. As we shall see, this example gives a surprising result based on the fact that, in this patient, the posterior rhythm happens to be completely synchronous and in phase in the P3 and O1 electrodes (which is not the case in most patients). Looking at the bipolar representation of this pattern,. Figure 4.52 shows the expected flat channel in Fp1-F3 as both of these electrodes are inactive. A comparison of the flat F3 electrode to the lower voltage sinusoidal wave in C3 shows a mirror-image reflection of that wave, with the peaks and troughs

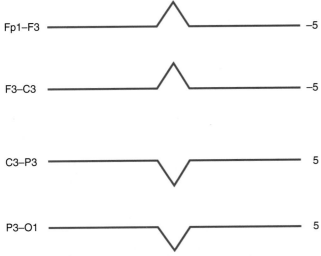

Figure 4.50 **Answer 7**. This figure shows the corresponding "positive phase reversal" with waves that point away from each other. Because the phases reverse at C3, this is the location of maximum positivity. The discharge should be compared to the discharge shown with the same field and the same intensity but opposite (negative) polarity in Figures 4.37 and 4.38.

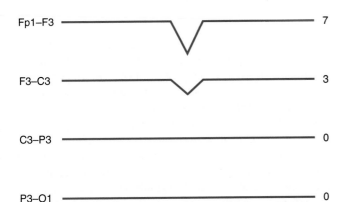

Figure 4.51 **Answer 8**. The downward deflections in the first two channels reflect the presence of a strong positivity in Fp1 with diminishing strength across the next two electrodes in the chain (Fp1 > F3 > C3). This pattern is consistent with eyeblink artifact caused by a sudden positive charge near the frontopolar areas related to upturning of the positively-charged front of the globe of the eye with eye closure (explained more fully in Chapter 6, "Electroencephalographic Artifacts").

flipped. The subtraction of P3 from C3 yields a similar result. As expected, at least mathematically, P3 and O1 cancel completely, and the P3-O1 channel is flat. This yields the paradoxical result of a posterior rhythm, strongest in the P3 and O1 channels in this hypothetical patient, that is not seen at all in the most posterior channel (P3-01) of the bipolar recording. In practice, this situation can occur in individuals in whom the posterior rhythm happens to be highly synchronous and "in phase" in the posterior channels (the peaks and troughs of the waves in P3-ref and O1-ref line up perfectly with one another). In most patients, however, the posterior rhythm representations in P3 and O1

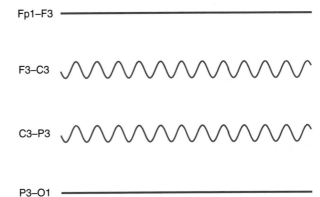

Figure 4.52 **Answer 9**. The bipolar display of these sinusoidal waves shows an unexpected and somewhat paradoxical effect in which the posterior rhythm is not evident in the most posterior electrode pairing (P3-O1) where one would expect it to be most prominent. This occurs as a result of a complete cancellation effect related to the posterior rhythm waves in P3 and O1 being perfectly in phase and of the same amplitude. In most patients, the posterior rhythm can be seen in the P3-O1 channel in a bipolar montage because the posterior rhythm expresses somewhat differently in P3 as compared to O1. In an occasional patient, however, the posterior rhythm waves are nearly identical in P3 and O1, yielding this surprising appearance of the posterior rhythm being absent from the most posterior channel of the bipolar montage (see text).

are somewhat out of phase with each other and have different amplitudes, so the subtraction of one from the other does yield a recognizable sinusoidal wave in P3-O1. Imagine that in the Figure 4.49 problem the wave in O1-ref were shifted one-half wavelength to the right with respect to the wave in P3-ref. In that case, the rhythm seen in the resulting P3-O1 channel of the bipolar montage would, indeed, have very high voltage.

PREDICTING THE APPEARANCE OF THE REFERENTIAL MONTAGE BASED ON THE BIPOLAR MONTAGE

In the problems above we have been looking at events in a referential montage and predicting their appearance in a bipolar montage. The reverse type of problem, starting with a bipolar montage and predicting how a page will appear in the referential montage, presents some unexpected challenges. The first such problem we will consider is shown in Figure 4.53, which shows a simple negative phase reversal in a bipolar montage. What will this look like in a referential montage? Going through each of the four channels, we develop a set of constraints: analysis of the bipolar tracing tells us that because Fp1-F3 is flat, so Fp1 and F3 must be of the same voltage. It seems most natural to assume that the voltages at Fp1 and F3 should be zero but, from the mathematical perspective, it also seems true that they could be any voltage, as long as it's the same value. By the same line of reasoning, P3 and O1 must be of the same voltage since P3-O1 is flat. Further, we know that the voltage of Fp1, F3, P3, and O1 must all be the same because the step-up of voltage from

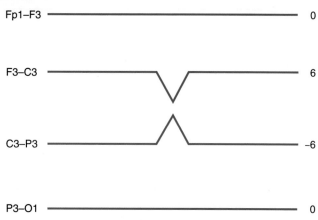

Figure 4.53 **Question 10**. Predict how this discharge, displayed in a bipolar montage, might appear in a referential montage. The figure depicts an isolated discharge with negative polarity and maximum in C3.

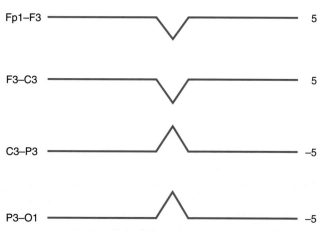

Figure 4.54 **Question 11**. Again, this discharge shows a negative voltage maximum (phase reversal with waves pointing toward each other) in C3. There is a smooth gradient of decreasing voltage surrounding the maximum. How might it appear in a referential montage?

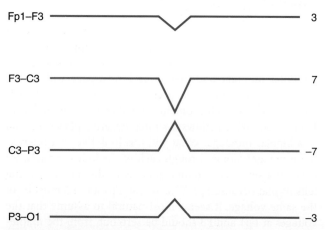

Figure 4.55 **Question 12**. Predict how this discharge, displayed in a bipolar montage, might appear in a referential montage. The figure shows a pattern that is quite similar to the previous example, with maximum negativity at C3; however, the second and third channels show a steeper drop-off of voltage than is seen at the outer (first and fourth) channels.

F3 to C3 is the same (6 units) as the step-down of voltage from C3 to P3. We know this because the height of F3-C3 is the same as, but opposite in direction to, the height of C3-P3, C3 must be more negative than those four electrodes by an amount equivalent to the heights seen in F3-C3 and C3-P3 (6 units). Any solution that meets these constraints is potentially valid. In summary, scanning down the four channels, the constraints can be summarized as: Fp1 is the same as F3, C3 is more negative than F3 by 6 units, P3 is less negative than C3 by that same 6 units, and P3 is the same as O1. Figure 4.56 shows three possible solutions to this problem.

Note that all three proposed solutions are equally correct from a "mathematical" point of view, fitting the constraints implied by the bipolar montage: Fp1 = F3 = P3 = O1, and C3 has a "more negative" voltage than those four electrodes by 6 units. However, certain of these solutions are more likely to be *plausible* solutions in clinical EEG than others. Indeed, the top trace showing the pure negative discharge in C3 is the most likely to occur in actual EEG recordings (and the pinpoint field of the discharge does suggest electrode artifact). The middle trace, in which there is a negativity seen across all electrodes but strongest in C3, remains a possible solution. It is less attractive from the physiological point of view because it requires Fp1, F3, P3, and O1 all to be of the exact same non-zero voltage, but still within the field of the negative discharge—a relatively unlikely occurrence (usually there would be some tapering of voltage away from the C3 maximum). The bottom trace of Figure 4.56 in which the surrounding electrodes are mildly positive but equipotential and C3 is mildly negative is also a mathematically sound solution (since Fp1 = F3 = P3 = O1, and C3 has a more negative voltage than the other four positions), but this solution is biologically implausible for similar reasons. It would require a central negativity surrounded by a large ring of positivity of precisely constant intensity (no gradient).

Differences in solving the conversion problem in the bipolar to referential direction include the fact that the bipolar trace has four channels but the solution, the corresponding referential trace, needs to have five channels. More important, when converting referential traces to bipolar traces, there was only a single correct solution. As was seen with the previous example, any given trace in a bipolar montage can correspond to an infinite number of possible solutions in the referential montage. The reason for this is akin to the fact that there is only a single solution to the problem: "5 − 3 = ?" —the answer must be 2. If we ask the "reverse" version of this question, "subtraction of what two numbers gives 2 as a result?" the answer is an infinite number of pairs, such as 5 and 3, 101 and 99, −6 and −8, and so on. This analogy holds up well because bipolar traces are analogous to a display of differences and referential traces to a display of "absolute values."

When there is a negative phase reversal at C3, what difference does it make in the shape of the electric field when the height of the waves surrounding the phase reversal is different in different examples? Figure 4.54 shows a similar negative discharge maximum in C3 as compared to Figure 4.53,

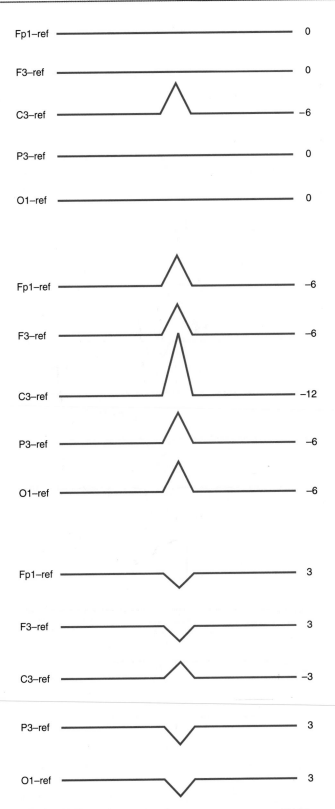

Figure 4.56 Answer 10. These are three of the many possible ways the discharge shown on the previous page may appear in a referential montage. All three of the solutions shown in this figure are mathematically possible, but the top solution is most likely (see text). All possible solutions will have in common the fact that the outside four channels, Fp1, F3, P3, and O1, are of exactly the same voltage and the middle channel, C3, is slightly more negative (by 6 units) in comparison to the other four. Think about why the middle and bottom solutions are mathematically correct, but are biologically implausible.

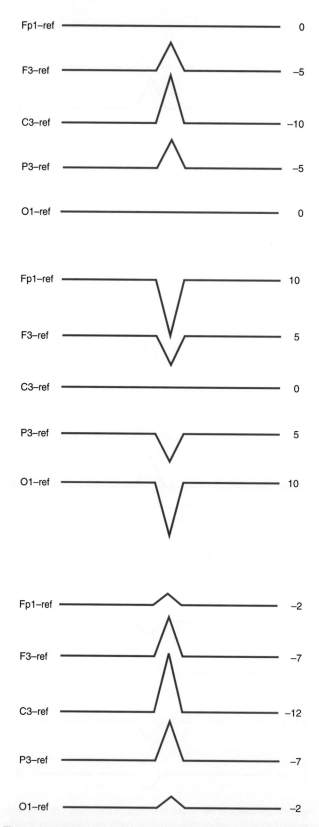

Figure 4.57 Answer 11. Possible representations in the referential montage of the discharge shown on the previous page in Question 11. The top and bottom traces depict the discharge as having a net negative charge, with decreasingly negative voltage as distance from C3 increases. The middle trace shows an alternative solution. This is a mathematically correct solution that shows C3 as neutral, surrounded by electrodes that become increasingly positive with distance; however, this solution is less physiologically plausible for reasons discussed in the text.

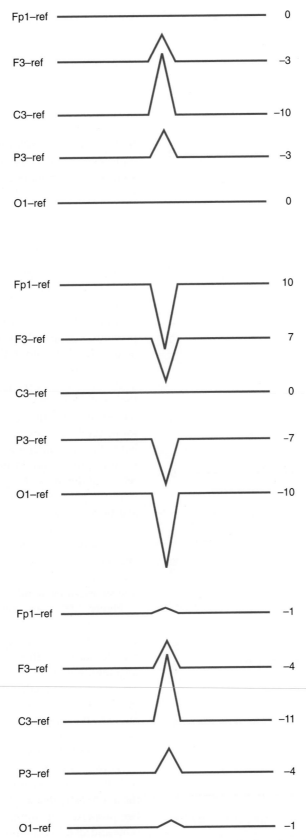

Figure 4.58 Answer 12. Possible representations in the referential montage of the discharge shown on the previous page in Question 12. The solutions are similar to those shown for the previous figure; however, the field in the immediately surrounding electrodes, F3 and P3, is weaker. Again, the top and bottom traces are most biologically plausible.

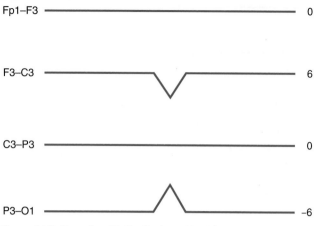

Figure 4.59 Question 13. Predict how this discharge, displayed in a bipolar montage, might appear in a referential montage. This figure depicts a phase reversal with an intervening flat channel. This type of pattern is also referred to as an isoelectric phase reversal.

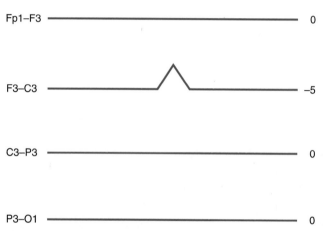

Figure 4.60 Question 14. Predict how this pattern, a bipolar tracing showing a single channel with an upward deflection in the middle of a chain, might appear in a referential montage.

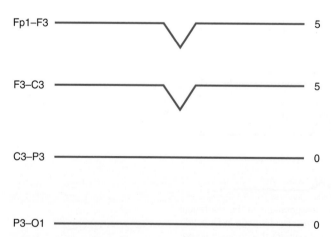

Figure 4.61 Question 15. Predict how this discharge, displayed in a bipolar montage, might appear in a referential montage. What type of commonly encountered EEG event does this pattern depict?

but this time with a more gradual gradient of decreasing voltage surrounding it going both in the anterior and posterior directions, as evidenced by the new deflections in the outer channels (Fp1-F3 and P3-O1). The possible solutions shown in Figure 4.57 are all potentially correct because they all show the most negative voltage in C3 with voltages that are gradually decreasingly negative in the surrounding electrodes. The top and bottom traces, however, are the most biologically plausible with a negative event maximum in C3 and a gradient of decreasing negativity as distance increases from C3. The middle trace is mathematically correct but biologically implausible. Although in the middle trace the "maximum negativity" among the electrodes remains in C3, this solution implies two concomitant positive events occurring in unison at each pole of the brain (frontal pole and occipital pole) having the exact same magnitude and gradient and a completely neutral area in the C3 region, an unlikely occurrence.

The discharge in Figure 4.55 again shows a spike with maximum negativity in C3, only subtly different from the previous example. In this example, however, the higher amplitude deflections in the two center channels, F3-C3 and C3-P3, imply a steeper gradient of voltage change near the C3 electrode. Can you predict how the small changes between the bipolar representations in Figures 4.54 and 4.55 will play out when converting to a referential montage? Figure 4.57 shows results that are similar to the solutions for Figure 4.58, but with small differences. Note that the relative heights of the waves in F3 and P3 are much less than the height of C3, reflecting the more abrupt drop-off in voltage with distance from the point of maximum (C3) in this example. The top and bottom traces are commonly encountered patterns for EEG events recorded on the scalp and are the most likely correct solutions for the same reasons given for the previous example—they are more biologically plausible compared to the mathematically correct but biologically implausible solution shown in the middle trace.

Figure 4.59 shows an example of a particular type of phase reversal, the isoelectric phase reversal that was discussed earlier. In this type of phase reversal, waves still reverse phase (in this case, changing from downgoing to upgoing), but there is an intervening flat channel. Figure 4.62 shows three mathematically correct solutions, although the top trace may be the most plausible of the three, followed by the middle trace. The bottom trace is a mathematically possible solution, but it requires a positive event to occur in Fp1, F3, and O1 at the exact same voltage across a relatively large area with an intervening area of negativity (C3 and P3)—a scenario that is unlikely to be produced by the brain. Note that all three of the solutions have the same two properties in common: the height of C3 and P3 is the same and all other channels are lower than C3 and P3 by the exact same amount.

Amplifier Artifact

The relatively simple tracing shown in Figure 4.60 initially appears straightforward but actually brings up a particular

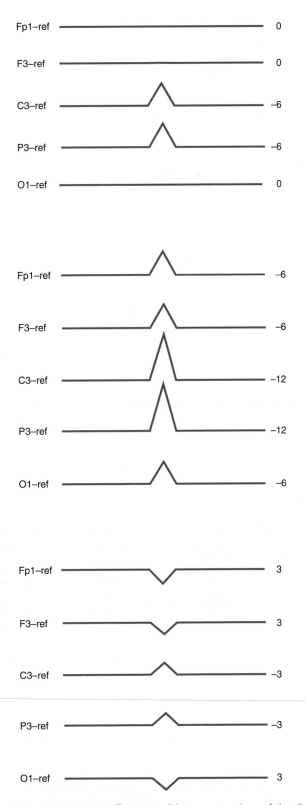

Figure 4.62 Answer 13. Three possible representations of the discharge shown on the previous page are shown in the referential montage. The top tracing is the most plausible solution to this problem, showing a discharge with a shared negative maximum in C3 and P3. Although the middle and bottom tracings are mathematically correct, they are less biologically plausible (see text). All of the solutions have in common the fact that C3 and P3 are of the same voltage and more negative than the surrounding electrodes, which are, in turn, of an equal but more positive voltage.

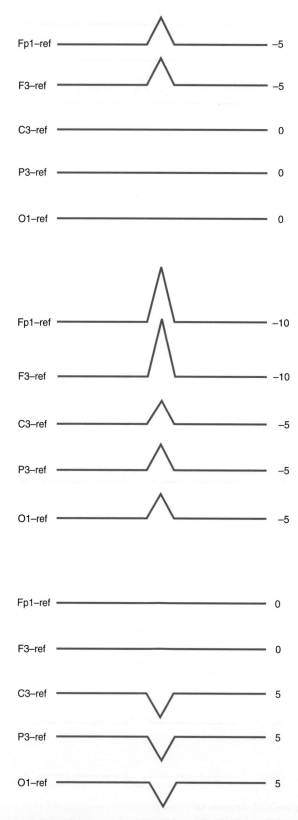

Figure 4.63 Answer 14. Possible representations of the discharge shown on the previous page in Question 14 are shown in the referential montage. The flat channels in the bipolar montage tell us that voltages at Fp1 = F3, and that C3 = P3 = O1, but at a more positive voltage. Although any solution that fits these constraints is mathematically valid, none is particularly plausible in terms of cerebral activity, and such patterns often represent an amplifier or channel artifact (see text and for further explanation).

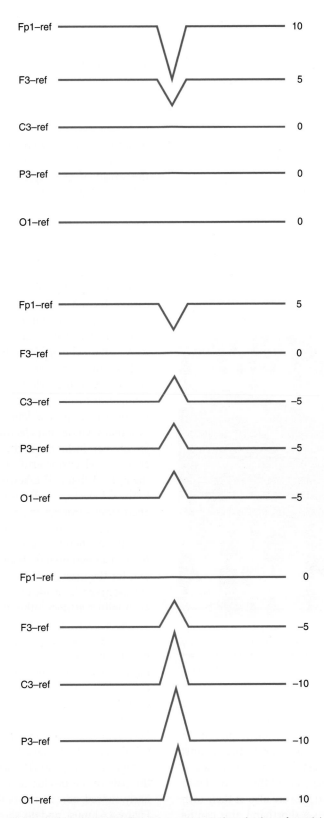

Figure 4.64 Answer 15. Possible representations in the referential montage of the discharge shown in Figure 4.61. The top tracing is the most likely solution, representing a positive event that is strongest anteriorly. The bottom tracing suggests a negative event posteriorly but is less plausible because C3, P3, and O1 would have to be negative but of exactly equal non-zero voltage (see text). This pattern of a large anterior positivity (the solution suggested by the top panel) is strongly suggestive of eyeblink artifact.

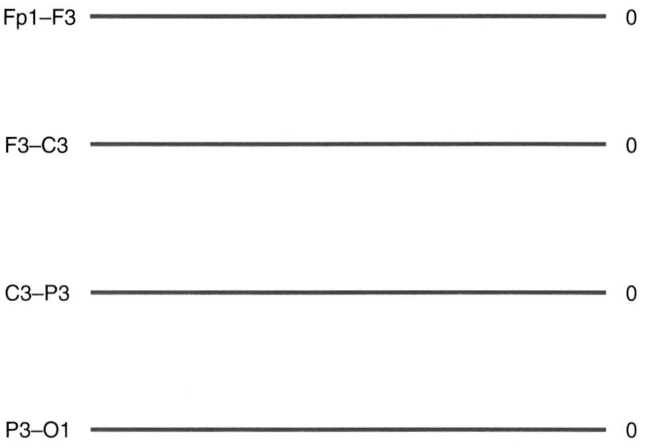

Fp1–F3 ———————————————————————— 0

F3–C3 ———————————————————————— 0

C3–P3 ———————————————————————— 0

P3–O1 ———————————————————————— 0

Figure 4.65 Question 16. Predict how this pattern, displayed in a bipolar montage, might appear in a referential montage. This example, showing four flat channels, is the simplest possible tracing but still has multiple possible solutions.

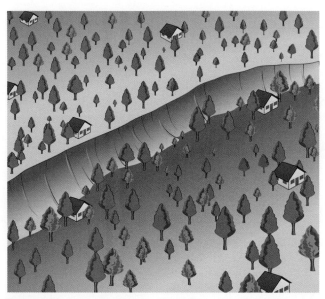

Figure 4.66 An escarpment is a long slope or cliff that separates a higher plateau from a lower plain. While you may occasionally encounter such geologic formations on earth, you would not expect to encounter the electrical counterpart of an escarpment on a patient's scalp.

problem in interpretation. A lone deflection is present in F3-C3, which implies that all the electrodes in the channel above it are at the exact same voltage (i.e., Fp1 and F3 are at one voltage because Fp1-F3 is flat), and all the electrodes in the channels below it (C3, P3, and O1) are also at their own exact same, but higher voltage. As a shorthand, this can be expressed as: Fp1=F3 < C3=P3=O1. The pattern suggests a plane of lower voltage anteriorly, a quick step-up between F3 and C3, and then a higher voltage plateau in the posterior electrodes. Why shouldn't it be possible for the front part of the brain to have an area of positivity and the back part of the brain to have an area of negativity as this pattern suggests?

The problem is the steep shelf of voltage change between F3 and C3, with absolutely flat voltage contours anterior and posterior to the single area of step-up. Going back to our analogy of electric fields looking like mountain ranges, what would this pattern look like topographically? The answer is, it would look like an escarpment. An escarpment is a steep cliff that separates a higher plateau from a lower plain. One of the best known examples of this geological formation is the Niagara escarpment over which Niagara Falls flows. Escarpments are occasionally found (but not too often) in the world of geography, but very rarely found in electric fields generated by the brain and measured on the scalp. It is very unlikely that the brain would produce two such large perfectly equipotential zones immediately adjacent to one another with an abrupt drop-off between the two (Figures 4.66 and 4.68). Figure 4.63 shows some of the possible mathematical solutions to this problem but, in reality, none of the solutions is particularly attractive for the reasons described earlier. Indeed, when a lone deflection such as this one is encountered in the middle of a chain in a bipolar recording, it is probable that it represents an electrical artifact in the F3-C3 channel *amplifier* rather than a true cerebral event.

Note the distinction between a single channel/amplifier artifact and a single electrode artifact. If there is an artifact in a single electrode (perhaps because the electrode is touched, is loose, or "pops"), a deflection will be seen in all the channels that include that electrode. Amplifier artifact looks different. For instance, if the deflection in Figure 4.60 were caused by electrode artifact in F3, why is it not also seen in the Fp1-F3 channel? Likewise, if it were caused by an artifact in the C3 electrode, why is it not seen in the C3-P3 channel? Such single-*channel* artifacts are considerably less common than single-electrode artifacts, but it is important to recognize them when they occur. Figure 4.63 shows possible solutions in a referential montage that are mathematically correct but, for the reasons discussed, none is biologically plausible, consistent with the idea that the single deflection is caused by an amplifier artifact rather than an electrocerebral event.

Figure 4.61 shows a pattern that can be interpreted either as increasing negativity going down the front of the chain caused by some negative event in the posterior head region, or increasing positivity going up the chain (through C3, F3, and Fp1) caused by some positive event anteriorly. If the former is the case (that the pattern comes from a posterior negative event), then there is again the problem that this negative event would have to be exactly equipotential in the bottom three electrodes: C3, P3, and O1. Because a negative event with the exact same voltage in C3, P3, and O1 does not seem plausible, the idea that this pattern was produced by a posterior negativity is much less likely. Indeed, note that all of the possible solutions suggested in Figure 4.64 must, and do, show the same voltage in those three electrodes. A simpler and more likely explanation is that this represents a positive event in the front of the head, as is seen in the top trace of Figure 4.64. The configuration of this discharge is again consistent with an eyeblink artifact as was described in Figures 4.61 and 4.64. The top "eyeblink" solution in Figure 4.64 also solves the problem of how the posterior three electrodes,

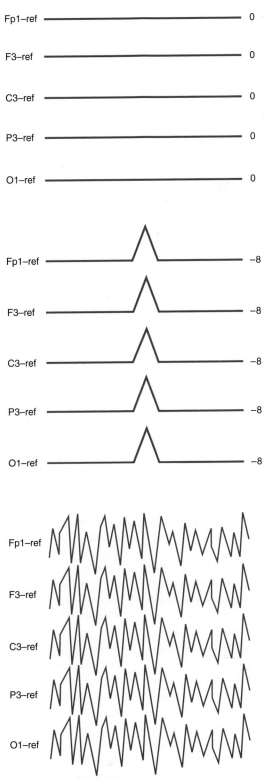

Figure 4.67 Answer 16. Possible representations in the referential montage of the pattern shown on the previous page. The top tracing depicts electrocerebral silence. The middle and bottom traces are also valid, representing electrical noise in all electrodes that canceled successfully in the original bipolar tracing. Any solution in which there is EEG activity with the exact same voltage in every channel is mathematically possible, but physiologically unlikely to have arisen from the brain since electrocerebral activity would be expected to show some degree of variation between scalp areas, which would, in turn, generate deflections rather than flat lines in a bipolar montage.

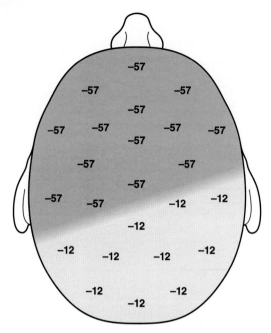

Figure 4.68 The implausible example of an "electrical escarpment." The purpose of this figure is to depict an imaginary situation where all voltages are exactly the same above a boundary, and exactly the same but with a different value below the boundary. This is the type of "electrical escarpment" that is implied by the single deflection shown in the bipolar montage in Figure 4.60, with a plateau of equal voltages in one area adjacent to a plane of a different but uniform voltages. This type of measurement is unlikely to occur in physiological systems. Instead, brain activity usually shows smoother and more gradual drop-offs when occurring across large areas. Single, isolated deflections in the middle of a bipolar chain as seen in Figure 4.60 are suspicious for channel or amplifier artifact rather than true electrocerebral activity.

C3, P3, and O1, can all be of the exact same voltage since their voltage is zero."

Figure 4.65 shows the simplest possible bipolar tracing with four flat channels. This exercise serves as a reminder of what might be hiding behind any bipolar recording, whether or not it consists of flat channels. The top trace of Figure 4.67 reminds us that this bipolar tracing may truly reflect electrical silence. The middle trace shows a spike that appears exactly the same in all channels and, therefore, likely represents electrical noise. Because like activity cancels across bipolar chains, the noise has been successfully suppressed by the bipolar recording technique. Such cancellation is a frequent occurrence, especially when the noise is from an external source that appears in all head areas in the same way. For instance, electrocardiographic (EKG) activity is always present throughout all head regions but is often not evident in bipolar displays. This is explained by the fact that the EKG potential may be of the same shape and amplitude across all the regions in question and will cancel in almost all channels of a bipolar recording (it will also cancel in a referential recording if the chosen reference happens to contain the exact same representation of the EKG signal). When there are slight differences in the way EKG artifact expresses in different head locations, slight amounts

of EKG artifact will be seen in those locations when the bipolar subtractions are made. Finally, the bottom trace of Figure 4.67 may be the most realistic solution of the group because large amounts of *common* electrical noise in the head can be cancelled out by the bipolar recording technique. It is always a good idea to keep in mind all the possibilities of what may be going on "behind the scenes" in a low-voltage bipolar tracing. Most often, the suppression of this common activity is seen as one of the principal advantages of the bipolar recording technique rather than as a loss of useful information.

A Summary of Scanning Technique for Understanding Voltage Contours in Bipolar and Referential Montages

Bipolar Montages

When you look at the image below, if you already have some experience in reading EEGs, you may immediately determine, "Aha, there is a negative spike in C3!"—and you would be correct. However, to understand the *voltage contour* the waves are suggesting, you will want to look at these four channels in a different way. Much as we imagined the farmer-in-the-field walking down his property with a rudimentary altitude-measuring instrument, now we will scan a bipolar montage as if we were an electroencephalographer-walking-down-the-head, from front to back. We want to imagine ourselves standing on the head at Fp1 (at the forehead) and walking down the chain, channel by channel, toward the back of the head. With each downward deflection, we imagine that "it's getting more negative" and with each upward deflection we imagine "it is getting more positive." When we see a downward wave that is big, we imagine "it's getting *a lot* more negative." When we encounter a small upgoing wave, we would imagine "it's getting *just a bit* more positive." In this way, we can now visualize not just the point of maximum, but also the contour of voltage the four channels are suggesting.

Referential Montages

Let's imagine the same experience walking down the same parasagittal chain, but now using a referential montage. The first difference is that five electrode contacts generate five channels, since each contact is compared to a reference (an ideal/neutral reference electrode for the sake of this example). Note that this referential montage has now been arranged horizontally rather than in the usual stacked vertical fashion. The height of each wave in the chain can be considered an absolute measurement of the height of the voltage, and the points of the peaks of each waves can be connected to see the contour of the voltage map across the chain. You can imagine that the height of each wave in a referential montage is the height of a telephone pole. You can now string a wire connecting the tops of each of the five telephone poles and that wire will mimic the contour of the voltage crossing the scalp—it is as simple as that!

Once you have mastered these concepts, you can look down any bipolar chain or any referential chain and imagine a voltage contour. Of course, there are multiple chains across the head in each montage, but how does each chain relate to the others? You can probably see what is coming next. In the AP bipolar montage, there are four long chains going down the head from left to right and a short midline chain (left temporal, left parasagittal, midline, right parasagittal, right temporal). Each of these five chains suggests a longitudinal voltage contour along a single line. But if we were to line the five contours up in parallel, how would we know how they relate to one another (Figure 4.69)? To get a more precise representation of the whole voltage map across the head, we can generate voltage contours in the perpendicular direction with a transverse montage. In theory, the contours from the transverse chains can be used to align the five anteroposterior bipolar contours to creating a mesh-like three-dimensional gradient map of the scalp for the event in question (Figure 4.70).

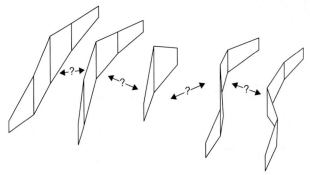

Figure 4.69 Note that each of the five bipolar chains gives us the up-and-down of the voltage contour in the front-to-back direction, but when we look at all five contours, it is not absolutely clear how each of the five chains relates to its neighbor in terms of relative height. For instance, from the AP bipolar montage, we have a good idea how F3 relates to C3 in voltage difference, and so on, based on the purely longitudinal comparisons we gain from this montage. But how does C3 relate to Cz? The answer is seen in the next figure.

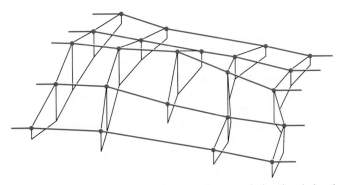

Figure 4.70 When we shift our focus to the transverse montage, analyzing the chains that cross the head from ear to ear, we now learn the relative voltage of C3 compared to Cz, and indeed the relative height position of all five front-to-back chains to each other. Note how the transverse montage voltage contours (in red) determine the relative position of the five longitudinal chains from Fig 4.69.

5

Electroencephalographic Electrodes, Channels, and Montages and How They Are Chosen

In electroencephalography, the term montage refers to the order and choice of channels displayed on the EEG page. Several decisions go into the design of a good display montage: which electrodes to use, how the electrodes should be paired to create each channel, and the ordering of the channels in a way that will render the tracing easy to interpret visually. Decisions of secondary importance include choice of the color in which to display each channel and placement of gaps or white space between groups of channels to allow easier visualization of groups.

Although a large number of montages is theoretically possible, a given laboratory ideally uses a relatively small set of montages. Smaller montage sets have the advantage of allowing the readers in a given laboratory to become more quickly familiar with each montage, offering more efficient and faster scanning of tracings. Therefore, one should hesitate before permanently adding a new montage to a laboratory's montage set that already includes the same electrode pairings, perhaps in another order, that are present in another member of the set; such a montage is redundant and may not really add a "new view" of the EEG.

In addition to scalp electrodes placed to record brain electrical activity, additional "monitoring" electrodes may be placed on nonscalp areas to record other physiologic activities including heartbeat, respirations, eye movements, contraction of certain muscles, including the respiratory muscles, and limb movements. The schema for the placement and naming of the EEG electrodes according to the international 10-20 system was described in Chapter 3, "Introduction to Commonly Used Terms in Electroencephalography." While considering the strategies used in different montage designs, the reader should consider how montage choice affects the reading process and also how new montages might be designed in special situations. Such situations could include a patient in whom part of the head is not accessible for one reason or another (e.g., a surgical bandage) or the occasional patient in whom accurate localization requires the placement of intervening electrodes.

CATEGORIES OF MONTAGES: REFERENTIAL AND BIPOLAR

Montages are generally divided into two large groups, *referential* and *bipolar*, denoting the technique by which EEG data are displayed. Because there are significant differences in the strategies used to interpret these two montage families, each is discussed in its own section. Localization techniques for

each of these montage categories were discussed Chapter 4, "Electroencephalographic Localization."

Recommended Montage Conventions

Although electrode channels can be presented in any order when creating a montage, certain conventions are encouraged (also see ACNS Guideline 6 referenced at the end of this chapter): in general, channels should be placed in a "left over right" configuration (electrode chains from the left side of the head are placed nearer the top of the page, and chains from the right side of the head are placed nearer the bottom of the page). More anterior electrodes should be placed before more posterior electrodes (front-to-back ordering of channels going down the page is encouraged). Interelectrode distances should be consistent (electrode positions should not be unpredictably skipped in electrode chains). Finally, the design should favor the simplest arrangement possible (Figure 5.1).

In the days of paper EEG recording, it was up to the EEG technologist to choose the montage in real time that would best demonstrate the patient's findings at any particular point in the tracing. If an EEG event happened to be recorded in a montage that was disadvantageous for interpretation, the ink had already dried on the page, and it was not possible to change settings retrospectively. Current digital EEG technology presents a new set of problems. Although the same EEG page can be viewed in a variety of montages during the course of interpretation, some readers may find that it takes less energy to leave the display in one montage for the whole tracing, usually choosing the montage with which they are most comfortable. Although scanning a whole EEG study in a single montage may allow for faster reading, occasionally an EEG finding may be seen well in one montage but only poorly seen, or perhaps not seen at all, in another. It is therefore best practice for the EEG technologist or the reader to cycle through a minimum set of montages during the course of each study. This will typically include some combination of longitudinal bipolar, transverse bipolar, and referential montages.

MONTAGE DESIGN

Referential Versus Bipolar Montages

Referential and bipolar recording techniques appear to use two distinct strategies for recording, but, as we shall see, there is considerable overlap between the two. A referential

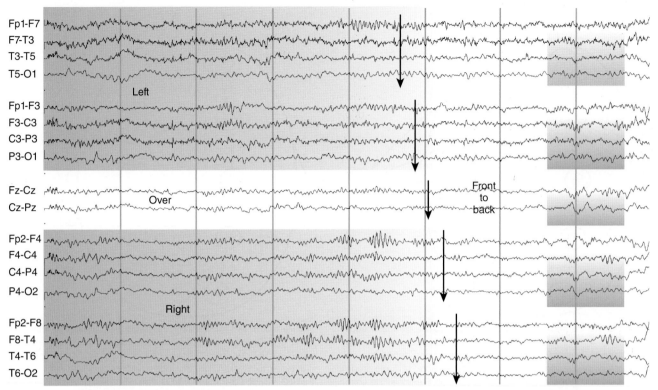

Figure 5.1 This page of EEG is shaded in a way that highlights the groupings and structure of a standard AP bipolar montage. The top two sets of four channels with shading (labeled LEFT) represent the left hemisphere and the bottom two sets of four channels with shading (labeled RIGHT) represent the right hemisphere. The middle, unshaded channels represent the midline. This montage therefore conforms to the general convention of placing left-sided channels over right-sided channels. Within each grouping of four channels, each chain of four runs from the front of the head to the back of the head (depicted by the gradient shadings on the right side of the figure). The downward-pointing arrows show how the eye scans from front to back through each four-channel (or two-channel) grouping. After this scheme is understood, it is possible to predict how each channel on the page corresponds to a location on the head based simply on its position in the groupings without needing to consult the channel labels.

montage compares each "point of interest" on the head (which may also be referred to as "the electrode of interest") to a reference point somewhere else on the body, perhaps still on the scalp, which it is hoped will be neutral or "indifferent." One of the main drawbacks of referential montage recordings is that no chosen reference point can be guaranteed to be completely neutral. Here is an example of the left parasagittal chain of five electrodes as it might be displayed in a referential montage:

Fp1–ref
F3–ref
C3–ref
P3–ref
O1–ref

The term *ref* as used here denotes a reference electrode such as the nose, the chin, the back of the neck, or the earlobes, another electrode on the scalp, or sometimes a combination of scalp electrodes. The specific choice used for the reference electrode is further discussed later in this chapter.

Considering the technique used to display the same group of five parasagittal electrodes in a bipolar montage, the following channel pairings would be used:

Fp1–F3
F3–C3
C3–P3
P3–O1

The term *bipolar* derives from the fact that, as can be seen from this chain, each channel represents the voltage difference between two "poles" on the scalp, and both electrodes in the comparison are potentially "electrodes of interest." Bipolar montages are occasionally referred to as differential montages because they display the difference between adjacent electrodes. Although the bipolar technique is a powerful recording technique and a favorite among many readers, bipolar montages also have their drawbacks, as discussed later. Figures 5.2 and 5.3 show a schematic of the difference between the way referential and bipolar montages are set up.

Note that, even the so-called *referential montage* is, in reality, "bipolar." Every channel must represent a comparison of two or more electrode positions—there are always two "poles" being compared. This is one of the criticisms of the term *bipolar montage*; it seems to imply that the counterpart term, *referential montage*, is not bipolar in some way. Indeed, there is no such thing as a truly "monopolar" montage, and technically

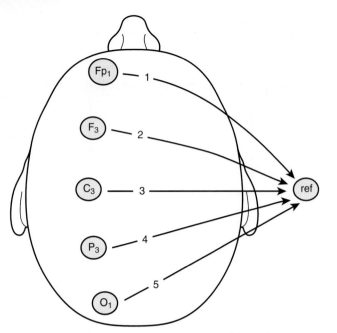

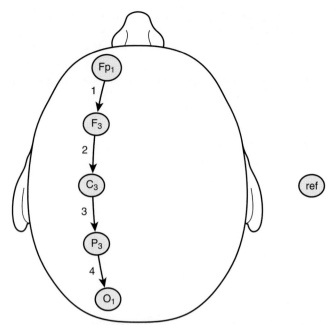

Figure 5.2 Referential montages are designed to compare each "electrode of interest" to a separate reference position that may be either close to or distant from the scalp electrodes depending on the montage design. For instance, the comparison "ref" electrode depicted on the right could actually be placed on the nose, the chin, the earlobe, or the back of the neck. Each arrow leads from the INPUT1 electrode, which is traditionally on the head, to the INPUT2 electrode and creates a channel derivation. This example shows a setup for part of a referential montage that would include the five electrodes in the left parasagittal chain: **Fp1-ref, F3-ref, C3-ref, P3-ref,** and **O1-ref.** Note that a referential montage designed to show readouts for five separate electrodes would generate five separate channels, labeled 1 through 5 in this illustration (compare to the situation in the next figure where the same five electrodes are displayed in a bipolar montage).

Figure 5.3 In this illustration, the same five parasagittal electrodes used in Figure 5.2 are connected to each other sequentially in a standard "bipolar chain." Again, each arrow points from an INPUT1 electrode to an INPUT2 electrode creating the following montage: **Fp1-F3, F3-F3, C3-P3,** and **P3-O1.** The reference position is not used. Each of the four channels generated with this technique represents the subtraction of an electrode from the previous electrode in the chain. Because the electrodes are paired to form each channel, the five electrodes generate four channels of output.

all montages are, at their root, "bipolar" because every channel displayed on the EEG page, be it part of a bipolar or referential montage, is a voltage comparison between at least two points.

Theoretical Strategies: How Can EEG Activity Best Be Recorded From a Single Point?

It is useful to consider the theoretical pros and cons of each recording technique by starting with a question that seems almost too simple to be worth asking. Imagine that your only interest is to accurately display the brain wave activity occurring under one specific electrode position on the scalp. For this example, let's consider the left frontopolar (Fp1) electrode which records at a point on the forehead above the left eye. Imagine that someone offers you a million dollar prize for finding a way to print out an EEG channel that shows *only* the brain electrical activity coming from the area under Fp1 and nothing else. This seems a straightforward and reasonable request, but what would be the best way to collect the prize money?

Recalling that our basic tool for creating an EEG channel is to print the amplified output of a voltmeter for which the needle sweeps one way or the other depending on the voltage difference between two points, there must always be two separate amplifier inputs, which we will call INPUT1 and INPUT2,

to make a comparison. A natural first step is to attach the "electrode of interest," Fp1, to the first pole of our voltmeter (INPUT1), but what would be the most advantageous choice of electrode(s) to attach to INPUT2, the comparison point? This comparison electrode is called the *reference electrode* and serves as the reference point against which the electrode of interest is compared (indeed, subtracted), remembering that all voltage measurements are differences rather than absolute values. As described in Chapter 4, "Electroencephalographic Localization" the voltage measured from whichever reference electrode we choose will be subtracted from the voltage measured at Fp1, and the resulting difference is the output for the channel that we will label as Fp1-ref.

It is clear that, at least mathematically, the choice of the reference electrode could have as big an impact on the appearance of the resulting output trace as the Fp1 electrode. At first glance, the channel label "Fp1-ref" may seem to imply that its output represents the voltage at Fp1 based on how we have named it. Note, however, that the "active electrode," Fp1, does not enjoy any privileged position by being attached to INPUT1 as opposed to INPUT2; the amplifier does not know that INPUT1 is the "important" electrode. The two voltages will simply be subtracted one from the other and displayed. Consider the possibility that Fp1 is relatively electrically quiet and the chosen reference electrode (let's say the left earlobe, A1) happened to be much more electrically active than Fp1. In this case, the output of an Fp1-earlobe channel would be dominated by the electrical activity in the earlobe—not the desired result. Put another way, if a spike discharge were seen in an Fp1-earlobe channel, it would not be immediately obvious whether any spike seen in this channel came from Fp1, from the earlobe, or perhaps from both. Clearly, the choice of the reference electrode in referential montages is important and requires thought, both at the time it is chosen and during the reading process.

Choice of a Reference Electrode

Considering different possible locations to place the reference electrode, because we might want a location with a "neutral" or "zero" voltage for comparison, one possible idea for placing the reference electrode to plug into INPUT2 would be an electrical ground. Possible ideas for grounds include the grounding prong from a three-prong wall outlet or a metallic cold water pipe that runs into the ground (in fact, many grounding points on electrical outlets are, indeed, eventually attached to long metal posts sunk into the earth or to one of the cold water pipes that serve the structure). In practice, what initially seemed like a good idea, attaching INPUT2 to an electrical ground for comparison to Fp1, is not feasible and yields poor results, mainly for two reasons.

First, electrical grounds, particularly those in large buildings such as hospitals, are not really electrically neutral. A variety of electrical devices throughout the building are attached to that same ground, and each connected device has the potential to spill electrical noise into the building's ground. Therefore, an Fp1-ground channel could include a terrific amount of noise from all of those distant devices, and the signal of interest, the microvolt-level brain electrical activity emanating from the region of the Fp1 electrode, could be easily overwhelmed by all of this electrical noise.

The second and perhaps less obvious problem is that the Fp1 electrode itself has a large array of electrical activity in it, but not all of that activity is brain wave activity. In addition to the very low-voltage activity that emanates from the left frontal pole of the brain (the activity from the Fp1 electrode that we hope to be paid for demonstrating), there is also a large amount of ambient electrical noise at that (and all) scalp locations. Some of this noise comes from the human body, including electrical activity given off by the frontalis muscle of the forehead, electrical activity from the heart (the electrocardiogram), electrical noise from movement of the eyes, and even electrical noise created during swallowing movements. Even more troublesome is the fact that, especially indoors, the environments we live in are full of electrical activity. You may be surprised to hear that, when indoors, large amounts of electrical noise from external sources flow through our bodies at all times, especially in electrically active environments such as hospital rooms or EEG laboratories where EEG recordings are usually performed. In these locations, we are virtually surrounded on all sides by electrical mains. As previously described, contamination of our bodies with 60 Hz signals from electrical outlets is especially common (this is a 50 Hz signal in many countries outside North America, depending on how electricity is supplied). Comparison of Fp1 to a completely indifferent electrode (such as an ideally quiet ground, if one were found) would do nothing to attenuate (or "subtract out") the large amount of electrical noise always

found in our bodies and in the vicinity of the Fp1 electrode in favor of the true brain wave signal in that area, which is an important goal. Therefore, paradoxically, *we do want some noise in the reference electrode*. Ideally, we would like the reference electrode to have the exact same noise signal that is present in the Fp1 electrode so that our differential amplifiers will subtract it out, leaving nothing but the brain wave activity under Fp1.

Considering these goals, choice of an ideal reference electrode becomes an interesting challenge. Instead of using an electrical ground as the reference electrode, consider the possibility of using an electrode placed on the foot. The choice of the foot electrode would be a vast improvement over using the ground because a recording electrode on the foot would detect a lot of the same electrical "body noise" as an electrode on the head (and also would lack the ground noise). Because the signals from Fp1 and the foot would be subtracted from one another in an Fp1-foot channel, electrical noise in the body common to both locations would cancel out and only the difference would appear in the resulting tracing. (Of course, we would have to ask the patient not to move the foot around!) The chance that the brain wave signal we seek under Fp1 would rise above the fray and be recognizable to us is now much higher.

Next, consider the idea of using an electrode position adjacent to Fp1 such as Fp2, the electrode over the right frontal pole, as the reference electrode. Subtracting Fp2 from Fp1 yields a signal that appears very much cleaner and will be of lower voltage compared with the Fp1-foot pairing. At first glance, this Fp1-Fp2 pairing would seem to be the most satisfactory solution yet because the amount of noise in the channel is minimized—any electrical noise in Fp1 is probably also present in Fp2 and that common noise should cancel out in an Fp1-Fp2 pairing. However, there is also a significant potential disadvantage that may not be obvious at first glance. If there is brain wave activity common to both the Fp1 and Fp2 electrodes, which is quite plausible, the subtraction of the Fp2 signal from Fp1 may actually cancel out some of that common brain wave activity, the activity we actually seek to record. The only signal displayed will be the difference between the two locations. If Fp2 includes some of the brain wave activity that we want to record at Fp1, which is easy to imagine, we will now only see a portion of the total brain wave activity at Fp1. The idea that there could be a lot of brain wave activity in common between Fp1 and Fp2 is plausible because there could be, for example, a frontal slow wave shared more or less equally by Fp1 and Fp2. The common mode rejection amplifiers used in our EEG instruments would cancel some or all of this common brain wave activity when the Fp2 activity is subtracted from Fp1. We would then have a tracing that appears to be "electrically clean" at the expense of losing some of the EEG activity we are looking for in Fp1. An additional problem with this solution is that if an interesting waveform such as a spike is recorded in the Fp1-Fp2 channel, it would not be immediately obvious whether the spike is present in Fp1 or Fp2 or both. Clearly the Fp1-Fp2 solution definitely will not win the million dollar prize.

Finally, consider the extreme example of moving the reference electrode so close to Fp1 that it is nearly in the same position as Fp1, just millimeters away. We can call this channel Fp1-Fp1'. This method should solve the noise subtraction problem well, and we also know that we are only recording activity from the Fp1 area (no worries that any spike seen comes from Fp2). In such an example, though, the signal in Fp1 and the Fp1' reference are so similar that when one position is subtracted from the other, the difference output will become nearly flat. A flat recording will not bring home the prize money. The succession of possible channel outputs for these different choices of reference is imagined in Figure 5.4.

Some generalizations then become apparent regarding the distance between the electrodes attached to INPUT1 and INPUT2 of a channel's amplifier. When two electrodes are moved closer to one another, there is greater commonality between what each detects in terms of both the noise signal *and* the brain wave signal. Therefore, as two electrodes become closer to one another, a channel comparing them will flatten. Conversely, as interelectrode distances increase, there is a bigger difference in both the noise signal and the brain wave signal and the channel's output voltage tends to increase.

Greater interelectrode distances are generally associated with higher voltage output signals.

Smaller interelectrode distances are generally associated with lower voltage output signals.

All things being equal then, channels with larger interelectrode distances are associated with higher voltages, and channels with smaller interelectrode distances are associated with lower voltages. This effect explains the recommendation that electrodes should not be skipped in bipolar montage chains (or stated another way, that interelectrode distances should be held constant). A channel pair with a large interelectrode distance will tend to produce a higher voltage channel, possibly giving the erroneous impression that there is more electrical activity in the vicinity of those electrodes than at other locations measured with standard interelectrode distances. Variation in interelectrode distances may occur in two ways: a montage design that skips an electrode position or a significant mismeasurement of electrode position during electrode application. Figure 5.5 shows the different impact of an electrode measurement error on bipolar and referential montages that is a reflection of this principle. So, what would the ideal reference electrode location be? Stated in brief:

The ideal reference electrode includes all of the noise, but none of the same brain activity as the electrode of interest.

It will come as no surprise that no such ideal reference electrode exists (and there is no way to collect the million dollar prize!). The goal is to find some compromise location for the reference electrode that will tend to cancel out noise fairly well but will not cancel out too much brain wave activity. The choice of a good reference electrode position represents a balance between wanting the electrode to be close to the "electrode of interest" so that it will share as much noise signal with it as possible, and wanting it to be distant enough from the "electrode of interest" so that there is not too much cancellation of the cerebral activity that is common to both electrodes. Finally, we don't want the reference electrode to be in an area that is itself intrinsically noisy. Commonly used

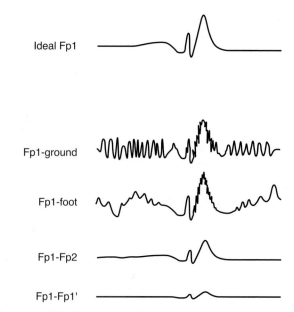

Figure 5.4 This figure summarizes the quest for the perfect reference electrode that we hope will allow us to display the "real" brain activity occurring under the Fp1 electrode. The top trace shows the idealized "truth" of what the brain is actually generating under the Fp1 electrode, a lone spike-wave discharge. The question is, what comparison electrode can we attach to INPUT2 of our amplifier to see this true brain electrical activity from under Fp1? In our first attempt, we attached the electrical building ground to INPUT2 to form an Fp1-ground channel in the hope that it will be electrically neutral and allow the true Fp1 activity to be displayed. To our dismay, we learn that the choice of ground has two major disadvantages: first, it is full of electrical noise from other electrical devices connected to it in our building, which displays prominently in the resulting output and, second, it also does not subtract out the specific electrical noise that contaminates the patient's head. The spike-wave discharge is all but lost in the sea of ground and patient noise. Using Fp1-foot, as shown in the third trace, is a significant improvement as much of the patient's electrical body noise is subtracted from Fp1, but because the noise pattern will still be moderately different between the head and the foot, there will still be a lot of residual body noise in this channel. For instance, EKG artifact would be expected to appear prominently in such a channel because EKG waves always express differently in the head compared to the foot. The fourth trace shows Fp1-Fp2, which generates a clean-appearing output, but the spike-wave complex will only be seen in this channel to the degree that it expresses *differently* in Fp1 compared to Fp2. A second disadvantage to this choice is that any brain electrical activity from Fp2 will appear as prominently as activity from Fp1. Because the two contacts are so close together, we see that the height of the spike-wave discharge is significantly diminished. Finally, moving the reference electrode just next to Fp1 to an Fp1' position to create an Fp1-Fp1' channel unfortunately cancels out nearly all electrical activity, both in terms of noise *and* activity from the brain.

reference points include the earlobes (A1 and A2) or mastoid areas (M1 and M2), the nose, the CS2 location, which is the skin overlying the most prominent spinous process of the cervical vertebrae (vertebra prominens or the C7 vertebra, which can be identified as the most prominent bony bump at the base of the neck), or more rarely the Cz electrode or another scalp electrode. More complex reference electrodes may be used as well, including techniques in which the arithmetic mean of some or all of the scalp electrodes is used as a

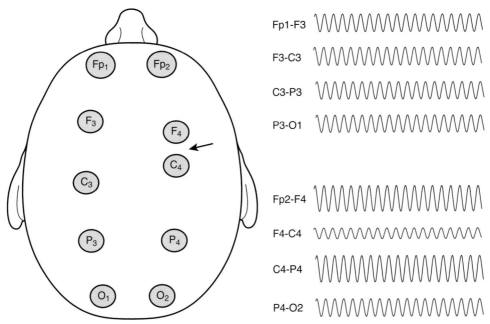

Figure 5.5 This figure illustrates the consequences of mismeasurement of electrode positions. The figure assumes that there is an idealized alpha rhythm of similar amplitude all over the brain surface. Note that the electrodes of the left parasagittal chain, starting with Fp1, are placed in the usual way with constant inter-electrode distances. The electrode positions of the right parasagittal chain, however, have been mismeasured so that the F4 and C4 electrodes have been placed too close together, resulting in an inadvertent increase in the interelectrode distance in the Fp2-F4 and C4-P4 electrode pairs, while the F4-C4 interelectrode distance is too small (arrow). The left parasagittal chain, whose output is represented by the top four channels on the right side of the page, correctly displays equal voltages in each channel. As a consequence of the mismeasurement in the right parasagittal chain, the channels for which interelectrode distances are too large, Fp2-F4 and C4-P4, show exaggerated, higher voltages, and the channel with the decreased interelectrode distance, F4-C4, shows a misleadingly decreased voltage. Note that if each of these chains had been displayed using a referential montage, the error in measurement in the right parasagittal chain would not be evident. Referential montages are less sensitive to this type of error in measuring interelectrode distances because, in such montages, the interelectrode distance in question is the distance between the electrode of interest and the reference rather than the distance between adjacent electrodes.

"virtual" reference electrode (the so-called *average reference*, discussed below in more detail). Each of these techniques is associated with its own advantages and disadvantages, which will also vary according to clinical circumstances.

Each potential reference location is prone to certain problems and advantages, and the goal is for the EEG reader to become an expert on what advantages and disadvantages are associated with the choice of each reference electrode in each particular recording situation and to be knowledgeable about how to take them into account during interpretation. No single reference electrode position will be ideal for all patients at all times. For instance, the earlobes often share a portion of the electrocerebral activity present in the adjacent midtemporal areas, causing both a cancellation effect and a contamination effect. This makes an earlobe reference a poor choice for a patient with a high-voltage midtemporal discharge because that discharge would then appear in every channel in which it is used as a reference. Also, the left earlobe in particular is often contaminated with EKG artifact because of the left-sided position of the heart. In other cases, if the patient's activity of interest is not very close to the earlobe, the earlobe electrode may be "quiet" and serve as an excellent reference point. In some patients, the nose reference may

be contaminated by a surprising amount of muscle artifact, whereas in other patients it can be electrically "clean." The cervical area can be contaminated by muscle artifact or EKG signal in some patients and may also be disturbed by movement when patients are lying on their backs, but in many the CS2 position is an excellent, quiet reference. The midline vertex electrode, Cz, is usually free of muscle artifact because of its location at the vertex of the scalp where there is no underlying muscle, however, Cz typically contains a large amount of electrocerebral activity, especially during sleep because vertex waves and spindles occur under it. In different individuals, any of these reference locations could generate satisfactory or unsatisfactory recordings at different times.

In the case of designing a referential montage, after the reference electrode has been chosen, there is little more to decide than the order to arrange the channels on the page. There are two general strategies for channel arrangement. One is to arrange the channels in left–right pairs so that each position on the brain can be compared with its homologous counterpart in the opposite hemisphere in the position immediately adjacent to it. This approach leads to a "left–right–left–right..." arrangement of channels (e.g., Fp1-ref followed by Fp2-ref, F7-ref followed by F8-ref, F3-ref followed by F4-ref, and so on). The alternative strategy for ordering the channels conforms to the "left-over-right" and "front-to-back" conventions mentioned above in which channels are "clumped" according to their location. Although each of the two systems offers specific advantages, neither is clearly superior to the other as each EEG electrode's channel will appear somewhere on the page with either system, only in a different order. The main difference between the two systems, one of which alternates left- and right-sided electrodes and the other of which groups left-sided electrodes in one area and right-sided electrodes in another, is the comparative ease of visual scanning for asymmetries.

Choice of one of these arrangements over the other is essentially a matter of preference. Figures 5.6 and 5.7 show examples of dramatic left-sided slowing displayed with each of these two common strategies. The latter system, which groups electrodes together by location, is seen to have certain advantages. Asymmetries that occur between hemispheres are not usually localized to a single electrode but to a regional group of electrodes. For instance, if a temporal slow wave is present, it may be recorded in multiple electrodes such as F7, T7, and P7.

When an abnormality such as a spike or a slow wave is present in multiple adjacent channels on a page, it tends to be easier to identify visually when the spatial clustering system is used. In the alternating left–right setup, the abnormality will only be seen in alternating channels. Another advantage of the clustering system is the ease of visualizing the topography of the discharge on the scalp. With this system, a region of the page corresponds to a region of the brain starting with the fact that the left hemisphere is represented on the top of the page and the right hemisphere is on the bottom. Grouping the channels by region, especially when gaps are used between electrode groups, as in the example illustrated in Figure 5.7, makes it simpler to know where a given channel is on the head at a glance, even without reading the channel labels. In contrast, when reading in a montage in which the left and right channels are alternated, it can be difficult to know the location of each electrode without consulting the channel labels. Proponents of the left–right alternating system like the fact that homologous channels are adjacent to one another, making individual interchannel comparisons easier. Considering these reasons together, the author prefers the clustering system (left over right and front to back),

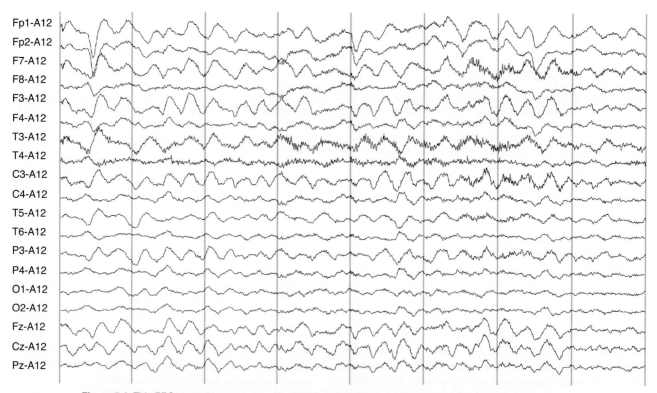

Figure 5.6 This EEG page shows an example of left hemispheric delta activity shown in a referential montage in which the channels are ordered on an alternating left–right basis. This commonly used arrangement has the advantage of allowing the reader to compare homologous areas of the brain in adjacent channels. For instance, the top two lines show channels comparing the left frontopolar area to the right frontopolar area, and so on. In this case, the reference used is an average of the A1 and A2 electrodes (placed on the left and right earlobes, respectively). Close observation reveals, at least on the top half of the page (and therefore over the anterior portion of the brain), that every other channel shows a more prominent delta wave, indicating increased slow wave activity over the left anterior hemisphere. Note that, because it is difficult to group channels according to head position with this montage setup, it is difficult to scan this montage without referring to the channel labels. When reading an alternating channel montage such as this, the eye searches for a pattern resembling "zebra stripes," which is the visual impression generated when a waveform is only present in every other channel.

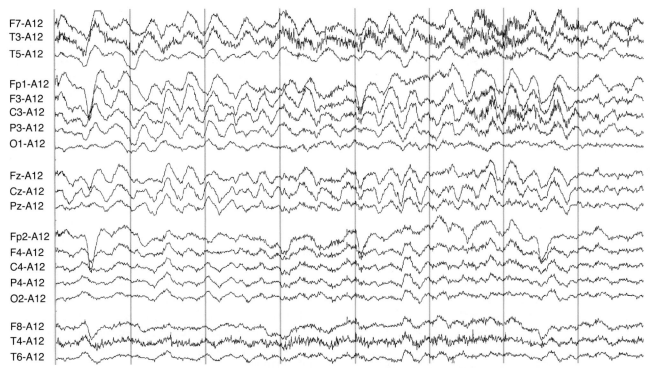

F7-A12
T3-A12
T5-A12

Fp1-A12
F3-A12
C3-A12
P3-A12
O1-A12

Fz-A12
Cz-A12
Pz-A12

Fp2-A12
F4-A12
C4-A12
P4-A12
O2-A12

F8-A12
T4-A12
T6-A12

Figure 5.7 This EEG page shows the exact same left-sided slowing as was seen in the previous figure; however, the channels are ordered in groupings of electrode chains so that the left hemisphere electrodes are shown on the top half of the page and the right hemisphere electrodes on the bottom. Starting at the top, channels are grouped on the page as the left temporal, left parasagittal, midline, right parasagittal, and right temporal chains (see channel labels). The same reference is used as in the previous figure, an average of the A1 and A2 electrodes. Note that, with nearby electrodes grouped together, it is visually much easier to appreciate the localization of the slowing over the left side of the brain (top half of the page). For this reason, this arrangement is favored by the author.

which should allow for easier and more accurate scanning and spatial visualization for most readers. However, the choice of either of these two arrangements is really a matter of laboratory or reader preference.

Bipolar Montages

In practice, most electroencephalographers do the bulk of their EEG interpretation using bipolar montages rather than referential montages, despite the potential disadvantages of the former. Bipolar montages are generally preferred because they produce "cleaner" tracings because of the proximity of the electrode pairs, which leads to more efficient noise cancellation. The clean appearance of the tracings and ease of reading does come at a potential price, however: the risk that the proximity of the electrode pairs has led to cancellation or an understated appearance of some of the brain wave activity, perhaps unbeknownst to the reader. When recording in a referential montage, if noise is present in the reference electrode, that noise may obliterate all the channels at once. Given the different strengths and weaknesses of each technique, it is best practice to interpret any given EEG study partly in a bipolar montage and partly in a referential montage.

Categories of Bipolar Montages

There are two principal categories of bipolar montages, the anteroposterior (AP) bipolar montage and the transverse bipolar montage. The two types differ in that, with AP bipolar

montages, electrode chains run from front to back (antero-posteriorly) down the head, and in transverse bipolar montages, the chains run from left to right (transversely) across the head. The fact that the reader has both of these montage families available for use raises the question of whether any particular discharge might only be visible in the AP bipolar but not in the transverse bipolar montage, or vice versa. Is it really necessary to use both AP and transverse bipolar montages for EEG interpretation, and, if so, what would be lost by not doing so?

It is true that the large majority of discharges seen in an AP bipolar montage will also be visible in a transverse bipolar montage; however, there are exceptions. Certain discharges may show a steep gradient in the AP direction and a shallow gradient in the transverse direction (or vice versa). Although such discharge topographies are relatively infrequent, examples of scalp events that are only evident in one type of bipolar montage but not the other do occur. As discussed in Chapter 4, "Electroencephalographic Localization" and illustrated in Figure 4.21, occasionally an electric field can be very steep and obvious when explored in one direction, but voltage changes may be more gradual when explored in the perpendicular direction, generating lower voltage and less obvious deflections.

Using a combination of these two montage types may also aid in localization. The AP bipolar montage will indicate the maximum of the discharge in the front-to-back direction, usually by the location of a phase reversal. Likewise,

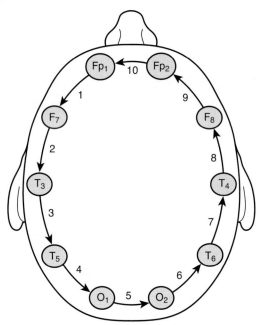

Figure 5.8 *This arrangement of a bipolar chain that encircles the head is called variously a circumferential, halo, or hatband montage in different laboratories. In the arrangement shown in this figure, the electrode chain starts with Fp1 and proceeds in a counterclockwise direction. In some versions of this montage, the circumferential chain can start and end with the occipital electrodes.*

the transverse montage will localize the maximum of the discharge in the left-to-right direction. Combining the two techniques allows localization of the maximum on a two-dimensional model of the scalp surface.

Circumferential Montages

Some laboratories also use a third ordering for bipolar electrode chains, one that makes a complete circumference around the head (Figure 5.8). This style of montage has been given a variety of names, such as a halo, circumferential, or hatband montage. Close examination of the electrode pairs used in the circumferential montages shows that almost every pairing is also present in the standard AP bipolar montage. The only electrode pairings that are unique to circumferential compared with AP bipolar montages are the Fp1-Fp2 and O1-O2 pairs. Because these two pairs are included in the transverse bipolar montages, circumferential montages are not a mandatory member of a laboratory montage set, although the decision to use such a montage is at the discretion of the electroencephalographer. For this reason, the use of a minimum of three montages—AP bipolar, transverse bipolar, and referential—is usually adequate to cover all necessary electrode pairings in routine EEG recording. Circumferential montages, when used, lend themselves to a particular technique for visual scanning. A visual axis is chosen and surrounding channel "layers" are compared (Figures 5.9 and 5.10).

Disadvantages of the Bipolar (Differential) Technique

We have already alluded to certain disadvantages of the bipolar montage strategy. These stem from the fact that we are looking at the display of the differences between electrodes pairs that are near (adjacent) to one another. Clearly, a significant amount of information can be lost using this technique. An analogy for how information is lost with the bipolar technique is illustrated by the following example of a weather report. Imagine that we are told about the weather during a 5-day period in the following fashion: "Between Monday and Tuesday, it got five degrees warmer, and on Wednesday it got another three degrees warmer. By Thursday the temperature dropped seven degrees from the previous day, and by Friday the temperature dropped another two degrees." Although there may be a lot of accurate information in these two sentences, the reader still cannot tell whether it is hot or cold outside. All of the information is given as subtractions, the difference between one day's temperature and the next. We don't know whether the temperature was below zero throughout this time period or whether these facts describe the temperature changes during a very hot week in July. All we know are the relative ups and downs of the temperature changes. Likewise, in a bipolar montage, when we note pen deflections telling us that voltages are getting more negative or more positive as we travel along a chain, we do not get absolute voltage information.

At first glance, if the bipolar montage recording system were as poor as the temperature reporting system given in this example in which we could not tell a hot day from a cold day, how is it that bipolar montages are useful at all? The answer is that, when we read an EEG page, we make an implicit assumption that the average baseline of everything that we see displayed is near neutral voltage (or "zero"). Indeed, because of the laws of electricity and charge, it is unlikely that all scalp areas will be either strongly negative or strongly positive for a prolonged period of time. Therefore, as we read, we are making a subconscious assumption that the average of everything that we see on the page is near zero. Nevertheless, we do lose absolute voltage information. We cannot know whether certain events may be slightly positive or slightly negative just by looking at the bipolar montage; we can only assert that an event is, for instance, "more negative" than the areas around it. For this reason, absolute measurements of voltage cannot be made as meaningfully as they can in a referential montage or, if they are made, they mean something different. When a reference electrode is used, we are making the implicit assumption for the purposes of measurement that the voltage at the reference electrode is neutral or near zero (although we might shy away from making this assumption at a time that there is clearly a lot of noise in the reference electrode). This assumption is shakier when made in a bipolar montage, a system in which we only see voltage differences between pairs of nearby points on the scalp rather than absolute voltage measurements.

This problem of not knowing the absolute magnitude of the voltage at any given point when reading in bipolar montages is related to a second problem that we have already discussed: the tendency for cancellation of like activity in adjacent electrodes with bipolar montages. Here, again, we can imagine a case in which there is a posterior wave more or less equally represented in the three posterior electrodes: C3, P3, and O1, as illustrated in Figure 5.11. In such an example, when recording with a

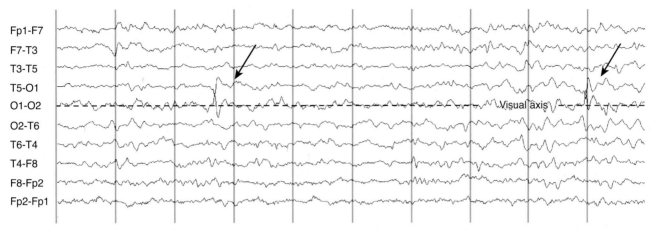

Figure 5.9 A circumferential bipolar chain is shown. Note the spike-wave discharges (arrows) phase-reversing in the O1 electrode. It is clear that the discharge represents an asymmetrical event because it is confined to one side of the visual axis, which is represented by a dashed line.

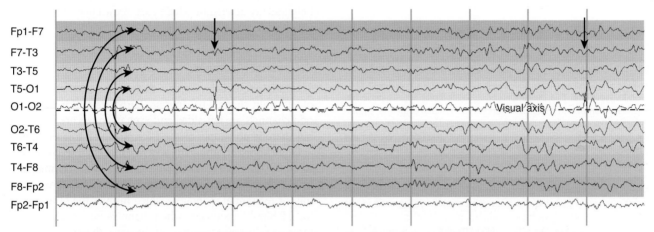

Figure 5.10 The same page of EEG material from the previous figure is shown with arrows and shading that suggest a method for visual scanning of a circumferential montage. Comparisons are made about the inner (unshaded) channel with the superimposed dashed line, which represents the "visual axis." Like-shaded areas represent homologous areas of the brain. For instance, higher voltage slowing in one dark red band compared with its counterpart on the opposite side would suggest an asymmetry of that slow activity between the hemispheres.

bipolar montage, this posterior slow wave could cancel itself out to a large extent in the areas where it is at highest voltage, simply because it happens to be *equally represented* between the pairs of electrodes being compared (e.g., C3-P3 and P3-O1). The example shown in Figure 5.11 uses the posterior rhythm, which is occasionally equally represented in those three electrodes, as an example of such inadvertent cancellation. This effect does not occur in referential montages.

This is one of the main disadvantages of bipolar recordings—that adjacent, in-phase activity tends to cancel out. This can cause a paradoxical effect: disappearance of a wave in an area where its voltage is highest and appearance of that wave only when a chain moves into an area where it begins to disappear. As shown in the figure, it is in the comparison of the area where the wave is present to the area where it disappears that the "difference" is best picked up by the bipolar recording technique, not necessarily the area in which the voltage is highest. Some of these effects are also illustrated in the exercises in Chapter 4, "Electroencephalographic Localization" on localization. Fortunately, in practice, this effect is not as

big a problem as it might seem to be, because like activity in adjacent electrodes is often out of phase (not perfectly lined up with the wave in the adjacent electrode) and therefore the subtraction does allow it to appear in the "correct" location in bipolar montages after subtraction. Still, it is important to confirm a mild voltage asymmetry noted in a bipolar montage by reexamining it in a referential montage to exclude this potential shortcoming of bipolar recordings.

Techniques for Visual Scanning of Montages
AP Bipolar Montages

Once you are familiar with the montage set used by your laboratory, it is useful to develop a visual scanning strategy for each montage in the set. This strategy will be a visual method or thought process for looking at each page of EEG that allows quick determination of interhemispheric or anterior versus posterior asymmetries. The first example we will look at is the standard AP bipolar montage used most frequently in the examples in this book. This AP bipolar montage conforms

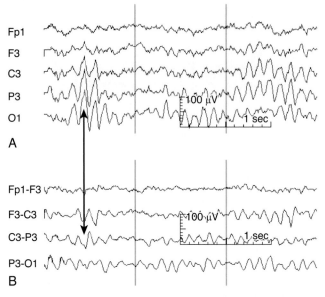

Figure 5.11 (A) EEG activity displayed in a referential montage (though the reference label was omitted from the channel marking for clarity) and (B) shows the exact same activity displayed in a bipolar montage. Panel A shows fairly prominent alpha activity, especially in the three posterior channels (C3, P3, and O1) during the first (arrow) and third seconds. Note that this posterior-predominant alpha activity is somewhat less dramatic in Panel B when the subtractions for the bipolar montage take place. The mathematical reason for this becomes evident when analyzing the alpha waves shown at the upper point of the double-headed arrow. Because the phase and shape of these waves are seen to be quite similar in the C3, P3, and O1 channels when viewed in the referential montage (Panel A) there is significant cancellation in the bipolar display shown (Panel B) when each is subtracted from the other. In fact, these waves can barely be recognized in the P3-O1 channel, even though they are strongly present in both P3 and O1. This is expected because the P3-O1 channel is a difference channel, only showing us what is different between P3 and O1. Because of effects such as these, it is preferable to confirm subtle voltage asymmetries seen in bipolar montages by checking a referential montage.

to the conventions suggested by the American Clinical Neurophysiology Society (ACNS) in that it uses the left-over-right and front-to-back conventions. Figure 5.12 uses shading to demonstrate the technique for detecting asymmetries. An axis should be imagined through the two midline channels, which have been left unshaded and represent the cranial midline. Next, the two inner (parasagittal) chains of four, which are lightly shaded in red, should be compared. Is there more slow activity or fast activity in one light red area compared with the matching light red area on the other side? If so, a parasagittal asymmetry is likely. Similarly, is there an asymmetry of activity between the more darkly shaded outer (temporal) chains? If so, a temporal asymmetry may be present.

Other laboratories may use the left parasagittal/right parasagittal/left temporal/right temporal ordering for the AP bipolar electrode chains. If so, the scanning strategy is adjusted accordingly. Figures 5.13 and 5.14 show a comparison of the two most common arrangements for the AP bipolar montage. Neither is technically superior to the other because both include the exact same set of channels, simply presented in a different order, and each will be commonly encountered in different laboratories.

Transverse Bipolar Montages

The transverse bipolar montage can be scanned in a fashion that is somewhat similar. Again, note the shading of each group shown in Figure 5.15. In this text, most illustrations of the transverse bipolar montage include a white space (a "gap") inserted between each chain, making it visually easier to scan, although the practice of inserting these gaps is not common to all laboratories. Gaps make it easier to see the groupings of individual electrode chains, but they sacrifice space on the page and therefore diminish the amount of line height that can be assigned to display each individual channel. The dashed lines in the figure suggest the axis around which each electrode chain should be visually scanned. If channels look different in the area above the axis compared with the area below it, this suggests a difference in that chain between the left and the right sides of the brain. The reader should practice visualizing the superimposition of this shading on the page to help quickly determine which part of the page corresponds to which part of the brain.

Referential Montages

Scanning referential montages that use the alternative method of left–right channel pairings are fairly straightforward in that odd channels are left-sided and even channels are right-sided, but there is no simple method for picking a line on the page and quickly ascertaining the area that that channel corresponds to on the brain surface without referring to the channel labels. This is one advantage of the second system of electrode ordering for referential montages, which mimics the ordering used for AP bipolar montages: when channels from each side of the brain are clustered together on the page, the brain location of any channel can be easily ascertained based on its position on the page (compare Figure 5.6 and 5.7 above).

Montages for Special Situations

The montage setups just described represent strategies useful for standard situations. When a patient has a surgical incision or some other impediment to electrode placement, the technologist must often decide how to rework a montage "on the fly" to make a useful display of the data despite the unavailability of certain electrodes. Standard montages must also be modified when additional electrodes are used. When doing so, keeping interelectrode distances consistent, if possible, can eliminate the effect in bipolar montages of a channel manifesting a higher voltage simply because of increased interelectrode distance. In some situations, though, variation of interelectrode distances may be unavoidable. The question of whether a voltage difference is the result of a variation in interelectrode distance can usually be resolved by analyzing referential montages, which are not sensitive to variations in interelectrode distance in the same way that bipolar montages are.

Regarding the use of additional electrodes, the most common "extra" locations added are the T1 and T2 electrode positions, which are designed to record from the anterior temporal lobe. The T1 and T2 names represent old nomenclature that is still in common use and correspond approximately to the FT9

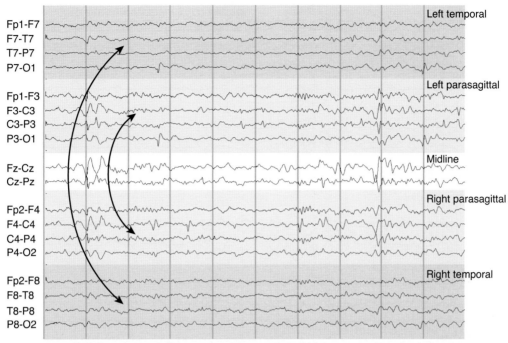

Figure 5.12 This schematic shows the visual scanning strategy used to compare homologous areas of the brain for the standard anteroposterior bipolar montage most commonly used in this text. The anteroposterior chain groupings progress from the left side of the brain to the right side of the brain as the eye scans down the page. The outer channel groups, shaded darker red, represent the temporal areas and the inner channel groups, shaded lighter, represent the parasagittal areas. The unshaded strip of two channels in the middle of the page corresponds to the midline of the head. Note that the sleep vertex waves in the second and eighth seconds manifest as bursts of sharp waves seen fairly symmetrically in both parasagittal areas and in the midline but do not involve the temporal chains, as expected for vertex waves of sleep. By contrast, nonsymmetrical scattered spikes are seen in other locations. Identify the low-voltage spikes at C3, O1, and C4.

and FT10 electrode positions of the modified 10-10 electrode system. They are sometimes referred to as subtemporal electrodes. A variety of methods can be used to incorporate these additional electrodes into a display montage. An example montage is shown in Figure 5.16. Use of these special temporal electrodes has largely supplanted the use of the more invasive sphenoidal and pharyngeal electrodes that were also intended to record from the temporal lobe.

The Choice of the Reference Electrode (Revisited): "More Important Than It Seems"

As described earlier, the choice of the reference electrode can have a large impact on the appearance of the resulting EEG tracing. Recall that, when looking at a channel labeled Fp1–reference (abbreviated as Fp1–ref in this text), there seems to be an implicit suggestion that the signal we are seeing represents activity from Fp1. In the best of all possible worlds, this would be true (because in the best of all possible worlds, the reference electrode is completely indifferent or neutral). It is worth keeping in mind, however, that Fp1 and the reference electrode have the same potential to contribute to the appearance of the final output channel; neither has any type of "mathematical" priority over the other. Each is connected to the amplifier in the same way, and the amplifier

subtracts one from the other without any type of favoritism for one over the other. The Fp1–ref channel only successfully represents Fp1 activity when the reference is quiet, and even better yet when it happens to include the same noise signal as Fp1 so that that noise signal cancels. Under what circumstances is the reference not quiet, and how might this affect our choice of reference for any particular patient in a given situation?

The importance of being aware of what reference electrode is in use at any given time when interpreting a referential montage cannot be overstated. There are several reasons for this, but two are particularly important. First, if there is noise in the reference electrode specific to that electrode, that noise will appear in every channel in which that reference electrode has been used. If that noise happens to resemble a spike, it is important not to mistakenly report it out as a "generalized spike" arising from the brain. However, the same would be true when an apparent single slow wave occurs across all channels of the EEG in a referential montage. When this occurs in a referential montage, it is most likely that the slow wave arose from the reference electrode rather than being a diffuse, identically-appearing slow wave occurring across all brain areas. Therefore, any deflection occurring across all channels identically in a referential montage likely is coming from the reference location, not from across the whole brain.

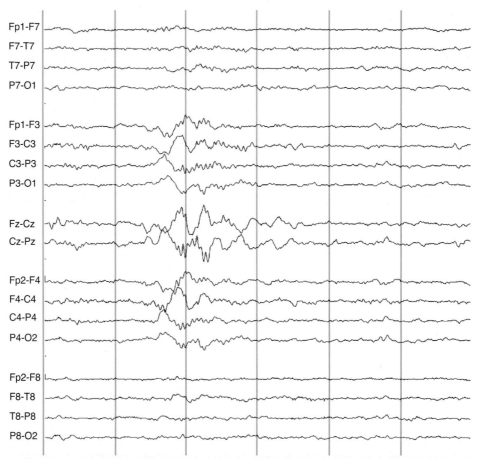

Figure 5.13 An example of vertex waves of sleep and sleep spindles is shown in the standard anteroposterior bipolar montage most commonly used in this text. The reader should appreciate that the topography of the page going from top to bottom corresponds to a left-to-right sweep across the head, as if from left ear to right ear. A main advantage of this system is that chains that are adjacent on the head are adjacent on the page.

Certain reference electrodes are more likely to generate certain types of artifact, and knowing which reference electrode is in use can aid in identifying certain waveforms as artifact. Usually, it is not difficult to identify a waveform as arising from the reference when an identical wave pattern of equal amplitude is seen in every channel that uses that reference (see Figure 5.17). When a similar wave is seen in all channels that use a particular reference, the reader will understand that either that wave is coming from every area of the brain with the exact same amplitude and at the same time (rarely a biologically plausible situation) or, more likely, that the wave is noise coming from the reference electrode. Artifacts common to specific references are listed shown in Table 5.1.

A second, more complex type of problem arises when the reference electrode itself is picking up brain wave activity. For instance, a commonly used reference electrode position, the earlobe, is well known to pick up a portion of the adjacent midtemporal lobe activity in many patients. This is to say that the A1 (left earlobe) electrode can pick up a large amount of T7 (left midtemporal) activity. How would this fact impact the display of a midtemporal discharge in a montage in which an earlobe reference is used? Two important effects occur: as you may have guessed, when the reference electrode is "active" or "contaminated" with a discharge, it will tend to at

least partially cancel that discharge in the temporal lobe channels when the subtractions take place (e.g., T7 minus A1); if this happens the resulting display will appear to understate the voltage of the discharge. In the most extreme example, if the discharge is picked up exactly to the same extent in the A1 earlobe reference as it is in T7, the discharge could conceivably be completely cancelled out in a T7-earlobe channel—the EEG display could show no discharge at all from the location at which it is maximum, T7! The second important effect is what neutral channels distant from the T7 discharge, such as Fp1-A1 or O2-A1, will look like when compared to an A1 reference that includes the discharge.

Figure 5.18 shows an example of just such a discharge, first as seen in a bipolar montage, which gives an excellent idea of this discharge's true location. The bipolar montage depicts a typical rolandic discharge in this example with highest voltage in T7 and with a field that includes C3. Note that the right hemisphere and midline are completely uninvolved. What would happen if we displayed this discharge in a referential montage using the left earlobe as the reference? In this example, the left earlobe (A1) is picking up a small portion of the T7 discharge. First, let's reconfirm that we know where this discharge "really is" with a clean referential montage. In this patient, the nose happens to be

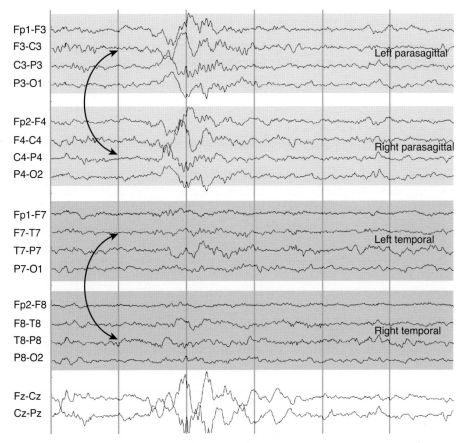

Figure 5.14 The same page of EEG as in the previous figure is shown in an anteroposterior bipolar montage using another common ordering of the chains. The shading and arrows imply visual comparisons of homologous areas. The top two sets of four channels correspond to the left and right parasagittal areas, and the bottom two sets of channels, shaded darker red, correspond to the left and right temporal chains. In this setup, the midline channels are at the bottom of the page. This system may facilitate comparison of like areas but requires the eye to jump around the page more to localize events because topographically adjacent areas are no longer adjacent on the page.

a very clean reference point at this moment (Figure 5.19). Note the distribution of the discharge and the true heights of the deflections for this spike. As expected, we see that the height of the discharge is maximum in T7, and a secondary maximum is seen in C3. The electrodes that flank T7 in the temporal chain, F7 and P7, also show the discharge to a lesser extent. Note that the discharge is completely absent from the right hemisphere and midline. Now let's look at this discharge displayed within an A1 reference (Figure 5.20). Several undesirable effects occur. First, the discharge is still well seen in T7, however the amplitude has been moderately diminished compared to when the nose reference was used. Because of the T7-A1 subtraction, the discharge's height should be diminished by the specific amount that A1 is picking up the discharge. The real problem comes when we look at the right hemisphere. The appearance of this EEG page suggests that this spike also involves the right hemisphere (though we know that that is not the case from having seen both the bipolar and the nose reference recordings in the previous two figures). The downward deflections seen across the right hemisphere represent the contamination in the

reference used (A1). For instance, we know that O2 is truly neutral and the spike does not at all involve that location, however, because O2 is being compared to the A1 reference, the spike is seen with its phase flipped upside down because A1 is attached to INPUT2 of the amplifier, and it is being subtracted from the uninvolved O2 electrode.

Figures 5.21 and 5.22 (Gradually Contaminated Spike) show schematic examples of this problem of the "contaminated reference," illustrating what might happen with increasing contamination or spillover into the reference electrode of an active discharge. The idea here is that not everyone's earlobe is exactly the same and the same T7 spike might flow into the adjacent earlobe to varying degrees in different individuals, varying from not at all to a lot. The figures show how this same T7 waveform would display only in the T7-A1 and O2-A1 channels depending on the amount of A1 contamination. These two channels are chosen for the figure because we know that the T7 electrode is a highly involved electrode and the O2 electrode is a completely uninvolved electrode.

An example of a third type of situation in which unrelated noise contaminates the reference electrode is shown in

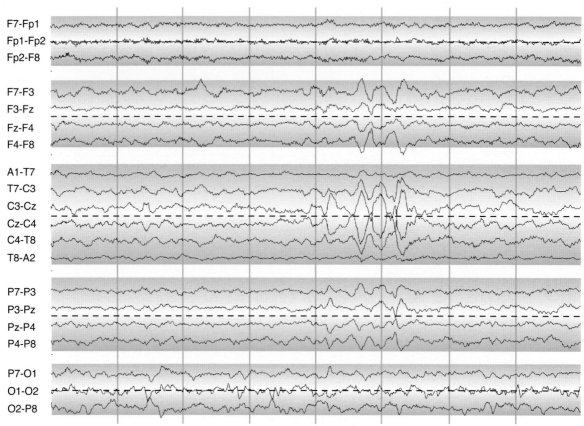

Figure 5.15 The figure shows an example of Stage II sleep displayed in a transverse bipolar montage. Each of the six chains is shown with gradient shading denoting the distance of each channel from the central visual axes, which are indicated by the dashed lines. In each grouping of channels, areas of like shading are compared with one another to establish symmetry. An event occurring above the visual axis but not below the axis in any grouping, be it a slow wave or a sharp discharge, suggests an asymmetry of that event between the hemispheres.

Figure 5.23 and is similar to what we saw in Figure 5.17. These examples emphasize this important idea: a waveform that has the same morphology in every channel in a referential montage likely arises from the reference rather than from the "electrode of interest." A simple example of this concept is shown in Figure 5.24.

The Average Reference: Strengths and Weaknesses

The "average reference" montage is a favorite among some electroencephalographers but disliked by others. The strategy behind this montage is the definition of a multi-electrode reference. Rather than using a single electrode as the comparison point, a "virtual" reference electrode is constructed that is composed of the average voltage of all the scalp electrodes at any given time. In practice, montages that use the average reference are neither "good" nor "bad"; in some circumstances they are very useful and render beautiful, informative recordings, whereas in others their disadvantages are so substantial that they can lead to serious reading errors and should not be used. You may be struck by the fact that the difference between "beautiful, informative recordings" and "serious

reading errors" is quite wide, which is why it is important for readers to understand and predict ahead of time which of these circumstances is likely to apply if a switch to the average reference montage is contemplated.

The concept of the average reference can be imagined in several ways. *Mathematically*, the average reference can be seen as a simple arithmetic average of the voltage of all the electrodes on the scalp chosen to be in the average. As you would expect, at any given moment the voltage value of the average reference can be calculated by summing the voltages measured by all of the electrodes used for the reference and dividing by the number of electrodes. Calculated in this way, this average voltage then serves as a comparison virtual electrode that is attached to INPUT2 of the amplifier just as a conventional electrode might be. Although the average reference can be defined to use all of the scalp electrodes, sometimes certain noisy electrodes may be excluded from the average, such as Fp1 and Fp2, which are often contaminated by high-voltage eyeblink artifact. Before the advent of the digital era, the average reference was not calculated numerically, but was created *electronically* in an analog fashion by connecting all of the electrodes chosen for the average together to one terminal using electrical connections to create the comparison

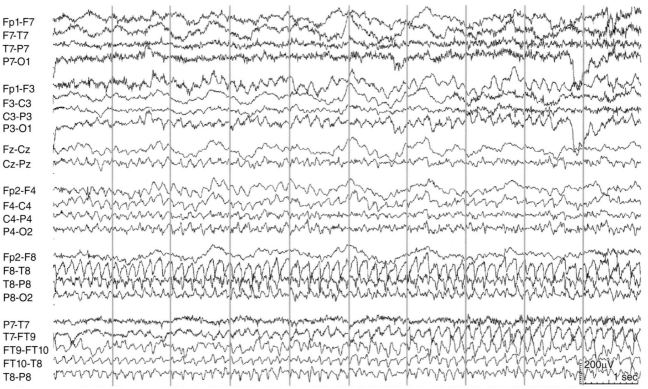

Fp1-F7
F7-T7
T7-P7
P7-O1

Fp1-F3
F3-C3
C3-P3
P3-O1

Fz-Cz
Cz-Pz

Fp2-F4
F4-C4
C4-P4
P4-O2

Fp2-F8
F8-T8
T8-P8
P8-O2

P7-T7
T7-FT9
FT9-FT10
FT10-T8
T8-P8

200 μV
1 sec

Figure 5.16 This EEG page shows an actual electrographic seizure discharge recorded with additional FT9 and FT10 electrodes (similar in position to the T1 and T2 electrodes used in many laboratories). The top 18 channels are identical to the standard anteroposterior bipolar montage used elsewhere in this text. The bottom five channels consist of a loop that includes the additional temporal electrodes. This seizure discharge is initially picked up well by electrodes at T8, P8, and FT10, as well as other nearby electrodes. The loop of five electrodes at the bottom of the page can be visually scanned imagining a visual axis through the middle FT9-FT10 channel. Note in this case that the seizure discharge begins below the axis defined by the FT9-FT10 channel (beginning of the page), implying that it has started on the right side of the brain. By the end of the page, the discharge is seen both above and below the axis, implying that it has become bilateral.

electrode. Alternatively, readers can estimate the average *visually* by looking at all the upsweeps and downsweeps of the pens on an EEG page at any certain moment, estimating what the average height would be at that instant (e.g., are there a lot more "up" waves than "down" waves?—if so, the average should be up) and, therefore, what the average reference being used for comparison should look like.

At first glance, using the average of all electrodes as the reference may seem to be a very clever strategy because there would seem to be a good chance that the voltage of all the electrodes averaged out at any one time may come out to something like zero. The hope is that, while some electrode voltages are going up, others are going down, and taken together the whole group of electrodes will average out to something near a neutral value, creating an ideal reference. Another potential strength of the average reference is seen when an identical noise signal is present in all electrodes, a situation that is not uncommon. In such cases, that signal will remain represented in the average reference and be available to cancel out that same noise signal in the "electrode of interest." For example, imagine that a 20 μV "spike" of electrical noise contaminates every scalp electrode; it will then average

to 20 μV in the average reference and, when it is subtracted from the electrode of interest in an average reference montage, the spike will be effectively removed. Sixty (or 50) Hz electrical artifact can cancel out in the same way in the average reference montage.

In practice, this situation where the average of all the electrodes adds up to a "near zero," or a neutral value, occurs often, but not all of the time. If the average of all electrodes always summed to zero, the average reference would, indeed, be an ideal reference, achieving a "holy grail" of electrical neutrality against which every other electrode's voltage could be measured. But how might it come to pass that the average of all EEG electrodes isn't zero all the time? After all, if a region of the brain becomes positively charged, wouldn't there have to be another region that becomes negatively charged to keep the whole system in charge balance, and the summation of all recording electrodes would necessarily average to zero? Indeed, it is true that the total net charge of the brain likely does not vary and always averages to zero, but the same cannot be said of all the scalp electrodes.

Thinking about it, it should not come as a surprise that the total average of the total charge measured by the scalp

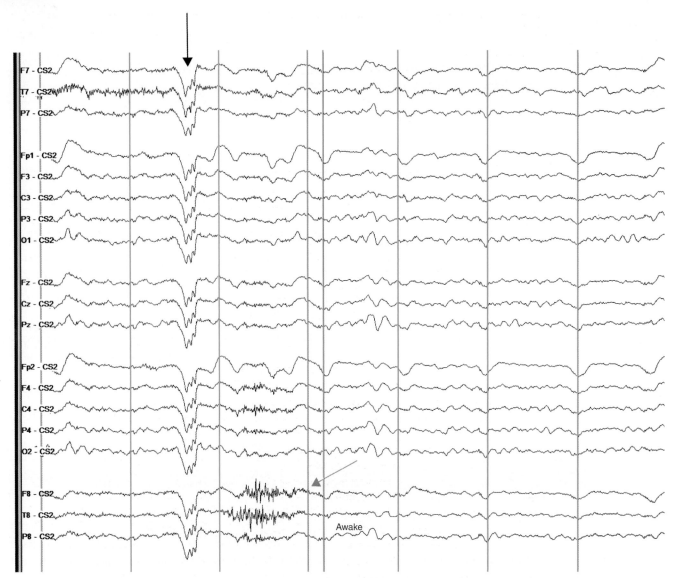

Figure 5.17 This referential tracing was created using a reference electrode placed over the back of the neck (CS2). The black arrow indicates a complex waveform that has an identical appearance in every channel. This pins down the source of the waveform to the reference electrode because it is the only contact used in every channel. It is extremely unlikely that the brain would create a waveform of the exact same shape and voltage over all areas at the same time. The gray arrow indicates some muscle artifact in the right central and temporal areas. Note that these waves are only present in a small subset of the channels and, therefore, cannot have arisen from the reference electrode.

TABLE 5.1 Advantages and Disadvantages of Different Reference Electrodes	
Reference Electrode in Use	**Type of Artifact/Contamination**
Earlobe reference	Often picks up midtemporal activity, left earlobe preferentially picks up EKG activity
Nose reference	Can partially pick up high-voltage frontal activity, such as high-voltage generalized spike-wave discharges, and can be noisy in some patients but quiet in others
Chin reference	Phasic and tonic muscle activity from mentalis muscle
CS2 (skin overlying C7 vertebra *or vertebra prominens*)	Motion artifact, EKG artifact, muscle artifact also can pick up high-voltage occipital activity, such as posterior spike-wave discharges.
Average reference	Any high-voltage activity in the EEG or any activity that is present in a large number of electrodes will contaminate the average reference.
Cz reference	This reference may have the least amount of muscle artifact in active patients (as there is no muscle at the scalp vertex), but in sleep this reference will be highly contaminated by vertex waves and sleep spindles.

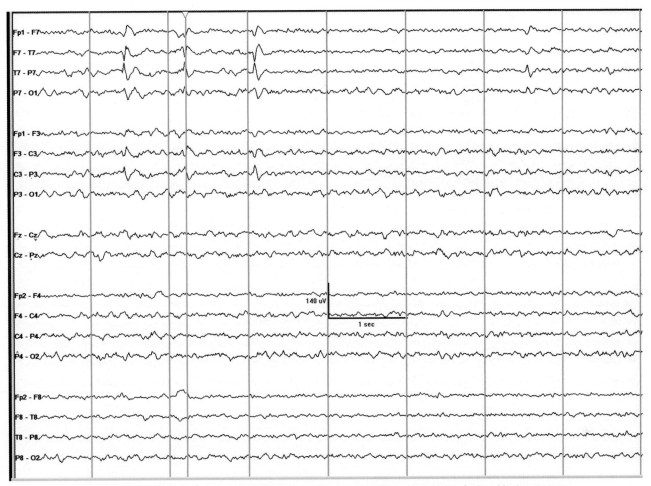

Figure 5.18 A pure left midtemporal (T7) discharge is seen with field spreading to C3 in a bipolar montage. Note that there is no involvement whatsoever of this discharge in the right hemisphere. The added vertical red line is placed on the second discharge for comparison to the following figures. Similar discharges can be seen in the seconds immediately before and after the discharge marked by the vertical line.

electrodes at any instant might be different from the total net charge of the brain. The main reason the two measurements are not consistently equivalent in practice is that our set of scalp electrodes only records the surface "shell" of the brain, and it is quite possible (and indeed occurs rather frequently) that the surface of the brain can achieve a net charge, positive or negative, and the counterbalancing charge is in deeper, unmeasured structures. As described at the end of Chapter 2, "Visual Analysis of the EEG: Wakefulness, Drowsiness, and Sleep," EEG electrodes sense charge in the extracellular space (and only near the very surface of the brain, at that). Because nerve cell membranes act as electrical insulators, the charge in the intracellular space is not measured by our scalp electrodes. Perhaps if we could have electrodes placed in all locations in the brain, inside and out, the average of all recording electrodes would average to zero, but this is far from the case with our setup of scalp-recording electrodes. For those reasons, it is not the case that the total of all our recording EEG electrodes sums to zero all the time. Figure 5.25 summarizes three theoretical counterexamples to the idea that the average of all scalp electrodes would be expected to be neutral all of

the time. The first example shows a diffuse, generalized negative spike. In this case, the scalp electrodes would experience a strong net-negative average because the counterbalancing positivity is deep to the scalp and unmeasured by surface electrodes. The second example shows an even simpler situation where there is a focal, but high-voltage negativity over one portion of the scalp, and the surrounding areas are neutral. If the magnitude of the negativity picked up by the subset of contacts is great enough, it will be noticeable as a negativity in the average. Finally, imagining the head as a globe, our scalp electrodes really only sample the "northern hemisphere" of the brain—the "southern hemisphere" (essentially the base of the brain) is not sampled.

When reading an EEG tracing in an average reference montage, it is a good strategy to visually estimate what the average reference signal should look like at any moment using some other type of montage (e.g., a bipolar montage). Considering all the channels together, the average reference can be visually estimated by mentally summing up the voltages of all the channels, noting the relative strength of upgoing waves compared to flat or downgoing waves and predicting what the average will

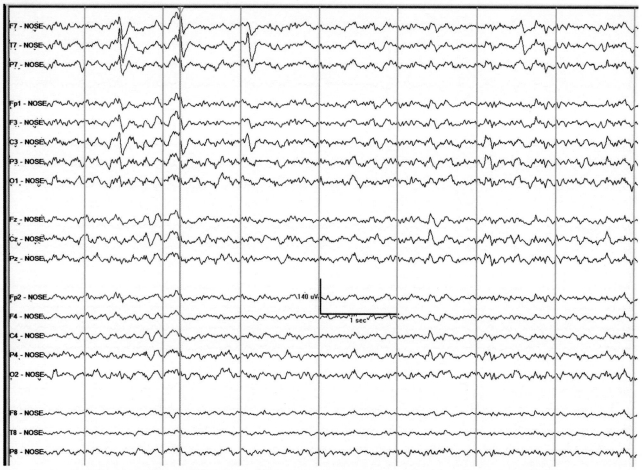

Figure 5.19 The same discharge is displayed in a referential montage using the nose as the location for the reference electrode. This montage yields an excellent representation of the field of this spike. The voltage is clearly highest in T7, but the field includes F7 and P7, and more medially, the C3 electrode is seen to be involved as well, as expected. Note again that there is no involvement of this spike in the right hemisphere.

look like. This process of "summing up" the voltages on a page of EEG can be done by either a visual or numerical estimation, perhaps in a bipolar montage as a first step.

It is clear that when most of the channels are of low voltage and there is not much activity, the average reference signal also will be of low voltage and relatively neutral. At such times, the average reference generally gives a clean and useful comparison. What happens, though, when there is higher voltage activity in the EEG? To model this problem, let's consider the simplified example of a 10-electrode set and, at one point, the reader notes that two of the channels measure -10 µV and the other 8 channels are flat (0 µV). This scenario is depicted in Figure 5.26 with an imaginary setup where there are 10 electrodes, numbered E1 to E10. The "true discharge" compared to an ideal neutral reference is shown on the left, and the same discharge as it would appear if switching to an average reference montage is shown on the right. The value of the average reference electrode at the time of the spike will be

$$\frac{-10+-10+0+0+0+0+0+0+0+0}{10}$$

or $-20/10 = -2$ µV. Therefore, the average reference would have the value of -2 µV when the -10 µV spike occurs at only two contacts. Once INPUT2 (the average reference) is subtracted from INPUT1 (each electrode of interest), of the 10 electrodes displayed in this example in an average reference montage, the 2 electrodes that are active with the -10 µV spike will be compared with the average -2 µV reference (-10 µV minus -2 µV $= -8$ µV) and display a -8 µV (upward) deflection, which is a fairly satisfactory approximation of the true -10 µV spike. The same subtraction also takes place, however, for each of the 8 inactive electrodes so that any inactive electrode's channel when compared with this average reference will show a small apparently positive (downward) deflection of 2 µV, even though these electrodes are, in reality, neutral (INPUT1 electrode $= 0$ and INPUT2 electrode $= -2$; INPUT1 more positive than INPUT2, so the pen goes down). This small amount of deflection may be tolerable, especially if it is expected by the alert reader who predicts that the average reference will be mildly negative at that moment based on seeing the negative spikes in two channels. A reader who does not take this effect into account could conceivably erroneously conclude that there is a low-voltage concurrent positive

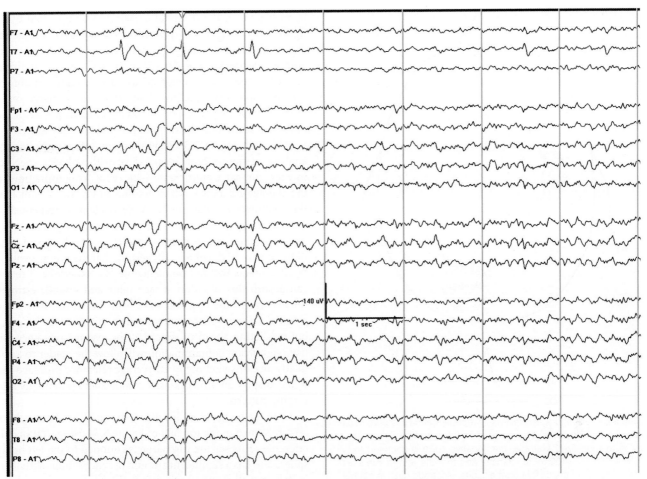

Figure 5.20 The same discharge as was shown in the previous two examples is now displayed in a referential montage using A1 (the left earlobe) as the reference electrode for all channels. Although it is still clear that the discharge's maximum is at T7, note that the discharge appears to manifest somewhat lower voltage. More problematic now are the large number of downward defections seen in all of the uninvolved channels, including the right hemisphere. In fact, the exact amount of contamination of the A1 electrode can be determined by looking at a completely uninvolved channel, such as O1-A1, and noting the height and shape of the deflection, which is reversed in phase (or "flipped") because A1 is attached to INPUT2 of the amplifier and subtracted from the relatively quiet signal in O1.

spike occurring broadly across the brain, which is not the case. Of course, the bigger the spike and the more channels it involves, the bigger these misleading downgoing deflections would be when using an average reference montage.

Although the presence of a 2 μV deflection in inactive channels does seem undesirable and misleading, there is a silver lining to the story. Assuming the reader knows that channels E4 through E10 are likely to be inactive (perhaps from previous review of the same spike in a bipolar montage), seeing these very similar deflections in these known inactive channels gives the reader an important tool in evaluating what the average reference signal might be. If the reader knows ahead of time that contacts E4 through E10 are highly likely to be inactive with this spike then these identical-appearing deflections in E4 through E10 actually demonstrate the specific amount of contamination of the average reference!

Figures 5.27 and 5.28 show an example of an effective use of the average reference. In this example, a spike in P8 is so focal and of low enough voltage that it does not contaminate

the average reference to any significant extent. In this example and for this discharge, the average reference montage displays an excellent representation of the field of the spike in Figure 5.28. Figure 5.29 shows an example of a seizure discharge with a broad field across the right hemisphere that is clearly restricted to the right side of the brain when displayed in a bipolar montage. Consider what this discharge might look like if displayed in an average reference montage. The alert reader will note that the discharge involves many electrodes and would thus be expected to be visible, at least to some extent, in the average reference. Figure 5.30 shows the same page displayed in an average reference montage. Because the average reference is subtly but definitely contaminated with the discharge, as expected, this montage gives the false impression that the seizure discharge is present on both sides of the brain.

Waves that are present in several electrodes, or of particularly high voltage, may also cause misleading phenomena. As an electrical scalp event rises in voltage or is present in an

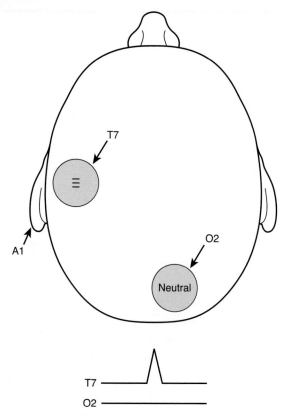

Figure 5.21 This figure shows a visual representation of a pure negative spike at T7 that will also be used in the following figure. Note that, in this idealized example, the negative spike is confined to T7. Imagine that it is -100 μV in intensity and that the rest of the scalp surface, including the distant right occipital electrode (O2), is neutral. The A1 (left earlobe) reference electrode is immediately nearby and may or may not pick up a portion of T7 spike's field, depending on the patient's particular "electrical anatomy." The consequences of what happens when increasing amounts of the T7 discharge are picked up by the A1 electrode and that electrode is used as the reference electrode are illustrated in the following figure.

increasing number of electrodes, it will have an increasingly large impact on the average reference. When discharges on the scalp make the average reference "active," it is important to remember that this activity will now be subtracted from every "electrode of interest" in the montage. When that subtraction is made from an inactive electrode, a "flipped" or upside-down version of the contamination will appear in inactive channels where a flat channel would otherwise be expected. Eyeblink artifact, which is typically of high voltage but confined to a minority of electrodes, provides a good example of this effect. You may wish to try to predict on your own what eyeblink artifact should look like in an average reference montage before examining Figures 5.31 and 5.32.

The more electrodes a discharge involves and the higher the voltage of that discharge, the more confounding the appearance of that event may be when displayed in an average reference montage. A schematic of an idealized posterior-maximum spike is shown along with its associated numerical voltages in Figure 5.33 to further illustrate the mathematics behind contamination of the average reference. The top half of the figure shows the "true" discharge, (a negative spike that

is maximum in the occipital areas). The bottom half of the figure shows what the display will look like if an average reference montage is used. What with all the deflections in the anterior electrodes, a reader who only sees the bottom display and who does not understand average reference montages may not appreciate the possibility that the discharge represents a simple negative spike involving only the posterior half of the brain and that the front of the brain is truly inactive.

Although Figure 5.33 shows a quantitative *mathematical* analysis of how a biposterior spike with voltages specified in each contact would create −30 μV of "contamination" in the average reference, while reading EEGs, we do not have the quantitative voltage of every electrode instantaneously at hand as it is provided in this figure. Instead, looking at the top panel, we can see that many contacts are involved and some of those with high voltage, suggesting that the average voltage of all contacts will not be negligible. An experienced reader can absorb this situation at face value and visually estimate the average of the upgoing waveforms based on their visual heights. Of course, the estimate does not have to be exact, but predicting ahead of time that the average reference will have significant contamination will allow the reader to know in advance of switching to an average reference montage that it may display an unnecessarily complex and potentially misleading pattern.

Note the image of an idealized, dramatic left-hemispheric seizure shown in the top half of Figure 5.34 using a clean chin reference. This seizure discharge is confined to the left hemisphere and has a significant amount of synchronous activity in fully half of all channels. Therefore, thinking ahead, it will not be a surprise that the average reference will be contaminated if we decide to display this seizure in an average reference montage. The degree to which the use of an average reference montage can confound the understanding of what is going on, however, may be surprising. The bottom half of the figure, displaying the seizure in an average reference montage, shows that we cannot even discern in which hemisphere the seizure has occurred. Although this is an idealized example, even in actual lab recordings the average reference can obfuscate the correct localization of a broad hemispheric seizure or other discharge. When many channels are involved with a waveform at significant voltage, we can expect that waveform to contaminate the average reference and potentially appear in all channels of the EEG.

The average reference can be contaminated by nearly any type of EEG activity, not just by abnormal discharges. In some patients, normal activity such as vertex waves of sleep and sleep spindles are of high enough voltage and have a broad enough field that they will affect all channels of an average reference montage, clearly an undesirable effect. Figures 5.35 and 5.36 show how even normal sleep activity can make a montage that uses the average reference confusing to interpret. Figure 5.37 shows the same page of EEG in an AP bipolar montage for comparison. The montage that uses the nose reference clearly shows the vertex waves and spindles in their proper locations, the midline and parasagittal areas; these waves are much less evident in the temporal chains, as

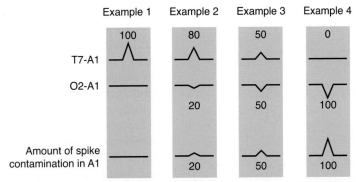

Figure 5.22 This figure shows how the -100 µV T7 spike discharge whose field was shown in Figure 5.21 will appear in a referential montage when an A1 electrode is used as the reference. For clarity's sake, rather than showing all 19 of the channels that would usually be shown for this montage, only the T7-A1 and O2-A1 channels are shown (top two lines). The four different examples are chosen to show how the T7-A1 and O2-A1 channels will appear depending on how much of the T7 spike is "sensed" or picked up by the A1 earlobe electrode. Note that through examples 1 to 4, we are imagining four separate patients whose "electrical anatomy" causes the A1 electrode to pick up an increasing amount of the T7-spike activity from patient to patient. **Example 1:** The example in this column depicts the simplest situation in a patient in whom the A1 electrode does not pick up any of the T7 spike. What with no contamination of the A1 electrode the two channels above (T7-A1 and O2-A1) give a completely accurate depiction of the fact that there is a negative spike in T7 and that there is no electrical event in O2. **Example 2:** In this example, the bottom row of the figure shows us that 20 µV of the T7 spike is picked up by the A1 electrode. Because this 20 µV is subtracted from what is seen in T7 by the channel amplifier (which only displays the difference signal), the T7-A1 channel's waveform height is decreased by 20 µV. Because the O2 electrode is neutral, however, when that A1 "contamination" is subtracted from O2 in the second row, this results in an apparent 20 µV downward (positive-appearing) deflection in this channel. **Example 3:** In this example, because of this particular patient's anatomy, the A1 electrode is picking up 50 uV of the T7-spike discharge. This results in the deflection in T7-A1 being decreased by 50% compared to Example 1, and a misleading apparent 50 µV "positive" deflection appearing in O2-A1, even though we know that, in truth, O2 is neutral based on Figure 5.21. In **Example 4**, the patient's electrical anatomy is such that the A1 electrode is picking up the spike in question just as well as the T7 electrode. This creates the completely misleading appearance of no discharge seen at all in the T7-A1 channel, and a big downward deflection suggesting a 100 µV positivity in O2, which we know is not really present. Clearly, if we know there is a discharge that significantly involves the midtemporal area, the adjacent earlobe electrode is not an ideal choice for the reference electrode.

expected. Because the spindles and vertex waves are widespread enough to contaminate the average reference, the average reference montage gives the mistaken impression that the field of the spindles and vertex waves extends strongly into the temporal areas, which it does not.

Clearly, a fair bit of thought needs to go into interpreting average reference montages. If a good, clean reference such as the nose, chin, the earlobes, or CS2 happens to be available, these will often produce excellent referential recordings without risking the confounding phenomena described above.

Clues to Contamination of the Reference Electrode in Referential Recordings

It is worth expanding our discussion of the upside down or "flipped discharge" that we just saw in the uninvolved channels of the left-sided seizure seen in Figure 5.34. A similar phenomenon will also occur in standard (nonaveraged) referential montages. This phenomenon occurs, in particular, when the reference electrode is so close to the vicinity of the discharge that it actually records a portion of that discharge. Indeed,

any type of activity picked up by the reference electrode, even noise, will be seen as a "flipped" version of that noise when the reference electrode is subtracted from an inactive electrode. From one point of view, these flipped discharges are misleading because, at first glance, they imply there is electrical activity occurring in locations where it isn't occurring. Ultimately, however, these flipped discharges can be informative. When asking what the extent and shape of contamination is in the reference electrode, seeking out a channel where we are confident that there is little or no electrical activity, we will expect to see a nice snapshot of the amount contamination of the reference, but in an upside down or "flipped" configuration.

A related version of the problem of the contaminated reference is seen in referential montages when the Cz electrode is chosen as the reference. In good electroencephalography laboratories, Cz is rarely chosen as the reference electrode for the referential montage for EEG scanning, particularly in sleep. Occasionally, however, Cz is the only available clean reference electrode in a very active patient because there is no scalp muscle to generate muscle artifact under this midline electrode. Although using a Cz reference can help avoid

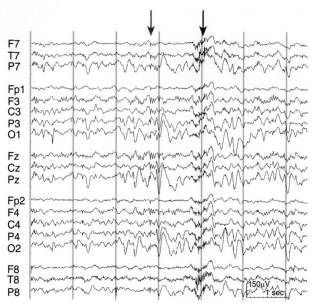

Figure 5.23 This EEG page is displayed in a referential montage with the nose used as the reference electrode. When there is electrical noise in the reference, it will appear in every channel in a more or less identical fashion. A burst of muscle artifact is seen in all channels (dark arrow), likely of nose origin because it is of similar morphology in all channels. The slightly higher voltage of this muscle artifact noted in the T7 and T8 channels probably represents a mixture of the contaminating muscle activity from the nose and additional muscle activity from the T7 and T8 electrodes (midtemporal contacts overlying the temporalis muscle). Looking at the Cz channel, because we know that there is no muscle at all in the scalp underlying the Cz electrode, this is additional strong evidence that most of this burst of activity does not arise from Cz, but instead from the reference. The light gray arrow indicates a single, low-voltage transient, the origin of which is also likely the nose. Note that this transient manifests the same shape and has similar polarity and voltage in all channels. Apart from the two brief examples of contamination of the reference described here, the majority of the page shows a beautiful EEG recording using a nose reference.

contamination with muscle artifact, what happens when the patient falls asleep? Sleep vertex wave activity is maximally represented in the Cz electrode and spindle activity is also plentiful there. For this reason, the sleeping patient in whom a Cz reference is used will manifest vertex waves and spindles in every channel (Figure 5.38). Such a tracing can be difficult to interpret and is essentially unsatisfactory for most purposes.

The Laplacian Reference

The Laplacian reference is based on mathematical expressions that attempt to model the spherical surface of the scalp. This type of reference is occasionally used in routine EEG recordings but has a number of disadvantages. The Laplacian reference is a type of average reference in which the weight of each electrode in the average is indirectly proportional to its distance from the electrode of interest. Electrodes that are closer to the electrode of interest (INPUT1 electrode) are

given more weight in the average, and more distant electrodes are given proportionally less weight. Because the more distant electrodes may only have a small impact on this type of weighted average, and also because the mathematical expression for the full Laplacian reference is relatively cumbersome to program into the EEG software (and differs for each electrode on the scalp), some labs use a simplified version of the Laplacian reference. In this abbreviated version, only the immediately surrounding electrodes (a maximum of four) are used in the average; the more distant electrodes only make small contributions to the Laplacian because of their reduced weighting, and for that reason and to save time, their values are discarded. Even this simplified technique has its weaknesses, such as the problem of how to handle electrodes that are on the edge of the electrode array such as O1 or Fp2 (typically only three electrodes are averaged in such instances). Likewise, noise in just one of the surrounding electrodes can have a fairly significant impact on this type of reference.

Although use of the Laplacian reference can produce some satisfactory recordings, there is a fundamental disadvantage to this technique. As stated earlier, a basic tenet of careful interpretation of the EEG is having a keen awareness of what is attached to INPUT1 and what is attached to INPUT2 of any EEG channel. Specifically, to really understand what is going on in a channel, we would like to have a precise awareness of the reference that is in use. The problem with the Laplacian reference is that the question of "what is the reference?" is a constantly moving target because for every scalp electrode, the reference attached to INPUT2 is different. The fact that each electrode has a different reference may either slow down a careful analytic process of EEG interpretation or give the reader the incentive not to consider what the true reference is for every given channel, possibly leading to sloppy interpretation of complex electrical events. What at first seemed attractive as a clever mathematical approach to creating a reference now becomes a barrier to precise interpretation. For these reasons, some feel that the Laplacian reference contributes little in the way of advantages over the average reference but presents a specific disadvantage to a careful reader who appropriately needs to know the composition of the reference for all channels at all times.

Using Colors in Montages

Digital computer systems offer laboratories the option of displaying different channels in different colors. For instance, some laboratories may choose to display all channels related to the left hemisphere in brown and all channels related to the right hemisphere in green. Although this may seem like a good idea at first, this information is already readily available based on channel position on the page. Because the eye is being trained to look for differences, the use of different colors may actually become a minor impediment given that the different colors create the appearance of a difference at the outset. To some, a darker color may look bolder during visual scanning, and therefore "bigger" than a lighter-colored channel, introducing an immediate bias toward one hemisphere. The author prefers montage setups in which a channel's page position rather than

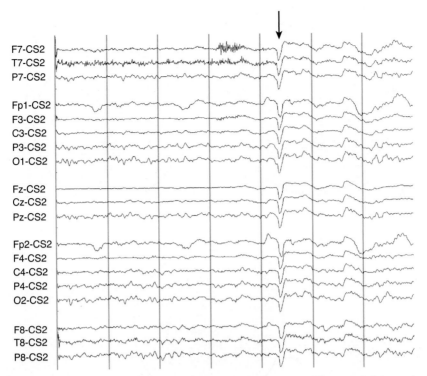

Figure 5.24 An identical downward deflection is noted in all channels in the fifth second of the tracing (arrow). When a waveform of identical shape and amplitude is seen in a montage in which all channels are compared to a single reference, the simplest explanation is that the deflection arises from the reference.

its color is the primary indicator of brain position, which is to say that all brain channels are displayed in the same color (usually black). Differing channel colors are most useful in the case of montages that alternate right- and left-sided channels (e.g., Fp1-ref, Fp2-ref, F3-ref, F4-ref...) because page location is more difficult to quickly associate with electrode position with those montages. In general, when colors are used in montages, like colors are preferred for like brain regions.

The Appearance of Standard EEG Features in Different Montages

Each standard EEG feature has a characteristic appearance in the different EEG montages. The following figures review the appearance of eyeblink artifact, lateral eye movement artifact, the posterior rhythm, vertex waves of sleep, sleep spindles, and focal spikes in a variety of montages.

Figure 5.39 shows the typical appearance of eyeblink artifact in the AP bipolar montage. Because eyeblink artifact is caused by a large transient positivity in Fp1 and Fp2 and nearby electrodes, the abrupt, downward-sloping waveforms seen in the four most anterior channels are characteristic of eyeblink artifact. The opposing phases seen in the anterior channels after the second eyeblink artifact are typical for lateral eye movements (see the figure caption for further

explanation). Now looking toward the posterior head regions, in this figure, the posterior rhythm is seen in the posterior channels and even reaches as far forward as the F3-C3 and F4-C4 channels. Does this imply that the posterior rhythm is actually present in F3 and F4? The answer is no—the posterior rhythm is seen in F3-C3 because it drops off and disappears *between* F3 and C3 in this patient. Because the two channels differ in that C3 picks up the posterior rhythm and F3 does not, the subtraction of the two channels still displays the posterior rhythm's waveform.

Practice Identifying Different EEG Elements in Different Montages

This same EEG page is shown in a variety of montages in Figures 5.40 through 5.46. It is worthwhile to take the time to practice identifying each of the main elements of the awake EEG in each of these montages. Figures 5.47 through 5.53 show the appearance of vertex waves, sleep spindles, and focal spikes from the same page of EEG recorded during sleep displayed in the various montages (see figure captions for additional description). The top half of the figures show the EEG without markings to allow the reader to practice identifying key features. The bottom panels show the same page with an "answer key" superimposed.

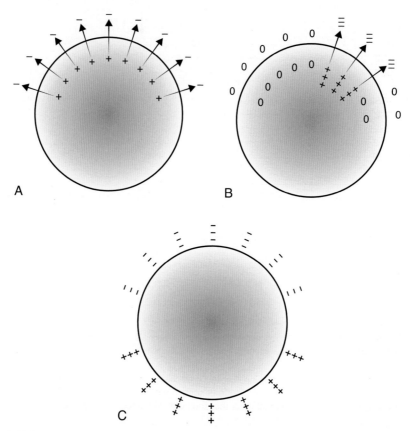

Figure 5.25 Unfortunately, there is no reason to assume that the average charge of all electrodes as measured on the scalp at any one time necessarily balances out to zero. Panel A shows the simplest and most dramatic counterexample to this idea. In the figure the head is modeled as a sphere and the surface is completely negative at this instant while the deeper areas are positive. The arrows represent electrical dipoles expressing on the scalp as negativities. The total of all charges for this sphere does average to neutral or "zero" (i.e., the number of pluses and minuses in the diagram are equal), but the average of the recording electrodes, which are all at the scalp surface, will be strongly negative. This occurs because the positivities go unmeasured by our recording electrodes because they are in a location deeper than they are able to measure. In Panel B, a bundle of radially oriented neurons (represented by three dipole arrows) shows a strong negative charge on the scalp balanced by a positivity of equal size deeper in the brain. The surrounding areas are neutral. In fact, physiological epileptic spikes often manifest this kind of electrical geometry: negative on the surface and positive deep. At the moment of this spike, the average reference electrode would clearly carry a negative value. Panel C shows a third counterexample. In this situation, the upper half of the brain ("northern hemisphere") may have a net negativity and the base of the brain ("southern hemisphere") could have a net positivity. Because we only sample the superior convexity of the brain with our scalp electrodes, the recording electrodes could experience an average negative charge even though the brain surface in its entirety could be neutral.

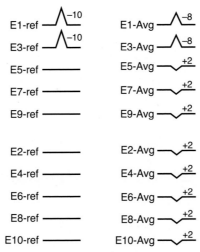

Figure 5.26 This is an idealized schematic of a 10-electrode set in which there is a high-voltage negative discharge in two of the contacts: E1 and E3. This scenario is illustrated on the left side of the figure, imagining that each of the electrodes E1 to E10 is being compared to an ideally neutral reference. Imagine that the odd-numbered electrodes are over the left hemisphere and the even-numbered electrodes are over the right hemisphere. The average voltage of all electrodes, which is to be used as the average reference, is -20 (the sum of the voltages of the ten electrodes) divided by 10 (the number of electrodes) = -2. Because the average reference is connected to INPUT2 of the amplifier, -2 is subtracted from every electrode of interest's value which, mathematically, has the same impact as adding 2 (remember that greater positivity in INPUT1 compared to INPUT2 yields a more downgoing deflection). When these 10 electrodes are set up in an average reference montage as shown on the right side of the figure, every electrode's voltage attached to INPUT1 will effectively have 2 units subtracted from it (for instance, for the E10–AVG channel, the average of -2 is subtracted from zero, resulting in a downward deflection of 2 units). Another useful way to look at the result of this montage is that every wave seen on the left side of the figure has been bumped downward by 2 units when displayed in the average reference shown on the right side. This appearance could lead to the potentially erroneous conclusion that there is a negative spike occurring focally on the left side of the head but that there is a simultaneous positive spike occurring everywhere else. The alert reader who understands how the average reference works may be able to tease out the fact that the identical downgoing 2-unit deflections over much of the brain simply indicate that the average reference is "contaminated" to that degree, and that these downward deflections do not necessarily signify that an electrical event is occurring in those areas.

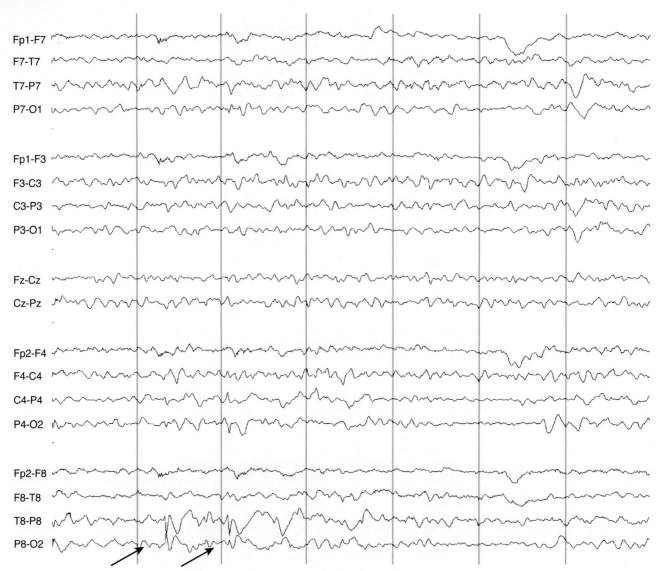

Figure 5.27 Two spike-wave discharges are seen phase-reversing in the bottom two channels (arrows). The technique of identifying the location of the phase reversal efficiently identifies the point of maximum of this discharge as P8, the electrode shared by the bottom two channels (T8-P8 and P8-O2). Because the waves' phases point toward each other, the spikes' phase reversal indicates a negative spike. A comparison to the appearance of the same discharge displayed in a referential montage is shown in the next figure.

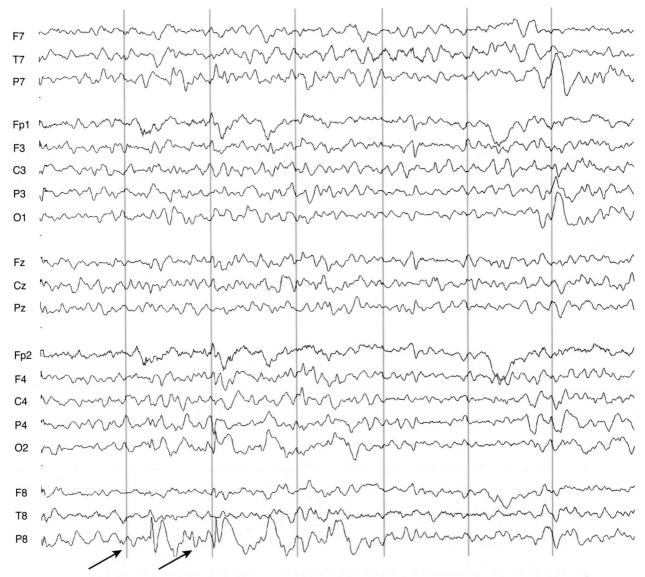

Figure 5.28 The same P8 discharges (arrows) from the previous figure are shown, this time in a referential montage in which the average reference is used. Because this is a referential montage, the localization technique of finding the maximum wave height is used and, therefore, the discharge's maximum is identified in P8, the bottom channel, because it is the tallest spike. Because the spikes are upgoing we can conclude that the spike is negative with respect to the reference. Because the discharge is so focal and not of particularly high voltage, it does not significantly affect the average of all the electrodes and the average reference is "clean." In this case, the average reference is a satisfactory choice of reference to display this discharge.

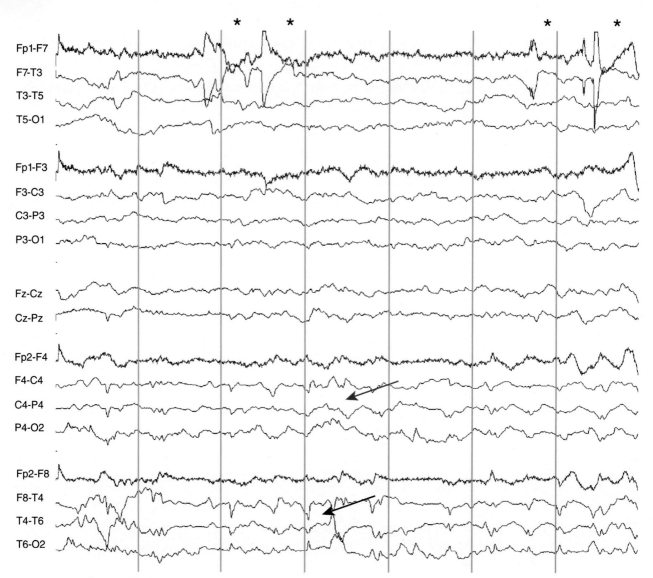

Figure 5.29 This figure shows a low-voltage, repetitive seizure discharge with maximum in the right mid- to posterior temporal area (black arrow). The field of the discharge spreads to include the right parasagittal area (gray arrow). Note that the discharge is not present in the left hemisphere (the top eight channels). Some high-voltage artifact can be seen arising from the F7 electrode (asterisks) related to a poor contact, seen in the top two channels and unrelated to the seizure discharge.

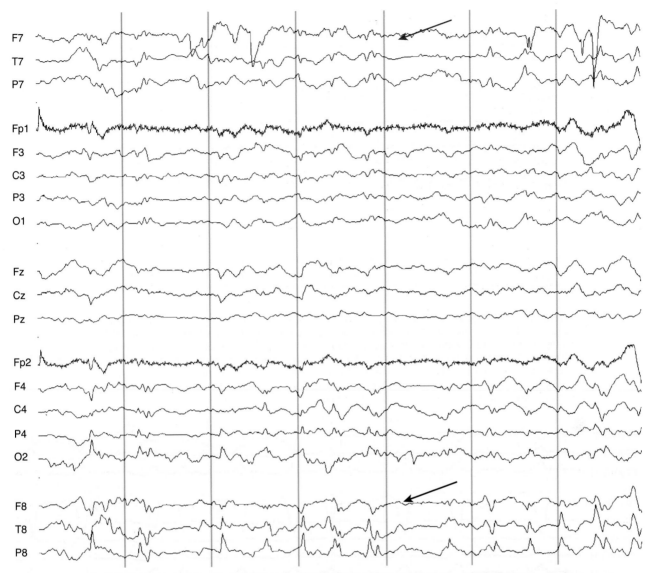

Figure 5.30 The same right posterior quadrant seizure discharge as shown in the previous figure is now displayed in a referential montage using the average reference. Because the discharge involves several channels, when all scalp electrodes are averaged, the discharge is actually noticeable in the average reference itself. Note that, even though the discharge is well seen in the channels in which we know it to be maximal, T8 and P8 (black arrow), and also to a lesser extent in the right parasagittal chain, the discharge now falsely localizes to areas in the opposite hemisphere, even in the left temporal chain where we know it not to be present (gray arrow) in addition to F3, C3, P3, Fz, and Cz. This occurs because the contaminated average reference is being subtracted from the electrodes in the inactive left hemisphere. A clue to the presence of this phenomenon is the "flipped" phase of the apparent seizure discharge in the left hemisphere. A reader who does not realize that the average reference is in use and contaminated by the discharge could erroneously report that this seizure discharge involves both hemispheres of the brain.

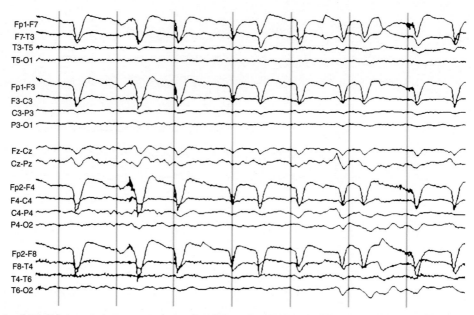

Figure 5.31 This image shows an awake tracing with copious eyeblink artifact. Importantly, and as expected, eyeblink artifact is confined to the anterior head regions. The eyeblink artifacts actually arise from big frontal positivities related to upward eye movement because the front of the eye carries a positive charge (see Chapter 6, "Electroencephalographic Artifacts" for a further discussion of the physiology of eyeblink artifact). These positivities are only recorded in the most anterior electrodes; the posterior electrodes are neutral during eyeblinks, which makes sense as they are distant from the eyes. Note that no deflections from the eyeblinks are seen in the posterior regions of the head.

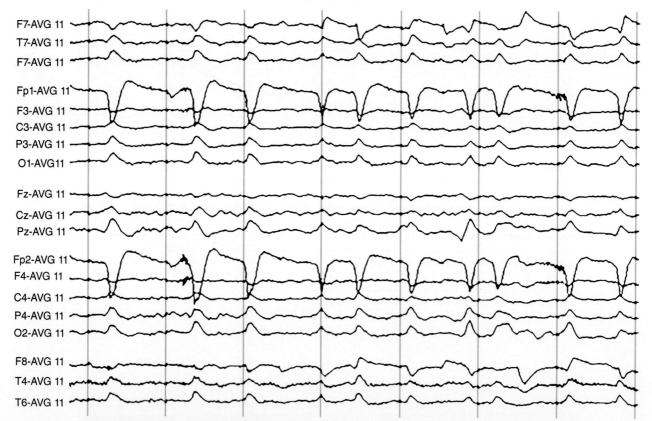

Figure 5.32 This is the exact same segment as seen in the previous figure, however displayed with an average reference montage. Because the eyeblink deflections are so large, it can be predicted that they will have a significant impact on the average reference. Once all of the electrodes have been averaged, a diminished version of the eyeblinks is still present in the average reference. When those deflections are subtracted from all channels, two things are noted. First, the amplitude of the representation of the eyeblink artifact seen frontally is reduced. More problematic is the fact that the eyeblink artifact is now present as "flipped" (upgoing) waves seen in the posterior, uninvolved electrodes.

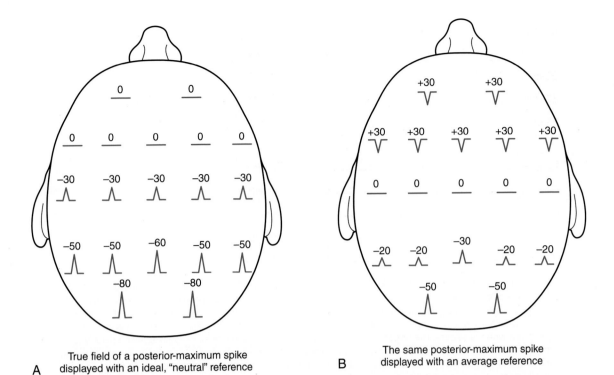

A   True field of a posterior-maximum spike
     displayed with an ideal, "neutral" reference

B   The same posterior-maximum spike
     displayed with an average reference

Figure 5.33 The top panel (A) illustrates the true field of a spike discharge that is maximal in the occipital areas with a field spreading forward to involve the posterior half of the head. The discharge does not, however, involve the anterior two rows of electrodes, which are shown in the diagram to measure zero voltage. The voltage measured at each electrode is given in microvolts. The bottom panel (B) shows what the exact same spike will look like displayed using an average reference montage. The resulting display can be predicted first by calculating the mean of the 19 recorded scalp electrodes, which comes to −30 μV (add all of the voltages in Panel A together and divide by 19), giving the voltage of the average reference. Because the average reference is attached to INPUT2 of the CMR amplifier, its value will be subtracted from that of each INPUT1 electrode. Arithmetically, the subtraction of −30 μV from each measurement is the equivalent of adding 30 μV (x − −30 μV is the same as x + 30 μV). Because of the convention of "pen-down = first electrode more positive," this subtraction results in each waveform being "lowered" by a height of 30 μV in every channel. Therefore, use of the average reference gives the unwanted effect of a broad apparent positivity in the neutral anterior electrodes (0 μV − −30 μV = +30 μV). It attenuates the apparent amplitude of the middle row of electrodes so that they appear neutral as shown, and also attenuates somewhat the values of the more strongly negative electrodes in the posterior two rows. The alert reader who analyzes this spike in an average reference montage must notice the unexpected "flipping" of the phase of the waveform between the front and the back of the head and consider the possibility that this atypical appearance may be related to a contaminated average reference rather than a discharge that is positive anteriorly, negative posteriorly, but neutral in between.

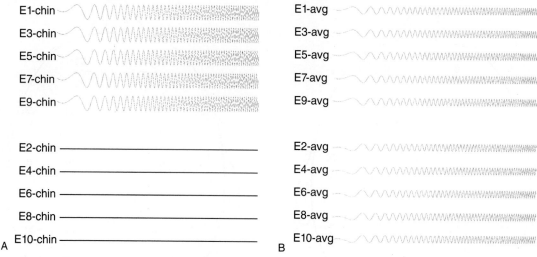

Fig 5.34 The top panel (A) shows an idealized seizure discharge in a simple montage, with electrodes labeled E1 to E10—odd-numbered electrodes over the left hemisphere and even-numbered electrodes over the right, as we are accustomed to. Each channel is compared to a clean chin reference. We can see that all of the left-sided channels show a synchronous decelerating seizure discharge while the right hemisphere is completely uninvolved with the seizure. The bottom panel (B) shows the same discharge as it would appear if displayed in an average reference montage. The most notable aspect of this average reference recording is that a reader who only saw the bottom panel (B) would have little idea which side this seizure even came from! Exactly what happened here is not difficult to piece together. Considering that half the channels have the identical seizure discharge and the other half are flat, the virtual average reference electrode signal will consist of the seizure discharge as seen in each channel of the left hemisphere of Panel A, but at half its height. This half-height waveform will now be subtracted from all channels, E1 to E10. When subtracting the half-height reference signal from the full-height discharge seen in the top panel, the waveform will now display at half its original height over the left hemisphere (e.g., any 100-μV wave will now be a 50-μV wave). When the half-height average reference signal is subtracted from the previously flat right-sided channels, we now see that half-height waveform flipped upside down because it was subtracted from zero-voltage flat channels.

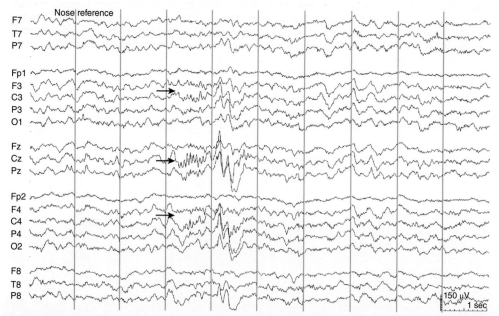

Figure 5.35 A page of EEG is displayed in a referential montage using the nose as the reference electrode. Stage II sleep is seen with vertex waves and spindles. Because the comparison electrode, the nose, represents a distant and indifferent reference point, this page gives an excellent representation of the field of both the spindles and vertex waves. As expected, the spindles are maximum in the central midline electrode, Cz, and also in the adjacent central C3 and C4 electrodes (arrows). The spindle field also extends forward to include F3 and F4. Likewise, the vertex waves seen in the following second have a similar field, maximum in the midline and in the parasagittal chains, but their field does not extend to the temporal chains to any great extent. Compare to the next figure.

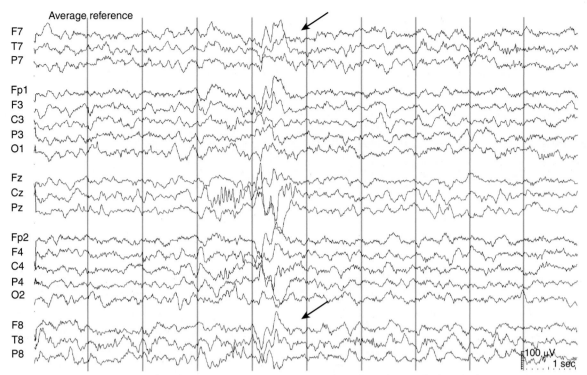

Figure 5.36 The same page of the EEG as shown in the previous figure is now displayed using an average reference montage. Although the spindles are still seen to be maximum in Cz, they now appear to have a much broader field and are even seen in the temporal chains. The reason for this misleading appearance is that the average reference is "contaminated" with the spindles. Even more misleading, the field of the vertex waves now appears to extend past the parasagittal areas to include the temporal areas (arrows). The apparent presence of the vertex waves and spindles in the left and right temporal chains represents a false localization, caused by contamination of the average reference with the vertex wave and spindle activity.

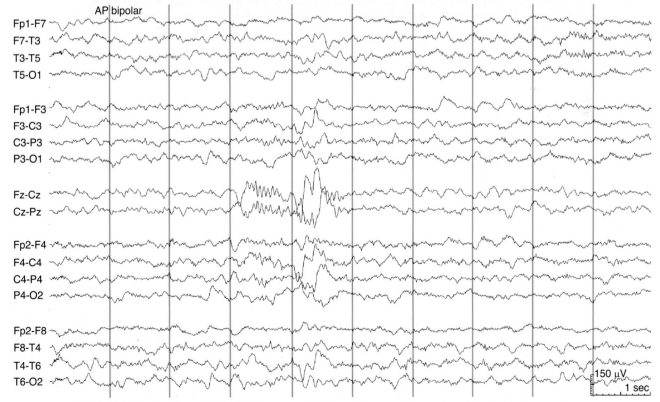

Figure 5.37 The same page of EEG as shown in the previous two figures is displayed this time with an anteroposterior (AP) bipolar montage. Note that on this page, the AP bipolar montage gives a fairly accurate representation of the fields of the vertex waves and spindles. The field of neither wave extends to the temporal chains (top four and bottom four channels).

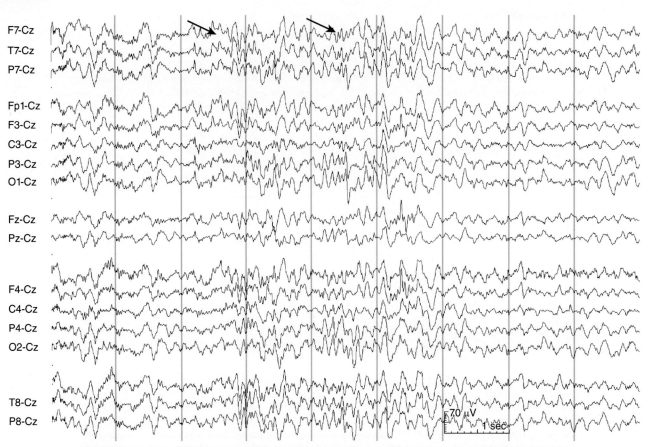

Figure 5.38 A page of EEG sleep is displayed using a Cz reference. Because the Cz electrode is active with spindle and vertex-wave activity during sleep, this electrode position makes a poor choice for the reference electrode. Note that spindles and vertex waves appear to involve all channels on the page (arrows). Ironically, because of cancellation effects, the spindles are least well seen in the channels where their fields are strongest, C3 and C4.

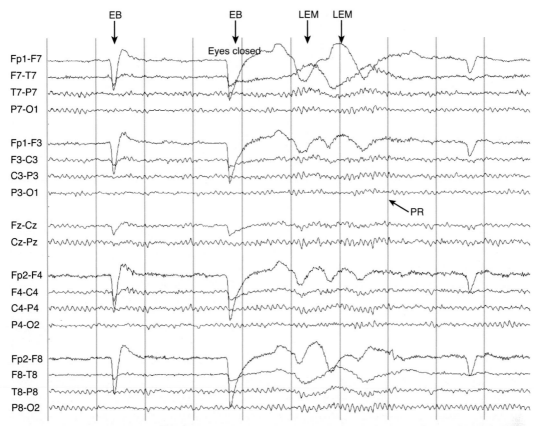

Figure 5.39 A page of wakefulness is shown in the anteroposterior (AP) bipolar montage. Eyeblink (EB) artifacts are the most prominent waveforms in this awake tracing, seen as dramatic downward deflections most prominent in the top channel of each grouping of four channels in the AP bipolar montage. A smaller but similar deflection is also seen in the first channel of the midline electrodes (Fz-Cz) because Fz senses the eyeblink as well, but Cz does not. Eyeblink artifact is caused by an upward bobbing of the eyes that reflexively occurs during eye closure or blinking (Bell's phenomenon). Because the anterior aspect of the eye is positively charged with respect to the posterior pole, eyeblinks result in a net positivity being thrust into the region measured by the most anterior electrodes. Because the gradient (voltage difference) is typically greatest for eyeblink artifact between the most anterior electrodes (Fp1 and Fp2) and those directly posterior to them (F7, F3, F4, and F8), the eyeblink artifact waveform is almost always of highest amplitude in the most anterior channels (e.g., Fp1-F3 and Fp2-F4) in bipolar montages, as seen in this figure. Typically, this artifact is also visible, but to a lesser extent, in the next more posterior channels (e.g., F3-C3 and F4-C4). Because of the anterior source of the eyeblink potential, it is unusual to see a deflection posterior to these channels. Indeed, as is seen in this figure, the eyeblink deflection is not picked up in channels such as C3-P3 or T8-P8. At the end of the sixth second, high-voltage waveforms show opposing phases on the left compared with the right (LEM = lateral eye movement). This type of artifact is caused by lateral eye movements and is discussed in more detail in Chapter 6, "Electroencephalographic Artifacts". PR = posterior rhythm.

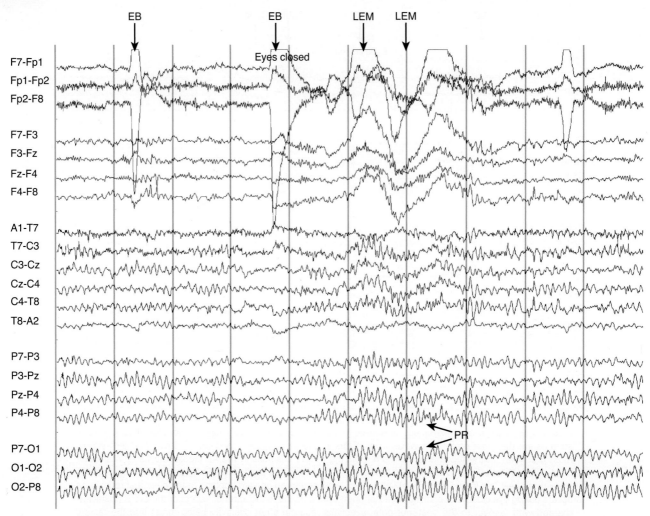

Figure 5.40 The same page of wakefulness as in Figure 5.39 is shown in the transverse bipolar montage. The eyeblink (EB) artifact is now essentially confined to the top three channels. Because the upward movement of the globes, which represents a net positive charge, is detected nearly equally in Fp1 and Fp2, the amount of deflection in the Fp1-Fp2 channel is minimal. The Fp1 and Fp2 electrodes are, however, closer to the positivity of the eyeball as it bobs upward compared to the F7 and F8 electrodes. For this reason, the net positivity picked up by Fp1 being greater than at F7, the first channel, F7-Fp1, deflects upward. Likewise, because Fp2 detects more positivity than the F8 electrode, the third, Fp2-F8 channel, deflects downward. The posterior rhythm (PR) is well seen in the bottom three channels as expected, and also in the four channels just above, which link the left and right posterior temporal areas together, and even in the chain that links the left earlobe to the right earlobe (middle group of six channels). Only occasional fragments of the posterior rhythm are picked up in the chain that links the anterior temporal electrodes, F7 and F8 (the fourth through seventh channels nearer the top of the page). LEM = lateral eye movement.

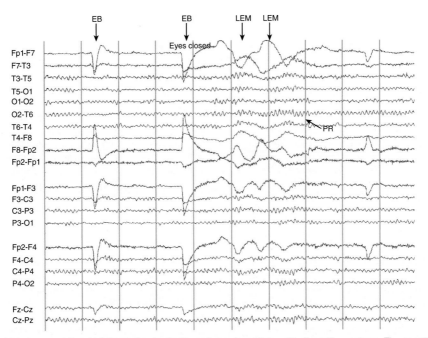

Figure 5.41 A page of wakefulness is shown in a circumferential or "hatband" montage. The top 10 channels represent the circumferential portion of the display. The posterior rhythm (PR) is best seen in the middle channels of the circumferential portion, because these pass through the occipital regions. This montage is most easily scanned for symmetry through the midline visual axis formed by the O1-O2 channel. Eyeblink (EB) artifact is seen in the expected positions at the ends of the circumferential chain, because these represent the frontal region. LEM = lateral eye movement.

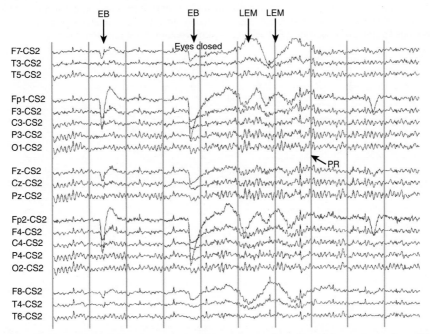

Figure 5.42 A page of wakefulness is shown in the anteroposterior referential montage using a CS2 reference (an electrode placed on the back of the neck). Recalling that in some patients electrocardiographic (EKG) artifact is present in the neck reference, rhythmic EKG artifact can be seen in all channels on this page. The fact that these "little spikes" appear with the same amplitude and morphology in every channel is a clue that they originate in the reference electrode rather than from the brain. In fact, on the basis of this artifact, the patient's EKG rhythm can be counted out at 66 beats per minute. The field of the posterior rhythm is well defined appearing, for the most part, in the posterior channels. Careful observation, however, shows that a small amount of the posterior rhythm (PR) is visible even in the most anterior channels. The astute reader will conclude that this is not because the posterior rhythm is actually present in the frontal areas but rather that the CS2 electrode is actually picking up the posterior rhythm to a small extent. This is not completely unexpected because the posterior rhythm's field is maximum in the occipital regions, fairly close to the position of this neck electrode. The limitations of the use of the CS2 electrode evident in this page do not apply to all patients; in some patients, EKG artifact and posterior rhythm contamination are not seen in the CS2 electrode. EB = eyeblink; LEM = lateral eye movement.

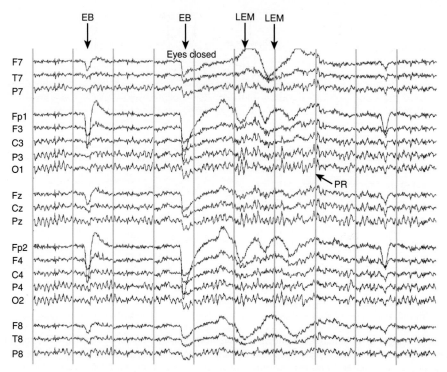

Figure 5.43 The same page of wakefulness is shown in the AP referential montage using the chin as reference. Because in this patient, the chin does not pick up electrocardiographic (EKG) artifact, we do not see the EKG spikes as in the previous figure. Instead, in this patient, there is a small amount of muscle artifact in the chin, which causes this artifact to appear in every channel of this tracing from time to time (this can be seen under the arrows for the LEMs). Note also that the posterior rhythm (PR) is appropriately completely absent from the Fp1 and Fp2 electrodes channels in this page (compare with the contamination phenomenon seen in the previous figure). EB = eyeblink; LEM = lateral eye movement; PR = posterior rhythm.

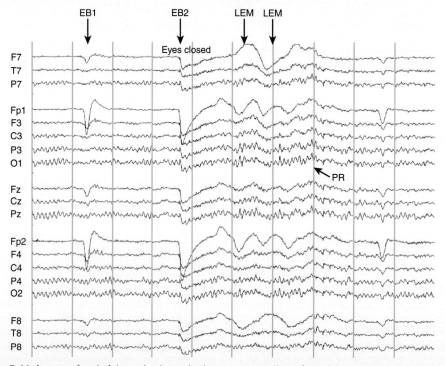

Figure 5.44 A page of wakefulness is shown in the anteroposterior referential montage using the nose as the reference. In this patient, the nose reference happens to be quiet, yielding an excellent quality tracing. Note the small spike-like artifact seen in the fourth second (under EB2 arrow). Because this small transient is similar in all channels, it can be identified as an artifact that originates in the nose reference. Again, eyeblink (EB) artifacts are seen confined to the anterior (Fp1, Fp2, F7, F3, F4, and F8) channels. The field of the posterior rhythm (PR) in this patient extends up to the C3 and C4 electrodes. Only occasionally are fragments of this rhythm seen as far forward as F3 and F4. As expected, the posterior rhythm cannot be identified in the frontopolar leads, Fp1 and Fp2. LEM = lateral eye movement.

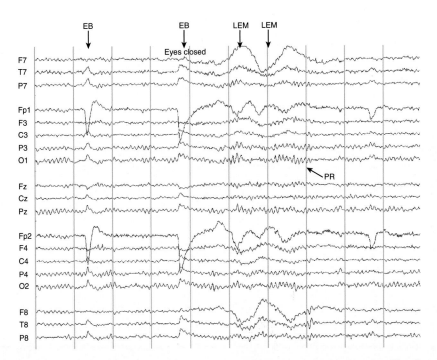

Figure 5.45 A page of wakefulness is shown in the anteroposterior referential montage using the average reference. Some of the advantages and disadvantages of the average reference are evident in this page. The average reference yields a clean display from the point of view of being free of muscle artifact. However, note that the eyeblink (EB) artifacts seen in the anterior channels are being "answered" with upgoing waves in the posterior channels. This is an artifact of contamination of the average reference by the high-voltage eyeblink deflections. Likewise, the posterior rhythm (PR) can be seen in all channels, again an artifact of the effect of contamination of the average reference by the posterior rhythm (see further description of these problems in the paragraphs on the average reference). LEM = lateral eye movement.

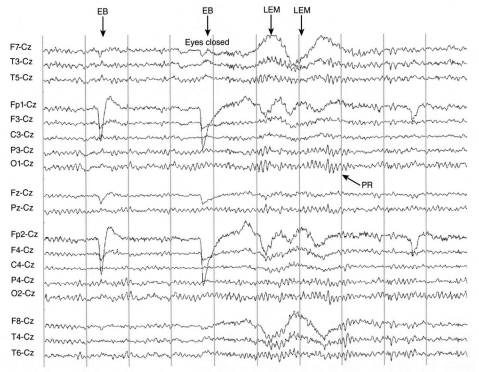

Figure 5.46 A page of wakefulness is shown in the anteroposterior referential montage using Cz as the reference. In this patient at this time in the tracing, the Cz electrode is relatively quiet. For this reason, this page appears to be of generally good quality, though note that the posterior rhythm can often be seen in all channels on the page, reflecting the fact that Cz is close enough to the back of the head that it intermittently picks up the posterior rhythm. This can be confirmed by looking at Figure 5.44 in which the posterior rhythm can often be discerned in the Cz-nose channel. Because all channels on this page are being compared to Cz, any activity that occurs in Cz has the potential to appear on every channel of the page. EB = eyeblink, LEM = lateral eye movement, PR = posterior rhythm.

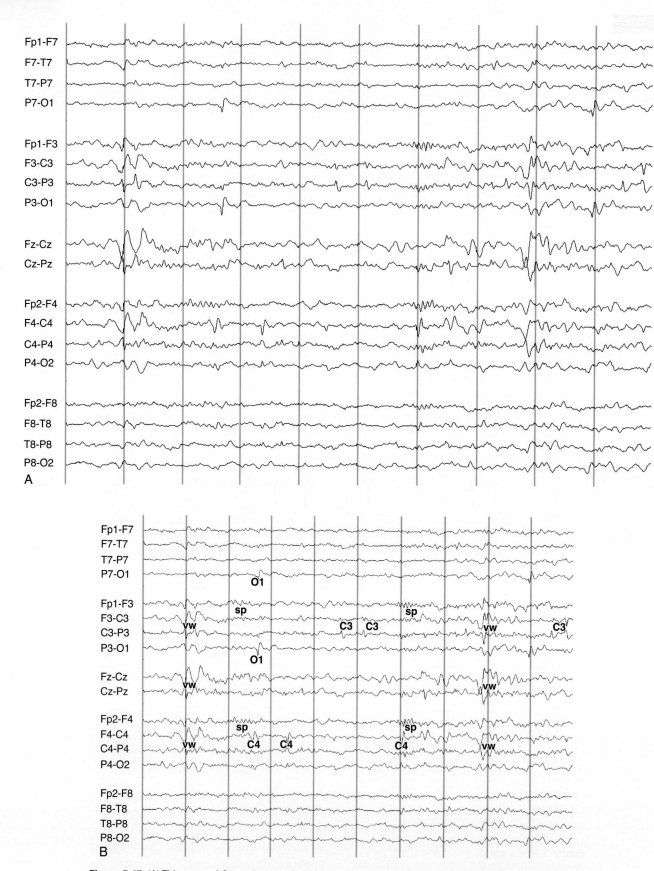

Figure 5.47 (A) This page of Stage II sleep displayed in an **anteroposterior bipolar montage** shows many features, including vertex waves of sleep, sleep spindles, a left occipital spike, and independent right and left central spikes. (B) The same page with labels: O1 = left occipital spike; sp = sleep spindle; vw = vertex wave of sleep; C4 = right central spike; C3 = left central spike.

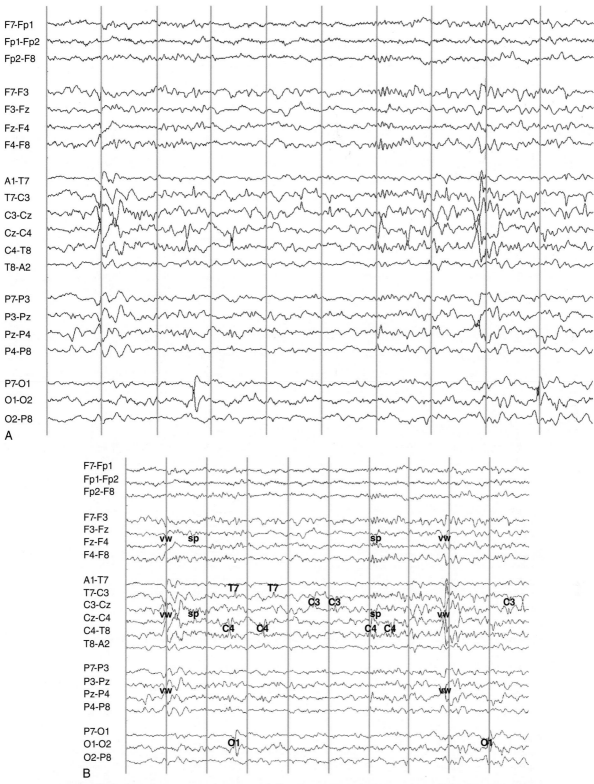

Figure 5.48 (A) The same sleep segment is displayed in a **transverse bipolar montage**. Identify all of the various features in this transverse bipolar representation. Note that the vertex waves phase reverse in the Cz electrode suggesting that their voltage maximum is in the midline as expected, rather than off to one side. In contrast, the C3 and C4 spikes show clear phase reversals in those electrodes "off the midline," clearly distinguishing them from the vertex waves. Likewise, the O1 spikes appear prominently at the bottom of the page. The spindles, which appear as low-voltage 14 Hz waves, clearly involve both the frontal and central areas. Because the spindle voltage falls off most steeply between F3 and F7 and between F4 and F8, the subtraction of these channel pairs shows the spindles well in F7-F3 and F4-F8. (B) The same page with labels: O1 = left occipital spike; sp = sleep spindle; vw = vertex wave of sleep; C4 = right central spike; C3 = left central spike.

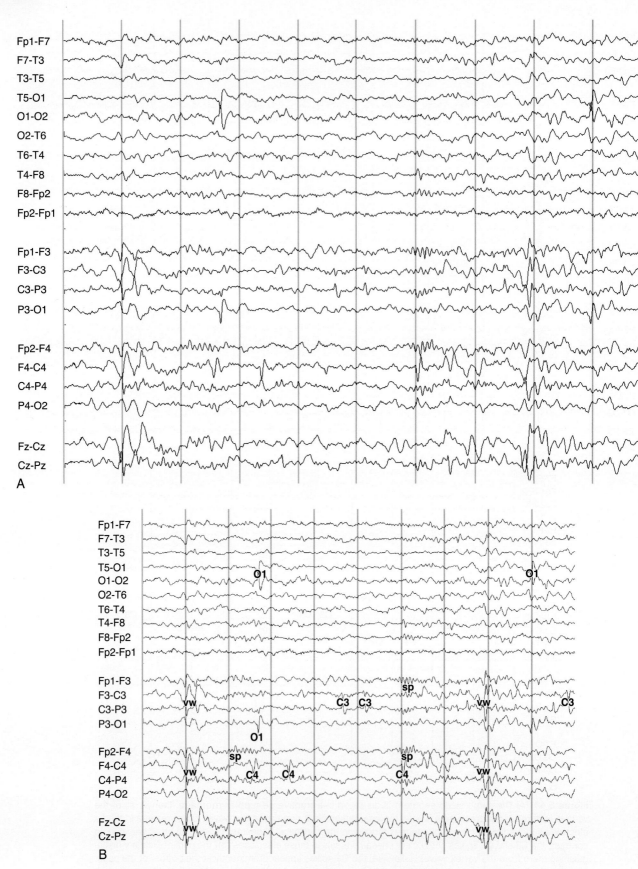

Figure 5.49 (A) The same page of sleep is displayed in a **circumferential bipolar montage**. The vertex waves and spindles are best seen on the bottom half of the page, which includes the parasagittal chains and the midline. The O1 spike appears prominently in the circumferential channels on the top half of the page. The C3 and C4 spikes are also evident. (B) The same page with labels: O1 = left occipital spike; sp = sleep spindle; vw = vertex wave of sleep; C4 = right central spike; C3 = left central spike.

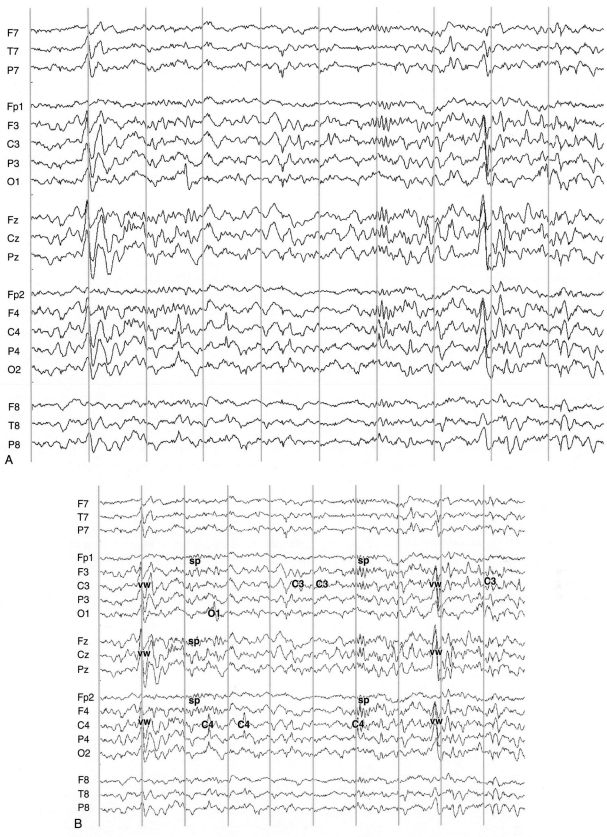

Figure 5.50 (A) The same page of sleep is displayed using an **anteroposterior referential montage using a nose reference**. In this patient, the nose is electrically quiet during sleep and performs as an excellent reference electrode. The O1, C3, and C4 spikes are seen as upward deflections, although they do not "jump out" from the background as much as they do in bipolar montages. The fields of the vertex waves and spindles can easily be appreciated in this montage. (B) The same page with labels: O1 = left occipital spike; sp = sleep spindle; vw = vertex wave of sleep; C4 = right central spike; C3 = left central spike.

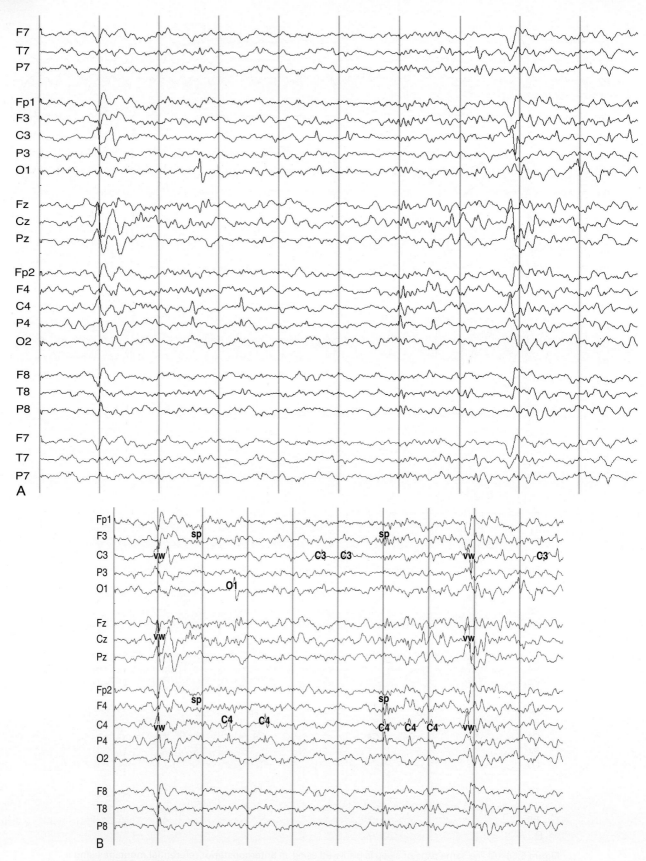

Figure 5.51 (A) The same page of sleep is displayed with an anteroposterior referential montage using the average reference. On this page the average reference gives a fairly good representation of EEG activity, but note that the spindle and vertex wave fields appear to be falsely broad because these waves have contaminated the average reference. In contrast, the O1, C3, and C4 spikes show up well against the background. (B) The same page with labels: O1 = left occipital spike; sp = sleep spindle; vw = vertex wave of sleep; C4 = right central spike; C3 = left central spike.

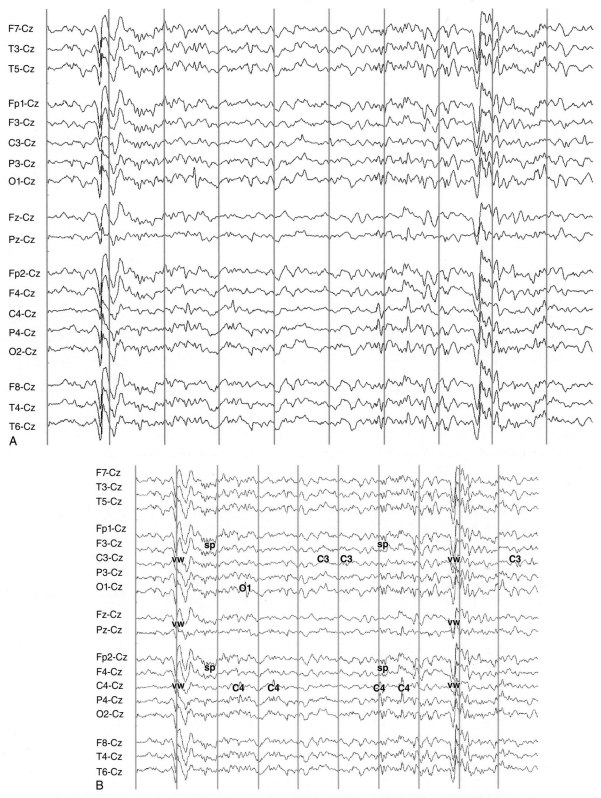

Figure 5.52 (A) **Anteroposterior referential montage to the Cz electrode**. Use of the Cz electrode as a reference is almost always a poor choice during sleep. Because sleep spindles, and especially vertex waves, appear strongly in the Cz electrode, this choice of reference spreads these waves across every channel, as is seen on this page. For example, the vertex waves appear in the temporal chains (top three and bottom three channels), although they are not really present in those locations. If one is able to ignore this effect, the location of some of the focal spikes can still be accurately discerned in this montage. (B) The same page with labels: O1 = left occipital spike; sp = sleep spindle; vw = vertex wave of sleep; C4 = right central spike; C3 = left central spike.

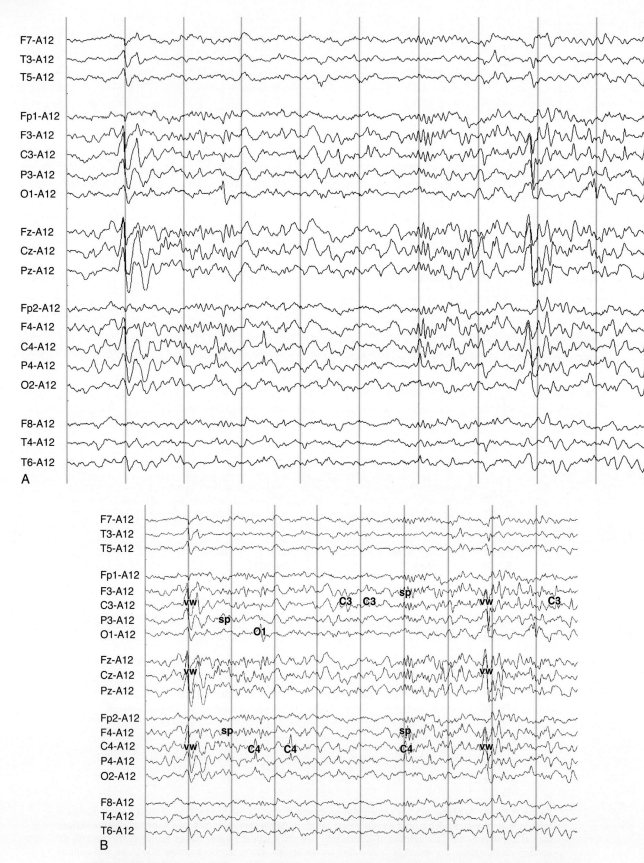

Figure 5.53 (A) This page shows a **referential montage using a "mixture" or average of the earlobe electrodes, A1 and A2,** as the reference. When the A1 and A2 electrodes are used as the reference electrodes, an alternative method used in some laboratories is to refer electrodes on the left side of the head to A1 and electrodes on the right side of the head to A2. (B) The same page with labels: O1 = left occipital spike; sp = sleep spindle; vw = vertex wave of sleep; C4 = right central spike; C3 = left central spike.

REVIEW QUESTIONS

1. Regarding montage types,
   a. an advantage of bipolar montages is that they show the true voltage of waves.
   b. referential montages have the advantage that their phase reversals are more obvious with long interelectrode distances.
   c. errors from mismeasured electrode placement are much more obvious with bipolar montages.
   d. a wave's peak voltage can be found by locating the highest voltage waveform in a bipolar montage.
2. In a referential montage,
   a. in general, the point of maximum voltage of an electrical event corresponds to the highest amplitude waveform for that event.
   b. bipolar montages measure voltages between two points, while referential montages measure voltage at a single point.
   c. the nose cannot be used as a reference because it is not over the brain.
   d. the ideal reference has no noise and no brain activity.
3. Small interelectrode distances
   a. have the advantage of common noise in each contact, which helps the noise to cancel out efficiently.
   b. are associated with higher voltage readouts.
   c. do not cancel common brain activity, yielding a cleaner tracing.
   d. All of the above
4. If a patient definitely has a posterior rhythm but it is not visible in the P3-O1 channel, then
   a. the patient's eyes must be closed.
   b. the patient may be in a dark room.
   c. it is probable that an error was made in the way the montage was programmed into the software.
   d. the patient's posterior rhythm may be present, but perfectly in phase and of similar amplitude between P3 and O1.
5. Regarding potential disadvantages of specific reference electrodes,
   a. earlobe references often pick up midtemporal activity.
   b. earlobe references often are contaminated by EKG activity.
   c. CS2 references can be contaminated by patient movement, and EKG activity in some.
   d. All of the above
6. Eyeblink artifact
   a. creates downgoing deflections in anterior channels in bipolar montages.
   b. creates upgoing deflections in referential montages.
   c. is formed from contraction of the eyelid muscles.
   d. All of the above
7. The ideal reference electrode
   a. would be electrically neutral.
   b. would have no noise or brain activity compared to the electrode of interest.
   c. would have the same noise but none of the brain activity of the electrode of interest.
   d. needs to be in a part of the body distant from the brain.

ANSWERS

1. ANSWER: **C.** Although it can be argued that neither referential nor bipolar montages show the precise voltage of EEG waves, referential montages, which strive to compare the electrode of interest to a neutral location, give the best estimate of wave voltages. Because bipolar montages subtract voltages from their neighbors, they will tend to give an underestimate of true voltage. In bipolar chains, when electrodes are mismeasured, pairs that are too close to each other will tend to manifest lower voltages than intended because of smaller interelectrode distances. Phase reversals are not used to locate voltage maxima in referential montages, only in bipolar montages. The voltage maximum of a wave is located by finding the highest amplitude waveform in a referential montage, but not so in a bipolar montage in which locating the phase reversal is key to identifying the point of maximum voltage.
2. ANSWER Answer: **A.** In referential montages, the point of maximum wave height corresponds to the location of maximum voltage. Both bipolar and referential montages measure the voltage difference between two different points. The nose can serve as an excellent reference point because it includes little brain wave activity but expresses the noise signal in the head, allowing it to be subtracted from the electrode of interest. The ideal reference electrode would have *all* of the noise, but none of the brain activity.
3. ANSWER: **A.** The main advantage of small interelectrode distances is that the noise signal is more likely to be similar, allowing for efficient cancellation. Unfortunately, smaller distances also allow for cancellation of brain activity as well. Because of the cancellation of like noise and brain wave activity, smaller interelectrode distances are associated with lower voltage readouts.
4. ANSWER: **D.** In a patient who is known to have a posterior rhythm, eye-opening (rather than closure) or a lighted environment that would allow for visual fixation

could both cause it to be suppressed. Although a montage programming error could cause apparent absence of the posterior rhythm, most montages are programmed once when the software is set up, and not once per patient, making this type of error very uncommon. Occasionally, however, electrodes may be incorrectly plugged in to the EEG machine (jack box). As discussed in the text, occasional patients have a posterior rhythm that is perfectly in phase in P3 and O1. In such cases, the posterior rhythm could become completely canceled in a P3-O1 channel displayed in a bipolar montage. The fact that the posterior rhythm is, indeed, present in these locations can be easily demonstrated by switching to a referential montage, in which case the P3-ref and O1-ref channels will demonstrate the rhythm.

5. ANSWER: **D**. All of these statements regarding reference electrodes are true.

6. ANSWER: **A**. Bipolar montages show the well-known downgoing waveforms of eyeblink artifact. Eyeblink artifact also creates downgoing waves in referential montages because the frontal electrodes experience a large positivity compared to the reference (INPUT1 more positive—pen goes down). Eyeblink artifact is not caused by movement of the eyelids, but by the fact that the eyes bob upward during eye closure (Bell's phenomenon) and the front of the eye carries a positive charge.

7. ANSWER: **C**. Although an electrically neutral reference would seem to be a good choice at first glance, such a reference would not aid in canceling out electrical noise from the head. For the same reason, a reference with no noise or brain activity would yield a noisy recording. A reference electrode location far from the brain is less likely to share a common noise signal with the electrode of interest and, therefore, would be less likely to efficiently cancel the noise signal compared to a location closer to the brain. A reference location close enough to the brain to share a common noise signal, but far enough that it does not sense brain wave activity, would be the ideal choice.

REFERENCE

Guideline 6: A proposal for standard montages to be used in clinical EEG. ACNS Guidelines, *J Clin Neurophysiol* 23:111–117, 2006.

6

Electroencephalographic Artifacts

An artifact is a waveform in the EEG that is not of cerebral origin. Those new to the world of EEG interpretation are often surprised to learn that at least half the challenge of EEG reading consists of identifying artifacts correctly so as not to mistake them for true EEG (cerebral) activity. This is quite different from other types of interpretation in clinical electrophysiology such as electrocardiogram (EKG) reading in which the problem of distinguishing electrical artifact from actual EKG waves is only occasionally a problem.

It is easy to see how the mistake of interpreting an electrical artifact as a true EEG wave can have important negative consequences. Reporting an innocent "electrode pop" artifact as an epileptiform spike is an error that can have serious clinical repercussions, perhaps even leading to the erroneous diagnosis of epilepsy in a patient. Unfortunately, mistaking an artifact for an EEG wave is not an uncommon type of error among inexperienced readers; even experienced readers can find the distinction between electrocerebral activity and artifact difficult at times. For these reasons, new readers should devote considerable energy to mastering the thought process used to distinguish artifacts from true EEG activity.

Some of the most common EEG artifacts are so distinctive in appearance that the experienced reader can rapidly visually screen them out without the need for close analysis. A good example of this is muscle artifact. Muscle artifact from the temporal, frontal, and occipital areas is so frequently encountered that, for some portions of the tracing, the challenge of interpretation is to read past these artifacts to see the true EEG activity. Eyeblink artifact is another example of an artifact easily identifiable by its shape and location.

Artifacts are not always a hindrance to EEG interpretation and, in fact, sometimes can yield valuable information. The presence of the same muscle artifact that obliterates the EEG from the temporal areas may also serve as a useful confirmation that the patient is moving and awake rather than asleep. Likewise, the presence of eyeblink artifact would not be expected in the sleeping patient and therefore helps exclude the possibility that the patient is asleep. Other types of eye movement artifact can help identify sleep stages. The presence of slow roving lateral eye movement artifact is often a useful marker of drowsiness. The presence of REM (rapid eye movement) sleep can be confirmed, as its name suggests, by the presence of REM artifact. Other types of artifact, however, can be a real hindrance to EEG interpretation. A patient who is constantly moving may generate a record so dominated by motion artifact that it is uninterpretable. In some patients, the motor activity associated with a

convulsion can generate so much muscle and motion artifact that the underlying EEG seizure discharge cannot be identified.

STRATEGIES OF ARTIFACT RECOGNITION

There are two main principles that are critical to the process of distinguishing what is "real" brain wave activity from artifact in the EEG record. The first is wave morphology, or using the shape of a wave to determine its nature; certain wave shapes and patterns are highly characteristic of certain types of artifacts. The second is the principle of "biologic plausibility"; electrical events of *cerebral* origin should show a distribution of intensity on the scalp surface that is plausibly consistent with brain wave activity. This means that the point of maximum voltage of a focal cerebral event is expected to be surrounded by a more or less gradual gradient of decreasing voltage as distance increases from its epicenter (i.e., as we say in EEG, the point of maximum should be surrounded by an electric field). In contrast, artifacts may show a topography of voltages that is bizarre and unpredictable, making it biologically implausible that the recorded signals come from the brain. When an event has a biologically implausible topography, this information guides the EEG reader toward interpreting the waves as electrical or motion artifact. We will expand on these concepts in the examples that follow.

Wave Morphology

Certain artifacts in the EEG have characteristic shapes, such as eyeblink artifact, muscle artifact, and some electrode pops. Some of these artifacts have such a specific appearance that their identification essentially consists of a "sight diagnosis" or pattern recognition. The conclusion that some waves represent artifact may require a combination of both techniques: wave pattern recognition and analysis of wave topography. Examples of various specific types of artifact are shown later in this chapter.

"Biological Plausibility" versus "Biological Implausibility"

Although some artifacts can be recognized on the basis of the shapes of their waves, the most powerful tool in distinguishing a true brain wave from an artifact is to establish its specific topography—where and how strongly it is positive or negative at each location on the scalp. Here, the major principle is that biological events recorded on the scalp tend to have a point of maximum voltage, with the surrounding measured voltages diminishing with varying steepness from the point of maximum (Figure 6.1).

The voltage gradients seen with electrocerebral events are expected to have some degree of "smoothness." In contrast, the electric fields of artifacts may have patchy and unpredictable contours (compare to Figure 6.2).

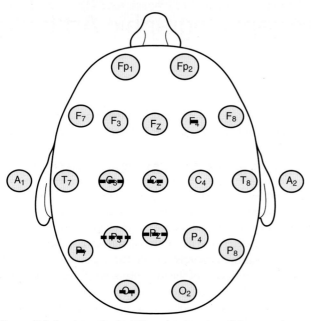

Figure 6.1 A schematic depiction of a pure negativity occurring on the scalp, maximum in the left parietal electrode (P3). Note that the intensity of the negative fields, denoted by the number of minus signs, dissipates gradually away from the maximum, but with varying "steepness" in different directions. This is what is expected of a "biological" field (as opposed to an electrical artifact), that the point of peak voltage is surrounded by a region of diminishing voltages.

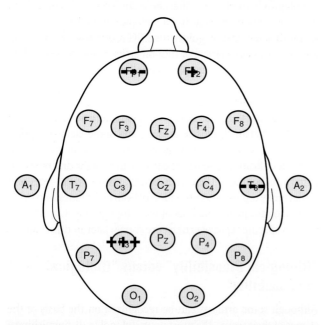

Figure 6.2 In contrast to the previous figure, the field of this discharge is scattered and patchy, showing different polarities in different locations. Electrodes that are measuring high voltages are not surrounded by a diminishing field. Negativities and positivities appear in haphazard locations on the scalp. The pattern of this scalp electrical event does not seem "plausible" for electrocerebral activity. Patterns such as these are most likely caused by electrical or motion artifact, perhaps a head movement that caused certain electrode wires to be tugged on.

A second principle is that the polarity of most discharges tends to be consistent. Most discharges, if negative at their maximum point, remain negative wherever they are detected on the scalp as shown in Figure 6.1. In general, negative events tend to be negative everywhere, and positive events tend to be positive everywhere. Exceptions to this rule exist, including the occasional examples of discharges that manifest a so-called *tangential dipole* (the example of the horizontal or tangential dipole is discussed in detail in Chapter 10, "The EEG in Epilepsy"). Even for the small minority of epileptiform events that manifest a simultaneous combined positivity and negativity, those areas of opposite charge are usually segregated in a simple and orderly fashion rather than showing a pattern of several separated regions of positivity and negativity (Figure 6.3). The respective positive areas and negative areas are contiguous. The negative/positive pattern occasionally occurs when a negativity is recorded on the scalp, but the "back end" or underside of the dipole (positive portion) is recorded elsewhere on the scalp. Even when such less common electrical events arise from the brain, we expect to see a "pool of negativity" and a "pool of positivity" as opposed to scattered and non-contiguous positive and negative electrodes.

Patterns with significant charge inconsistencies are not expected from biological systems. The example of an apparent

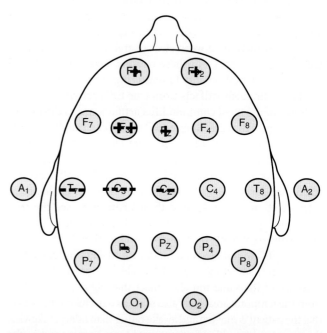

Figure 6.3 A schematic of a "horizontal dipole" is shown, a relatively uncommon finding outside of benign rolandic epilepsy and related syndromes. In contrast to most epileptiform discharges that show a single polarity on the scalp at any one time (usually negative), in this example, a negative charge and a positive charge are recorded on the scalp simultaneously. Even though both polarities are present, the transition between the two has a reasonable geographical and electrical pattern, and both the positivity and negativity are surrounded by a plausible electric field. The configuration shown here of a negativity in the centrotemporal area and a positivity in the anterior head regions is characteristic of the so-called *rolandic spike with a tangential dipole* (simultaneous scalp negativity and positivity), discussed in more detail in Chapter 10, "The EEG in Epilepsy."

discharge with strong negativities in the left posterior quadrant and the right anterior quadrant but no measured voltage change in the intervening areas as depicted in Figure 6.4 is not likely of cerebral origin. Because this is not a "biological" pattern, there would be a strong suspicion of motion or some other type of artifact having affected two distant electrodes and giving rise to this appearance. This pattern and the pattern that was seen in Figure 6.2 may be produced by the haphazard jostling of electrodes during patient movement. The main clue is that the negative areas and positive areas are not at all contiguous.

Whenever analyzing any wave on the EEG page, the reader should be able to visualize the voltage topography of the wave to confirm that there is a distribution of charge that is potentially consistent with cerebral activity, asking, "Does this make biological sense?" Usually with a bit of practice this can be done quickly. Discharges with bizarre or unpredictable electrical fields likely represent artifact. The importance of localization skills cannot be overemphasized, and it is for this reason that the techniques of localization discussed in Chapter 4, "Electroencephalographic Localization," should be mastered before moving on. One of the main skills that marks experienced electroencephalographers is the ability to understand when an apparent discharge's field looks electrically inconsistent and recognizing it as an artifact rather than mistaking it for a cerebral wave.

How do such "biologically implausible" artifacts arise in the first place? Many artifacts are related to head motion. When the patient's head moves, some combination of electrodes are tugged on or moved. The pattern of wires that is pulled on with a head movement is often unpredictable and may not follow any particular logical spatial pattern on the scalp. Disparate and distant deflections on the scalp, especially with varying polarities, are much more suggestive of motion artifact than of electrocerebral activity.

A type of motion artifact that may more reliably follow a spatial pattern is head rolling or rocking. In such instances, the electrodes lying against the bed are most susceptible to motion artifact, but of course others may be pulled on too by the movement. For example, if the back of the patient's head is in contact with the bed, head motion artifact will tend to be most dramatic in the posterior electrodes. Likewise, if the patient is lying on the left side of the head, the left temporal electrodes will be most prone to motion artifact. Artifact may appear in these or other electrodes with voluntary head movements, or even with the low-amplitude head movements associated with the patient's respirations. For example, a slowly repetitive waveform in the O2 electrode that matches the respiratory channel probably indicates that the patient is lying on the back of the head and that breathing motion has caused the head to rock very slightly on the electrode(s) in contact with the bed. This can often be confirmed by checking the patient's head position on video, if available.

Some significant EEG diagnostic challenges occur when patients are referred for the question of whether sudden movements, including head, limb, or torso jerks, are epileptic. The question the electroencephalographer is trying to answer is whether or not there is an epileptic discharge (such as a polyspike) in the EEG that is driving the movement. The diagnostic problem is made more difficult by the fact that the patient's movement may generate a quick burst of motion or muscle artifact, and these brief motion artifacts can sometimes resemble polyspike discharges. The EEGer is thus often confronted with quick movements associated with quick EEG deflections and is asked whether the deflection is an epileptic discharge (in which case the movements are brief epileptic seizures) or just motion artifact (in which case the movements may represent something not seizure-related, e.g., a tic or perhaps a benign sleep movement). There are several concepts that can be used to help separate the two situations when a body movement and an EEG deflection occur at the same time.

When there is a body movement and a simultaneous EEG burst, the question is easier to answer if the movement is confined to a limb, because a simple limb movement would not be expected to cause motion artifact in the scalp electrodes. But if the movement involves the head or perhaps a limb that causes a whole-body movement and there is a simultaneous deflection in the EEG, it may be more difficult to tease apart whether the movement caused the wave (and is an artifact) or the wave caused the movement (and is an epileptic discharge). The initial approach to this problem takes into account that when the head moves, is turned on the pillow, or is subject to some other type of external movement, the

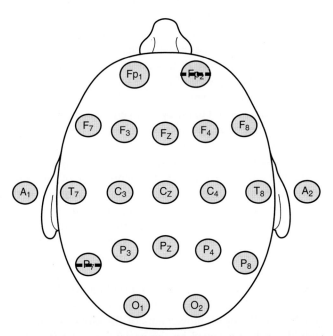

Figure 6.4 A localized negativity is seen in the left posterior temporal area simultaneously with a strong negativity in the right frontopolar area. The intervening areas are electrically neutral. This field does not seem consistent with the biology of the brain. Rather, this pattern, which lacks a gradient and only involves two individual but distant electrodes, is much more suggestive of electrode or motion artifact than a true discharge of cerebral origin.

pattern of electrodes that are disturbed tends to be more random with inconsistent fields, as described above. Artifacts caused by electrode motion or head motion tend to show a nonregular distribution or inconsistent voltages like those shown in Figures 6.2 and 6.4. In comparison, the patterns associated with electrocerebral activity are expected to show more consistent polarities and a voltage gradient that tapers with distance from the point of maximum.

A second approach to this problem is to analyze the way in which the EEG discharge is time-locked to the movement. When a movement is epileptic and caused by an EEG burst that is driving the movement (e.g., epileptic myoclonus), there is always a slight time lag between the EEG burst (possibly a polyspike) and the body movement it generates because it takes some amount of time for the cortical signal to be transmitted through the nervous system and down to the muscles. This latency between the burst and the movement may be confirmed either by a synchronized video recording of the patient or by analyzing the timing of muscle artifact that may appear in some of the EEG electrodes (muscle artifact created by the movement can help mark the exact time of the onset of the movement in the EEG). Using the video, the reader asks, "Which do I see first, the EEG deflection or the patient moving?" The EEG should deflect first if it is an epileptic event because that deflection is *causing* the (slightly) later movement. Using any muscle/movement artifact that may be seen in the EEG electrodes and/or the video to time the movement, the EEG burst would appear first, *followed by* the muscle burst or movement in the video (usually with a lag of about a tenth of a second or 100 msec) if the movement is an epileptic event. If an apparent EEG burst is just an example of motion artifact not related to epilepsy, the two are generally seen to occur exactly simultaneously (the EEG burst does not lead the movement), or the body movement may even start before the EEG deflection.

Finally, deflections that are motion artifacts from body movements tend to have some variation from deflection to deflection. Imagine a repetitive head movement not related to epilepsy. Chances are, each time the head moves, the movement may be slightly different and a different grouping of electrodes will be jostled, causing the pattern of the artifact to vary from example to example. Epileptic discharges themselves, such as a polyspike that is driving a body movement, are more likely to have a stereotyped appearance from discharge to discharge. Although this is not an entirely reliable method to distinguish motion artifacts from epileptiform discharges, it can be used as a factor in deciding about difficult cases (see the example of hiccup artifact later in this chapter which provides a minor exception to this rule).

SPECIFIC TYPES OF EEG ARTIFACT

Artifacts Associated with Eye Movements
Eyeblink Artifact and Bell's Phenomenon

Electroencephalographers know that when individuals close their eyes, the globes of the eyes deviate upward. This comes as a surprise to some because when we watch a person casually blink or close the eyes, this upward movement of the globes is usually completely hidden from view by the closed eyelids. It is only in special situations that this reflex upward eye movement that accompanies eye closure, termed *Bell's phenomenon*, is readily observable. Bell's phenomenon becomes strikingly evident in the case of individuals who suffer from Bell's palsy. In the disorder *Bell's palsy*, the patient develops a paralysis of one side of the face because of dysfunction of the facial nerve (cranial nerve VII), one of whose functions is to close the eyes by contraction of the orbicularis oculi muscles that surround the eyes. The nerves that move the globe of the eye up and down and left and right (cranial nerves III, IV, and VI) are unaffected in persons with Bell's palsy. Therefore, Bell's palsy patients have normal eye movements but cannot close the eyelid on the affected side. Thus, the facial nerve paralysis caused by Bell's palsy literally uncovers Bell's phenomenon—we can see what the globe of the eye is doing during intended eyelid closure on the affected side. Bell's palsy patients have normal eye closure on the unaffected side, but when blinking or closing the eyes, the globe of the eye can be seen to deviate upward on the side of the paralysis because the globe is no longer hidden by the eyelid. As it happens, this usually hidden phenomenon of the globes bobbing upward during eyeblinking makes quite a splash on the EEG.

The type of artifact that an upward movement of the globes might cause during eye blinking or eye closure is not intuitively obvious without knowing that the globe of the eye has a particular distribution of charge. As it happens, the cornea (the front of the globe of the eye that covers the iris and pupil) carries a net positive charge and the posterior pole of the globe carries a net negative charge, forming a dipole. Because of the presence of this positive charge on the cornea, the bobbing upward of the eye with eye closure is easily detected by EEG electrodes. Figure 6.5 illustrates how the EEG electrodes closest to the eye "perceive" an eyeblink. With upward eye deviation, the electrodes closest to the globes, Fp1 and Fp2, perceive the strong positivity of the corneal surfaces. The F3 and F4 electrodes, which are immediately posterior to the Fp1 and Fp2 electrodes, also sense some of this positivity, but to a lesser degree compared to Fp1 and Fp2. With Fp1 being more positive than F3 and Fp2 being more positive than F4, the Fp1-F3 and Fp2-F4 channels show the characteristic sharp, downward-sweeping waveforms of eyeblink artifact (Figure 6.6). A similar type of artifact is seen with eye fluttering (Figure 6.7).

A useful general rule regarding eyeblink artifact is that it should not be detectable in the electrodes of the posterior half of the head; movements of the globes of the eye should not be perceived by the parietal or occipital electrodes because they are too distant. Eyeblink artifact is only occasionally picked up by the central electrodes, C3 and C4, and when it is it should be of low voltage (Figure 6.8). Waveforms that resemble eyeblink artifact but are present in more posterior electrodes may not be eyeblink artifact at all.

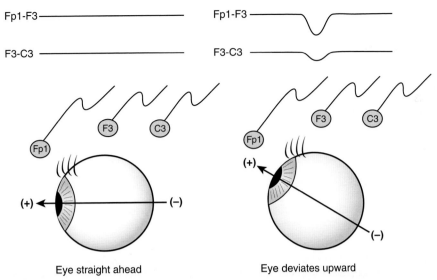

Figure 6.5 This figure shows how the dipole across the globe of the eye leads to the appearance of eyeblink artifact on the EEG. The cornea of the eye carries a net positive charge relative to the posterior pole of the eye, which carries a net negative charge. When the eyes are blinked or closed, the globes of the eye deviate upward under the closed eyelids (Bell's phenomenon). This results in the exposure of the Fp1 electrode in the diagram to the net positivity of the cornea. The F3 electrode, which is more distant from the cornea, also picks up some of the positivity, but to a lesser extent. Thus, when the eyes bob upward as shown in the right panel, the Fp1-F3 channel deviates downward (Fp1 is more positive than F3). When the F3 electrode is compared with the C3 electrode, the smaller amount of positivity picked up by the F3 electrode is compared to the neutral C3 electrode (C3 is too distant from the cornea to detect this event), and the F3-C3 channel shows another, smaller downgoing wave. More posterior channels in AP bipolar chains would not be expected to show deflections from eyeblink artifact.

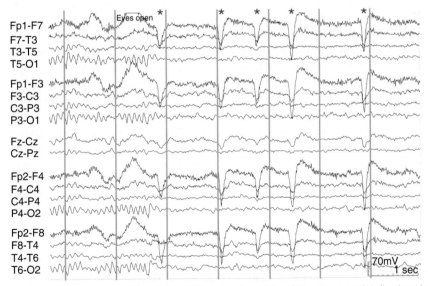

Figure 6.6 The typical appearance of eyeblink artifact showing high voltage downward deflections in the top two channels of each four-channel chain of the standard anteroposterior bipolar montage. Asterisks at the top of the page denote the timing of each eyeblink artifact. Note that, in each set of four channels, the deepest deflection is seen in the top channel. A less intense deflection is seen in the second channel, just below the top channel in each group of four. Eyeblink deflections are not seen in the more posterior channels. The presence of repetitive eyeblink artifact usually indicates that the eyes are open and the patient is awake. This is consistent with the observation in this figure that the posterior rhythm disappears at the time the eyeblink artifact makes its appearance, suggesting a transition from an eyes-closed to an eyes-open state. The technologist has made a notation confirming this.

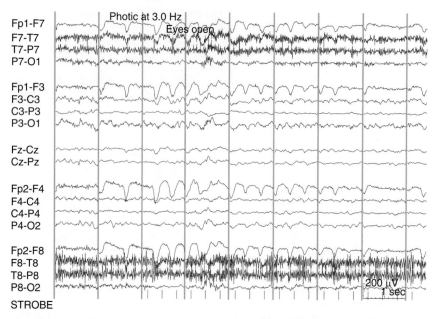

Figure 6.7 An artifact similar to eyeblink artifact is seen during eye fluttering. In this example, the eye flut-tering is caused by the patient's reaction of surprise to the repetitive flashes of the strobe light during photic stimulation (note strobe flashes in the bottom channel marked by vertical lines). Occasionally, eye fluttering or eye bobbing artifact can be difficult to distinguish from frontal slow-wave activity. In such cases, special electrodes placed below the eyes can help distinguish between the two possibilities. Muscle artifact is seen in each temporal area, especially in T7 and T8, the electrodes located over the temporalis muscles.

Lateral Eye Movement Artifact

An extension of this same phenomenon involving the motion of the positive charge on the anterior aspect of the globe is used to understand the appearance of lateral eye movement artifact. In the case of lateral eye movements, the anterior temporal electrodes, F7 and F8, are the electrode contacts best placed to perceive the positivity of the cornea as the eyes move from side to side in the horizontal plane. For example, when a patient gazes to the left, the F7 (left anterior temporal) electrode picks up a net positivity. Also as the eyes gaze to the left, the F8 (right anterior temporal) electrode picks up a net negativity from the posterior pole of the globe of the right eye (Figure 6.9). This results in a characteristic pattern seen with a simultaneous "positive phase reversal" in the anterior temporal electrode on the side to which the eyes have turned and a "negative phase reversal" in the anterior temporal electrode on the side away from which the eyes have turned. In the case of more rapid voluntary saccades or REM sleep, these lateral eye movement artifacts can have a squared-off or triangular appearance at wave onset. During drowsiness, slow roving lateral eye movements may be seen in which the artifact shows a more rounded appearance (Figure 6.10). Therefore, iden-tification of both eyeblink and lateral eye movement artifact requires a combination of wave pattern recognition and local-ization of the electrical events to their characteristic locations. The presence of eyeblink artifact almost always suggests that the patient is awake.

Slow Roving Eye Movements of Drowsiness and Sleep

Slow roving eye movements of drowsiness mentioned earlier represent an important example of lateral eye movement arti-fact. This type of eye movement shows an electrical pattern that is similar to other lateral eye movements, with a "positive phase reversal" at the anterior temporal electrode on the side to which the eyes are moving and a "negative phase reversal" at the opposite anterior temporal electrode. The slow roving version of lateral eye movements has a distinctively rounded, more prolonged shape (see Figure 6.10). In contrast, lateral eye movements occurring during wakefulness or during REM sleep tend to be quicker and have a more squared-off onset. Correct identification of eyeblink artifact and the various lat-eral eye movement artifacts can be quite helpful in determin-ing sleep stage.

Nystagmus Artifact

Nystagmus is a quick, repetitive, motion of the eyes, most often seen in the horizontal plane. Nystagmus artifact is a spe-cial example of lateral eye movement artifact, identifiable by its rhythmicity. It is easy to distinguish from repetitive wave-forms of cerebral origin based on its characteristic polarity in the anterior temporal electrodes (F7 and F8). Figure 6.11 shows a repetitive, rhythmic waveform for which the polarity of the phase reversal is opposite on the left and right sides at any given moment, indicating a repetitive lateral eye move-ment consistent with nystagmus.

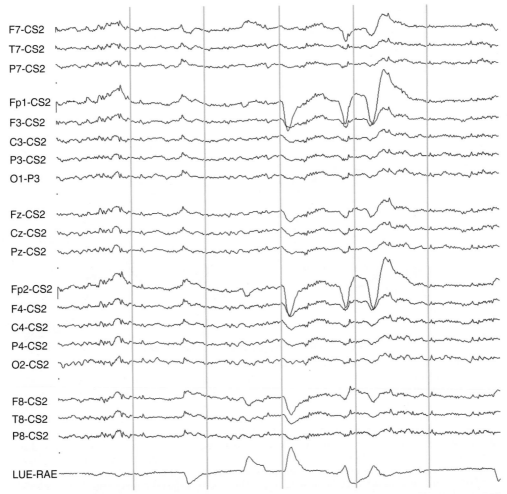

Figure 6.8 Three apparent eyeblink artifacts are shown in a referential montage, with each active electrode compared to a CS2 reference, a location on the back of the neck and distant from the eyes. The artifact is of high voltage in the Fp1 and Fp2 channels and is picked up to a lesser extent in F7 and F8. More posterior channels are neutral. Low-voltage EKG artifact can be seen in all channels indicating that it is being picked up by the CS2 reference electrode. The alert reader may have noted that the first artifact does not have a deflection in the F7-CS2 channel and it is accompanied by a simultaneous upgoing wave in the LUE-RAE channel. Deconstructing this pattern, the first eye movement is likely up and to the right as the upward deflection in the LUE-RAE channel suggests that the RAE electrode is experiencing a positivity. LUE = Left under eye, RAE = right above eye.

Lateral Rectus Spikes

In addition to the types of lateral eye movement artifacts described earlier, lateral eye movements may also cause an artifact that appears as a sharp transient in the anterior temporal area with each lateral eye movement (Figures 6.12 and 6.13). This type of artifact is important to recognize so as not to mistake these sharp transients for true epileptic spikes. It is hypothesized that these sharp transients represent electromyogram (EMG or muscle) artifact from activation of the lateral rectus muscle during lateral eye movements.

Electrode Pops and Other Single Electrode Artifacts

Electrode Pops

Electrode pops may occur because of a buildup of static charge in an individual electrode followed by a quick release of that charge. Sometimes an electrode pops because it has been poorly applied, but frequently there is no clear explanation for electrode popping. Electrode pops often have a distinctive shape (Figure 6.14), although the morphology of electrode pops may vary.

The key attribute of the electrode pop is the strict localization of the event to a single electrode. Because, by its nature, an electrode pop is confined to a single electrode, it is said to "have no field." This is an important concept in artifact identification. A "biological" (brain wave) event usually manifests some amount of an electric field in at least some of the surrounding electrodes—the voltage of the event tapers away from the point of maximum in a more or less gradual fashion. However, if a wave is caused by a problem in a single electrode, be it a "pop" or a problem with the contact, the field of the event will be restricted to that single electrode; the adjacent electrodes perceive nothing at the moment of the "pop." Therefore, the pure electrode "pop" appears as a single discharge isolated in the wilderness of electrodes. Even turning

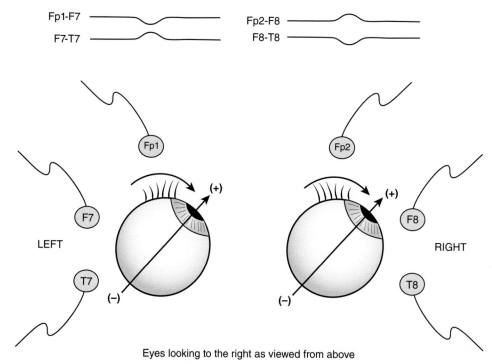

Fp1-F7

F7-T7

Fp2-F8

F8-T8

Fp1

Fp2

F7

F8

LEFT

RIGHT

(+)

(+)

(−)

(−)

T7

T8

Eyes looking to the right as viewed from above

Figure 6.9 Lateral eye movements create a specific type of artifact in the EEG. The diagram here shows the example of both eyes gazing to the right, as seen from above. Because the cornea holds a net positive charge and the posterior pole of the eye a net negative charge, a lateral eye movement creates opposing situations for each pair of frontopolar and anterior temporal electrodes (Fp1 and F7 compared to Fp2 and F8). When the eyes move to the right, the right anterior temporal electrode (F8) is exposed to the positive charge of the cornea of the right eye. With F8 being more positive than Fp2, the "positive phase reversal" depicted above the right eye results. At the same time, the left anterior temporal electrode is exposed to a net negative charge by the medial movement of the left eye, as shown in the figure. This results in a simultaneous "negative phase reversal" appearing at the left anterior temporal electrode (F7). Lateral eye movements are therefore identifiable by the very characteristic simultaneous appearance of a "negative phase reversal" in one anterior temporal electrode and a "positive phase reversal" in the opposite anterior temporal electrode. Another way of putting this is that if you see a simultaneous "bulging apart" of the channels in one anterior temporal area and see a simultaneous "hourglass" pattern over the other temporal area as shown in this figure, a lateral eye movement artifact is likely and the eye movement is in the direction of the waves that "bulge apart."

up the amplifier gain should not reveal involvement of adjacent electrodes.

Figure 6.15 shows an example of an electrical event completely restricted to a single electrode, T3. Careful scrutiny of surrounding electrodes reveals no evidence of an electric field or gradient in any of the adjacent electrodes (F7, T5, or C3). Another way of proving the isolation of this event is to ask whether, if the two channels that include the T3 electrode were to be erased from the EEG or covered by your finger, would it still be possible to identify the moment of the would-be spike? In this example, not even the smallest deflection in the adjacent channels can be seen, establishing this as a single electrode event representing an electrical artifact rather than an electrical event of cerebral origin.

Although electrode popping often occurs as an isolated event, sometimes highly repetitive popping can occur which can resemble seizure activity. Figure 6.16 shows an example of repetitive electrode popping in the P4 electrode. Note that the adjacent electrodes, O2, C4, and T6, show no evidence of

the deflection. The same effect is seen in Figure 6.17, a deflection that has some resemblance to a spike-wave discharge in T4 is seen to be an electrode pop on closer analysis. Figure 6.18 shows a high-voltage, complex waveform confined to the Fp2 electrode. Again, because this waveform is of moderately high voltage but cannot be detected in the adjacent channels (Fz-Cz, F4-C4, and F8-T4), these deflections are correctly interpreted as an artifact in the Fp2 electrode.

As with most rules, exceptions exist. Is it possible for a true cerebral event to be detectable only in a single electrode? True cerebral events isolated to a single electrode may occur, but they are relatively rare. The phenomenon is most likely to occur with a low-voltage event. Turning up the amplifier gains aggressively can help identify small deflections in adjacent electrodes if they are present. Events localized to a single electrode are more common in newborns than in older children or adults. The higher the voltage of a true cerebral event, the less plausible that it is localized to a single electrode.

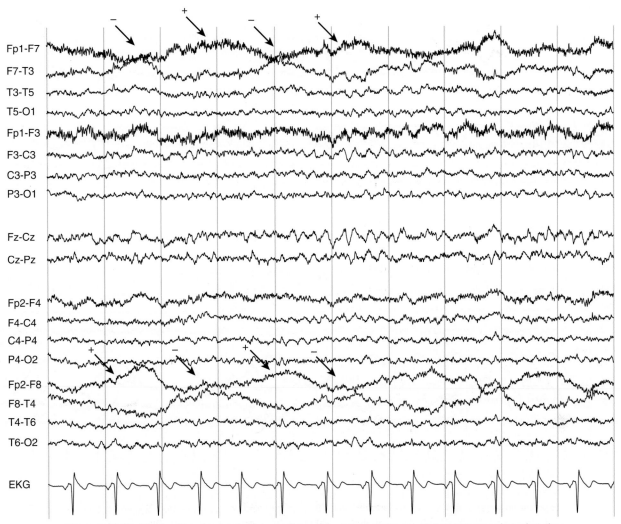

Figure 6.10 Slow roving lateral eye movements of drowsiness have a characteristic appearance based on the polarities seen with lateral eye movement artifact, as described in the previous figure. In this example, "negative phase reversals" are seen in the F7 electrode at the same time as "positive phase reversals" are seen in the F8 electrode (arrows). Each electrode experiences positivities and negativities of more or less equal duration, reflecting sequential slow shifting of the eyes to the left and then to the right under closed eyelids. This differs from voluntary saccadic movements, which manifest sharper waveforms and also do not necessarily give equal time to the leftward and rightward phases of the movements. Depending on the patient's individual physiology, slow roving lateral eye movement artifact may be subtler/lower voltage than the large amplitude waves shown in this tracing, but the pattern will be distinctive and similar.

The Single "Bad Electrode"

A poor electrode contact can cause a distinctive, high-voltage pattern in which adjacent channels in a bipolar montage appear to mirror one another (Figure 6.19; also see 6.16). In this example, the high-voltage pattern seen in the F3-C3 channel is mirrored in the C3-P3 channel, implying a poor electrode contact at C3. It is especially useful to recognize the patterns caused by a poor electrode contact when it only occurs intermittently in a tracing. Knowing that there is a poor contact in C3, the alert reader immediately becomes suspicious of any high-voltage deflection that may be seen at a later time in the recording in that electrode, realizing that it could represent electrode artifact from the poor contact.

OTHER TYPES OF ARTIFACT

Muscle Artifact

Muscle artifact is one of the most commonly encountered artifacts in the EEG and is especially common during wakefulness. Muscle artifact is recorded most often by electrodes that overlie the muscles of the scalp: the frontalis, temporalis, and occipitalis muscles. For that reason, it is the frontopolar and midtemporal electrodes, Fp1, Fp2, T7, and T8, that are most affected (as was seen in Figure 6.7), but most others can be affected as well. Because there is almost no muscle over the vertex of the skull, muscle artifact is usually not seen in the midline (Cz and Pz) electrodes. In fact, this fact can provide a

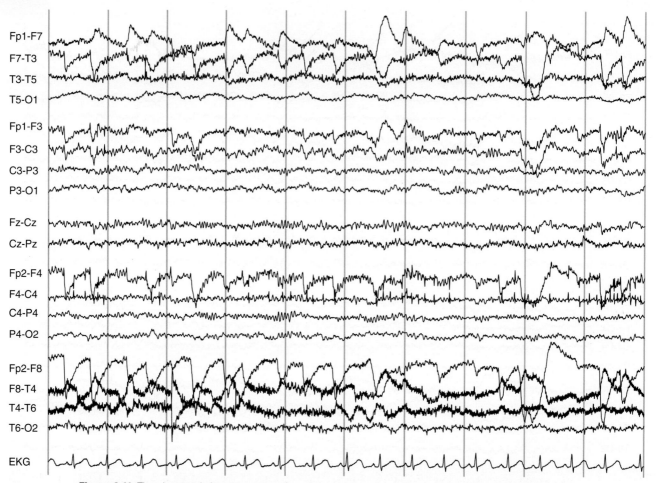

Figure 6.11 The characteristic appearance of nystagmus is seen here in the form of repetitive lateral eye movement artifact with sharp contours, maximum in the anterior temporal electrodes, F7 and F8. Note the opposite polarities at any given time in the F7 and F8 electrodes and compare the more jagged contours of the eye movement artifact seen here with those of the slow roving lateral eye movements in Figure 6.10.

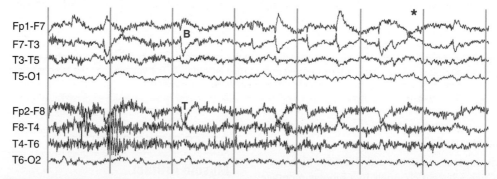

Figure 6.12 Lateral rectus spikes are seen in the left anterior temporal electrode, F7. The timing of the lateral eye movements can be discerned by the presence of a "positive phase reversal," seen at the same time in F7 as a "negative phase reversal" is seen in F8. Lateral eye movements are identified by seeing one anterior temporal channel "bulge apart" (B) at the same time as the opposite channels' traces "come together," (T). A sharp transient is seen at the onset of each positivity in F7. Although this transient does resemble an epileptic spike, the fact that it occurs at the onset of each lateral eye movement helps identify it as a lateral rectus spike artifact on gaze to the left. Although most of the eye movements in this image are to the left, a single slow movement to the right is noted, indicated by the asterisk.

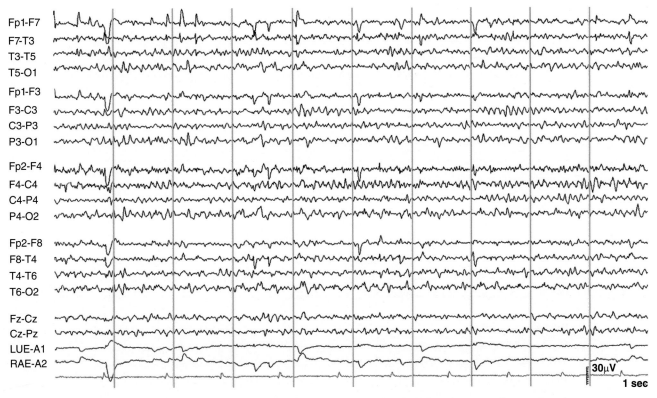

Figure 6.13 The spikes shown on this page are not as easy to identify as lateral rectus spikes compared to the examples shown in the previous figure. The two eye-monitoring channels, LUE-A1 ("left under eye"–left earlobe) and RAE-A2 ("right above eye"–right earlobe), clearly establish that the apparent spikes seen in the F7 electrode correspond to lateral eye movements.

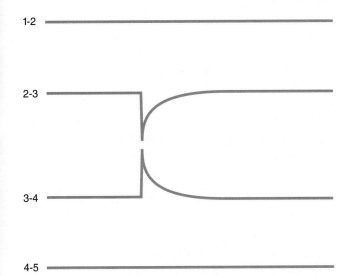

Figure 6.14 A schematic representation of an electrode pop shown in a hypothetical bipolar chain formed from five adjacent electrodes, "1," "2," "3," "4," and "5." The two most characteristic features of an electrode pop artifact are evident in the shape of the discharge and the fact that it is isolated to a single electrode. The shape shown in this figure with a fast upswing and a slow decay is highly suggestive of electrode popping, although electrode pops may assume other shapes as well. This schematic of a high voltage event in Electrode "3" with no voltage change whatsoever in the adjacent electrodes is characteristic of this type of artifact.

nice way to confirm that widespread muscle artifact is, indeed, that (as opposed to diffuse, rapid spikes). If the pattern is diffuse muscle artifact, it should still be relatively underrepresented or absent in the midline electrodes, especially Cz.

Muscle artifact appears as a very fast wave that appears to "turn the channel black." Occasionally muscle artifact can be difficult to distinguish from a train of rapid spikes, although certain characteristics help make the distinction. Muscle artifact usually fires at a fast, uncountable rate, and it can be difficult to appreciate a specific wave morphology from within this rapidly firing, heterogeneous mixture of waves. Muscle artifact usually consists of a mixture of spike-like potentials with variable shape and height. An interesting exception to this rule is the repetitively firing isolated motor unit. This type of artifact appears as a repetitive, low-voltage monomorphic (always the same shape) spike that has a stuttering firing frequency and may persist for varying lengths of time. Although the firing rate does vary, it does not show sustained trends toward speeding up or slowing down as seizures tend to do (Figures 6.20 and 6.21). Motor unit spikes usually do not have an electric field; that is, they are highly confined and not seen in adjacent electrodes. When seen over the temporalis muscle, they may be terminated by asking the patient to relax the jaw, although the firing of an individual motor unit may not be easily under the patient's control.

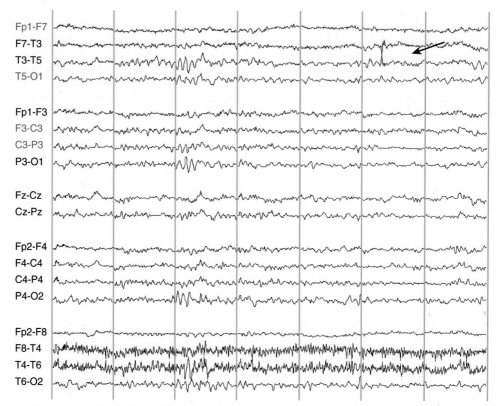

Figure 6.15 A single electrode artifact is noted in the T3 electrode (black arrow). Morphologically, this sharp transient could be difficult to distinguish from a true epileptic spike. The main clue to its noncerebral origin is the complete lack of an electric field in the surrounding electrodes (F7, F3, C3, P3, and T5). This is confirmed by the absence of any simultaneous deflection in the channels that include these electrodes: Fp1-F7, T5-01, F3-C3, and C3-P3 whose channel labels are shaded red.

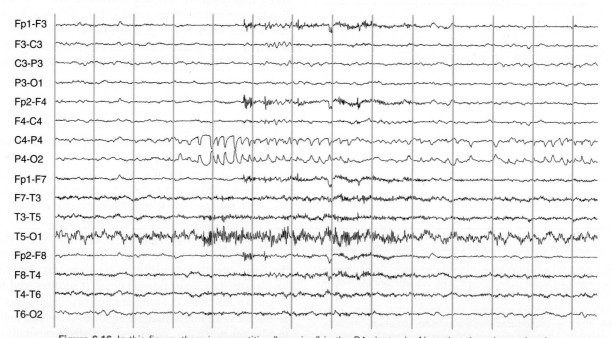

Figure 6.16 In this figure, there is a repetitive "popping" in the P4 electrode. Note that there is no electric field surrounding this event, confirming that it is an artifact; the surrounding electrodes, T6, C4, and O2 are seen to be quiet. (Pz is another adjacent electrode, but does not happen to be included in this montage so it cannot be checked in this example.) If the field of the P4 discharge extended to any of those adjacent electrodes, we would see some deflections in T6-O2, F4-C4, or T4-T6, which are all completely quiet. This could be further confirmed by turning up the amplifier gains aggressively and showing that no simultaneous deflections appear in adjacent channels. Given the repetitive nature of this artifact, it would be possible to mistake it for a seizure discharge. The fact that this waveform is restricted to a single electrode is the clue to its noncerebral origin. The "mirror image" configuration of the C4-P4 and P4-O2 channels is also characteristic.

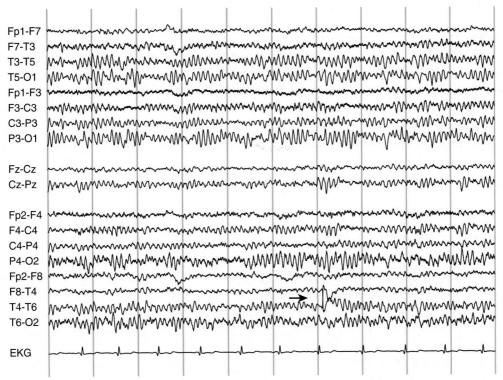

Figure 6.17 The discharge seen in the seventh second of this page in the T4 electrode has a morphology potentially suggestive of a spike-wave complex (arrow). Note that even though the spike deflection is fairly large, there is no evidence of the discharge whatsoever in the adjacent electrodes (C4, T6, or F8). The presence of this relatively high-voltage event in a single electrode helps confirm that it is an electrode artifact rather than a spike-wave complex.

Sweat Artifact

A patient who is sweating may manifest an artifact that consists of long duration, high-voltage potentials recognizable by their distinctive, prolonged shape (Figure 6.22). This slow, swaying artifact is caused by electrolyte bridges that form between adjacent electrodes because of excess sweating. Sweat artifact can be eliminated by anything that stops the patient from sweating, including cooling the room where the EEG is being performed.

EKG Artifact

EKG artifact is usually easy to identify. Its most distinctive features are its shape and its rhythmicity. Most EEG tracings are recorded with a dedicated EKG channel. Suspicion that a spike seen in the EEG is really an example of EKG artifact can be confirmed or excluded by trying to match the timing of the deflection in question with the QRS complex in the EKG channel. This can be done with the vertical cursor. Also, the width of EKG artifact should be similar to the width of the QRS complex in the EKG channel (Figure 6.23A and B).

EKG artifact tends to occur in certain contexts. Because in most individuals the heart is on the left side of the chest cavity and the left ventricle with its thicker muscular wall makes a bigger electrical contribution to the QRS complex than the right ventricle, the left temporal electrodes are most likely to pick up this type of artifact. Patients with higher voltage QRS complexes from ventricular hypertrophy may have greater degrees of EKG contamination in the scalp; in those with right ventricular hypertrophy, the EKG artifact may be more prominent on the right side of the head. Also, patients with wider necks tend to transmit EKG artifact more readily to the head. (If you think of the neck as an electrical wire, the thicker the wire, the more easily EKG signal will be transmitted to the head.) Finally, the height of the EKG complexes as measured on the scalp tend to vary with the respiratory cycle.

Given the fact that EKG signal is present everywhere on the scalp, it is worthwhile to consider why EKG artifact is not seen in every channel. Because almost exactly the same amount of EKG signal is present in adjacent scalp electrodes, the EKG complex efficiently cancels itself out in bipolar comparisons of nearby electrodes. Even many reference electrodes have similar amounts of EKG signal compared with the scalp, yielding EKG-free referential tracings (although the choice of certain references may add an undesirable amount of EKG artifact to the tracing—an effect that is electrode position and patient-dependent).

The unexpected appearance of EKG artifact in a lone electrode can serve as a clue to a poor electrode contact. When two electrodes that have been applied well and have good impedances are subtracted from one another, the EKG

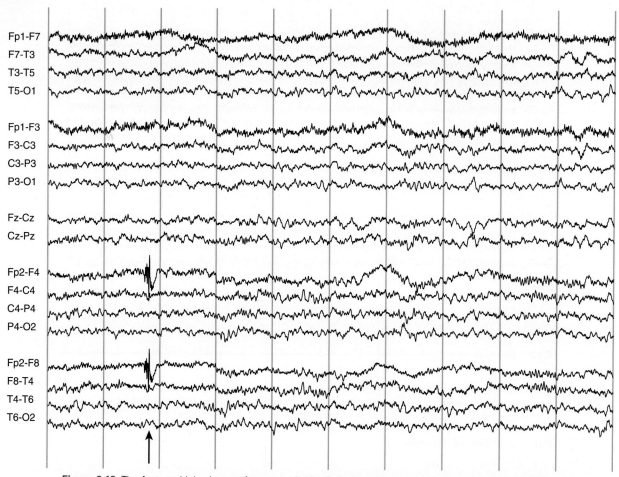

Figure 6.18 The fast, multiphasic waveform seen in the Fp2 electrode (arrow) is more complex than what has been seen in previous examples and clearly represents an example of electrode artifact. Once again, the key feature is that the event is restricted to a single electrode. The cause of such artifacts is not always clear. Possible explanations include a poor electrode contact, the patient touching the electrode, or some other momentary electrical contamination of the electrode. Also note the longer duration artifact in Fp1, which is a clue to a poor contact.

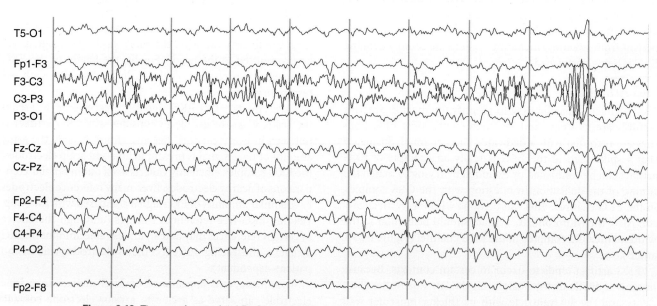

Figure 6.19 The waveforms of the F3-C3 and C3-P3 channels mirror each other and are of higher voltage than their neighbors. Note that, notwithstanding this high voltage activity mirrored activity in these two channels, the adjacent channels (e.g., Fp1-F3 and P3-O1) seem "oblivious" to it. This characteristic pattern is caused by a faulty electrode contact at C3. In the meantime, true spike activity can be seen in C4.

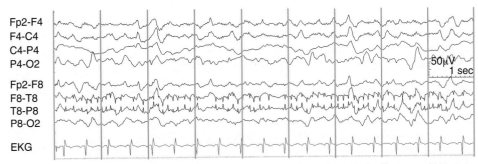

Figure 6.20 A spike-like discharge is seen in the T8 electrode and represents an artifact caused by a repetitively firing motor unit. The discharge does not maintain a trend toward speeding up or slowing down but has a sputtering characteristic. No electric field is detected by adjacent electrodes.

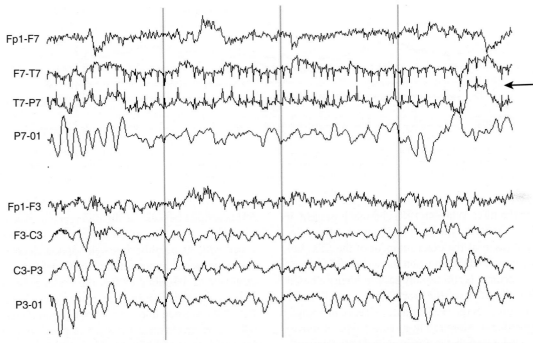

Figure 6.21 A continuously firing motor unit is seen in the channels shared by the T7 electrode (arrow). The unchanging morphology and the lack of a sustained tendency toward speeding up or slowing down help identify this as a motor unit artifact. One way of demonstrating that these repetitive spikes have no adjacent field would be to cover up the F7-T7 and T7-P7 channels so they cannot be seen. Without them, would you have any idea when the spike is firing from the channels that remain visible, even if you increased the amplitude of all the channels by turning up the amplifier gains?

artifact cancels out efficiently. When there is a poor electrode contact, however, the poorly applied electrode picks up the EKG signal to a different extent than its properly applied neighbors. When the signal from the good electrode is subtracted from the signal from the bad electrode, there is a net difference in the amount of EKG picked up by the two, and the net difference will appear in the display as EKG artifact.

Apart from the situation of poorly applied electrodes, EKG artifact would be expected to appear when any two regions of the scalp are compared that carry different amounts of EKG signal for anatomical reasons. The most common example of this is seen in the transverse bipolar montage in the channel where the left earlobe is compared with the left midtemporal electrode (A1-T7). For anatomical reasons, the left earlobe carries less EKG signal than the left midtemporal area in most patients. Because of the left-sided orientation of the heart in most individuals, the same effect is seen but less dramatically on the opposite side when T8 is compared with A2 (see Figure 6.23). Among all the electrode pairs in standard bipolar chains, these pairings are the most likely to manifest EKG artifact in normal patients with well-applied electrodes.

Pulse Artifact

Pulse artifact is seen when one electrode happens to be placed directly on an artery in the scalp (often the temporal artery), creating an artifactual waveform related to the pulsations. This type of artifact has also been called the *hemoballistogram* or *ballistogram*. In this case, a wide pulse artifact is seen in

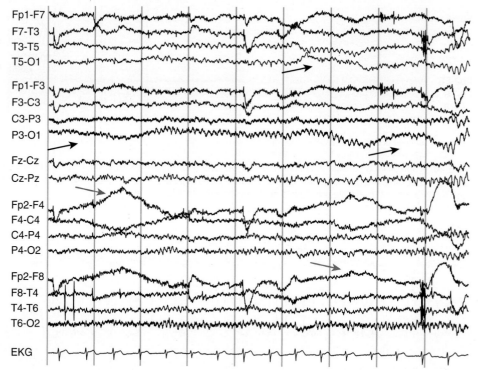

Figure 6.22 Sweat artifact usually appears as slow, wandering deviations of a channel's baseline. In this example, sweat artifact can be seen in the posterior channels on the left (black arrows). Anteriorly, the large deflections may be caused by a combination of some eye movement artifact and sweat artifact (gray arrows).

synchrony with the EKG. When an EKG channel is present, it is easy to link this artifact to the heart rate (note that the pulse artifact does not occur at the exact moment of the EKG but follows it by a set interval). Even when there is no EKG channel, this type of artifact is still usually easy to identify based on its heartbeat-like rhythm, the fact that it is much wider than the QRS complex of the EKG, and its presence in a single electrode (Figure 6.24). More rarely, a related type of movement artifact may be seen that is synchronized to the patient's EKG in cases in which the patient's body makes a low-amplitude rocking movement with a hyperdynamic heartbeat.

60 Hz (50 Hz) Artifact

The problem of 60 Hz artifact is discussed in more detail in Chapter 7, "Filters in the EEG," as a specific filter is available to help suppress this type of artifact. It may be surprising to hear that small but easily measurable amounts of AC current from the power mains that surround us flow through the patient's body in indoor situations (like EEG laboratories) all of the time, accounting for this type of artifact. (In countries that use line frequencies of 50 Hz, 50 Hz artifact is seen instead.) Because this small amount of 60 Hz current is present in similar amounts throughout the body in most recording environments, this signal is usually canceled out by the subtraction process used by the common mode rejection amplifiers in the same way that EKG artifact is canceled out as described above. Here again and similar to the case of EKG artifact, a poorly applied electrode is more likely to manifest

60 Hz artifact because of the difference between the amount of 60 Hz activity the poorly applied electrode picks up compared with its neighboring well-applied electrodes. As with the unexpected appearance of EKG artifact in an isolated electrode as described earlier, the presence of 60 Hz artifact only in channels that include a particular electrode suggests that that electrode may have a poor contact (Figures 6.25 and 6.26). The mechanism by which a poor contact may cause the appearance of 60 Hz (or EKG) artifact is summarized in Figure 6.27A and B.

Electrical Artifacts from External Equipment

Many machines used in medical settings give off a variety of electrical signals. Fortunately, it is the nature of most of these devices to give off signals in a highly regular fashion. Electronic intravenous fluid pumps are a well-known source of repetitive electrical artifact. Mechanical ventilators and electric hospital beds are other possible sources of interference (see Fig 6.28A and B). A waveform that occurs with precise regularity is almost never of biological origin. Even though the electrocardiogram is generally considered a regular wave, when carefully measured, small variations are always seen between beats. When electrical complexes are seen in the EEG with strict regularity (no variation in the interval between the complexes), these almost always represent signals from medical devices. Repetitive, highly stereotyped, complex waveforms (i.e., unusually-shaped waves that have the exact same appearance every time) are also

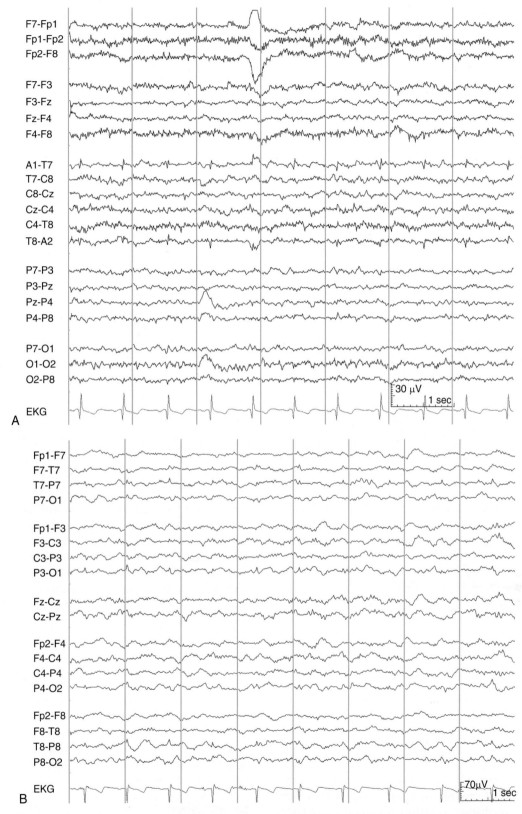

Figure 6.23 **(A)** Electrocardiogram (EKG) artifact is seen in the A1-T7 and T8-A2 channels. This spike-like artifact lines up with each QRS complex in the EKG channel. Because the amount of EKG signal differs between the earlobe and the midtemporal electrode, these two channels are a common location for EKG artifact to appear. Unlike in this example, in most patients the artifact is often of higher amplitude on the left compared with the right. Also note the appearance of eyeblink artifact in a transverse montage in the top three channels at the end of the third second. Can you work out why an eyeblink causes the Fp1-Fp2 channel to be generally flat, while the F7-Fp1 channel goes up and the Fp2-F8 channel goes down? **(B)** Even without the aid of the EKG channel, the regularity of the low amplitude spike-like artifact seen in multiple channels makes it readily identifiable as EKG artifact.

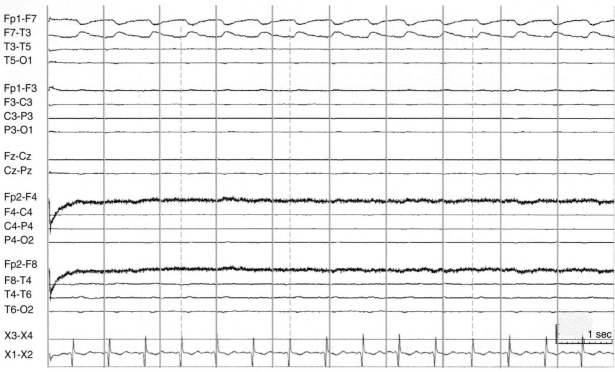

Figure 6.24 The regular, rounded deflections in the top two channels of this otherwise suppressed EEG represent pulse artifact in the F7 electrode, which likely lies on the temporal artery. Note that the EKG complexes consistently line up with the same "bulging" phase of each wave (denoted by the broken vertical lines). Although pulse artifact will be synchronized with the EKG, note that the shape of the artifact with its slow, rounded waveform is quite different from the spike-like appearance of EKG artifact. A poor contact in Fp2 causes the appearance of 60 Hz artifact in the two channels that include that electrode.

suspicious for electrical artifact. Other electrical devices that patients may have in use, such as cell phone chargers, and so forth, may occasionally cause electrical artifact in the EEG.

Special Types of Motion Artifact

Certain types of motion artifact are seen fairly frequently in the EEG. Respiratory artifact occurs when breathing motions cause a gentle rocking of the head with each breath, especially in the sleeping or comatose patient. Usually, the electrodes in contact with the bed (often the occipital or temporal electrodes) are preferentially involved. Linking the occurrence of what is usually a broad artifactual wave to the respiratory cycle can definitively establish the source of this type of artifact. This task is made considerably easier when a respiratory channel is in use. Ventilator artifact can be considered a subset of either respiratory artifact or motion artifact; wave artifacts may be created by body movements induced by the ventilator. A special case of ventilator artifact is seen with high-frequency oscillating ventilators, which can cause high-frequency motion artifacts (see Figures 6.29 and 6.30).

Patting artifact occurs most frequently in children but is also seen in adults. When the patient's back is patted, a repetitive and regular motion artifact may appear in the EEG (see Figure 6.31). Chest physical therapy artifact may also cause a similar appearance. Usually, patting rhythms are maintained fairly regularly throughout their duration; it is uncommon for a caregiver's patting rate to increase or decrease substantially throughout its course, and abrupt pauses are common (Figure 6.32). This differs from seizure activity, which tends to gradually evolve in frequency throughout its course. The implied polarity of patting artifact waves usually is not "biologically plausible" for electrocerebral activity.

Hiccup Artifact

Hiccup artifact is a special type of motion artifact associated with hiccupping. Because each hiccup usually causes a similar movement in the patient, the EEG artifact caused by hiccupping is often fairly stereotyped (Figure 6.33). Occasionally, hiccup artifact may resemble a polyspike discharge, but the field of the artifact is usually irregular enough that the distinction is not difficult.

Breach Rhythm

The breach rhythm is a distinctive rhythm that can be considered an artifact of a skull defect, usually from a previous neurosurgical procedure (a breach in the skull is a gap in the skull). Defects in the skull tend to allow preferential

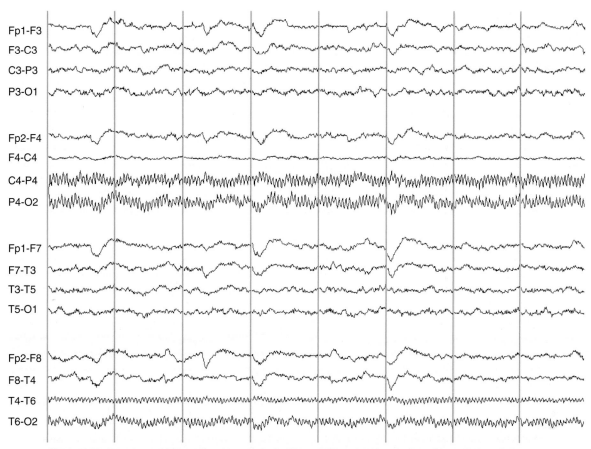

Figure 6.25 Prominent 60 Hz artifact is seen in the P4 and T6 electrodes. At first glance, 60 Hz artifact can be mistaken for muscle artifact, but the highly regular, sinusoidal pattern of the waves in these channels is not consistent with muscle activity. Sixty-hertz artifact may be seen at exactly 60 Hz, or as a subharmonic of 60 Hz. In this example, the artifact has a frequency of exactly 20 Hz. Sixty-hertz artifact can often be eliminated after the fact with the use of a 60 Hz notch filter (see Chapter 7, "Filters in the EEG"). Use of the 60 Hz notch filter may also produce a subharmonic of 60 Hz when 60 Hz contamination is high. It is important to keep in mind, however, that even though it may be easy to eliminate this artifact with the notch filter, the presence of the artifact tells us that P4 and T6 have poor contacts (bad impedance), making it more likely that they will generate spurious (artifactual) waveforms elsewhere in the record.

transmission of high-frequency activities. For this reason, higher voltage fast rhythms may be present over the area of a previous craniotomy site. Breach rhythms are discussed in more detail in Chapter 11, "Normal Variants in the EEG."

Chewing and Bruxism Artifact

Chewing artifact is usually easy to recognize, appearing as brief, repetitive muscle bursts from the jaw muscles, maximum in the temporal areas (Figure 6.34). Chewing artifact can be seen while the patient is eating but sometimes occurs as a "nervous habit" even when the patient has nothing in his or her mouth. Chewing artifact may also be seen associated with chewing automatisms during focal seizures with impaired awareness. Bruxism (tooth grinding) usually occurs during sleep, but may also be seen during wakefulness, especially in individuals with intellectual disability. Its appearance is similar

to chewing artifact because both involve rhythmic tensing of the jaw muscles. Bruxism artifact is of longer duration and occurs at a slower pace than chewing artifact (Figure 6.35).

Glossokinetic Artifact

Glossokinetic artifact is generated by movements of the tongue, which also has a net dipole (much like the globe of the eye), with the tip of the tongue being negative relative to the base. If necessary, the appearance of this artifact in a tracing can be confirmed by having the patient reproduce it on the EEG by request. The patient is asked to move the tongue forward in the mouth repetitively by repeating syllables such as "la-la-la" or "ta-ta-ta." The field of glossokinetic artifact can extend over the whole scalp in some patients and can be recorded at highest voltage by electrodes placed on the face (Figure 6.36).

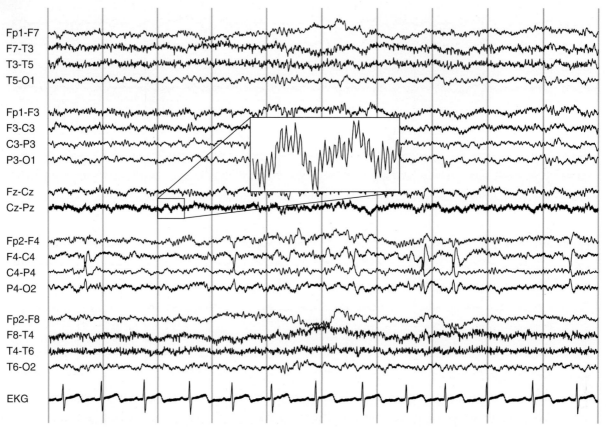

Figure 6.26 Sixty-hertz artifact in the Cz-Pz channel magnified to show the shape of the wave. Unmagnified, the channel simply looks "dark," but close inspection reveals a 60 Hz sinusoidal wave. The magnified area represents one half second. Because 30 waves are counted within the half-second area, the artifact's frequency is 60 Hz.

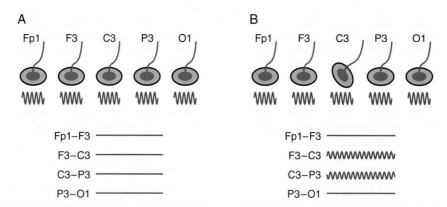

Figure 6.27 Panel **A** of this figure shows the real-life example of 60 Hz artifact being present under each of the scalp electrodes, Fp1, F3, C3, P3, and O1 in this example. Because bipolar montages only display the difference between each electrode and its neighbor, if the 60 Hz activity is the same under each electrode and each electrode is applied in the same way, this activity will completely cancel out in all of the bipolar pairs, yielding the clean tracings shown at the bottom of the panel. In Panel **B**, we can see that the C3 electrode either was not applied correctly or became loose during the recording. Now C3 is picking up the 60 Hz artifact differently than its neighbors. When C3 is compared to F3 in F3-C3, or to P3 in C3-P3, when the subtractions are made the difference in the signals picked up by those electrode pairs causes the artifact to appear in those channels. Because of this effect, the presence of 60 Hz artifact usually implies an impedance problem in the involved electrode(s).

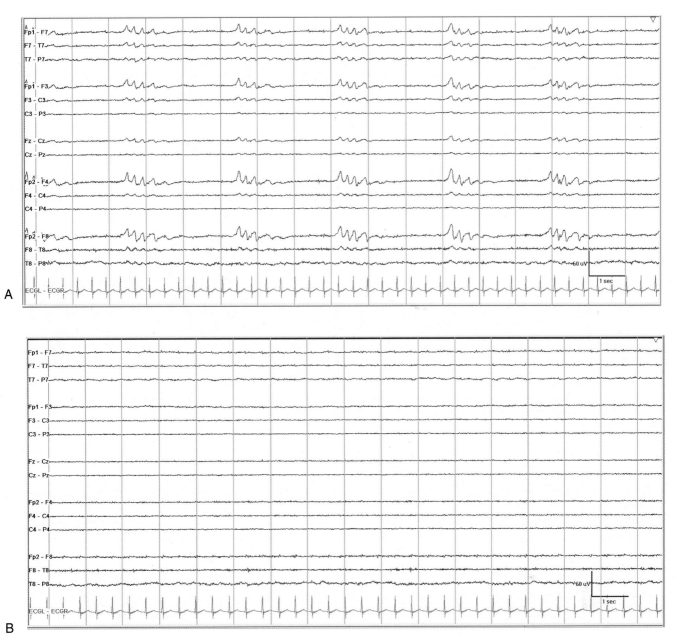

Figure 6.28 Panel **A:** This unusual and repetitive artifact was seen in a ventilated patient with a severe traumatic brain injury and a very low voltage EEG. The possibility that the repetitive pattern could represent an epileptiform discharge or a periodic pattern should be considered, but the stereotyped nature of the waveform makes it suspicious for artifact. Panel **B:** This wave was proven to represent ventilator artifact as it disappeared completely after the patient's endotracheal tube was suctioned. The small rippling waveform was caused by "gurgling" of fluid inside the patient's endotracheal tube before suctioning.

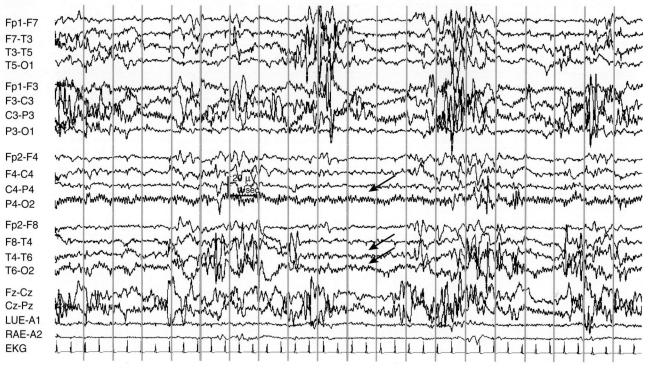

Figure 6.29 Motion artifact related to a high-frequency ("HiFi") ventilator is seen in three channels (arrows). The highly regular waveform is an indicator that this waveform is of mechanical rather than cerebral origin. Based on the electrodes that are involved, can you guess this baby's head position?

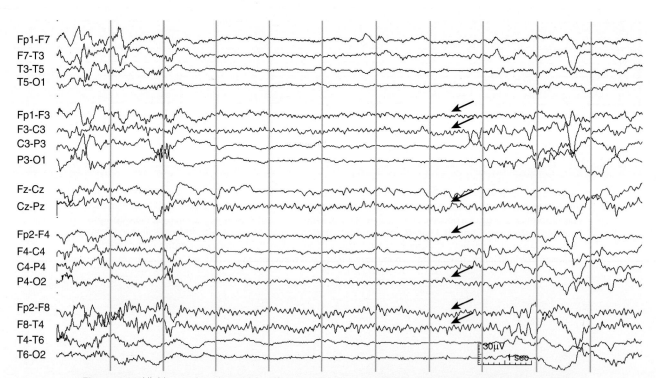

Figure 6.30 Highly regular, sinusoidal artifact caused by an oscillating ventilator can be seen in multiple channels (arrows). The long duration, "patchy" localization, and lack of frequency evolution help distinguish this waveform from a seizure discharge. If there is a question about whether these waves could be of cerebral original, asking that the patient's head be repositioned will likely clarify that this is an artifact related to ventilator-associated head motion. Moving the patient's head may cause the artifact to disappear from some channels and reappear in others.

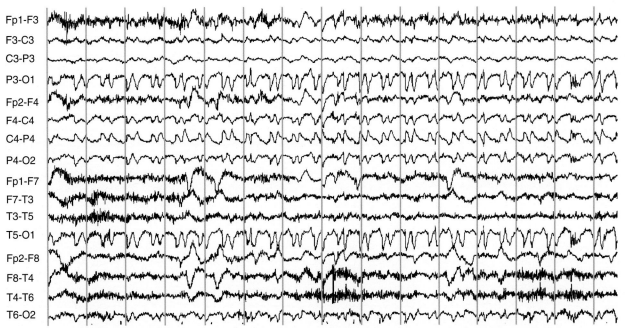

Figure 6.31 Rhythmic discharges are seen in several channels of this EEG, some of which resemble spike-wave complexes in morphology. Close analysis of the waveforms shows that the discharges do not make "topographic sense." Negativities are seen adjacent to positivities, and high-voltage deflections are seen in certain electrodes, while immediately adjacent electrodes are silent. These waves represent patting artifact rather than seizure activity.

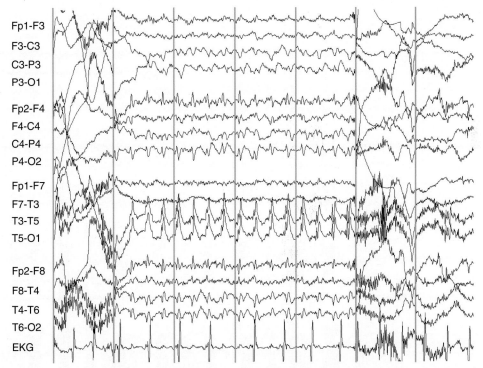

Figure 6.32 The large amount of motion artifact seen in the first second of this page is related to the patient crying. The Rhythmic, high-voltage deflections that neither speed up nor slow down and do not have a plausible electric field represent patting artifact. After the patting stops, high voltage artifact in the last two seconds of the page indicate that the baby has resumed crying.

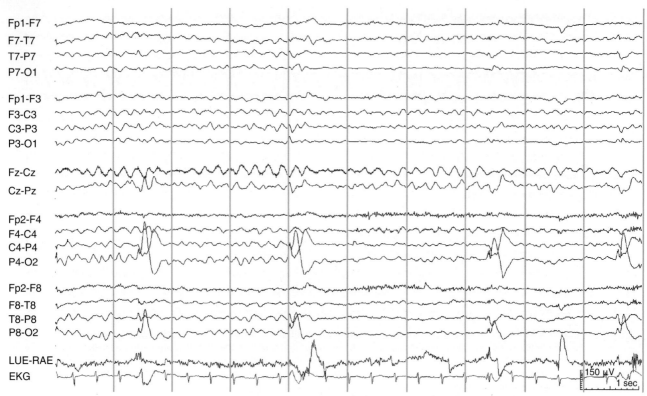

Figure 6.33 The four high-voltage deflections seen over the right posterior quadrant represent hiccup artifact. The patient is lying with her head turned to the right so that each hiccupping movement creates a relatively stereotyped pattern of motion artifact from the electrodes lying in contact with the bed.

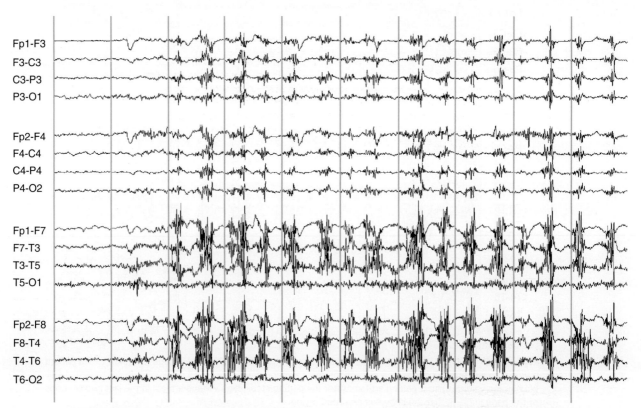

Figure 6.34 Chewing movements create rhythmic bursts of muscle artifact, maximum over the temporalis muscle. Note that in this montage, the temporal chains are arranged at the bottom of the page, which is why most of the artifact is seen in the bottom eight channels.

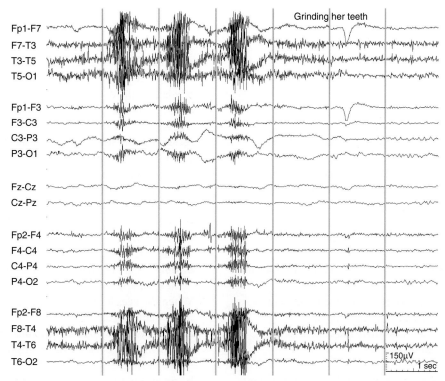

Figure 6.35 The bursts of temporal muscle artifact seen with bruxism are often of slightly longer duration and have longer intervals than chewing artifact. Note that, despite the high-voltage muscle activity seen in the temporal areas, the midline electrodes (Fz, Cz, and Pz) are free of artifact because of the relative absence of scalp muscle in these areas.

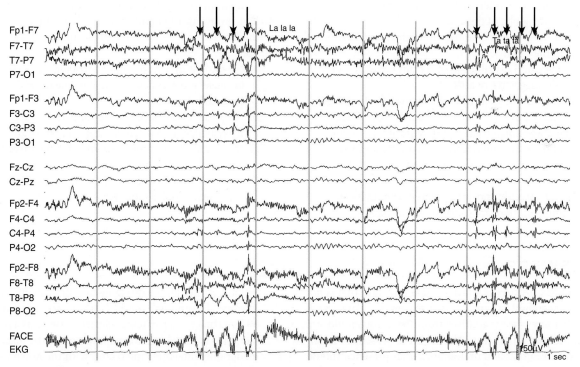

Figure 6.36 Glossokinetic artifact is caused by motion of the tongue, demonstrated in this case by asking the patient to speak repetitive syllables (arrows). The artifact may also appear spontaneously during tongue movements associated with speaking or swallowing. The glossokinetic artifact may have both slow wave and spiky components, as in this example. Characteristically, this type of artifact has a broad field across the scalp and especially over the face, as demonstrated by the placement of a face electrode and displayed in the second channel from the bottom labeled "FACE," which the technologist applied to prove that this was an example of glossokinetic artifact. Courtesy of Maria DeBurgo, R. EEG T.

REVIEW QUESTIONS

1. Regarding artifacts in the EEG,
   a. a good reader screens out and ignores artifacts because the point of EEG interpretation is to read the brain waves.
   b. REMS should not be considered an artifact because they indicate to the reader the onset of REM sleep
   c. if a wave comes from the brain, it should not be considered an artifact.
   d. EEGs that have a lot of 60 Hz artifact should always be recorded using a 60 Hz notch filter to render the EEG readable.

2. EKG artifact
   a. should not appear in the head because the head is distant from the heart.
   b. may indicate a poor electrode contact if it only appears in a single scalp electrode.
   c. is generally more effectively eliminated in referential montages as compared to bipolar montages.
   d. cannot be identified unless there is a concurrently recorded EKG channel.

3. Eyeblink artifact
   a. is caused by the positive charge on the eyelids moving up and down during blinking.
   b. arises from the eyeblink center in the frontal lobes.
   c. will still occur on both sides of the EEG when the patient blinks even if the patient is missing one eyeball.
   d. is related to the differential charge on the front and back of the globe of the eye.

4. Which of these is not true regarding the identification of artifact in the EEG?
   a. The shape and distribution of certain waves can be strongly suggestive of artifact.
   b. Figuring out the polarity and location of a discharge in the EEG is a first good step to identifying artifact.
   c. When a waveform has a region of positivity in one area of the scalp and negativity in another, this is inconsistent with electrocerebral activity and the wave should be labeled an artifact.
   d. Areas of abruptly appearing charge without a surrounding gradient are suggestive of artifact.

5. The best way to identify an electrode "pop" is to
   a. establish that the discharge is only appearing in a single electrode.
   b. identify the distinctive shape of a "pop".
   c. ascertain that the waveform is associated with a patient movement on the video.
   d. identify the wave in multiple electrodes at one time.

6. Hemoballistogram artifact
   a. should occur at the exact same time as the EKG, because it is pulse-related.
   b. resembles the QRS complex because it is from the heartbeat.
   c. sometimes is time-linked to the EKG, and sometimes it is not.
   d. only occurs by chance when an electrode is applied near an artery.

7. When the eyes look to the right, the associated lateral eye movement artifact
   a. does not allow the reader to discern if the eyes are moving to the left versus the right without checking the video.
   b. manifests a negativity in F7 and a positivity in F8.
   c. manifests a positivity in both F7 and F8, because both corneas have a positive charge.
   d. can be seen if it is from a rapid eye movement during dream sleep, but not if it is just a voluntary gaze movement to the right during wakefulness with eyes open.

8. You review an EEG and there is EKG artifact confined to the C4 electrode in the AP bipolar montage. You conclude that
   a. the patient may have right ventricular hypertrophy because in patients with a normal heart, EKG artifact is usually seen on the left.
   b. the patient may have an unusually thick neck because EKG artifact is not usually seen in that location.
   c. there is likely an impedance mismatch between the C4 electrode and the other electrodes.
   d. the EKG artifact will disappear if you switch to the transverse bipolar montage.

ANSWERS

1. ANSWER: **C.** An artifact is defined as any wave that is not of electrocerebral origin. For that reason, the converse is true, that any wave that arises from the brain should not be considered an artifact. Although the presence of artifact in the EEG is often undesirable, their presence should not be ignored because artifacts often convey useful information. The simple presence of muscle artifact or eyeblink artifact suggests that the patient is awake. Other eye movement artifact, such as slow roving eye movements of drowsiness and REMS may also be informative in defining the current sleep state, but they should still be considered artifact. Although the 60 Hz notch filter can go a long way toward "cleaning up" the EEG, the presence of increased 60 Hz artifact in a particular electrode suggests a poor contact. This is valuable information that can be missed if the reader only interprets the record with the notch filter "in." The notch filter should always be "out" (off) at the start of reading an EEG study. Once the pattern of 60 Hz artifact has been appreciated, it may be desirable to use the notch filter. If the notch filter is in use, it may be useful to turn it off from time to time to confirm that there are no new problems with electrode contacts.

2. ANSWER: **B**. In fact, EKG artifact is present throughout the whole body, including the head and limbs. For that reason, it may come as a surprise that one does not see EKG artifact in every channel all the time. The strategy used by bipolar montages helps suppress EKG artifact. Because adjacent electrodes in a chain should have similar amounts of EKG artifact, the artifact should disappear when one electrode is subtracted from an adjacent electrode. However, in a bipolar chain, when there is a single poor contact, the amount of EKG picked up by neighboring electrodes may differ because of a poor electrode application. When the subtraction is made, the difference between how much EKG is picked up by the "bad" electrode and the "good" electrode will be displayed in the channel. Because bipolar montages subtract adjacent electrodes (which will have similar amounts of EKG artifact), these are generally more effective in canceling EKG artifact than referential montages. This is because referential montages may use a more distant reference/comparison electrode which, because of its greater distance from the scalp-recording electrode, may pick up EKG artifact in a slightly different way, and that difference will appear in the EEG. Although it is more challenging to do so, EKG artifact usually can be identified even without a separate EKG channel to match up the complexes. EKG artifact should be narrow, similar to an EKG QRS complex. It should also appear in a regular fashion at a rate consistent with the patient's expected heartrate.

3. ANSWER: **D**. Eyeblink artifact is caused by the positive charge on the cornea of the eye. Eyelid movement is actually not a major factor in creating eyeblink artifact. Eyeblinking unto itself is not associated with a measurable change in frontal lobe activity on the EEG and the EEG waves seen during eyeblinking do not come from the brain. Because eyeblink artifact is generated from the globe bobbing up and down during eyeblinking, patients who lack one globe will only manifest unilateral eyeblink artifact.

4. ANSWER: **C**. The shape and distribution of a wave can be highly suggestive of artifact. For example, eyeblink artifact consists of high voltage positivities seen in the frontal areas, which cause downgoing deflections in the frontal channels in both AP bipolar and referential montages. Muscle artifact consists of very fast activity seen maximally in the scalp areas that have the most muscle (temporal, frontal, etc.). Identifying the combination of wave shape and wave location can be very useful in determining the nature of a wave. One of the most powerful methods in identifying artifacts is establishing the polarity and location of a wave on the scalp. Because certain patterns are so complicated and abrupt that they are not biologically plausible, this will help determine that they represent artifact. Although the appearance of a simultaneous negativity and positivity on the scalp is not common, it does not necessarily indicate that a wave is an artifact, and this specific pattern is well-known to appear, for instance, in children with benign rolandic epilepsy and trait. Discharges with a

horizontal or tangential dipole may manifest just this pattern (see Figure 6.3).

5. ANSWER: **A**. An electrode pop will generally occur in only a single electrode at a time. Electrode pops do not have a surrounding field, which helps identify them. Although electrode pops often have a distinctive shape, sometimes the morphology of popping artifact varies and its shape cannot be used, in and of itself, to confirm with certainty that a waveform is an electrode pop. The fact of single electrode involvement is, therefore, the most useful tool in identifying an electrode pop. Electrode pops usually occur spontaneously, and are not necessarily associated with patient movement. A discharge that occurs in multiple electrodes at one time is unlikely to represent an electrode pop. Reapplying the electrode and observing disappearance of the electrode pop can confirm its nature as an artifact.

6. ANSWER: **D**. The hemoballistogram artifact does not occur at the exact same time as the EKG, but rather follows it with a fixed time lag. This is because there are time lags between the electrical EKG impulse, the squeezing of the heart muscle, and the subsequent transmission of the pulse up to the head. Hemoballistogram artifact does not resemble the EKG complex at all (which tends to be narrow and spiky in appearance), but rather has a rounded and longer contour. This is because the artifact is not related to an electrical complex, but rather is a motion artifact related to movement of the arterial wall by the pulse, which in turn causes the movement of the overlying electrode if it happened to be placed near an artery.

7. ANSWER: **B**. The direction of a lateral eye movement is easily discerned from the artifact that it produces. With a movement of the eyes to the right, the right cornea presents a positive charge to the F8 electrode and the posterior pole/retina of the left eye can be thought of as presenting a negative charge to the F7 electrode. This results in a simultaneous "negative phase reversal" on the left (F7) and a "positive phase reversal" on the right (F8) when the eyes move to the right. Lateral eye movement artifact has the potential to be equally well seen during wakefulness (e.g., searching or voluntary eye movements), drowsiness (slow roving eye movements of drowsiness), and sleep (REMS).

8. ANSWER: **C**. Although it is true that right ventricular hypertrophy (or right axis deviation) would make it more likely that EKG artifact would appear on the right side of the head, it would not explain the isolated appearance of the artifact in the C4 electrode. As mentioned in the text, EKG artifact is most likely to be evident in the T8-A2 pairing in the transverse bipolar montage as compared to A1-T7 in individuals with greater right-sided cardiac forces, but this would not explain the presence of the artifact only in C4. Although it is also true that having a thick neck facilitates the transmission of EKG artifact to the head and scalp as a whole, again, it would not account for its appearance in a single electrode. The best explanation for this situation is that the C4 electrode has a poor contact and its impedance differs from its

neighbors. For that reason, when the EKG contamination in C4 is subtracted from the EKG contamination in adjacent electrodes, there will be a difference in the EKG signals when the comparisons are made and it will appear at the position of the poor contact in bipolar recordings. The presence of artifact in a single electrode warns the reader ahead of time that any unusual signals at that location may be caused by a poor contact. The phenomenon of isolated EKG artifact only in channels involving C4 will also be seen in a transverse bipolar montage for the same reason it is seen in the AP bipolar montage, so switching to that montage will not eliminate the artifact or solve the problem.

7

Filters in the Electroencephalogram

The use of filters in recording and displaying EEG data is an indispensable tool in producing interpretable EEG tracings. Without filters, many segments of EEG would be essentially unreadable. As we shall see in this chapter, the use of filters can affect the EEG signal in ways that range from the subtle to the dramatic. The main benefit of filters is that they can appear to "clean up" the EEG tracing, making it easier to interpret and generally more pleasing to the eye. Certain filter settings can also be used to accentuate particular types of EEG activity that might otherwise be hidden in other activity. Filters can, however, be used improperly at times leading to unintended consequences, the most problematic being changing the shape of a wave, which might otherwise clearly represent an artifact when unfiltered, into something that can easily be mistaken for a real brainwave. During routine EEG interpretation, it is not always necessary to choose filter settings consciously, as almost all laboratories have a standard set of filter settings that are put in place at the beginning of every EEG recording. It is up to the reader to adjust these as needed during the reading process.

Some consider the study of how filters work an inherently dry topic. The purpose of this chapter is to provide a simple technical overview of how EEG filters work so that they can be used appropriately by the EEG technologist and reader. Keep in mind, however, that as you learn about filters there are two levels at which you might decide to understand the topic. The first and most practical level is developing an understanding of the impact a change in filter settings will have on the *visual* appearance of the EEG. The second level is to understand filters at the electronics or mathematical level. That second, more sophisticated level of understanding is perhaps not always necessary for day-to-day EEG interpretation, but it will enrich the reader's understanding of the whole matter. Those who do wish a deeper understanding of the topic or who would simply enjoy a review of electric circuits may benefit from the basic discussion of circuits and filters that follows later in this chapter, as these circuits form the basis of the behavior of filters that we use in modern EEG machines. Also, some EEG certifications that the reader may seek may require this knowledge. Therefore, identify your goals as you read this chapter, distinguishing your progress in understanding the visual impact that filters have on the EEG, which is important to all readers, from the mathematical behavior of filters, which will only a be of interest to some readers. There follows a basic discussion of electronics and simple circuit design for analog EEG filters, a topic that has traditionally been a part of electroencephalography training. The basis of some of the digital techniques used to filter EEG signals is also introduced.

Figures 7.1 and 7.2 illustrate the impact of filters on a fairly messy page of EEG, as may be encountered from time to time in daily recordings. The first figure (Figure 7.1) shows an EEG recorded during a moderate amount of patient movement, a "raw" EEG trace displayed without the explicit use of filters. The second figure (Figure 7.2) shows the same page displayed with typical filter settings. Note that, even though muscle artifact still obliterates portions of the top four and bottom four channels of the EEG (the temporal areas), in the filtered example the amplitude of that muscle artifact is reduced, making it easier to see adjacent channels. Indeed, in the filtered example, the tracing is improved enough that the presence of certain waveforms can be intermittently recognized within the areas of muscle artifact (caused by contraction of the underlying temporalis muscles) that otherwise would not have been detectable. Also note that the baseline of each channel is flatter, allowing for easier interpretation—each channel is more likely to stay within its own horizontal area after the filters are used. The bottom channel of the tracing, T6-O2 (among others), is a good example of this effect. Instead of flying up and down and even crossing the EKG channel as it does in the unfiltered example, it is now restricted to its own "alleyway" and is more interpretable. We refer to the "explicit" use of filters here to remind us that, even when no specific filter settings are specified, our electroencephalograph's hardware and software do have certain limitations in terms of what they are able to record and display. For instance, if there were a 2,000 Hz signal coming from the brain, our EEG setups would not be able to reproduce that waveform. This reminds us that all electronic recording systems may be filtering out some types of activity based on the architecture of the electronics and software in use.

There are also potential pitfalls in choosing filter settings. When using filters on a page of EEG that has a cluttered appearance, one might think that if a given filter setting works moderately well, then even more aggressive settings might work even better. With filters, however, the strategy of "more is better" often does not hold true because implicit to the act of filtering the EEG signal is the potential for loss of information. Overzealous filter settings can overly "clean" the EEG, resulting in the filtering out and disappearance of waveforms that may otherwise have been of interest to the reader. As we shall see, some filter settings can even change the shape

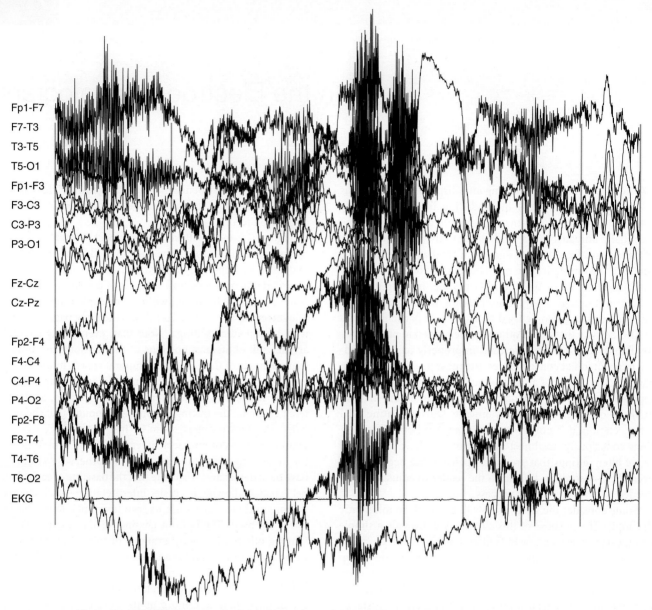

Fp1-F7
F7-T3
T3-T5
T5-O1
Fp1-F3
F3-C3
C3-P3
P3-O1

Fz-Cz
Cz-Pz

Fp2-F4
F4-C4
C4-P4
P4-O2
Fp2-F8
F8-T4
T4-T6
T6-O2
EKG

Figure 7.1 This EEG page was obtained without the explicit use of filters. Muscle artifact obliterates much of the temporal chains (the top four and bottom four EEG channels). The baselines of certain channels fluctuate so widely that they often obliterate other channels. Note that the bottom two channels even dip below the EKG channel. Most of these high voltage deflections are caused by patient movement. Compare to Figure 7.2.

of brain waves in a way that might suggest the presence of waveforms that are not really there.

BANDPASSES AND THE BASIC STRATEGY BEHIND CHOOSING FILTER SETTINGS

The most "ideal" filter design would be one that removes all the electrical noise or artifact from the EEG and only allows true cerebral activity to pass through. Unfortunately, no such "smart" filter exists. Filters are not "reading" the EEG and making decisions about what is what, like you or I do; they can only remove waves according to rigid mathematical rules. Luckily, there are good rationales for filtering out certain components of EEG signals using fairly simple mathematical assumptions. The core assumptions are based on the idea that

the brain only generates EEG waves within a certain range of frequencies and that any activity outside that range (unusually slow activity and unusually fast activity) is not likely to be of cerebral origin. Indeed, one of the basic assumptions of EEG filter design is that waveforms well below 1 Hz and well above 35 Hz do not arise from the brain and likely represent electrical noise or movement or other artifact. Like many assumptions, this claim is substantially true but not completely true, as there is renewed interest in very slow and very fast activity in the EEG. Conventional interpretation of routine EEGs still does proceed on the assumption that the frequency of almost all brain electrical activity of interest for routine interpretation lies within this particular, relatively narrow bandwidth. EEG filters are then typically paired so that one filter rejects the majority of very high-frequency activity and another

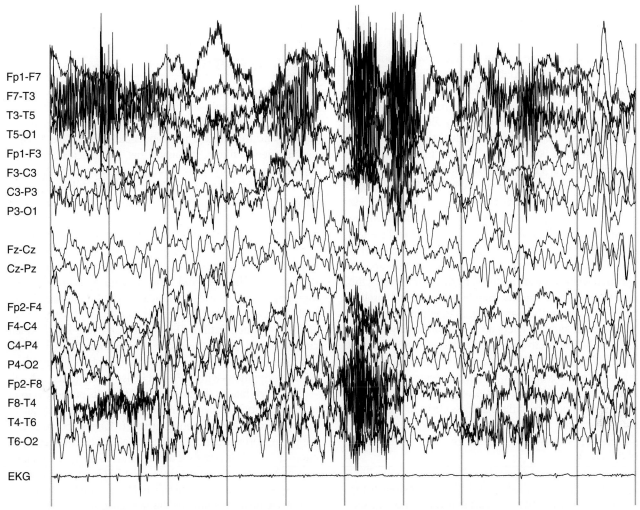

Fp1-F7
F7-T3
T3-T5
T5-O1
Fp1-F3
F3-C3
C3-P3
P3-O1

Fz-Cz
Cz-Pz

Fp2-F4
F4-C4
C4-P4
P4-O2
Fp2-F8
F8-T4
T4-T6
T6-O2

EKG

Figure 7.2 This is the same 10-second EEG page that was displayed in Figure 7.1 except that now the low-frequency filter is set at 1 Hz, and the high-frequency filter is set at 70 Hz, standard filter settings used in many laboratories. Note that the baselines of each channel are flatter. Also, the amplitude of the muscle artifact is significantly reduced throughout, though still present. Although there is still a large amount of artifact present on this complex page, the use of standard filter settings has rendered this page considerably more readable.

filter rejects the majority of very low-frequency activity. The band of frequencies between these unwanted high and low frequencies that is allowed to "pass through" the filter setup is referred to as the bandpass. The way that different filter setups can be used to create different bandpasses is illustrated here.

An example of an *idealized* (though not real-world) bandpass curve is shown in Figure 7.3. A bandpass curve shows the percentage of activity at any given frequency that would be allowed to "pass through" and be seen by the reader. Assuming a filter-designer believed that only wave activity with frequencies between 1 and 35 Hz were worth seeing, this bandpass curve would be ideal. The shape of the curve implies that all activity below 1 Hz and above 35 Hz would effectively be eliminated from the displayed EEG signal, which would seem reasonable if you believed that that activity definitely did not come from the brain. Now let's see how this idealized bandpass setup would behave if it functioned according to the Figure 7.3 diagram. We have a patient who, in reality, has a beautiful 5 Hz brain wave but, as it happens, this beautiful sine wave is partly obscured by both slow and fast artifacts (Figure 7.4). The fast activity riding

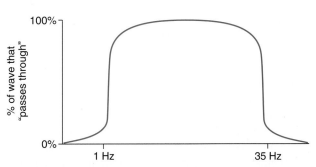

Figure 7.3 This is the graphical representation of an idealized pair of filters creating a bandpass of 1 and 35 Hz, meaning that all wave activity between 1 and 35 Hz would be displayed, and all activity below 1 Hz and all activity above 35 Hz would effectively be removed from the output waveform. The y-axis shows the percentage of activity of any particular wave frequency (x-axis) that this bandpass would allow to "pass through" onto our display screens. As it happens, real-life filters do not have such sharp cutoffs for their bandpasses, and the effect of cutting off frequencies above or below the nominal bandpass frequencies is much more gradual, as is seen in the figures below.

on this wave is just noise occurring at about 40 Hz. Similarly, the true 5 Hz brainwave arising from the brain has a perfectly flat baseline, but the patient's rocking movement just under 1 Hz is causing this wave's baseline to drift up and down about once per second. Applying a perfect 1 to 35 Hz bandpass pair of filters should clean up both of these problems beautifully. A 35 Hz high-frequency filter (HFF) should eliminate the unwanted 40 Hz fast activity and a 1 Hz low-frequency filter (LFF) should be able to eliminate the rocking artifact that is just below 1 Hz. We decide to combine both of these idealized filters, which will eliminate all activity at 1 Hz and below and all activity at 35 Hz and above, allowing only frequencies between 1 Hz and below 35 Hz to "pass through" (which is, in this case, the pure 5 Hz sine wave). The slow motion rocking artifact component we are eliminating with the LFF is illustrated in Figure 7.5 and the fast 40 Hz noise component we are eliminating with the high filter is shown in Figure 7.6. When the low-frequency motion artifact and high-frequency noise are removed by this pair of filters, the pristine 5 Hz wave now appears smooth and on a flat baseline (Figure 7.7). Of course, these are idealized examples because, as we shall see, high and low filters do not unfortunately remove one 100% of their respective activities and leave the 5 Hz activity completely unchanged. These examples are given in order to illustrate an *idealized goal* of how a bandpass setup might work. Part of the idealized nature of this example is reflected by the steepness of the shoulders of the bandpass curve in Figure 7.3, a situation that is not attainable with real filters. The shoulders of real-life bandpass curves roll off more gradually as we will see later in this chapter.

Some strategic uses of filters can aid in reading the EEG not just by rejecting presumed artifacts, but also by removing some true brain wave activity. Occasionally, it can be advantageous to filter out known high-voltage brain wave activity in order to render other activity more easily visible to the eye. Using this strategy, the electroencephalographer may, for instance, purposely attenuate the slow activity in a record (even though it represents true cerebral activity) to accentuate or "bring out" fast activity that would otherwise be lost in high-voltage slow waves. Examples of such specific filtering techniques (which are not necessarily used to read most EEG records) are illustrated in Figures 7.8 and 7.9. These figures show how aggressive use of the LFF can be used to bring out the presence of spike-wave discharges in this example.

Typical filter settings with which many routine EEGs are initially recorded include a pairing of an LFF set at 1 Hz and an HFF set at 70 Hz. Taking into account the fact that the roll-off characteristics for these filters are relatively gradual, it is no surprise that a fair amount of EEG activity with frequencies above and below the nominal frequencies of 1 Hz and 70 Hz still may appear in the recording. Figure 7.10 shows two possible bandpass setups, one with LFF = 1 Hz and HFF = 70 Hz, and the other with LFF = 5 Hz and HFF = 70 Hz. Figure 7.11 illustrates the same bandpass setup, but plotting the curves with the frequency on a linear scale for comparison. Figure 7.12 illustrates the bandpass curve that uses a more aggressive HFF setting of 35 Hz. Note that, comparing the Figures 7.10 and 7.12, the shapes of the curves are similar, and the portions of the curves on the left (representing the low frequencies) are nearly identical. The portions of the curves on the right (representing the higher frequencies) show more attenuation when the HFF is set to 35 Hz rather than 70 Hz.

TYPES OF FILTERS

The three commonly used filter types in clinical EEG are low-frequency filters, high-frequency filters, and notch filters. The purpose of a low-frequency filter is to filter out low-frequency activity and to leave higher frequencies as they are. Because low-frequency filters attenuate low frequencies and allow high frequencies to "pass through," engineers often refer to low-frequency filters as high-pass filters. Likewise, high-frequency filters are designed to filter out high-frequency activity and allow low-frequency activity to pass through and are sometimes referred to by engineers as low-pass filters. Although the use of the terms high pass and low pass to name filters is more common in the world of electrical engineering, these are not the preferred terms in clinical electroencephalography. In the world of clinical EEG, the alternate terms high-frequency filter (HFF—filters *out* the high frequencies) and low-frequency filter (LFF—filters *out* the low frequencies) are used, while the shorter terms high filter (HF) and low filter (LF) can be used as shorthand abbreviations. Thus, HF is synonymous with HFF and LF is synonymous with LFF.

The notch filter is the third type of filter. Its purpose is to filter out activity at a specific frequency (rather than a frequency range). Because the alternating current (AC) in standard electric outlets in North America oscillates at 60 Hz, electric fields produced by the 60 Hz activity that surrounds us in our indoor environments frequently contaminates the EEG. Sixty-hertz notch filters (filters designed specifically to filter out 60 Hz activity) are used to attenuate or eliminate this unwanted signal. In the many countries where the frequency used in the electrical mains is 50 Hz, 50 Hz notch filters are used for the same purpose.

HOW FILTERS ARE NAMED

There are two different naming schemes for high- and low-frequency filters. A filter can be named after a frequency (e.g., a "5 Hz low filter") or after its time constant (e.g., a "low-filter with time constant of 0.1 seconds"). When a filter is named after a particular frequency, this is referred to as the nominal frequency (nominal meaning the frequency for which the filter was named) or the cutoff frequency of the filter. Whether the filters on a particular EEG machine are named according to the filter's cutoff frequency or its time constant is the decision of the manufacturer. Because referring to filters by their cutoff frequencies is becoming more common, and also because cutoff frequencies are more intuitive, we will discuss how a filter's electrical characteristics relate to its cutoff frequency first and time constants will be discussed later.

Low-Frequency Filters

The term cutoff frequency conjures up the image of an all-or-nothing effect at the frequency named. For example, a class may have a particular cutoff grade for passing or failing—one point below the cutoff grade and the student does not go on. An amusement park may have a particular height cutoff to go

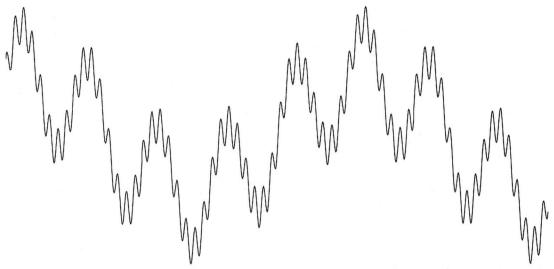

Figure 7.4 This idealized waveform is meant to represent a recording obtained from a patient who in reality has a pure 5 Hz frequency coming from the brain. Unfortunately, the patient's 5 Hz brainwave activity is partially distorted by two sources of artifact. The first is electrical noise that is causing the fine sawtooth pattern to be superimposed on the wave. The second is a slow oscillating artifact caused by the patient making a rocking motion that causes the baseline of this wave to waver up and down about once per second like a roller-coaster. The purpose of this illustration is to see how a pair of idealized or "perfect" pair of filters with a very steep bandpass of 1 Hz to 35 Hz would help "clean up" this wave.

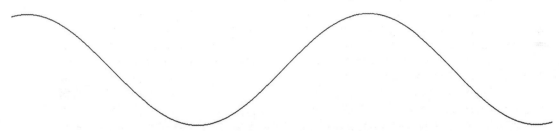

Figure 7.5 This wave of about 1 Hz shows the isolated slow component of the motion artifact that has been mixed into the wave above, caused by the patient's rocking motion.

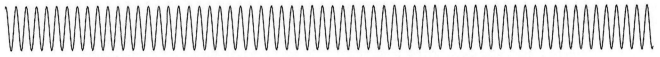

Figure 7.6 This is a look at the fast, noisy component at about 40 Hz that is also superimposed on the 5 Hz wave in Figure 7.4 that we are relying on our bandpass filter setup to "clean up." This noise could represent some type of electrical or muscle artifact. Because it is outside our ideal 1 to 35 Hz bandpass filter setup, we expect our filters to eliminate it.

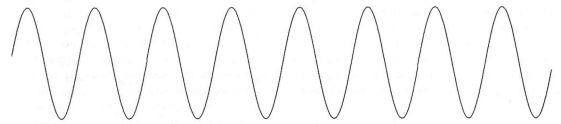

Figure 7.7 Applying the idealized bandpass setup from Figure 7.3 to the wave we recorded in Figure 7.4, the 1 Hz and 40 Hz components are eliminated by these idealized bandpass filters and the pristine 5 Hz brain wave is displayed. Of course, filter setups in real life with real EEG waves do not do such a complete job of removing unwanted activity outside the bandpass frequency range, but the purpose of these figures is to show an idealized example of what we are striving for with our filter setups.

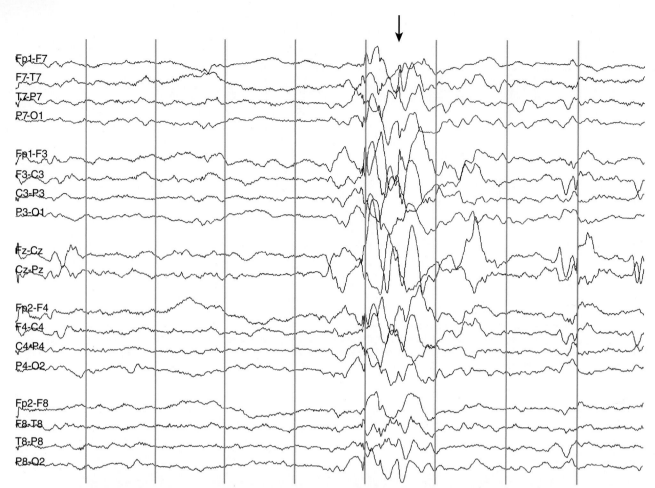

Figure 7.8 This recording is made during a transition from Stage I to Stage II sleep using the standard low filter setting of 1 Hz. A burst of high-voltage slowing is seen during the sixth second (arrow). Inspection of the burst suggests the possibility that some spike activity may be intermixed, but a definite determination as to whether spike activity is truly present is difficult. Compare to same EEG signals displayed with different filter settings in Figure 7.9.

on certain rides—all individuals below that height are excluded from the ride. The behavior of low-frequency filters in terms of their cutoff frequencies is not at all so absolute as the behavior of classroom teachers or amusement park staff. In fact, it may be surprising to learn how little a filter affects activity at its cutoff frequency. When a low-frequency filter encounters a sine wave that happens to be exactly at its cutoff frequency, it cuts down the amplitude of that wave by approximately 30% (which means that 70% of the wave is still there!). Sine waves at frequencies somewhat below that frequency are reduced by somewhat more than 30%—the farther the wave's frequency is below the filter's nominal (cutoff) frequency, the more it is attenuated. Perhaps more surprising, sine waves at frequencies somewhat above the cutoff frequency are also reduced in size by the filter, although by somewhat less than 30%. Again, the more the sine wave's frequency exceeds the low-frequency filter's nominal frequency, the less it is affected by the filter.

Visual Effects of Low-Frequency Filters

When standard LFF settings such as a cutoff frequency of 1 Hz or below are used for the LFF, the main effect is to help each EEG channel stay within its own horizontal area, eliminating large drifts upward or downward into the areas of adjacent channels. LFFs create this desirable effect because any baseline drifting represents a very low-frequency wave, usually well below 1 Hz. LFFs are especially useful for filtering out certain artifacts caused by patient motion. Motion artifact from patient movement may generate a high-amplitude wave that spans several seconds and, therefore, is well below 1 Hz. For that reason, such waves that might shift a channel's baseline slowly are handled by filters as very low-frequency activity and LFFs can do a very good job of reducing this type of very slow artifact, helping to return large deflections to the channel's baseline.

More aggressive use of the LFF (such as raising the LFF cutoff frequency to 3 Hz or 5 Hz) may have the effect of beginning to attenuate some slower frequencies that could very conceivably be of interest to the reader. Even higher cutoff LFF frequencies could almost completely eliminate the ability to see some slow activity. Switching the LFF frequency to these higher cutoff frequencies sometimes has the advantage of bringing out other features in the EEG (Figures 7.13 through 7.17) that may have previously been masked by underlying slow activity. Examples of how different LFF settings might affect a simple trace of the posterior rhythm

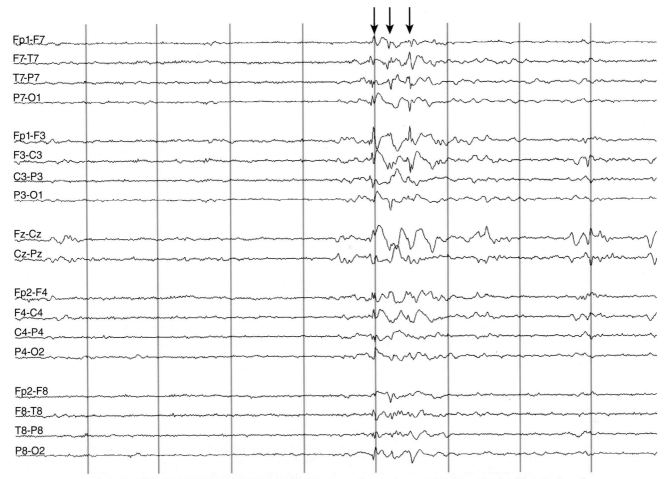

Figure 7.9 The same EEG page as shown in Figure 7.8, but this time with an aggressive low-filter setting of 10 Hz. Note that the bulk of the slow activity is suppressed (all the baselines are much flatter) and because the slow activity is less prominent, faster activity, and the spikes in particular, are accentuated. With this filter setting, it is clear that there are three repetitive spikes with a broad field (below arrows) mixed into this slow-wave burst. If there was a question as to whether the initial slow-wave burst represented some type of motion artifact, the presence of these three embedded, rhythmically repetitive spikes with organized topography increases the likelihood that this represents an example of a diffuse, repetitive spike-wave discharge rather than motion artifact. Once the nature of the burst is better understood with the aggressive use of the LFF, the reader will likely return the filter to its standard setting.

are shown in Figure 7.18. Note that when successively more restrictive settings are used for the low filter, the baselines of each channel become straighter, like a ruler, but faster activity is relatively preserved. Use of aggressively high LFF settings for this purpose is usually temporary to check for hidden activity, after which the cutoff frequency may be returned to more standard settings.

Roll-off Characteristics

The graph in Figure 7.19 illustrates an example of how a real-world 5 Hz LFF would handle sine waves of varying frequencies. The curve describes what percentage (y-axis) of a pure sine wave at any given frequency (x-axis) would be allowed to pass through the filter. Considering the example of this 5 Hz LFF in more detail, the curve shows that a 5 Hz sine wave presented to this filter will lose 30% of its amplitude after passing through the filter. (Why the amount of reduction at the cutoff frequency is specifically 30% is explained below in the

paragraph on decibels.) If the original 5 Hz wave presented to the filter has an amplitude of 100 µV (the input wave), then the filter's output wave would be a 5 Hz wave of 70 µV. But what does the 5 Hz LFF do with waves just above and just below a 5 Hz frequency? The roll-off curve for a filter answers this exact question. This roll-off curve for the filter shown in this figure indicates that a 4 Hz sine wave would be attenuated by 33%, but a 6 Hz sine wave would only be attenuated by 26%. The type of curve shown in Figure 7.20 that shows how a given filter processes pure sine waves of different frequencies is called the roll-off characteristic of the filter. It shows the percentage of a wave of a particular frequency that the filter in question allows to pass through (in the case of this figure, a 5 Hz LFF). Figure 7.20 shows how a 5 Hz LFF handles input waves of 10 Hz, 5 Hz, 2 Hz, and 0.5 Hz, all of the same amplitude, attenuating the lowest frequency waves in its output dramatically but only causing a mild reduction in the amplitude of the 10 Hz wave. The exact amount of reduction

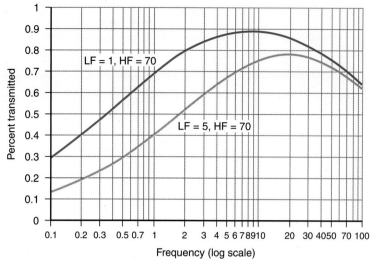

Figure 7.10 When a high filter and a low filter are combined, a particular middle range of frequencies is favored and higher and lower frequencies outside of that range are relatively excluded. This type of setup is called a *bandpass*. Two curves showing the bandpass characteristics generated by combining a 1 Hz low-frequency filter (LFF) and 70 Hz high-frequency filter (HFF; top curve), and a 5 Hz LFF and 70 Hz HFF (bottom curve) are shown. The height of the curve indicates the percentage of activity at any particular frequency shown on the x-axis that will be allowed to pass through the filter setup. Because the difference between the two bandpasses illustrated is caused by a change in the LFF used, the left sides of the curves that describe the filters' effect on low frequencies differs, while the right side (high-frequency) portion of the curves is similar. Note that both bandpasses (especially the 1 Hz LFF/70 Hz HFF example) generally favor the frequency range of greatest interest in clinical EEG, the frequencies between 1 and 35 Hz.

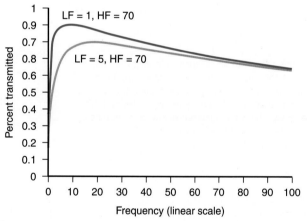

Figure 7.11 For the sake of comparison, the same two bandpass curves as are shown in Figure 7.10 are plotted on a linear frequency scale.

at each frequency is given by the roll-off characteristic shown in the previous figure. Figure 7.21 shows the roll-off characteristics of example LFFs with nominal frequencies of 0.1, 1, 5, and 10 Hz, respectively. Knowing that an LFF attenuates the height of a wave at its nominal frequency by 30%, we expect to see the roll-off characteristic curve for each filter to intersect the 70% transmission level at its nominal frequency.

Of course, when filters are applied to real EEG signals, the waves presented to the filter consist of mixed frequencies rather than perfect sine waves. One of the main principles of how filters handle waves of mixed frequencies is that they handle *each frequency component* of a wave according to the rule of the filter's roll-off characteristic for that frequency as if they were separate waves, *even in wave mixtures*.

The steepness of the roll-off characteristic of a filter is sometimes described in the units of decibels per octave. The term octave is best known in the music world, describing the difference between two notes such as "middle C" and "high C." In both the world of music and the world of electrical signals, an octave represents a doubling or a halving of a wave frequency. Therefore, 4 Hz is one octave above 2 Hz (and "middle C" on the piano is the tone at 256 Hz, whereas the note one octave above, "high C," is the tone at 512 Hz). Simple LFF response curves "roll off" at a maximum of 6 dB per octave, which corresponds to the steepness or shallowness of the roll-off curves shown in these figures (although this roll-off rate is not constant across the entire frequency band). The decibel unit is described below.

High-Frequency Filters (HFFs)

High-frequency filters also have a roll-off characteristic but, logically, their curves roll off in the direction opposite to the roll-off curves for LFFs, falling off toward the right (the direction of the higher frequencies). Just as was the case for LFFs, an HFF attenuates a sine wave at its nominal (cutoff) frequency by 30%; higher frequency waves are attenuated by even more than 30%, and lower frequency waves are attenuated by less than 30%. Figure 7.22 shows examples of roll-off characteristics for theoretical 70, 35, and 15 Hz HFFs. High-frequency filters are especially useful for filtering out muscle artifact and other high-frequency noise. Overly aggressive use of HFFs, however, will not only attenuate the height of high-frequency waves but can also change wave shape giving misleading results, as discussed later in the discussion of time constants.

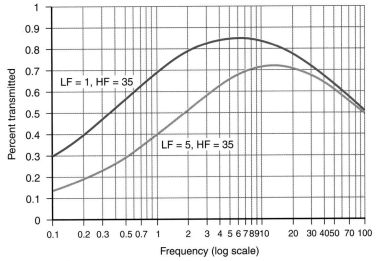

Figure 7.12 These curves illustrate the bandpasses resulting from pairing a 1 Hz LFF with a 35 Hz HFF and the pairing of a 5 Hz LFF with a 35 Hz HFF, respectively. Frequency is plotted on a logarithmic scale. Note that the right side of the curves falls off more steeply compared with the curves shown in Figure 7.10 because of the more aggressive (lower) HFF cutoff frequency used.

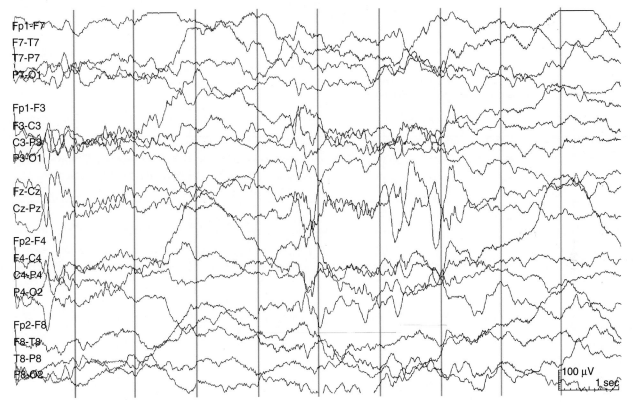

Figure 7.13 An example of Stage II sleep recorded with a conservative low-frequency filter setting of 0.1 Hz. Note that the baselines of several channels wander into the areas of adjacent channels making the tracing more difficult to read. Some of the largest and broadest slow-wave deflections may represent artifact rather than true electrocerebral activity.

DECIBELS: THEY MIGHT NOT BE EXACTLY WHAT YOU THINK

The term *decibel* is probably best known in the context of measuring sound. When people say that a rock concert reached 130 decibels, this gives the impression that the unit is an absolute measure of sound, but it is not. Rather, the decibel is more like a percentage change or ratio measurement.

If someone says a sound increased by so many decibels, they are actually saying by so many percent (or alternatively, by a factor of some number). When the term *decibel* is used to describe the change in sound or electric power, it turns out that halving the *power* of a wave is equivalent to a decrease of 3 decibels (dB), and why this is the case is explained below. Filters are named for the frequency at which they reduce the *power* of the input wave by half (and therefore also by 3 dB).

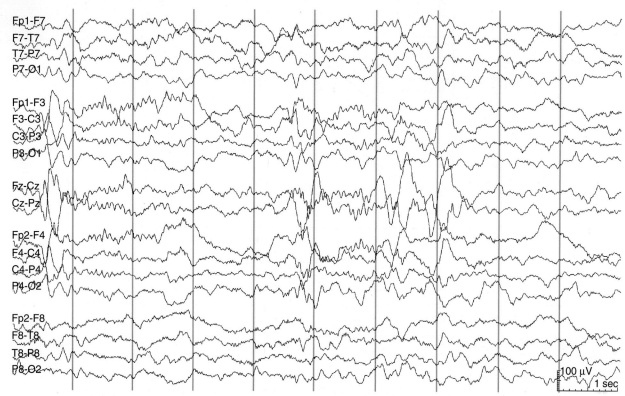

Figure 7.14 The same page of Stage II sleep from the previous example is shown, now displayed with a standard LFF setting of 1 Hz. The wide deflections in the baselines of each channel seen in Figure 7.13 are no longer present, making the page more readable.

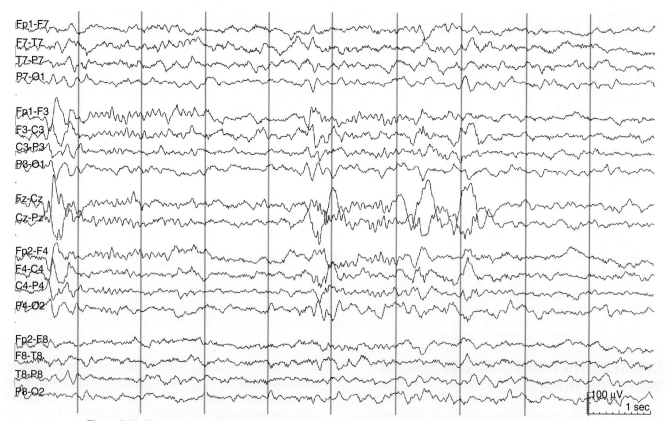

Figure 7.15 The same page of Stage II sleep from the previous examples is shown, now with an LFF setting of 3 Hz. The amount of slow activity detail is further decreased, but fast activity, such as the spindles and vertex waves, is still easily seen. Note that the slower, roller coaster-like wandering of the channels seen in the previous figure has now been significantly reduced.

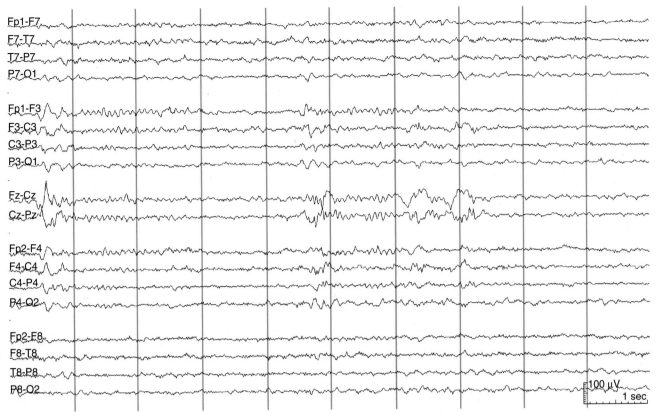

Fp1-F7
F7-T7
T7-P7
P7-O1

Fp1-F3
F3-C3
C3-P3
P3-O1

Fz-Cz
Cz-Pz

Fp2-F4
F4-C4
C4-P4
P4-O2

Fp2-F8
F8-T8
T8-P8
P8-O2

100 μV
1 sec

Figure 7.16 The aggressive LFF setting of 10 Hz used to display this same page of Stage II sleep is only occasionally used in routine EEG interpretation. Note that, now, most of the slow-wave activity is no longer evident. For instance, even the vertex waves, whose wavelengths indicate approximately 3 Hz activity (because, visually, we can see that approximately three such waves could fit into 1 second) are considerably reduced in amplitude. Faster activity such as the spindles and the vertex waves in reduced form can still be appreciated. If there had been an asymmetry of slow wave activity between the right and left hemispheres, however, the ability to appreciate it would likely be lost with this LFF setting.

Interestingly, the unit of the bel was named after Alexander Graham Bell when a unit was needed to describe increases and decreases in electrical power in telephone lines. Currently, the bel unit is almost never used, but instead the decibel (dB), which is one tenth of a bel, is the unit in most common use today. To understand how decibels work, it is important to recall how logarithms work.

What is the common logarithm of a number? The answer is: the power that you would have to raise 10 to in order to get that number. To figure the log of a particular number:

Log of "a particular number" = $10^?$

If I can figure out what '?' is,

then that is the log of "a particular number."

Some of the answers to these questions are easy, such as what is the log of 100? Because you need to raise 10 to the power of 2 to get 100 (which is 10^2) the common log of 100 is 2. It then follows that the log of 1,000 is 3 (because 10 has to be raised to the third power—10^3—to get to 1,000), and so on. Numbers in between the powers of 10 (10, 100, 1,000...) are, of course, harder to guess and easiest to determine with a calculator. For instance, the log of 50 is the number that would solve the problem 10^x = 50. You would expect the answer would be between the log of 10, which is 1, and the log of 100, which is 2, and the answer

is, indeed, approximately 1.7, which makes sense: $10^{1.7}$ = ~50. Another way to think of it is that the common log of a number effectively reflects the order of magnitude of a number.

As mentioned above, the original definition of the bel was defined to describe the proportion of power increases in telephone lines when the power changed, for instance from $power_1$ to $power_2$. The formula is simply:

$$bel = \log\left(\frac{power_2}{power_1}\right)$$

Considering the example of an increase in power from 10 milliwatts to 1,000 milliwatts (a 100-fold increase):

$$\log\left(\frac{1,000\,mW}{10\,mW}\right) = \log(100) = 2\ bel = 20\ db$$

As mentioned, the bel is not in common usage and the *decibel* is the common unit used today. A decibel (dB) is defined as 1/10 of a bel (i.e., there are 10 decibels in a bel), so the formula to give the result in dB multiplies the result of the initial formula for bels by 10 so the answer comes out in decibels and becomes:

$$dB = 10 * log\left(\frac{power_2}{power_1}\right)$$

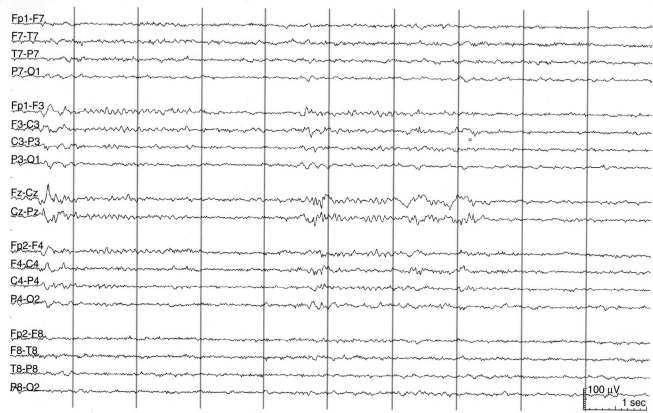

Figure 7.17 The LFF setting of 15 Hz used to display this same sample of Stage II sleep was chosen for illustrative purposes and is rarely used during routine EEG interpretation. The vertex-wave activity, most prominent at Cz, is now dramatically attenuated because it can be seen as the equivalent of approximately 3 Hz activity. This aggressive low-filter setting now even begins to attenuate amplitude of the 14 Hz spindle activity. This setting eliminates a lot of important detail from the EEG tracing and is therefore seldom used during conventional EEG interpretation.

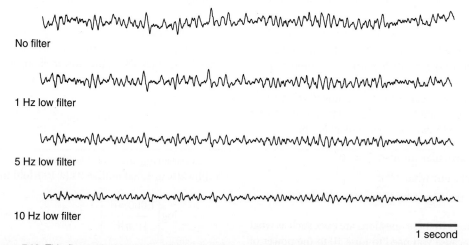

Figure 7.18 This figure illustrates the effects of different low filter settings on the same sample of the posterior rhythm. Although an adult posterior rhythm generally does not represent an example of slow activity, subtle amounts of slow activity are often intermixed with the posterior rhythm to a greater or lesser extent. Note that as the cutoff frequency of the low filter is steadily increased, the mild "waviness" of the baseline flattens, especially as the 5 Hz filter is used. Some amount of wavering of the baseline of the top, "no filter" trace can be seen, while the bottom "10 Hz low filter" trace has a very straight backbone that you could draw a straight pencil-line through with a ruler. After the cutoff frequency rises into the zone of the posterior rhythm itself, such as when the 10 Hz low filter is used, the filter begins to attenuate the waves of interest significantly (compare the amplitude of the posterior rhythm waves in the bottom line with those in the top line).

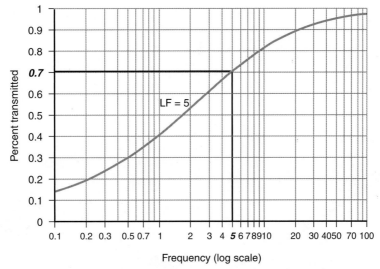

Figure 7.19 This curve describes the roll-off characteristic of a theoretical 5 Hz low-frequency filter. The graph shows the percentage of a pure sine wave that is allowed to pass through the filter (y-axis) as a function of its frequency in hertz (x-axis, plotted on a logarithmic scale). Note that waves at frequencies well below 5 Hz are attenuated substantially but waves at frequencies above 5 Hz are also attenuated to some extent, although the amount may be relatively minor. The curve shows that a sine wave of exactly 5 Hz is attenuated by 30% (heavier bars). For an explanation of why wave amplitude is specifically attenuated by 30% at the filter's nominal frequency, see discussion in text.

This implies that a 100-fold increase in power is an increase of 20 dB. If we wished to determine how many dB a 10-fold increase in power would be, we could plug in 100 for power$_2$ and 10 for power$_1$ into the formula above and, and because $\log(10) = 1$, we get:

$$10 * \log\left(\frac{100}{10}\right) = 10 * \log(10) = 10 db$$

One of the more useful relationships for us to remember is how many dB represent a doubling or halving of power, because this is the number used to define cutoff frequencies for filters (more on the 30% figure mentioned earlier in a moment). For this we need to know the log of 2, because the formula we want to solve for doubling of power (for instance for a change of power$_1$ to power$_2$ being a change from 5 to 10) could be: dB = $10 * \log(10/5)$, or $10 * \log(2)$. Because log 2 is approximately 0.3 (and that is the answer in bel), according to the decibel formula above, doubling the power of a wave is the same as increasing it by 3 dB. And this works in both directions: halving the power is a reduction of 3 dB. Considering the reverse example where the power drops from 10 to 5, knowing that the log of 0.5 is approximately –0.3, we get: $10 * \log(5/10) = \sim -3$ dB.

Therefore,

A 3 dB increase in a wave represents a doubling of power and a 3 dB reduction in a wave represents a halving of power.

The Relationship of Power to Voltage

Now we need to throw a slight curve into the story to transition from the world of telephony to electroencephalography. So far, we have been talking about comparative reductions in power because that is what the telephone company engineers were

most interested in. As EEGers, we are usually most interested in changes in the wave's voltage (or height, or amplitude—all the same) because that is what we see on the page. When we see the voltage of a wave swinging back and forth in a wire or on an EEG page, this is not the same as the power of that wave (power is defined as energy per second). In fact, the voltage of a wave has to be squared in order to calculate its power. What this means is that if the voltage (or amplitude) of a wave doubles, power actually goes up four times. If you asked the power company to double the height of the voltage wave in your electric outlets, you would be asking for four times the power, and you will likely be asked to pay accordingly. The company would have to use four times the coal or gas or solar power or wind turbines to satisfy your request, but now you will be able to burn four lightbulbs instead of one lightbulb at the original intensity to illuminate your home.

The previous paragraph explained how halving the *power* of wave is the same as a 3 dB reduction. The question we now have to ask is, if power is related to the square of the amplitude, by what percent does the amplitude of an EEG wave visually go down on an EEG page when the power is halved, (i.e., reduced by 3 dB reduction, which is the same). We want to know this because this is the amount of *amplitude* decrease that will be expected at the cutoff frequency of the filter. So, what ratio of amplitudes, A$_2$ to A$_1$, if squared, will give a ratio that reflects a 50% reduction (in power)? This is the same as asking, what is an example of two numbers, A$_2$ and A$_1$ that, if squared, will yield a ratio of 2:1 of their squares? A good example answer is a reduction in the amplitude from 10 to 7 (which is a 30% reduction in wave height). Here is why, and notice that we have picked power values that are perfect squares to make the math easier. To make this problem easier to visualize, we will choose a power reduction from 100 to 49, which is basically a halving of the power.

EFFECT OF 5 Hz LOW FREQUENCY FILTER

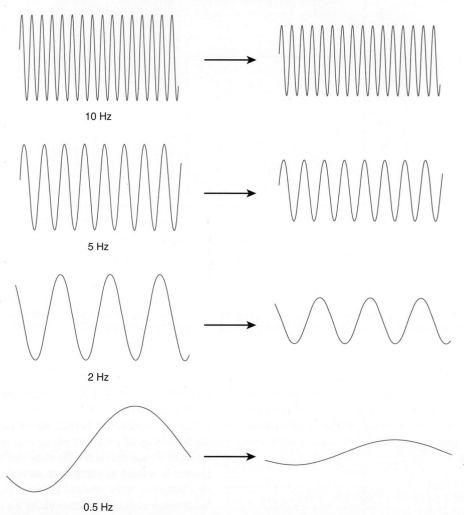

Figure 7.20 This figure shows how the wave of different frequencies shown on the left will be handled by a 5 Hz low-frequency filter (LFF). The output of each wave on the right shows how waves of increasingly lower frequencies are attenuated to increasing degrees by a 5 Hz LFF. Note that the sine waves shown on the left are all of the same amplitude, but descend in frequency, and are to be presented to a 5 Hz low-frequency filter represented by the arrow, with the respective outputs shown on the right. Note that the 10 Hz sine wave shown at the top, even though above the filter's nominal frequency, is transmitted by the filter with a slightly decreased amplitude. The 5 Hz sine wave's amplitude is attenuated 30% by the 5 Hz LFF, as expected. Amplitudes of 2 and 0.5 Hz waves are reduced even more substantially.

If amplitudes/voltages have to be squared to get power differences, what two numbers A_2 and A_1, if squared, will have a ratio of 2:1? An excellent answer will be 10 and 7 because, when those to numbers are squared, we get a drop from 100 to 49. Therefore, a 50% power drop, from 100 to 49, corresponds to a 30% voltage drop (i.e., from 10 and 7).

$$\text{If } \frac{\text{amplitude}_2}{\text{amplitude}_1} = \frac{10}{7}$$

Because power is related to the square of the amplitudes, the amplitude ratio needs to be squared to get the power ratio:

$$\frac{10^2}{7^2} = \frac{100}{49} = \frac{\text{power}_2}{\text{power}_1} = \sim 2$$

Thus, a power drop of 50% corresponds to a voltage drop of only 30%. To bring decibels back into the story, recalling the decibel formula from above:

$$10 * \log\left(\frac{10^2}{7^2}\right) = 10 * \log\left(\frac{100}{49}\right)$$

$$\cong 3\,\text{dB} \left(\dots \text{because } \log 2 =\sim 0.3\right)$$

To summarize, a voltage drop of 30% corresponds to a power drop of 50%, which corresponds to a 3 dB drop—all are equivalent and all correspond, by definition, to the degree a filter attenuates a wave at its nominal frequency. However, between amplitude, power, and decibels, the one that we see on the EEG page is the 30% amplitude drop.

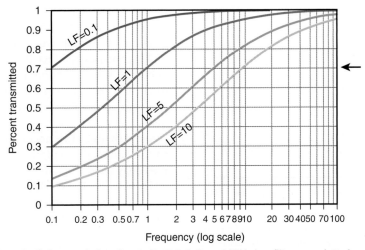

Figure 7.21 The roll-off characteristics of example 0.1, 1, 5, and 10 Hz low filters are plotted on a semilog plot. Note that a low filter setting of 0.1 Hz barely affects the frequency range of brain wave activity most commonly seen in conventional EEG recording: 1 to 35 Hz. The 10 Hz low-frequency filter, however, has a major impact on frequencies in this range. Note also that the graph line representing 70% transmission (i.e., 30% reduction) passes through each roll-off curve at each filter's nominal frequency (arrow).

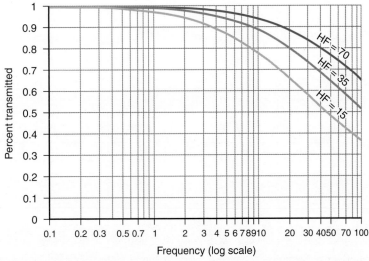

Figure 7.22 Roll-off characteristics for theoretical high-frequency filters (HFFs) with cutoff frequencies of 70 Hz, 35 Hz, and 15 Hz. Note that, as was seen with the low-frequency filters, each roll-off curve passes through the point of 70% transmission at its respective cutoff frequency. Higher frequencies are attenuated more dramatically, and frequencies lower than the cutoff frequency are attenuated by less than 30%. In this example, the 70 Hz HFF allows 90% or more of frequencies below 20 Hz to be passed through the filter, thus affecting activity between 1 and 35 Hz very little.

You may still be asking, what about the 130-decibel rock concert? If decibels always refer to percentage differences, how is it that the intensity of environmental sounds are always quoted in dB? The answer to this question is that any use of decibels to measure sound must always do so in implicit comparison to some reference level of sound pressure. The most common reference level chosen is a sound intensity that is just at the threshold of human hearing.

50 HZ AND 60 HZ NOTCH FILTERS

Unlike HFFs and LFFs, which have a gradual roll-off curve, the purpose of a notch filter is to exclude a *single* frequency from the EEG signal. These notch filters are most useful when

the electric field of the AC current from the electrical wiring, outlets, and machines that surround the patient is contaminating the record. The ideal notch filter's transmission curve would show a flat response for all frequencies, except for the nominal frequency of the filter, where there is a notch in the curve denoting near complete attenuation of any waves at that particular frequency but no others (Figure 7.23). Of course, in the world of working EEG, notch filters may not operate as perfectly as this description implies, but they typically do a good job of suppressing unwanted AC line voltage artifact. Figure 7.24 shows a sample of EEG with 60 Hz contamination in multiple channels. Figure 7.25 shows detail of the 60 Hz artifact. The reader should become adept at identifying the fine 60 Hz sine wave that comprises the fine structure of this

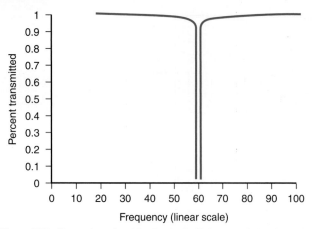

Figure 7.23 Illustration of an idealized roll-off characteristic of a 60 Hz notch filter. The goal of the notch filter is to allow all frequencies to pass except for activity exactly at the nominal frequency. In this case 60 Hz activity would be rejected completely.

type of artifact. Figure 7.26 shows the same page of EEG with the 60 Hz notch filter "in" (applied or "on").

Some of the imperfections of notch filters can be overlooked, such as the fact that a 60 Hz notch filter will also attenuate some adjacent frequencies, such as 59 Hz and 61 Hz to a very small extent. The good news is that the electroencephalographer is rarely interested in these nearby frequencies because they are in a range much faster than the cerebral rhythms that are of interest during routine analysis, so this minor shortcoming is rarely noticed. Also, a notch filter may have difficulty suppressing very large amounts of 60 Hz activity. The 60 Hz notch filter is useful in countries in North America and other locations where AC electricity is supplied at 60 Hz. The 50 Hz notch filter is used in the many countries where the line frequency is 50 Hz (in North America, the 50 Hz notch filter would serve no useful purpose).

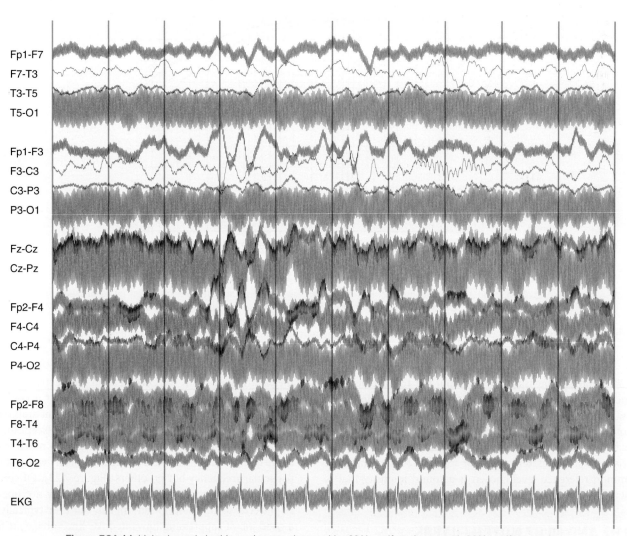

Figure 7.24 Multiple channels in this tracing are obscured by 60 Hz artifact. In general, 60 Hz artifact can be distinguished from muscle artifact by its highly regular, though very compressed, sinusoidal appearance. Close examination of the waves often allows a 60 Hz wave to be discerned, which in this example has the appearance of vertical ribbing or an extremely fine-toothed comb. Also, notice that the amplitude of the artifact tends to stay steady in each channel. Compare to Figure 7.26.

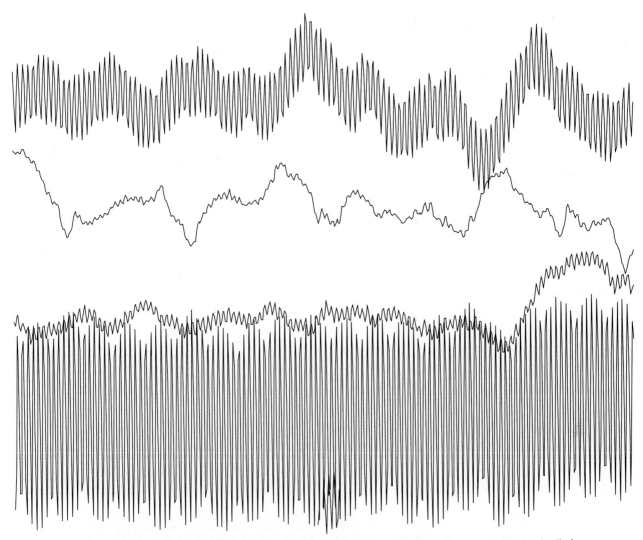

Figure 7.25 An enlargement of the top four channels from the previous figure is shown, revealing the detail of regular, well-formed 60 Hz sine waves. Each of the four channels shows different amounts of 60 Hz contamination. This artifact represents contamination of the patient's body with the alternating current sources that surround us in modern indoor environments, and also possibly impedance mismatches between compared electrodes.

ELECTRODE IMPEDANCE PROBLEMS

EEG technologists must perfect the art of applying EEG electrodes so that they can make an accurate recording of brain wave activity through the scalp. The procedure involves measuring the correct electrode location accurately followed by preparation of the skin, often by rubbing with an abrasive compound. Electrolyte solution or paste may be applied under the electrode to facilitate recording of electrical currents. After application but before the study begins, electrode impedance is measured for each electrode to assess how well the electrodes have been applied and to identify problem electrodes. Impedance is a measure of resistance that is partially dependent on the frequency of the wave being measured (discussed subsequently). Generally, electrode impedances should be under 5 kΩ (killiohms). It is good practice to recheck impedances both during and after the recording to document that electrodes have stayed well applied throughout.

Because it would never seem desirable to have 60 Hz artifact present in the EEG tracing, you may wonder, why not keep the 60 Hz notch filter in at all times? In fact, it is best technique to use the 60 Hz notch filter only when necessary (when 60 Hz artifact has already been seen to be contaminating the tracing). One reason for this is that the presence of 60 Hz artifact in one or more electrodes serves as a clue that there is an impedance problem in the electrodes in which the artifact is seen. Apart from being a good example of 60 Hz artifact obscuring a tracing, the dramatic appearance of the EEG in Figure 7.24 is also a red flag indicating that multiple electrodes have poor contacts. (This effect of an electrode with a poor contact showing 60 Hz artifact was also illustrated in Figure 6.26 in the previous chapter.)

Why is the presence of 60 Hz artifact in an electrode an indicator of a poor electrode contact? Consider that there is generally 60 Hz activity present all over the head, which is an

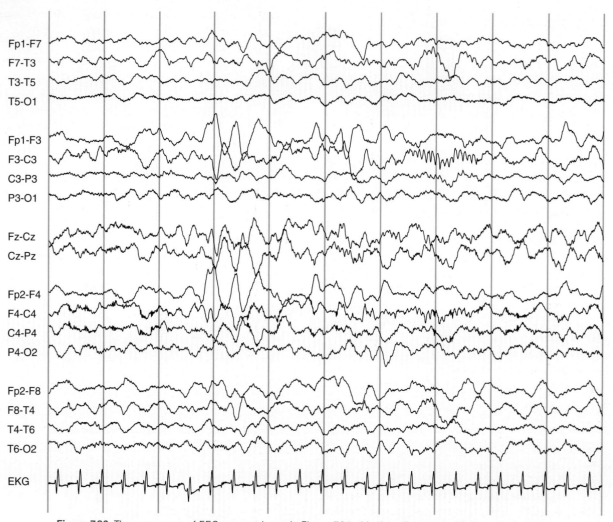

Figure 7.26 The same page of EEG as was shown in Figure 7.24, this time displayed with the use of a 60 Hz notch filter. The notch filter has dramatically "cleaned up" the EEG tracing, and the page now looks fairly unremarkable and easy to interpret. Now that the page has been filtered, there is little to suggest to the reader that several of the electrode contacts probably have impedance problems.

unavoidable situation. The good news is that there is generally *the same amount* of 60 Hz activity under each scalp electrode—there is no reason for it to differ in any significant way from place to place on the head. The reason we often do not see any 60 Hz activity at all in a tracing is that the common mode rejection amplifiers used in our EEG instrument subtract the signal between the compared electrodes. For instance, if the two electrodes being compared are Fp1 and F3, each will have the same amount of 60 Hz artifact under it. When the Fp1-F3 subtraction takes place, this omnipresent 60 Hz signal is subtracted away, and it disappears when we display the Fp1-F3 channel—we may even forget that it is there.

Impedance Mismatch

Now imagine that one of the electrodes in the Fp1-F3 pair is attached much better (has a much lower impedance) than the other. In that case, the two electrodes will "read" the 60 Hz activity to different degrees, even though there's really the same amount under each electrode. In the case of a poor

contact, when F3 is subtracted from Fp1, the 60 Hz artifact will be visible even after the subtraction because there are *different amounts* of 60 Hz activity picked up by each electrode because they have been attached differently. For this reason, the presence of 60 Hz artifact in an electrode is a clue to the possibility that that electrode may have a poor contact with the scalp. This is important to know because an improperly attached electrode may also have a tendency to show voltages that are too high or too low and may also be more prone to include other noise or transient activity caused by its poor attachment. Being alert to the fact that there is a poor electrode contact may prevent the reader from making the error of thinking that an abrupt electrode deflection represents true electrocerebral activity (such as a spike) when it really is caused by a poorly attached contact. Good practice is to keep in mind which electrode contacts showed the 60 Hz artifact before "cleaning up" the EEG with the 60 Hz notch filter, thereafter having a higher level of suspicion regarding any unusual waves that appear to come from those contacts.

CIRCUITS FOR FILTERS

If you were asked to imagine how to design a circuit that could filter the low-frequency component or high-frequency component out of a complex waveform, the task would seem quite daunting. However, you may be pleasantly surprised to see how easy it is to design circuits that perform these functions! The good news is that the circuit designs used to create high-frequency and low-frequency filters are quite simple. In their simplest forms, the circuits have one resistor and one capacitor. Electrical circuits with a combination of resistors and capacitors are called "*RC circuits.*" What follows is a simple review of the basics of RC circuits. Please note that knowledge of RC circuits and the circuit diagrams presented below for high and low filters may not be necessary for the day-to-day reading of EEG, but understanding these circuit designs may give you some extra insights into why filters behave the way they do. This material also explains the rationale behind calibration tests and square-wave responses and how and why they change with different filter settings. If these topics are not of particular interest to you, you may choose to defer reading this section and focus on the more clinically oriented chapters in this text. Alternatively, you may wish to skim the topics in this chapter and read those that may be of particular interest to you.

Basic Circuits and Ohm's Law

The simplest circuit to imagine would be one with a source of voltage (e.g., a flashlight battery) and a resistor, (e.g., a light bulb; see Figure 7.27). The battery is the source of electromotive force in the circuit. You can tell from the structure of the word "electromotive" that this is the circuit element that gives the *electrons* the urge to be in *motion* around the circuit. The battery does this by being positively charged at one end (the cathode) and negatively charged at the other end (the anode). The electrons, as negatively charged particles, have the urge to "run away" from the negative end of the battery and to run toward the positive end. This is the electromotive force set up by the battery, and the strength of this force between any two points is measured in volts. (Although the battery looks like a single object, the trick of its creating a voltage difference between its poles is that there are different chemical reactions

going on in two separated compartments/cells in the battery, one cell creating positive charge at one pole and the other cell creating negative charge at the opposite pole). The more strongly positive the positive side and more strongly negative the negative side, the more strongly electrons will be "urged" to flow around the circuit. A nine-volt battery will cause the electrons to flow through the lightbulb 50% more exuberantly than a 6-volt battery. The flashlight battery set up in Figure 7.27 is a simple, constant source of electromotive force and induces a direct current (DC), a stream of electrons that flows in one direction through the lightbulb. In later examples, we will be replacing the battery/voltage source here with something a bit more complicated, such as a voltage source that wavers left and right (an alternating current or EEG wave), but we will consider the DC examples first.

The lightbulb in the circuit is a source of resistance. It is also considered a "load" in the circuit because it is doing some type of work. In the circuitry diagram, it is symbolized by a resistor. The lightbulb provides resistance to electron flow. Two things happen here worthy of note. First, the electrons have to slow down to get through the resistor. Imagine the electrons as children running through an alleyway. All of a sudden, they encounter the tight zigzag pathway of the resistor. This slows them down. You can think of a lightbulb as offering resistance or friction to the children's ability to run through this pathway, and the resistor/lightbulb gives off heat or light in exchange for slowing down the electrons. Every time they are slowed down by a "zig" or a "zag," they lose energy, which is essentially transferred into making light. In a resistor, the amount of friction or resistance offered by the resistor to the flow of electrons is measured in ohms (the symbol for ohms is Ω). In the Figure 7.27 example, the energy is given off in the form of light and heat in the lightbulb, but you could imagine that the load in this circuit could be some other type of device, such as a motor, a speaker, a popcorn maker, etc. It is intuitive that the bigger the load or resistance you put in the circuit, the more slowly the current will flow. The bigger the voltage (or battery) in the circuit, the faster the current will flow, and the load will be able to do more work. If you had already guessed these relationships then you have essentially already intuited Ohm's law. Ohm's law captures these relationships in a simple mathematical expression: $V = IR$.

How Do You Remember Ohm's Law?

Because Ohm's law is such a key relationship, it is good to have a way to memorize it. If you happened to have studied Latin, or even if this mnemonic just makes things easier for you, you might like to first write Ohm's law as $V = IR$. In Latin, the word *vir* means "man" (e.g., "virile"). In Ohm's law, V stands for voltage (in volts), I stands for current (in amps), and R stands for resistance (in ohms). All of the forms in which you might want to write Ohm's law are easily derived from remembering this $V = IR$ expression. For instance, if you divide both sides of the equation by 'R' you get the form that we use the most here:

$$I = \frac{V}{R}$$

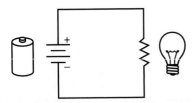

Figure 7.27 A simple circuit with a battery powering a light bulb, using the symbols for a battery and a resistor. The chemical reactions set up in the separate cells of the battery cause its top pole to carry a positive charge and the bottom pole a negative charge. Electrons have the urge to flow counter-clockwise through this circuit, toward the positive pole of the battery. In this circuit, the load is a light bulb, but many different types of loads can be imagined. All loads will cause resistance to electron flow, and are symbolized by a resistor in this diagram.

Which is to say that:

$$current = \frac{voltage}{resistance}$$

This is probably the most intuitive way of writing Ohm's law. This form of the expression shows you how fast the current will flow (i.e., how fast the electrons are moving around the circuit) with any combination of voltage and resistance in a circuit, including the one depicted in Figure 7.27. Ohm's law says that the current, in amps, will be higher if the voltage (V) goes up, but lower if the resistance (R) goes up, and that these changes are all proportional. For instance, if you have a 6-volt battery and a 3-ohm lightbulb, the flow through the circuit will be 2 amps. If you now replace the battery with a 9-volt battery, flow through the circuit will increase, to 3 amps.

$$2\ amp = \frac{6\ volt}{3\ ohm}$$

...changing to a bigger battery $$3\ amp = \frac{9\ volt}{3\ ohm}$$

So that same lightbulb will burn more brightly with a bigger battery because the current will be flowing through it 50% faster and doing that much more work. You can also see that if you put a bigger lightbulb that has a higher resistance into the circuit, this will increase the number of ohms in the 'R' part of the formula and the current will slow down, which makes sense because the electrons have to do more work to get through the higher-resistance lightbulb.

Incidentally, current is measured in amps (or amperes). In basic chemistry, we all had to learn that a "mole" of particles is 6.02×10^{23} particles. If you consider a mole of electrons, each of which holds a very small negative electrical charge, the total charge on a mole of electrons is defined as one *coulomb* of charge (i.e., a coulomb is the total charge on 6.02×10^{23} electrons). An amp is defined as the passage of one coulomb (or one mole—take your pick) of electrons per second. Not to worry, moles do not reappear in this discussion—suffice it to say that an amp implies a fixed number of electrons (current) flowing past a particular point per second.

Measuring Voltage around a Circuit

Now that we have our simplest circuit with a battery and a source of resistance, it is important to get used to using a voltmeter to test the Ohm's law relationships around our circuit. A standard voltmeter has two prongs. Touching both prongs of the voltmeter simultaneously to two different points in a circuit gives you a readout of the voltage drop between those two points (in volts) from the voltmeter. Note that touching a single prong to a single point in a circuit is meaningless—implicit in the concept of voltage is voltage *difference between two points*. Even referring to a 9-volt battery, we are naming the voltage difference between the two battery poles. Touching just one prong of a voltmeter to a point in a circuit (no matter

what is happening at that point) without doing anything with the other prong will not produce a useful number.

How a voltmeter will respond to testing any pair of points in a circuit is a key concept in understanding how filters work because, as we shall see below (spoiler alert!), filter outputs are just the voltmeter outputs at different pairs of points in RC circuits. If you gain an intuitive understanding of what a voltmeter output would look like when different pairs of points are compared in the simple RC circuits below, then you will have gained a good understanding of basic filter electronics, because these different voltmeter outputs will end up being the filter outputs.

Returning to the simple circuit in Figure 7.28 and using the expression of Ohm's law to predict the current in the circuit, the battery is a 6-volt battery and the resistor is 3 ohms. Ohm's law tells us that the current running around this circuit would be 2 amps (6 volts/3 ohms = 2 amps), and this would apply equally at all points in the circuit, A, B, C, and D. If we care to measure the voltage of this circuit, we could put a voltmeter with its prongs across the battery at points C and D and, no surprise, the voltmeter will read 6 volts because, after all, we did buy a 6-volt battery. If we measure the voltage across the resistor at points A and B, we also get 6 volts. Even though it does somehow seem conceptually different to measure the voltage across the battery compared to the voltage across the resistor, it becomes clear from looking at the circuit diagram that this is really the same measurement. Sliding the voltmeter prong from point C to point A doesn't change anything because there is nothing in the circuit between the two points (likewise between point D and point B). Another way of stating this is that points C and A are *equipotential*, which is to say that there is no potential (voltage) difference between them. You could prove this by putting the voltmeter prongs on C and A, which would register "0."

Now let's look at a slightly more complicated circuit with two resistors and make them of different sizes. The resistors in Figure 7.29 are attached head-to-tail, also said to be attached *in series*. This circuit has a 2 ohm resistor and a 1 ohm resistor connected in series. You can also visualize this as a circuit with a bigger light bulb on the top and a smaller light bulb on the bottom. Now let's use a voltmeter

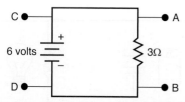

Figure 7.28 Measuring the voltage drop across the battery (placing the voltmeter prongs at points C and D) and measuring the voltage drop across the resistor (comparing points A and B) give the same reading because points C and A, like points D and B, are equipotential because there is nothing between them but an ideal resistance-free wire. Ohm's law tells us that the current flow through this circuit will be (6 volts/3 ohms) = 2 amps. Note that the lines connecting A, B, C, and D to the main circuit are not formally part of the circuit, but just show points where a voltmeter's prongs might be applied to the main circuit to measure voltage drops between pairs of points.

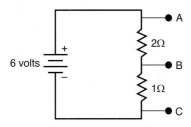

Figure 7.29 A circuit with a 2-ohm and a 1-ohm resistor connected in series with a 6-volt battery. It is no surprise that, similar to the previous circuit in Figure 7.28, measuring the voltage drop from A to C yields 6 volts, because this measurement is equivalent to reading the voltage across the battery. Measuring from A to B, then from B to C, shows what portion of the 6-volt voltage drop is used up by each resistor. The total resistance of the two loads in series can simply be added ($2\Omega + 1\Omega = 3\Omega$), so Ohm's law tells us that the current again will be 2 amps everywhere in this circuit. Ohm's law also tells us that 4 volts is used up measuring from A to B across the 2Ω load, and 2 volts measuring from B to C across the 1Ω load. Intuitively, it makes sense that two thirds of the voltage drop is used up by the bigger resistor and the remaining one third by the smaller resistor.

to measure voltage drop across each part of the circuit. It is no surprise that measuring across A and C gives a value of 6 volts because we are measuring across a total resistance of (2 ohms + 1 ohm) = 3 ohms, much as we did with the previous example, so we get the same result as with the previous circuit: 6 volts. Also, we have a 6-volt battery and, according to the same logic as described above, the A to C measurement is equivalent to measuring across the 6-volt battery. Using Ohm's law, the current flow running around this circuit equals 6 volts divided by the total 3-ohm resistance of the circuit leaving (6 volts/3 ohms) = 2 amps, the same as in the last problem. When a circuit follows a circular track as in this example, the current value is the same in all locations in the circuit—there are no slow or fast regions of current flow—it is 2 amps everywhere.

The voltage measurements become a little more interesting when we measure the voltage drop across just the 2-ohm resistor (comparing point A to point B) and then across the bottom 1-ohm resistor (point B to point C). This can be figured out in two ways, either mathematically using Ohm's law, or by intuition. Solving for voltage will be easiest using the original expression of Ohm's law: $V = IR$. We know the current across both resistors is 2 amps from the previous calculation (and that the current is the same everywhere in a circular circuit). The resistance of the load between A and B is 2 ohms. Ohm's law tells us then that there is a 4-volt drop across this resistor: *4 volts* = 2 amps × 2 ohms. Using Ohm's law to calculate the voltage drop across the second, 1-ohm resistor, $V = IR$ gives us a voltage drop of 2 volts because *2 volts* = 2 amps × 1 ohm. This is a harmonious outcome because the total voltage drop across both resistors (4 volts + 2 volts) is 6 volts, which we have previously established is the total voltage drop across the whole circuit (both resistors).

An important concept here is that, when you have a string of loads attached in series, the sum of the voltage drops across

each of the loads must equal the total voltage drop across all of the loads, which for this circuit totals 6 volts. If you prefer the mathematical expression of this, you could say that $V_1 + V_2 + V_3 \ldots = V_{total}$ for one, two, three, or more loads attached in series along a circuit. Now imagine the circuit shown in Figure 7.29, but instead of each resistor having a fixed value, such as 1 and 2 ohms in the diagram, each resistor had a knob that would allow you to vary its resistance—let's say between 1 to 1,000 ohms. No matter what settings you would choose for the knobs, if you had a voltmeter (V_1) measuring from A to B and a second one (V_2) measuring from B to C, the sum of the two voltages from these voltmeters ($V_1 + V_2$) would always equal 6 volts in this circuit, no matter how you might spin the knobs. This principle that, whatever the resistance values of the two loads are, $V_1 + V_2$ will always sum up to the total battery voltage is a key concept to understanding how RC circuits work to create filters. Convince yourself that $V_1 + V_2$ is always true, imagining that you have turned the resistor knobs to all types of different values between 1 and 1,000 ohms. When trying different examples, remember that the current around the circuit, I, is calculated by using Ohm's law, $V = I \times R$, using the total of all resistors in the circuit for R and that the calculated current, I, will be the same at all points in the circuit. The general lesson here is that circuit elements with large resistances will have large voltage drops across them, and smaller resistances will be associated with smaller voltage drops.

Capacitors and RC Circuits

We will now introduce the second key element of the RC circuit, the capacitor, and consider how it behaves when placed in our simple circuit attached to a 6-volt battery. A capacitor consists of two flat plates stacked right next to each other, much like a stack of two pancakes, but the two plates are separated from one another by an insulator that electrons cannot jump across. They can look much like the symbol of parallel lines used in circuit diagrams to represent them as in Figure 7.30. Considering the idea of putting a capacitor into one of our DC circuits, your first reaction might be that capacitors would be worthless in DC circuits run by a battery because they would act like a brick wall that would simply stop current flow. Although in certain circumstances, especially with DC currents, their behavior does resemble that of a brick wall, we will see that they display interestingly different behaviors with oscillating currents. Note that flipping the switch closed to allow the DC circuit to run in Figure 7.30 causes the battery current to start flowing and the capacitor becomes charged. Think of the positive pole of the battery attracting electrons off the top plate of the capacitor so that the top plate becomes positive. Likewise, the negative pole of the battery pushes electrons onto the bottom plate so it becomes negative.

What does current flow look like when the switch is closed and the battery starts charging up the capacitor? You can visualize the capacitor plate as a shallow beach along a river bank, about 100 feet wide and 10 feet deep. Access to the riverbank is by a narrow passageway that allows the children from our previous example to run onto the narrow beach.

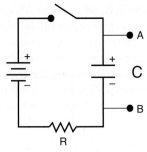

Figure 7.30 A simple RC circuit with a battery, a capacitor, a resistor, and a switch. When the switch at the top of the diagram is closed, at first current will flow quickly because the capacitor is empty of charge and offers little resistance to flow, but then increasingly slowly as the capacitor accumulates charge. The length of time it will take the capacitor to reach a fully charged state is a function of the resistance, R, of the resistor and the capacitance, C, of the capacitor. The bigger the resistor, the more slowly the capacitor will fill with charge. The bigger the capacitor, likewise, the longer it will take to fill with charge. This is consistent with the idea that the time constant of a circuit, $\tau = R \times C$, describes how quickly the capacitor fills with charge. Imagine placing a voltmeter across the capacitor, at points A and B. Try to guess what the voltage curve might look like after the switch is closed. The explanation appears later in the text.

Once the switch is closed allowing current to flow, children can start running down the passageway and fill the narrow beach along the river. When the first kids run across the passageway, they encounter an empty beach and the speed they run is just as fast as they were running even before they got to the beach entrance because, from their point of view, there is nothing but a big empty expanse of beach ahead and nothing to slow them down. Of course, as time passes the beach progressively fills with children and each one will have more difficulty finding a space on the beach. Because of the progressive crowding effect, as time passes the speed with which children can continue to run down the passageway steadily decreases. Eventually, when the riverbank beach is 99% full, the flow in the passageway falls almost to zero children per second because there is really no more room (though there is always some child very slowly trying to cram onto the beach, even when it appears full to everyone else!). Just how hard the kids are crammed onto the riverbank, of course, depends on how big the voltage of the battery is in the circuit that is pushing them onto this limited beach area. If you replace the 6-volt battery with a 12-volt battery, you will be able to cram twice as many kids onto this capacitor–beach.

How does one describe the *capacitance* of a capacitor? If you go to the capacitor store and speak with a capacitor salesman, he will boast of each capacitor's capacitance as follows. This is an excellent capacitor! If you put just 1 volt across this 1-farad capacitor, it will charge up and hold a whole coulomb of charge. But this bigger, 2-farad capacitor, if you put that same 1 volt across it, will charge up to and hold 2 coulombs of charge! It seems logical then that the unit of capacitance, the *farad*, is defined as the number of coulombs of charge a capacitor will hold per volt put across its terminals. Therefore, a farad is 1 coulomb/volt. The bigger the capacitor, the bigger its capacitance, which makes sense because it

is as if the facing beaches along the river are bigger. It is also not a surprise that if you double the voltage of the battery used across the same capacitor, it will be able to hold twice as much charge. So capacitance is how much charge per volt the capacitor can hold: C (in farads) = charge (coulombs)/voltage (volts).

Capacitors and Alternating Current

The magic of the role of capacitors in filter circuits becomes obvious when we consider what happens when the battery is replaced with an alternating current. In fact, in electronics, alternating currents are more commonly encountered than direct currents. AC is the type of current that is supplied by the electrical mains in our buildings and houses, and how electricity is transmitted through power lines. Voltages supplied through our electric outlets resemble a sine wave. Instead of driving the electrons always in one direction as is done with a simple DC battery setup, instead the electrons are caused to go back and forth, back and forth, without a net flow in one direction or another. There is no reason to be disappointed that there is no net flow of electrons around the circuit. Energy can still be easily harnessed from this back-and-forth motion. Imagine that, instead of constantly rubbing one hand against the other in a single direction (e.g., left hand going up and right hand going down), you rub your hands back and forth for a period of time. Both methods would cause the palms of your hands up to heat up. Running electrons back and forth through a light bulb filament can work just as well as running a direct current through a light bulb filament in order to make light. Flashlights work with the direct current from a battery, while our household lights use the alternating current method, and both can make an incandescent lightbulb shine. The alternating current example we are interested in the most, however, is not what comes out of our electric outlets, but the fact that EEG signals also resemble alternating currents in that they look more like sine waves than straight lines. When you start to consider the behavior of RC circuits when presented with an alternating current rather than a direct current, things start to get interesting.

So what does a capacitor think of an alternating current? Let us imagine an alternating current that alternates very, very quickly (i.e., has a high frequency) and has a relatively low amplitude. In essence, this current causes the electrons to simply quickly "jiggle" back and forth in the circuit, jiggling left and right just a small amount, but very fast. What does the jiggling wave do when it encounters the capacitor? When we first switch on this fast, jiggling AC signal, the capacitor starts out uncharged. The first electrons start to flow onto the capacitor's plate, but as soon as they arrive, they are immediately "called back," and asked to go the opposite direction, vacating the plate. You can see what happens—because the capacitor plate is nowhere near filled up with electrons at the time the electrons are made to turn back, it presents almost no resistance to the flow of this type of wave. Far from being a brick wall, with a low amplitude, fast-jiggling sine wave, the capacitor is almost invisible to this type of electron flow!

Now we will imagine the same experiment, but instead of a fast jiggling current, we will use a wave that fluctuates at a very slow rate (a slow wave). In this example, the capacitor plate will, indeed, fill up with electrons, slowing down the flow of the current before it reverses direction. If the frequency of the wave is very, very slow, the experiment actually begins to resemble the case of the DC battery, trying to charge the capacitor completely. In this example, with *very* low frequencies, the capacitor can, indeed, act like a "brick wall" for the advancing electrons. Intuitively we can see that the amount of resistance a capacitor presents to an alternating current becomes less and less as the frequency of the current increases—very fast frequencies are less slowed down by a capacitor and very slow frequencies are very much impeded by the capacitor. Of course the second factor will be how big the capacitor is. If the capacitor has a lot of "space" for electrons on the plate (i.e., has a high capacitance), it will offer less resistance to current flow at any particular frequency. Small-capacitance capacitors will offer more resistance to flow at any particular current frequency. This is the big difference between resistors and capacitors. Although resistors always offer the same amount of resistance to current flow independent of current frequency, the amount of resistance a capacitor offers varies, and is a function of the frequency of the wave it encounters. Instead of resistance, a capacitor is said to have a certain *impedance*, which is symbolized by the letter 'Z.' Impedance is the resistance to current flow offered by a capacitor. As we worked out intuitively above, impedance will vary upward with slower frequencies and will be lower the bigger the capacitor. The formula for the impedance Z of a capacitor will then not come as a big surprise:

$$Z = \frac{1}{2\pi f C}$$

where Z is the effective impedance in ohms, f is the frequency of the signal, and C is the capacitance of the capacitor given in farads. Note that the formula predicts, just as we expected, that with higher frequencies f, the impedance to current flow that the capacitor provides, Z, becomes smaller. At extremely high frequencies (f very high), the capacitor might provide little, if any, resistance to flow in the circuit. Likewise, as the capacitance of the circuit's capacitor rises (C very high), the impedance also will become very low, as we predicted. You can see where this is going—basic filter design is based on this general principle that capacitors preferentially block flow to more slowly oscillating currents and are much more liberal in allowing higher frequency alternating currents to remain undisturbed. The size of the capacitor and resistor in the circuit will help "tune" how aggressively the filter will handle different frequencies.

HIGH-FREQUENCY FILTERS, LOW-FREQUENCY FILTERS, AND RC CIRCUITS

Now we have all the pieces and concepts required to make high- and low-frequency filters out of the simple RC circuit in

Figure 7.31. Returning to the idea that when two loads are in series, we recall that the voltage drop across the first load plus the voltage drop across the second load must always equal the voltage drop across the whole circuit: $V_1 + V_2 = V_{total}$. For the RC circuit in Figure 7.31, the same concept holds true: the voltage drop across the resistor plus the voltage drop across the capacitor must always equal the battery voltage: $V_R + V_C = V_{total}$. What is the voltage drop across each element? Calculating V_R seems straightforward. Recalling Ohm's law, $V = IR$, because the resistance of the resistor doesn't vary, the voltage drop across the resistor is simply $I \times R$, as shown in Figure 7.32. Clearly, V_R is a simple function of the current flow because R does not change. When there is current flowing through the resistor, V_R will be a certain value depending on the amount of current, and as the current falls toward zero, if that happens, a voltmeter across the resistor will also fall toward zero. What the voltmeter across the capacitor, V_C, will measure will depend on the frequency of the wave the capacitor is dealing with. Consider a very fast "jiggling" current. Knowing that the capacitor offers very little resistance to flow for that type of signal, V_C will be low (remembering that voltage drops across a circuit element only to the extent that the element offers resistance to current flow). For *slowly* oscillating currents, the capacitor does have time to accumulate charge and a charged capacitor resists flow, so V_C will have a greater value. Don't miss what just happened here, we just invented a high-frequency filter! A voltmeter measuring V_C continuously across the capacitor won't see almost any voltage change if there is a very high-frequency signal in the circuit. Its readout will just look like a flat (or near-flat) line (i.e., the "jiggle" has been filtered out). On the other hand, if the circuit has a very low frequency signal, charge will keep accumulating on the capacitor plates as the wave sweeps slowly back and forth, resulting in resistance to current flow. The voltmeter will then measure an oscillating voltage drop across

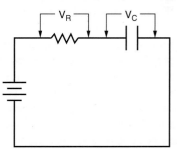

Figure 7.31 In an RC circuit with one resistor and one capacitor, the sum of the voltage across the resistor, V_R, and the voltage across the capacitor, V_C, will always equal the battery voltage. This means that the total voltage drop of the circuit can be thought of as being passed back and forth or shared between V_R and V_C. When the battery is initially attached, the flow of current through the resistor will be fast as will be the filling up of the capacitor with charge. Fast flow through the resistor implies that V_R will be high ($V_R = I \times R$) and lack of resistance to current flow into the capacitor means V_C will be low. Eventually, as the capacitor becomes nearly full, current flow through the resistor slows to near zero, so V_R will approach zero, and the voltage across the capacitor, V_C, will rise toward battery voltage as it fills with charge and the current drops to zero.

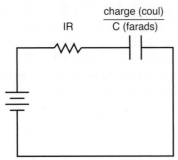

Figure 7.32 This is the same circuit as in the previous figure, but now with the output voltages expressed as their respective mathematical expressions. The voltage across the resistor, V_R, is a direct function of the amount of current flow, I, because the R-value for the resistor is fixed ($V_R = I \times R$). Voltage across the capacitor, V_C, is a function of how much the current flow is impeded by charge having filled up the capacitor ($V_C = $ charge/C). These examples are given with a DC battery, but the next step is to replace the DC battery symbol with an oscillating wave, such as an EEG wave. The total voltage of the oscillating wave will also be shared by each of the two circuit elements, depending on the extent to which the capacitor impedes current flow. The capacitor impedes the flow of current a lot with slower wave activity because the capacitor has time to fill with charge and resist current flow (V_C is higher). With faster frequencies, the capacitor is never anywhere near full, so it resists current flow less (V_C is lower). The opposite is happening to V_R, because it is simply a function of current flow. When the capacitor is impeding current flow because there is a low frequency signal (V_C is high), V_R is low because the current flow is low, and the opposite apportionment of voltage occurs with a high-frequency wave. This is how the total voltage of the wave is "shared" between V_R and V_C.

the capacitor accordingly, outputting a slow-wave signal. The slower the slow wave, the more the capacitor resists flow and the more that slow wave's contour will appear in a voltmeter that spans the capacitor (V_C). Because a capacitor is less likely to offer resistance to current flow with high-frequency waves, so a voltmeter across the capacitor will reflect little, if any, of a very fast wave.

There is also another way to estimate the voltage across the capacitor based on the definition of the farad as given above. One farad of capacitance (C) was defined as the ability to hold one coulomb of charge per volt put across the capacitor, implying that C = charge/volt, or C = charge/V_C. We can actually turn the tables on this equation and use it to "read" the voltage across the capacitor, V_C, by rearranging it as: V_C = charge/C. Because the capacitance of our capacitor in the RC circuit in Figure 7.32 does not change, this is another way of saying that the voltage across the capacitor, V_C, is proportional to the amount of charge on the capacitor at the moment of the measurement. And we have already seen that the capacitor might charge up quite a bit if there is a very slow wave, but very little if there is a fast wave.

The circuit in Figure 7.33 represents a high-frequency filter. Imagine that, instead of a DC battery in the position on the left side of the circuit, we replaced this with an oscillating input signal to be "processed" into the voltage output at the B and C points that flank the capacitor, an output will be obtained that resembles the input signal, but with the high frequencies filtered out.

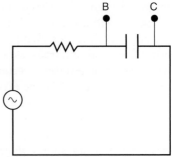

Figure 7.33 This is the schematic for a high-frequency filter. The input wave (e.g., an EEG wave) is presented to the left side of the circuit where the new alternating current symbol is. The output signal is obtained from the B and C poles, which flank the capacitor and output V_C. You can imagine that, for a "jiggling" high-frequency wave the capacitor provides little resistance to current flow and, therefore, a voltmeter measuring across points B and C will measure very little voltage change. If a slow wave is run through this circuit, however, charge will repeatedly build up in the capacitor as the slow wave cycles, providing resistance to current flow and, therefore, a voltage drop across the capacitor will be repeatedly seen. With a slow wave input, the voltage measured across points B and C will show most of the slow wave oscillation.

Now we will consider what the voltage drop across the resistor, V_R, will look like, again comparing its behavior with fast waves versus slow waves. It will come as no surprise that the output of the V_R voltmeter is going to be the output of a low-frequency filter. First, let's consider a very fast wave in the circuit in Figure 7.34, but now with the voltmeter prongs placed across the resistor at points A and B. As we worked through above, with a quickly "jiggling" fast wave, the voltage drop across the capacitor, V_C, will be very low because the capacitor provides little resistance to current flow with this type of wave. In the extreme case of a very fast wave and/or very big capacitor, the capacitor behaves similarly to an open wire (in fact, if you want to, at these extremes you could visually erase the capacitor from the circuit). In this case, V_C is zero, and a voltmeter across the resistor in the circuit will reflect a readout of the fast wave accurately. Remembering that $V_R + V_C = V_{total}$, so if V_C is near zero for the very fast wave, then the equation tells us that V_R will effectively reflect the total voltage of the input wave, which is the fast wave in this case. Thus, the output at poles A and B in Figure 7.34 will transmit a fast wave nicely, just as we would expect from a LFF. In the case of a very slow wave, the opposite happens. The capacitor fills with charge and provides much more resistance to flow, so V_C is high which implies that V_R will be low to balance the $V_R + V_C = V_{total}$ equation. What really makes V_R low? In the case of the slow wave, the capacitor is slowing the current down and, remembering that Ohm's law tells us that the voltage across the resistor $V_R = $ IR, we can see that with slowed down currents, the IR term will be lower with slow wave activity. The capacitor's filling up with charge and slowing down the current, I, in the circuit makes the V_R reading across the resistor lower, effectively filtering out slow wave activity, but favoring fast wave activity. Thus, we have seen that a voltmeter (at poles B and C in Figure 7.33) across the

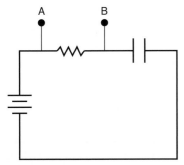

Figure 7.34 This is the schematic for a low-frequency filter, similar to the setup in Figure 7.33 but now with the output voltage measured across points A and B (V_R), flanking the resistor. When a slow wave is presented to this circuit, the wave's oscillations are slowed down by the capacitor which, in turn, causes slowed current flow through the resistor. With little current flow through the resistor there is little voltage drop across the resistor (because $V = IR$), so a voltmeter output at this position effectively filters out slower oscillations when measured from points A and B. In contrast, a fast "jiggling" wave will not be impeded by the capacitor, so the current will likewise "jiggle" through the resistor and be reflected accurately by a voltmeter at positions A and B.

capacitor in an RC circuit will filter out high frequencies. A voltmeter (at poles A and B in Figure 7.34) across the resistor in an RC circuit will filter out low frequencies.

The examples we gave in this discussion were for pure slow waves or pure fast waves. It is worth noting that, in the case of waves of mixed frequency such as EEG waves, these RC circuits handle the high- and low-frequency components of mixed waves as if they were presented to the filter circuit separately, much as was illustrated in Figures 7.4 through 7.7 that showed the action of filters on a wave with mixed frequencies.

THE IMPACT OF FILTERS ON THE FAST COMPONENT AND SLOW COMPONENT OF SQUARE WAVE INPUTS

Before an EEG recording begins, the technologist can confirm that the different filter setups on the machine are behaving as expected by sending calibration pulses through the machine consisting of square waves. When filters are functioning properly, they will change the shape of the square wave in a predictable fashion. Measurements can then be made in the changes in the square wave output that can confirm the proper functioning of the filters. Why is it that a square wave is a good choice to check that the instrument's amplifiers and filters are functioning properly and similarly across all channels? Square waves hand the recording system extreme examples of both fast wave and slow wave activity. The essentially vertical upswing of the square wave can be seen as representing very, very fast activity—a fast transient. The horizontal portion of the slow wave represents very, very slow activity, essentially a DC shift of electricity (the slowest of all slow waves) held at a specific voltage. It makes sense then that we will expect the HFF to change the shape of the upswing of the square wave

KEY POINTS IN UNDERSTANDING HOW RC CIRCUITS CREATE HIGH-FREQUENCY AND LOW-FREQUENCY FILTERS

1. The sum of the voltage across the resistor (V_R) and the capacitor (V_C) always equals the total voltage across the circuit (V_{TOTAL}). That total voltage is determined by either the battery or the oscillating EEG waves shown on the left side of the circuit diagrams.
2. The amount of voltage drop each of the two circuit elements, the resistor and the capacitor, contributes to the total is proportional to the degree that each presents a barrier to current flow: no barrier—no voltage drop, high barrier—high voltage drop.
3. The output of the voltmeter placed across the resistor (V_R) is the output of the LFF.
4. The output of the voltmeter placed across the capacitor (V_C) is the output of the HFF.
5. Capacitors present little barrier to the flow of quickly oscillating currents, so these currents do not show up in the V_C readout, resulting in high frequencies being filtered out at V_C—the HFF. Because the capacitor does not slow down quickly oscillating currents through the circuit, these fast currents continue to oscillate back and forth through the resistor and appear in V_R ($V_R = IR$ for the resistor)—the LFF.
6. Capacitors present a large barrier to the flow of slow waves, so slow waves appear readily in the V_C readout—the HFF. Because capacitors slow down the current flow of slow waves everywhere in the circuit, little of the slow wave currents passes through the resistor either, so they do not appear in V_R (again, $V_R = IR$ for the resistor)—the LFF.

and the LFF to change the shape of the horizontal portions of the square wave (see Figure 7.36). The method by which a square wave response can be analyzed to confirm proper function of HFFs and LFFs and how the square wave changes shape for these filters are described in the following sections.

High-Frequency Filter Handling of Square Waves

First, in the case of the high-frequency filter, what will the output wave be when the input voltage is a square wave? Remember that the output voltage of a high-frequency filter is essentially the measurement of the voltage across the capacitor in the RC circuit shown in Figure 7.33. Running a square wave through our HFF is equivalent to introducing a square wave voltage generator at the battery position in the circuit, and replacing that input with whatever is output from voltmeter connected to the B and C poles in the circuit diagram. In order to mimic the nearly vertical upswing of the square wave, we can imagine simply closing the switch on the circuit if a plain battery were still in the circuit. Once the switch is closed on a circuit with a battery, you can imagine that the "input voltage" will jump vertically up to 6 volts, which will have the same shape as the upstroke of the square wave. At the *initial* moment of connection of the battery and upsweep of the square wave (imagine the first millisecond of current flow), the capacitor is empty of charge. Because it is empty, it effectively provides no resistance to current flow and our high-frequency filter (which is the same as the output voltage of a voltmeter connected to poles B and C) registers zero because V = I × R, and *R* for the capacitor is initially zero. As the capacitor continues to charge rapidly it begins to provide resistance to current flow and an increasing voltage drop can be measured across it. If the first part of the square wave were allowed to continue vertically forever, the capacitor becomes fully charged (and eventually behaves as a "brick wall" to current flow), the maximum voltage difference across its poles would be attained, and the output voltage curve seen in Figure 7.35 would result. In practice, only the very first part of the filter output shown in Figure 7.35 is seen because the square wave only rises to a specific voltage, 6 volts in our example, and is held there. Based on this explanation, we expect that an HFF will round out the *upswing* (vertical portion) of a square-wave pulse as seen in the bottom portion of Figure 7.36. Remember that the quick step-up of the input voltage at the beginning of the square wave can be seen as a type of very high-frequency activity, akin to a "spike," or the quick up and down of waves seen with muscle artifact, or some other very high-frequency wave. In summary, in addition to attenuating the voltage of high-frequency waves as discussed earlier in this chapter, high-frequency filters also tend to "round out" the shape of the rapid (close to vertical) upswings and downswings in these fast waves (fast transient activity). This is why very aggressive use of an HFF (setting it to increasingly lower cutoff frequencies) tends to round out the up and down component of very fast, spikey waves (such as muscle artifact), potentially creating an unwanted change in wave shape that can make muscle artifact more difficult to recognize. Aggressive use of a HFF can give muscle artifact a

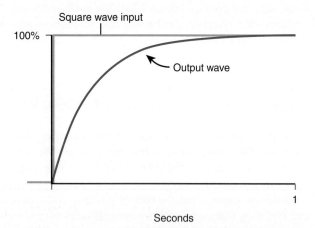

Figure 7.35 This figure shows a magnification of the upper left corner of a square wave input (the lighter red vertical line at the left side of the figure continuing to the horizontal line at the top of the figure), showing the output assuming that the square wave were run through a 1 Hz **high-frequency filter** (the curved, darker red line)—compare to the bottom portion of Figure 7.36. The exaggerated HFF setting of 1 Hz shown in this example is not used in clinical EEG but is used here for illustrative purposes. Imagining that the upswing of the red square wave on the left side of this example represents a very fast spike in the EEG, the HFF would tend to round its shape considerably ("Output wave"). Aggressive use of HFFs can misleadingly round out activity that would otherwise have a "spiky" shape (for example, turning muscle artifact into output that appears more sinusoidal).

more rounded appearance, making it look more sinusoidal, and more similar to fast brain wave activity, which it is not.

The tendency of the high-frequency filter to round the shape of a fast transient (such as the very quick upswing component of the square wave) as illustrated in the idealized curve shown in Figure 7.35 can also be seen in changes in the shape of EEG waves recorded in practice. Figures 7.37 through 7.39 show the effect of increasingly aggressive HFF cutoff frequencies on a page of EEG. Note in particular the change of the appearance of the muscle artifact in the right temporal channels at the bottom of the page (F8-T8 and T8-P8). The use of aggressive HFF settings transforms what was obvious "spiky" muscle artifact into a wave that is sinusoidal in appearance and could easily be mistaken for brain wave activity.

An additional type of distortion produced by RC filters is phase shifting, which is a displacement of a wave to the left or to the right from its original position along the time axis. Although phase shifting is usually minor and does not present a practical problem in clinical electroencephalography, the phase shifting effect can be more important in other applications, such as evoked potentials, in which absolute wave latencies are measured.

Why doesn't the HFF affect the shape of the horizontal component of the square wave? During the horizontal part of the slow wave, the voltage in the circuit is held at a single value, such as the 6-volt value of the original simple battery circuit we started off with. At this point, the capacitor has acquired its charge and creates a non-varying resistance to flow. The voltage drop across the capacitor (points B and C) then remains steady, maintaining the horizontal component of the square wave.

Low-Frequency Filter Handling of Square Waves

Because the horizontal component of the square wave is the (very) slow component, we will expect to see the LFF affect the shape of that portion of the square wave. For the LFF, the filter output is now the voltage across the resistor as depicted in Figure 7.34, and a converse type of behavior is seen. Keep in mind that the total voltage change across the circuit (which, in this example, is essentially the voltage of the square wave input at any given instant) must be the sum of the voltage drop across the capacitor and the voltage drop across the resistor. Given the LFF design, the output wave is synonymous with the voltage change, V_R, across the resistor as shown in Figure 7.34 (i.e., the output voltage that compares poles A and B). At the initial instant of the step-up in voltage of the square wave, the capacitor is uncharged and thus provides no resistance to current flow, so current flow through the circuit and the resistor is at a maximum at the beginning (upswing) of the square wave. Consequently, according to Ohm's law, there is initially no voltage drop across the capacitor ($V_C = 0$). With the voltage across the capacitor out of the equation, at the moment of the square-wave upswing, the voltage drop across the resistor accounts for the total voltage drop across the circuit and is equal to the voltage of the square wave input—the filter output wave nearly exactly parallels the upswing of the square wave. Another way of thinking of this is that, at the moment of the upswing of the square wave, because the capacitor is

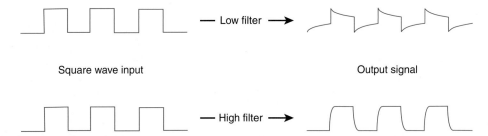

Figure 7.36 This figure depicts the separate effects of a low-frequency filter (LFF) and a high-frequency filter (HFF) on a square wave input. Note the transformation of the square wave brought about by the LFF in the top part of the figure. The vertical portion of the square wave is unchanged (because it really represents very fast activity) but the horizontal portions of the wave tend to "sag" or "float" back toward the baseline. LFFs tend to filter out any horizontal (DC) portion of a square wave that is away from the baseline by causing it to drift toward "zero" voltage. In contrast, the vertical component of the square wave can be thought of as a very fast wave and is not changed by an ideal LFF. The lower portion of the figure shows the effect of an HFF on a square wave. Now note that the upswings and downswings of the square wave (the vertical components) are slurred and rounded off. The tendency of HFFs to curve or round off the fast or near-vertical components of a waveform can transform spike-like waves into waveforms that appear more rounded or sinusoidal. This effect is accentuated by more aggressive use (setting lower cutoff frequencies) of HFFs. As expected, the HFF does not affect the horizontal (DC) component of the square waves.

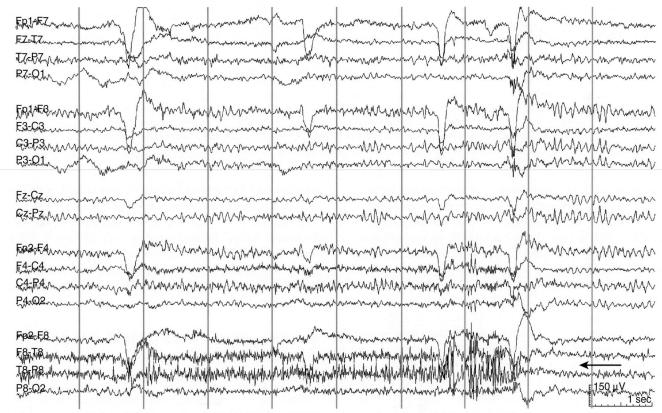

Figure 7.37 This page of EEG recorded with a standard high-frequency filter setting of 70 Hz shows an awake pattern with a posterior rhythm that is well seen and multiple eyeblink and eye-movement artifacts. The varying, spiky, and sputtering nature of the fast activity as is seen in the F8-T8 and T8-P8 channels (arrow) and its location are strong clues that these waves originate from muscle rather than brain. The effect of lowering the HFF cutoff frequency on these waves is examined in the following figures.

empty of charge and offers no resistance to current flow, you could erase it from the circuit diagram. It is now easy to see that the voltage measured across poles A and B is the battery or square wave voltage, at least at that initial moment (just as it was in the simpler Figure 7.27). This formula $V_R = I \times R$ is simply telling us that the output voltage of the filter, V_R, is a

simple reflection of how much current, I, is running through the resistor at that initial moment. This explains why the LFF has no impact on the vertical component of a square wave.

As the capacitor begins to charge, however, it begins to offer increasing resistance to current flow and the voltage drop measured across it increases. Because the sum total of the voltage

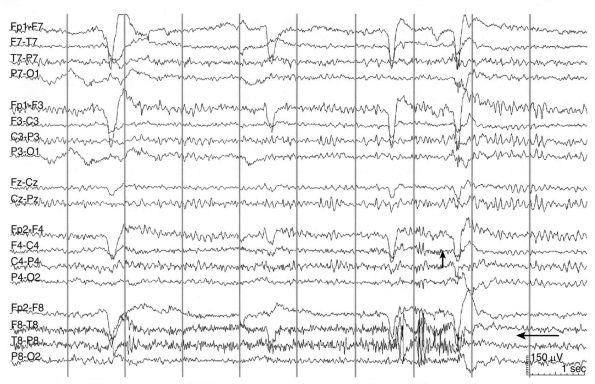

Figure 7.38 The same page of EEG shown in the previous figure is displayed with a more aggressive high-frequency filter setting of 35 Hz. Compare the appearance of the muscle artifact in the right temporal area to the previous figure. The ragged, spiky appearance of the right temporal muscle artifact is now less pronounced, though, for the most part, the activity can still be recognized as arising from muscle rather than from brain (arrow). Also note changes caused by the filter, sometimes subtle, elsewhere on the page. For instance, the muscle artifact seen in the middle of the eighth second of the page in the F4-C4 and C4-P4 channels is now not so obviously an example of muscle artifact (vertical arrow).

drops offered by the capacitor and the resistor must remain a constant, (V_{total}, the square wave input voltage, always equals V_R +V_C), it is clear that as the voltage increases across the capacitor as it is acquiring more charge (and providing more resistance to current flow), the voltage across the resistor must concomitantly fall. It is logical that V_R will continue to fall because current flow is slowing down as the capacitor charges, and the voltage drop across the resistor, $V_R = I \times R$, falls. This accounts for the sagging curve of the LFF filter output seen in Figure 7.40. If the square wave is held at peak voltage long enough, the capacitor will eventually become completely charged and current flow in the circuit will completely stop. If there is no current flow across the resistor, there will be no voltage change across the resistor (per Ohm's law, $V = I \times R$), and the output wave curve of the LFF in Figure 7.40 eventually drops to the zero-baseline, as shown.

Therefore, in addition to decreasing the amplitude of slow-wave activity as discussed earlier in this chapter, low-frequency filters also change the shape of low-frequency activity. LFFs create a tendency for a wave that otherwise would have been "horizontal" in shape, but hanging above the channel baseline or sunken below the channel baseline, to veer back toward the zero-baseline. The square wave input depicted in Figure 7.40 "wanted" to stay hanging up at the 100%-line, but LFFs tend to make such persistent channel deflections "sag" back down to or "float" back up to the

zero-baseline. One advantage of the action of LFFs is that, by causing the output voltage to sag or float back toward zero, they help keep EEG channels from straying far outside their horizontal "alleys" for prolonged periods of time, bringing them back toward the center of the channel. A disadvantage is that, should there actually be a prolonged DC current (voltage held above or below zero for a significant period of time) arising from the brain, the LFF would tend to mask it.

Measuring Square Wave Calibration Pulses to Confirm the EEG Instrument is Functioning Correctly: Filter Time Constants

Confirming the effect of high and low filters on square wave inputs is the method we use to confirm that an electroencephalograph is operating properly and according to the stated filter settings. The effect that high- and low-frequency filters are expected to have on square waves is determined by the filter's time constant.

Let's pause for a moment and ask the question: how long does it take for a capacitor to become fully charged in an RC circuit? Looking at the capacitor in Figure 7.30, we can think about this question intuitively. First, the bigger the capacitor's capacitance, "C," in farads, the longer it should take to charge. This makes sense because there's a bigger "beachfront" to fill up with electrons, so it will take longer to fill up. The second

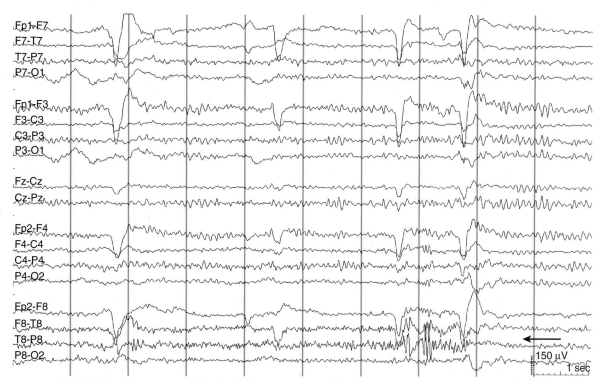

Figure 7.39 The same page of EEG as shown in the previous two figures is now displayed with a very aggressive high-frequency filter (HFF) setting of 15 Hz. This very low HFF cutoff frequency is rarely used in clinical practice because of its profound effect on wave shape but its effect is shown here for illustrative purposes. The HFF's tendency to round the shape of fast activity has converted the previously spiky muscle artifact into a sinusoidal waveform (arrow). It is no longer obvious that the source of the right temporal activity is muscle rather than brain activity. With these filter settings what we know to be muscle artifact could now conceivably be mistaken for right temporal spikes. The rounding of these waves is based on the phenomenon of rounding out of a square wave by a HFF as shown in Figures 7.35 and 7.36.

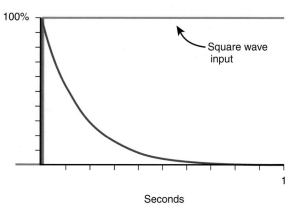

Figure 7.40 Like Figure 7.35, this figure shows the upper left corner of a square wave input (again, the lighter vertical red line at the left side of the figure continuing into the lighter horizontal red line at the top of the figure), comparing it to the output of the square wave after a 1 Hz **low-frequency filter** has been applied (a magnification of the corners of the waves in the top portion of Figure 7.36). The output wave shows how the fast initial upsweep portion of the square wave is not affected by the low-frequency filter, but the filter then causes the horizontal portion of the square wave to "sag" toward zero. The filter handles the horizontal portion of the square wave, which is a step-up of voltage to a constant level held for a period of time, akin to very low-frequency activity. The horizontal part of the square wave can also be thought of as a direct current with a frequency of zero.

factor is the resistance, "R," of the resistor in the circuit. Intuitively, the greater the resistance offered by the resistor, the more slowly the electrons will be able to flow around the circuit to charge the capacitor. So, both a higher R value and a higher C value will extend the amount of time it takes to charge the capacitor. In fact, the formula for the time to charge a capacitor in an RC circuit is quite simple, and is the *product* of the resistance and the capacitance of the circuit, $R \times C$, which is also called the *time constant* of the circuit. It is really a considerable convenience that deriving the time constant of a filter is as simple as multiplying the resistance and the capacitance of the circuit together. The time constant is sometimes also symbolized by the Greek letter tau: τ, as in:

$$\tau = R \times C$$

The time constant gives the time that it takes the capacitor to reach 63% of its full charge after the switch to a circuit is closed (the reason for the 63% figure is explained below). If asked to imagine the graph of what the current flow would look like for the capacitor as it is charging, you would probably imagine the current at an initial top value, which would then proceed to fall as if it were going down a ski slope, first steeply, then gradually and eventually slowing toward zero, but never quite getting exactly to zero as the capacitor attains its full charge (see Figure

7.40). In fact, there is a nice formula that demonstrates this ski slope shape, and it is as follows:

$$I = I_o e^{\frac{-t}{RC}}$$

This equation may look complicated, but it really is not. The equation tells you what the current, I, will be after any amount of time, t, in seconds has elapsed. Plug in any time for t, and you will get the current, I, at that time point. All of the other terms in the equation are constants, which simplifies matters. I_o stands for the maximal initial current seen the moment the switch is closed to allow current flow, 'e' is the natural log base (which is approximately 2.71), and R and C are our old friends, the resistance of the resistor and the capacitance of the capacitor in the circuit, which are set to specific numbers depending on which filter design we have chosen. Rewriting this equation with more English terms:

the current at time elapsed (t in seconds)

$$= initial\ maximal\ current \times 2.71^{\left(\frac{-time\ elapsed}{resistance \times capacitance}\right)}$$

Remembering that RC is the time constant, τ of the filter, we could have written this equation even more simply as

the current at any time elapsed (t in second)

$$= initial\ maximal\ current \times 2.71^{\left(\frac{-time\ elapsed(t)}{time\ constant(\tau)}\right)}$$

When encountering an equation like $I = I_o e^{-t/RC}$, it is good practice to test it out with a few numbers to make sure it makes sense and performs as expected. When using this formula, remember that when an exponent is negative (e.g., 2^{-7}); this is handled by raising 2 to the power of 7 but putting the expression in the denominator of a fraction (i.e., taking its reciprocal), so that $2^{-7} = \frac{1}{2^7}$.

First, let's test what the formula gives for current at time = 0, as soon as the switch is closed. Letting $t = 0$, the formula becomes $I = I_o e^0$. Remembering that any number raised to the power of zero equals 1, the formula reduces to $I = I_o \times 1$, which gives us the result that the current I is I_o when $t = 0$, just what we would expect because that is the definition of I_o, the initial maximal current at the moment the switch is closed. Now let's explore what happens to the current when the switch has been closed for a long time, for instance when $t = \infty$. Setting t to ∞, the term becomes $I_o e^{-\infty/RC}$. Because $e^{-\infty/RC}$ essentially becomes $1/e^{\infty/RC}$, which tends toward zero, the current I after "∞" seconds becomes zero. This, too, makes sense because the capacitor is full and electrons essentially aren't flowing anymore after waiting an infinite amount of time.

The last check we'll do is calculate the current after t seconds where t is the time constant (in seconds) of the circuit. Plugging in RC or τ for t in the original equation causes an interesting result: the exponent of e becomes -1, and the result is $I_o \ x\frac{1}{e}$. Because $1/e = \frac{1}{2.71} = 0.37$, this is to say that, after "time-constant" seconds or τ seconds, the current will have fallen to 37% of its original value. Another way of saying this is that the current has fallen by 63% (100% to 37%), which is a familiar number! This is the origin of the definition given above, that the time constant of an RC (filter) circuit is the number of seconds that it takes the capacitor to achieve 63% of its full charge.

This fact that a square wave should fall to 63% of its maximum value after τ seconds is the basis for the procedure used to measure and check a calibration signal. An example of the measuring technique for checking low filters is shown in Figure 7.41. When looking at the calibration pulse in this figure, one would do the following:

1. Measure the total height of the pulse, then
2. Calculate what 37% of that height is and put a tick-mark at that point on the y-axis.
3. Extend a line from the tick mark toward the right until it intercepts the descending pulse, then
4. Drop a perpendicular line to the x-axis to see how many seconds it took for the output curve to drop to that 37% value.

This measurement gives the apparent time constant of the current filter setup in seconds. Considering that filters can be named either according to their cutoff frequencies or time constants, each has certain advantages. If you are most interested in measuring calibration signals and confirming that

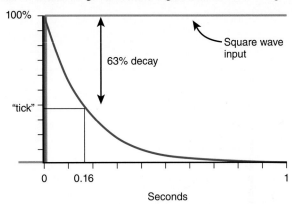

Figure 7.41 Proper behavior of the filter settings in use can be confirmed by measuring the changes in square wave calibration pulses. The time constant of a **low-frequency filter** is defined as the amount of time it takes for the horizontal component of a square wave pulse passed through the filter to fall by 63% of its original value (i.e., to 37% of its original value). The square wave pulse generated by the instrument is shown in light red. The reader measures the height of the calibration pulse and identifies the point at which it has fallen by 63%. The amount of time in seconds that it has taken for the wave to fall to this point is measured on the x-axis, in this example, 0.16 seconds, and represents the filter's time constant. The value of the time constant, τ, can be plugged into the equation which gives the relationship between the cutoff frequency and the time constant $f_{cutoff} = (1/2\pi\tau)$, which equals 1 per second (1 Hz) in this case. Therefore, the measurement of this calibration pulse implies that a low-frequency filter with a time constant of 0.16 seconds (equivalent to a cutoff frequency of 1 Hz) is in use.

the time to rise or decay equals the time constant, then having the time constant at hand may be more useful. Knowing the cutoff frequency of a filter tells us the wave frequency that the filter will attenuate by 30%, which is probably more practical information for the daily EEG reader.

The Relationship between Time Constant and Cutoff Frequency

If some EEG machines use filter cutoff frequencies to name filters and others use time constants, what is the relationship between the two? The time constant, τ of a filter, can be easily derived from the filter's cutoff frequency and vice versa by means of the following simple formula:

$$f_{cutoff} = \frac{1}{2\pi\tau}$$

or, exchanging the positions of the cutoff frequency and the time constant:

$$\tau = \frac{1}{2\pi f_{cutoff}} = (0.16)\frac{1}{f_{cutoff}}$$

The 0.16 term comes from taking $1/(2\pi)$ term out of the fraction on the left side of the equation. For example, for a 5 Hz low-frequency filter, using the formula above, the corresponding time constant is $(0.16) \times (1/5 \text{ per second}) = 0.032$ seconds (Figure 7.42). Likewise, for the example of the 1 Hz filter, the time constant will be 0.16 seconds. The equations:

$$\tau = \frac{1}{2\pi f_{cutoff}} \qquad f_{cutoff} = \frac{1}{2\pi\tau}$$

can be used interchangeably to convert cutoff frequencies to time constants and vice versa. Major cutoff frequencies and their associated time constants are shown below.

Frequency (Hz)	Time constant (sec)
0.5	0.32
1	0.16
5	0.03
10	0.016

A comparison of the effects of high- and low-frequency filters is summarized in Table 7.1.

DIGITAL FILTERS

The complex science of digital filter design belongs to the field of digital signal processing and the details are beyond the scope of this text and the mechanics of how digital filters work is not required to learn to record or interpret EEGs. However, it may be interesting to get a glimpse of some of the basic techniques in digital filtering to have a general idea of

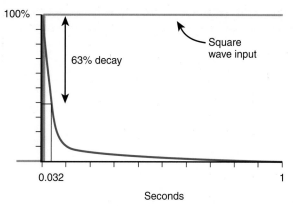

Figure 7.42 Here, the same square wave pulse (shown in light red) is passed through the instrument. In this example, the pulse falls to 63% of its original value after only 0.032 seconds. When this time constant, τ, is plugged into the equation $f_{cutoff} = (1/2\pi\tau)$, we get the result $f_{cutoff} = 5$ per second, implying that a 5 Hz low-frequency filter is now in use.

the workings of these filters. The RC circuits described earlier are designed to work on real (analog) electrical currents and are therefore analog devices. Indeed, before the big shift from analog to digital machines around the turn of the last century, modifications of the RC circuits described above were exactly what the EEG machines that printed EEGs out with paper and ink used for filters.

The advent of computerized digital EEG instruments has completely changed the methodologies used to design filters. It is very easy to forget that the curves of the EEG waves that we interpret on the EEG screen are not really curves at all but that each is, in reality, a long list of numbers. Although two of the electrodes plugged into the EEG machine's connection box can make an analog voltage measurement between two points, the magic of the digital EEG machine is that it converts this analog voltage wave into a stream of numbers, each representing an instantaneous measurement of the height of the analog wave. This process is called *analog-to-digital conversion*. Depending on the sampling rate set up in the software, the measurement of the incoming wave height could be taken, for example, 500 times per second (i.e., once every five-hundredth of a second). Our original smooth analog voltage curve has now been converted into a stream of positive and negative numbers, each representing the height of the curve, positive or negative, at intervals every five-hundredth of a second. You can imagine this successive string of numbers as the tops and bottoms of histograms above or below the x-axis, as shown in Figure 7.43. This wave was depicted with a purposely chosen low sampling rate in order to exaggerate the raggedy appearance of a wave that is sampled at a low sampling rate. It is clear that, the higher the sampling rate, the smoother and more accurate our displayed curves will look. Also, note that, even with low sampling rates, we can get a good idea of the shape of slow-wave curves. However, if we wanted to see the detail of any fast activity that may or may not be overlying the curve in Figure 7.43, we would need to

TABLE 7.1	**Effects of High- and Low-Frequency Filters**					
	Synonyms	Attenuation	Advantages	Effect on Wave Shape	Pitfalls of Use	Possible Standard Setting
Low-frequency filter	Low-filter, high-pass filter	Attenuates a sine wave at cutoff frequency by 30%	Helps keep waves near the zero-baseline, reduces very low-frequency activity, which is often artifact	Causes waves to "sag" or "float" back toward the baseline	Reduces ability to appreciate slow waves and asymmetries in slowing	1 Hz
High-frequency filter	High-filter, low-pass filter	Attenuates a sine wave at cutoff frequency by 30%	Reduces very high-frequency activity, which is often electrical noise, muscle, or other artifact	Overly aggressive use causes rounding of shape of fast transients (vertical elements) making them resemble brain waves	Makes high-frequency noise (e.g., muscle artifact) look more like sine waves (brain waves)	70 Hz

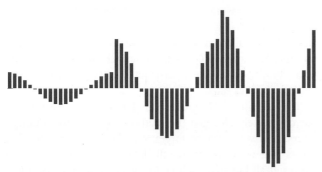

Figure 7.43 The waves that appear on the EEG display represent a graphical depiction of digital data, even though those data were originally analog at the time they were gathered. Typically, the EEG is sampled at a rate approximately between 200 and 500 times per second. Each sample or "bin" of data is then plotted and displayed graphically creating a curve. This figure shows how discrete digital data points (albeit obtained at a low sampling rate and creating a raggedy appearance for the sake of illustration) can be displayed as histograms and resolved into a curve.

use a much higher sampling rate—the detail of any overlying fast activity has been lost at this low sampling rate.

This problem of capturing higher frequency activity with lower sampling rates brings up the concept of the *Nyquist frequency*. The Nyquist frequency is the highest frequency that can be captured effectively at any particular sampling rate and is simply one half the sampling rate. This is to say that at a sampling rate of 500 Hz, the Nyquist frequency for that sampling rate would be 250 Hz (i.e., 250 Hz activity can be effectively captured with a 500 Hz sampling rate). Sampling rates used for conventional EEG recording are typically well above the Nyquist frequency (necessary sampling rate) for the waveforms 70 Hz and below that we typically look for in routine EEGs. The sampling rate becomes more of a concern in more specialized reading applications, such as analyzing "fast ripples" (very high-frequency EEG waves) in the EEG. Note that the *Nyquist rate* is the sampling rate required to capture

a particular frequency, and the *Nyquist frequency* is the highest frequency that can be captured at any particular sampling rate. Obviously, the two terms are tightly associated with one another, with the Nyquist rate being twice the Nyquist frequency. In the example above, the Nyquist rate for an application in which one would want to capture 250 Hz activity is 500 samples per second. The Nyquist frequency for a machine sampling at 500 samples per second would be 250 Hz.

Take a look at the stream of numbers in Table 7.2. Do you see any epileptiform activity? Is there a slow wave component? Of course, this table of numbers seems overwhelming and few people could look at the column of numbers and guess what this wave really looks like. As it happens, these are the samples that define the waveform shown in Figure 7.44. Each of the small dots on that curve corresponds to a number in the table that represents a wave height. This table of numbers is included to remind us that our EEG software does not see the world in terms of spikes or slow waves at all, but rather as a simple stream of numbers. If only given this stream of numbers, you would be able to recreate the curve shown in the figure by joining each point together to create a curve, turning the number stream back into a visual EEG wave on a computer display, which is exactly what EEG software does.

Looking at the wave shown in Figure 7.44, a reader who is accustomed to analyzing EEG waves may see a faster wave riding on a slow wave, but it is important to remember that what we see on the display screen and what the computer is manipulating are entirely different. Rather than the shape of the wave the human eye appreciates, or the jiggling electrons an RC circuit processes, the software that runs the digital EEG instrument has nothing more available to it than the stream of numbers that define the wave in question. Every time we make an adjustment in the settings on the EEG instrument, the software is carrying out a mathematical manipulation on multiple streams of numbers, and only "at the last minute" after all the mathematical manipulations of the filters and

TABLE 7.2   Digital Data for Waveform Shown in Figure 7.44

0.200	0.487	-1.607	-0.291	-0.777	-1.824	0.203	-0.770	-0.459	1.369	-0.091	1.067	1.661	-0.120
0.395	0.631	-1.468	-0.172	-0.780	-1.849	0.110	-0.947	-0.598	1.201	-0.233	1.030	1.636	-0.052
0.580	0.777	-1.315	-0.032	-0.755	-1.845	0.040	-1.109	-0.732	1.025	-0.391	0.968	1.583	-0.011
0.752	0.919	-1.151	0.126	-0.705	-1.811	-0.004	-1.250	-0.856	0.846	-0.562	0.884	1.501	0.004
0.906	1.053	-0.983	0.299	-0.631	-1.749	-0.022	-1.368	-0.966	0.669	-0.741	0.781	1.393	-0.009
1.038	1.175	-0.813	0.482	-0.537	-1.659	-0.012	-1.461	-1.058	0.499	-0.924	0.662	1.260	-0.049
1.146	1.280	-0.648	0.671	-0.425	-1.544	0.024	-1.526	-1.128	0.339	-1.104	0.532	1.107	-0.114
1.228	1.365	-0.492	0.861	-0.301	-1.406	0.088	-1.562	-1.174	0.195	-1.279	0.395	0.936	-0.203
1.281	1.427	-0.349	1.047	-0.168	-1.249	0.175	-1.570	-1.194	0.069	-1.443	0.256	0.751	-0.313
1.306	1.462	-0.223	1.225	-0.032	-1.076	0.286	-1.549	-1.185	-0.035	-1.591	0.120	0.558	-0.441
1.303	1.470	-0.118	1.389	0.104	-0.892	0.415	-1.500	-1.148	-0.114	-1.721	-0.008	0.361	-0.583
1.271	1.449	-0.036	1.536	0.234	-0.701	0.560	-1.427	-1.082	-0.166	-1.827	-0.125	0.164	-0.734
1.214	1.399	0.020	1.662	0.354	-0.508	0.717	-1.331	-0.989	-0.191	-1.909	-0.225	-0.028	-0.890
1.133	1.321	0.050	1.764	0.459	-0.318	0.880	-1.216	-0.870	-0.189	-1.963	-0.306	-0.209	-1.046
1.032	1.216	0.052	1.840	0.546	-0.136	1.046	-1.086	-0.728	-0.160	-1.988	-0.364	-0.376	-1.198
0.915	1.087	0.027	1.888	0.612	0.034	1.209	-0.946	-0.567	-0.105	-1.983	-0.397	-0.525	-1.340
0.784	0.936	-0.024	1.906	0.653	0.187	1.366	-0.799	-0.389	-0.026	-1.950	-0.404	-0.652	-1.469
0.646	0.766	-0.100	1.895	0.668	0.321	1.510	-0.650	-0.199	0.073	-1.888	-0.382	-0.754	-1.580
0.503	0.582	-0.198	1.855	0.655	0.432	1.638	-0.505	-0.002	0.189	-1.800	-0.333	-0.830	-1.669
0.363	0.388	-0.314	1.788	0.614	0.518	1.747	-0.368	0.199	0.318	-1.688	-0.257	-0.879	-1.734
0.228	0.189	-0.445	1.696	0.545	0.576	1.832	-0.243	0.397	0.457	-1.556	-0.155	-0.899	-1.773
0.104	-0.010	-0.587	1.583	0.450	0.607	1.892	-0.134	0.588	0.600	-1.407	-0.030	-0.891	-1.783
-0.006	-0.205	-0.736	1.450	0.330	0.610	1.924	-0.045	0.768	0.742	-1.245	0.115	-0.856	-1.764
-0.097	-0.392	-0.886	1.303	0.188	0.585	1.927	0.021	0.932	0.880	-1.075	0.277	-0.796	-1.716
-0.166	-0.564	-1.032	1.146	0.028	0.535	1.900	0.062	1.077	1.007	-0.902	0.452	-0.714	-1.640
-0.211	-0.720	-1.171	0.983	-0.148	0.462	1.845	0.076	1.199	1.121	-0.730	0.635	-0.612	-1.537
-0.230	-0.854	-1.298	0.819	-0.334	0.367	1.762	0.063	1.296	1.216	-0.564	0.822	-0.495	-1.409
-0.222	-0.964	-1.408	0.659	-0.527	0.256	1.653	0.022	1.365	1.290	-0.409	1.008	-0.367	-1.261
-0.186	-1.048	-1.498	0.508	-0.721	0.132	1.521	-0.045	1.406	1.340	-0.269	1.188	-0.232	-1.094
-0.122	-1.105	-1.565	0.370	-0.911	-0.001	1.369	-0.137	1.418	1.362	-0.147	1.358	-0.094	-0.913
-0.033	-1.133	-1.605	0.248	-1.093	-0.137	1.201	-0.251	1.401	1.357	-0.048	1.513	0.040	-0.723
0.080	-1.132	-1.618	0.147	-1.263	-0.273	1.022	-0.385	1.358	1.323	0.028	1.648	0.167	-0.529
0.214	-1.104	-1.602	0.070	-1.415	-0.404	0.835	-0.535	1.289	1.260	0.077	1.762	0.283	-0.335
0.365	-1.050	-1.557	0.017	-1.547	-0.524	0.647	-0.697	1.198	1.170	0.099	1.850	0.382	-0.145
0.531	-0.973	-1.483	-0.009	-1.656	-0.630	0.460	-0.865	1.088	1.054	0.094	1.911	0.462	0.035
0.706	-0.875	-1.383	-0.007	-1.738	-0.718	0.281	-1.037	0.963	0.914	0.062	1.944	0.519	0.200
0.886	-0.760	-1.257	0.022	-1.792	-0.784	0.114	-1.206	0.826	0.754	0.004	1.947	0.551	0.348
1.066	-0.633	-1.109	0.077	-1.817	-0.825	-0.037	-1.369	0.683	0.578	-0.078	1.921	0.556	0.475
1.242	-0.497	-0.943	0.156	-1.812	-0.840	-0.169	-1.520	0.539	0.389	-0.180	1.866	0.534	0.578
1.408	-0.358	-0.762	0.258	-1.779	-0.828	-0.278	-1.655	0.398	0.192	-0.300	1.785	0.483	0.654
1.560	-0.220	-0.570	0.378	-1.719	-0.787	-0.362	-1.770	0.264	-0.009	-0.433	1.681	0.405	0.703
1.694	-0.087	-0.373	0.514	-1.634	-0.719	-0.420	-1.863	0.142	-0.207	-0.575	1.555	0.302	0.724

Continued

TABLE 7.2   Digital Data for Waveform Shown in Figure 7.44—cont'd

1.807	0.035	-0.175	0.661	-1.527	-0.623	-0.449	-1.930	0.037	-0.400	-0.722	1.413	0.175	0.716
1.896	0.142	0.020	0.814	-1.401	-0.503	-0.451	-1.969	-0.048	-0.581	-0.868	1.257	0.027	0.683
1.957	0.231	0.205	0.969	-1.260	-0.360	-0.426	-1.979	-0.111	-0.747	-1.009	1.093	-0.138	0.624
1.990	0.298	0.378	1.121	-1.108	-0.198	-0.375	-1.960	-0.149	-0.895	-1.141	0.926	-0.316	0.542
1.994	0.341	0.534	1.265	-0.951	-0.020	-0.301	-1.911	-0.160	-1.019	-1.259	0.759	-0.503	0.441
1.969	0.357	0.669	1.397	-0.793	0.168	-0.206	-1.835	-0.143	-1.119	-1.359	0.599	-0.695	0.325
1.914	0.347	0.781	1.513	-0.638	0.363	-0.094	-1.733	-0.099	-1.192	-1.437	0.448	-0.885	0.197
1.833	0.308	0.866	1.608	-0.492	0.560	0.031	-1.607	-0.028	-1.236	-1.491	0.313	-1.070	0.063
1.727	0.242	0.924	1.681	-0.358	0.754	0.165	-1.462	0.067	-1.252	-1.518	0.195	-1.245	-0.074
1.600	0.150	0.954	1.727	-0.241	0.940	0.303	-1.300	0.186	-1.239	-1.517	0.099	-1.406	-0.208
1.454	0.034	0.956	1.745	-0.145	1.114	0.440	-1.126	0.324	-1.199	-1.488	0.028	-1.547	-0.335
1.294	-0.103	0.930	1.735	-0.071	1.271	0.572	-0.944	0.478	-1.135	-1.429	-0.018	-1.667	-0.450
1.125	-0.258	0.878	1.696	-0.023	1.409	0.693	-0.760	0.645	-1.047	-1.343	-0.036	-1.762	-0.549
0.950	-0.428	0.803	1.627	-0.001	1.522	0.801	-0.578	0.819	-0.941	-1.230	-0.027	-1.830	-0.629
0.775	-0.607	0.708	1.532	-0.006	1.610	0.890	-0.403	0.996	-0.819	-1.093	0.009	-1.869	-0.686
0.605	-0.792	0.595	1.411	-0.039	1.670	0.958	-0.240	1.171	-0.686	-0.936	0.070	-1.879	-0.718
0.444	-0.978	0.470	1.268	-0.098	1.701	1.001	-0.091	1.340	-0.547	-0.762	0.155	-1.860	-0.723
0.297	-1.159	0.336	1.105	-0.182	1.703	1.018	0.038	1.497	-0.406	-0.575	0.261	-1.813	-0.700
0.166	-1.331	0.199	0.928	-0.288	1.676	1.007	0.144	1.639	-0.268	-0.379	0.385	-1.739	-0.649
0.057	-1.489	0.062	0.740	-0.413	1.622	0.967	0.226	1.762	-0.137	-0.180	0.522	-1.641	-0.570
-0.029	-1.630	-0.068	0.545	-0.553	1.543	0.899	0.282	1.861	-0.019	0.019	0.668	-1.522	-0.466
-0.089	-1.750	-0.189	0.349	-0.704	1.442	0.805	0.309	1.935	0.084	0.211	0.819	-1.386	-0.337
-0.122	-1.845	-0.295	0.157	-0.863	1.322	0.685	0.309	1.982	0.167	0.393	0.970	-1.237	
-0.127	-1.914	-0.382	-0.028	-1.023	1.187	0.542	0.283	1.999	0.227	0.560	1.117	-1.079	
-0.106	-1.954	-0.448	-0.200	-1.180	1.041	0.379	0.230	1.988	0.262	0.709	1.253	-0.917	
-0.058	-1.966	-0.490	-0.355	-1.330	0.889	0.201	0.154	1.947	0.270	0.835	1.376	-0.756	
0.014	-1.947	-0.505	-0.490	-1.469	0.736	0.011	0.058	1.878	0.251	0.937	1.481	-0.601	
0.108	-1.901	-0.493	-0.602	-1.591	0.586	-0.185	-0.056	1.782	0.204	1.011	1.565	-0.455	
0.221	-1.827	-0.452	-0.688	-1.692	0.445	-0.384	-0.183	1.664	0.130	1.058	1.624	-0.324	
0.349	-1.728	-0.385	-0.746	-1.771	0.315	-0.581	-0.319	1.525	0.031	1.077	1.657	-0.211	

amplifiers have been done, converts the final stream of numbers to a visual wave on the display. Some of these manipulations are easy to visualize. For instance, if the reader halves the sensitivity setting, say from 10 μV/mm to 5 μV/mm, the software can double each element of the stream of numbers that determines the height of the displayed wave. Other changes, such as an adjustment in filter settings, will require a much more complex mathematical manipulation of the number stream.

We might ask, how does a digital EEG machine filter out the slow component, or the fast component, of the wave shown in Figure 7.44? But that is not the specific question we should be asking. The real question is, how does the EEG machine filter out the slow component, or the fast component, of the wave shown in Table 7.2? Clearly, the challenge

of creating a filter that might remove either the fast activity or the slow activity from the stream of digits that comprises this waveform represents a completely different type of problem from that of designing an RC circuit for the same task with analog waves. Whereas analog electrical signals can be passed through RC circuits of the types depicted above, a completely different technique will have to be used to design an HFF or a LFF for the stream of numbers.

Digital HFFs

First, we consider a simple algorithm to filter out fast activity from this digital waveform. The technique used here is similar to the technique referred to as "moving averages." (The technique of moving averages is also used by some financial analysts to track the historical movement of a stock's price

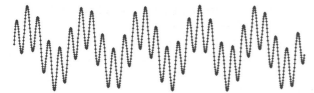

Figure 7.44 You may be wondering what the table of numbers on the previous page represents. Table 7.2 shows the digital stream of data that underlies the complex waveform shown above. The individual data points from Table 7.2 used to generate this wave are shown as small diamonds superimposed on the waveform allowing the graphical form of the curve to be generated. Each diamond represents a data point from the table. A visual analysis of this waveform would suggest an approximately 5 Hz wave superimposed on a 1 Hz wave. The examples that follow show how the 5 Hz and then the 1 Hz components of this mixed wave can be partially filtered out using the simple digital algorithms described in the text.

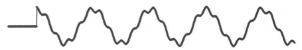

Figure 7.45 When the simple digital "moving average" technique is applied to the data points in Table 7.2 and their corresponding waveform shown in the previous figure, the curve above is generated. In this technique, each point is converted to the arithmetic average of the previous 99 data points from the original wave table. This technique helps to smooth out the high-frequency oscillations and is a simple version of a digital high-frequency filter.

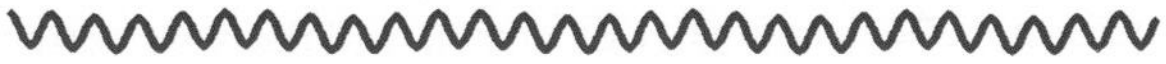

Figure 7.46 The wave shown in this figure is the result of replacing each data point from Table 7.2 with the subtraction of adjacent data points as described in the text. The original wave is shown in graphical form in Figure 7.44. This simple technique removes most of the low-frequency oscillation and leaves the bulk of the high-frequency component intact, though a very slight wavering of the baseline can still be appreciated representing a vestige of the original slow-wave component.

over time with the goal of damping out quick fluctuations.) With this technique, a digital wave, consisting of a stream of numbers or "bins," is transformed by replacing each bin in the number stream with the average of a set number of the previous numbers/bins before it. In the example that follows, the wave shown in Figure 7.44 has been transformed by replacing the 100th point by the average of the previous 99 points (points 1 through 99). Likewise, the 101st point is replaced by the average of points 2 through 100, and so on. Applying this technique to the stream of numbers shown in Table 7.2 that created the wave shape seen in Figure 7.44, the new wave seen in Figure 7.45 is generated. Note that the fast component of the wave is considerably attenuated, although it is still recognizable. The slow component of the wave has been preserved and is now its most prominent feature. By choosing different figures for the number of previous bins averaged before the current number, different amounts of fast wave attenuation will be seen.

Digital LFFs

A simple digital algorithm for filtering out slow activity involves subtracting adjacent bins and replacing the original values with the differences. Using this technique, the second

point would be replaced by the difference between the second point and the first point, the third point would be replaced by the difference between the third point and the second point, and so on. The wave depicted in Figure 7.46 shows the result of using this simple algorithm on our original digital wave from Table 7.2. Note that the slow activity is nearly completely filtered out, and the fast activity remains. The only remnant of the slow activity is a slight wavering of the baseline, which is still, but just barely, discernible.

Of course, the digital filtering algorithms used in commercial EEG instruments are much more complex and sophisticated than the simple algorithms used in the previous examples, which show obvious defects. These examples are given to remind the reader that digital filtering involves complex mathematical manipulations on streams of digits as opposed to the outputs of analog circuits. Digital filters are designed to mimic the behavior of the RC circuits they have replaced. Digital filters have their own inherent imperfections depending on the specific filtering algorithms used.

REVIEW QUESTIONS

1. If *no* low-frequency filter is in use, the most likely visual impact on the EEG would be
   a. excessive 60 Hz artifact.
   b. excessive muscle artifact that may obliterate true brain waves, especially in the temporal areas.
   c. an increase in broad high voltage deflections that may intrude into adjacent channels, especially with patient movement.
   d. a false sense of increased slow activity in the tracing.

2. The impact of a high-frequency filter on a wave at its nominal (cutoff) frequency (e.g., the impact of a 70 Hz high-frequency filter on a 70 Hz wave) is that it would
   a. reduce the wave at the nominal frequency by 70%.
   b. reduce the wave at the nominal frequency by 30%.
   c. reduce the wave at the nominal frequency by 63%.
   d. This cannot be predicted because it depends mainly on what other frequency waves are mixed into the EEG signal at the time.

3. The type of filter most likely to change the appearance of muscle artifact into something that could be mistaken for a sinusoidal brain wave is
   a. the high-frequency filter.
   b. the low-frequency filter.
   c. the notch filter.
   d. All of the above.

4. Which statement is true?
   a. A high-frequency filter set at 35 Hz will even reduce 80 Hz activity, but only a little.
   b. A low-frequency filter set at 1 Hz will decrease activity below 1 Hz by more than 30%.
   c. A 60 Hz notch filter will suppress 50 Hz electrical contamination, but only partially.
   d. Using both a high-frequency filter and a low-frequency filter at the same time can cause unwanted interference and unpredictable results on the appearance of the EEG.

5. A filter that reduces a waveform by 3 dB will
   a. reduce wave power by 30%.
   b. reduce wave amplitude by 30%.
   c. not have an effect because decibel reductions are used for sound rather than EEG waves.
   d. cannot be discerned because decibels are only meaningful if a reference point is specified.

6. The extent to which a capacitor provides a barrier to current flow is
   a. best represented by the concept of resistance rather than impedance because resistance considers the frequency of the wave presented to the capacitor.
   b. lower when the capacitor is empty because electrons cannot jump across empty capacitor plates.
   c. lower when there is a high voltage drop across the capacitor.
   d. higher when there is a lot of charge on the capacitor plates.

ANSWERS

1. ANSWER: **C**. Low-frequency filter settings have little, if any, impact on the presence of 60 Hz artifact in the EEG. Because muscle artifact is essentially a high-frequency phenomenon, low-frequency filters have little effect on the appearance of this type of artifact. Answer C. is correct because high voltage artifact from patient motion is most commonly in the low-frequency range, and use of a low-frequency filter can be helpful in avoiding large deflections away from the channel baseline caused by such artifacts. When such a deflection occurs, the low-frequency filter helps bring these deflections back toward the baseline. Low-frequency filters only reduce the amount of low-frequency activity displayed. Failure to use a low-frequency filter would not, however, add low-frequency or slow-wave activity to the tracing.

2. ANSWER: **B**. A high-frequency filter will allow 70% of a wave at the nominal frequency to pass, which is to say that it reduces the wave by 30% (greater reductions for waves lower than the nominal frequency and lesser reductions for waves above the nominal frequency). The 63% figure refers to the amount of attenuation expected after the "time constant" number of seconds. High- and low-frequency filters filter out activity based on individual frequency components in waves, even if they are of mixed frequency.

3. ANSWER: **A**. A high-frequency filter can "round out" muscle artifact so that it could be mistaken for fast activity of cerebral origin. Low-frequency filters and notch filters will have little impact on the visual impression of muscle artifact.

4. ANSWER: **A**. Although a 35 Hz high-frequency will suppress a 35 Hz wave by 30%, the roll-off characteristic curves for these filters show that even frequencies well above the cutoff frequency will experience some degree of attenuation, but perhaps so little that it may not be visible to the eye. A 1 Hz low-frequency filter does attenuate slow activity below 1 Hz even more than 30%, but it never *increases* wave amplitude at any frequency. A 60 Hz notch filter will have no discernible effect on 50 Hz electrical artifact, and vice versa. High-frequency filters and low-frequency filters are customarily used as a pair to create a bandpass, and do not interfere with each other.

5. ANSWER: **B**. A 3 dB reduction by a filter is associated with a decrease in wave power of 50% and of wave amplitude by 30%. The concept of decibel changes works equally well for sound waves as it does for EEG waves, which indeed have many similarities. Wave attenuation stated in dB denotes a percentage decrease, so no reference point needs to be specified for that use of the decibel unit. In order for the concept of decibels to be meaningful to indicate an *absolute* amount of power (or sound intensity), a reference point does have to be specified.

6. ANSWER: **D**. It is the concept of impedance rather than resistance that takes wave frequency into account in terms of how much of a barrier a capacitor represents to current flow. When the capacitor plates are empty, it is easier (rather than harder) for current to flow onto the capacitor. When a capacitor is empty, there is a low voltage drop across the capacitor and this is the condition when current flow is easiest. A high voltage drop across a capacitor implies that it is holding charge, and therefore further current flow onto the capacitor plates will be impeded. This idea is also reflected by the expression $V = q/C$ (that the voltage across a capacitor is equal to how many coulombs of charge, q, are held on the capacitor per farad of capacitance, C). It is harder for current to flow onto a capacitor that is near full.

8

The Structure and Philosophy of the EEG Report

The essential purpose of preparing an EEG report is to efficiently communicate the information you have gleaned from the EEG tracing to the referring provider to aid in the patient's ongoing care. In an ideal world, perhaps the electroencephalographer might review the actual pages of every EEG with the referring provider in person, pointing out any interesting waveforms in the EEG and discussing the nuances of their clinical implications. Indeed, from time to time, sharing the visual picture of the EEG directly with the referring clinician is possible, but most of the time such in-person explanations of the EEG results are just not practical. Even when a face-to-face interpretation is given, there still needs to be a permanent record of the EEG interpretation in the medical record for others to access from a distance or in the future. The ideal EEG report then could be seen partly as a stand-in for the type of in-person discussion you might wish to have with the provider as you would page through the EEG together, but in a more formal format. However, considering that the EEG report often becomes the de facto permanent record of the study, the report must also contain a lot of basic description of what the EEG actually looks like for readers of the report who will never see the actual tracing. Information surrounding the patient and the technique of the recording also need to be conveyed. For these reasons and others, considerable thought should be put into the content and wording of the EEG report, which is typically divided into a number of sections as described below.

IDENTIFYING INFORMATION

The EEG report generally starts with clinical identifiers, including the patient's name and date of birth, the name and location of the laboratory performing the study, the date and time of the study, and the name of the ordering provider. Next, a brief clinical history is given that includes the indications for which the study was ordered. This brief summary may include a combination of the clinical information that has been obtained from the patient or family by the EEG technologist, possibly supplemented by additional information from review of the medical record. The technologist obtains this brief additional history from the patient to complete this portion of the report, but this brief history-taking also has additional advantages. It may be a first step in establishing a conversational relationship between the technologist and the patient or family. It also may alert the EEG technologist

to the necessity of using specific recording techniques. For instance, if absence seizures are suspected, the technologist may concentrate particularly on the hyperventilation portion of the EEG, perhaps even performing it twice if negative the first time. If temporal lobe epilepsy is suspected, the technologist may choose to place additional special electrodes over the temporal areas. The medications taken by the patient and the date of the most recent seizure may also be given, if applicable. This history is usually recounted in a concise fashion:

> This 60-year-old woman is referred because of episodes of confusion lasting 1 to 2 minutes that started approximately 1 month ago. There is a history of a left-sided stroke 3 years previously. This EEG is requested to help rule out seizures.

The clinical history may also may help the EEG reader tailor the discussion in the "Clinical Correlation" paragraph at the end of the report. For example, if the referring physician suspected temporal lobe epilepsy, the reader may choose to include additional pertinent negatives that directly address the clinical question posed, such as a comment that no epileptiform was seen and that there was no slow-wave activity noted in the temporal areas. Finally, the clinical history may also alert the technologist and the reader to special situations such as skull defects from previous surgeries, areas of the scalp that are inaccessible because of a bandage or recent surgical incision, or perhaps the fact that this is the fourth EEG in a sequence obtained on a patient in a coma.

TECHNICAL DESCRIPTION

Next, a technical description of the procedure used for the recording is provided. Because in any given laboratory most EEGs are recorded using the same technique, this descriptive paragraph is usually standardized and only requires revision when there are deviations from the laboratory's routine procedures. Because the technologist is responsible for the recording procedure, this paragraph is typically produced by the technologist. An example of a procedure description for a routine EEG is as follows:

A 21-channel digital electroencephalogram was performed with simultaneous video recording in the Clinical Neurophysiology Laboratory of *The Particular Hospital* at a sampling rate of 512 samples per second. The 10-20 international system of electrode placement was used and both bipolar and referential electrode montages were monitored. Additional electrodes were placed at the T1 and T2 positions and an additional reference electrode was placed on the chin. The patient was sleep-deprived. No sedation was administered. The patient was recorded during the waking, drowsy, and sleep states. The total recording time was 41 minutes.

The next three sections represent the core of the EEG report and are produced by the interpreting electroencephalographer. These include a Description of the appearance and findings of the EEG, a summary of the findings or Interpretation of the EEG (which may include an "abnormality list" for EEGs that are not normal), and a Clinical Correlation paragraph discussing the clinical implications of the findings. Each of these sections is now discussed in more detail.

EEG DESCRIPTION

Here the electroencephalographer provides a concise description of the appearance of the EEG. Precise technical terms may be used in this part of the report, including electrode names from the international 10-20 system and technical EEG terminology may be used and need not be avoided. The purpose of this portion of the report is to allow another electroencephalographer to visualize the appearance of the recording without actually having seen the original tracing. Provided with an *ideally* written description, another electroencephalographer could read your description and draw the EEG exactly as it was recorded. Moreover, the reader of the description would be able to produce the same abnormality list and clinical conclusions as if the EEG tracing had been personally reviewed. To provide this level of detail, the technical description paragraph may include EEG terminology that is not necessarily easily understandable to an internist or other general physician, or even in some cases to a neurologist who does not specialize in electroencephalography. Although this ideal description may be difficult to achieve, it does provide a practical bar to reach for in EEG description. You may choose to reread the description you have written and ask yourself what EEG pattern another person would draw based on your report. If it would differ significantly from what you actually saw on the EEG page, how could you improve your description to narrow the gap?

A good description allows a second electroencephalographer either to confirm the identifications of waveforms given in the interpretation paragraph or perhaps even disagree with them. For instance, if low-voltage sharps waves seen in the occipital areas in sleep with positive polarity were described as epileptiform activity, this description may lead a second (more experienced) electroencephalographer to reject this interpretation and suspect that these waves are actually POSTS (positive occipital sharp transients of sleep), a normal variant (see Chapter 11, "Normal Variants in the EEG," for further discussion of POSTS). Formally, the description paragraph should consist of a pure description of the visual appearance of the EEG; conclusions as to whether a described wave is normal or abnormal are not absolutely required in

this paragraph and would usually appear in the interpretation section. In practice, for clarity's sake, some readers will flag findings as normal or abnormal in the description, especially if there are multiple findings, so that the message of the report is as clear as possible.

If appropriate to the EEG, the description is organized according to sleep state. Separate paragraph descriptions may be written for wakefulness, drowsiness, and sleep as needed. In this way, these sequential paragraphs can serve as a continuous narrative of what the EEG looked like as the recording proceeded and the patient fell asleep. In the paragraph describing wakefulness, it is customary to quote the frequency and reactivity of the posterior rhythm, assuming it is identifiable. The amount of fast activity present during wakefulness is also commented on. A sleep paragraph would generally describe the presence of vertex waves and spindles if these are present. Any additional findings in each state would also be included in these sections. A typical description of normal wakefulness and sharp waves in sleep might include the following:

AWAKE

A moderate amount of 11 to 12 Hz medium-voltage rhythmic waves are seen posteriorly that suppress with eye opening. A small amount of symmetric 18 to 30 Hz low-voltage fast activity is seen anteriorly bilaterally. Medium voltage rhythmic 3 to 4 Hz delta waves are seen continuously in P8 and T8.

ASLEEP

Stage II sleep is seen with vertex waves and a moderate amount of 14 Hz bicentral sleep spindles. Low- to medium-voltage sharp waves are seen occasionally in P8. The slow wave activity seen in P8/T8 during wakefulness persists in sleep.

These two paragraphs describe the background activity during wakefulness and the presence of normal sleep elements. It is also clear that the right posterior temporal sharp waves were seen in sleep but not during wakefulness. This could be useful information if a future EEG is recorded awake-only and no P8 sharp waves are seen—they may be absent not because the patient's epileptiform activity has abated but simply because the patient did not sleep.

INTERPRETATION

This paragraph generally starts by clearly stating whether the EEG is considered normal or abnormal, assuming that this determination can be made. Terms such as *probably normal* or *probably abnormal* should be avoided whenever possible as they limit the usefulness of the report and are often found frustrating by the clinician who receives the report. Such noncommittal terms should only be used in the small minority of cases in which a determination of normality is not possible. If appropriate, the terms *mildly abnormal, moderately abnormal*, and *severely abnormal* may also be used.

At this point in the report, it is also useful to give an abnormality list, an example of which follows:

This EEG is abnormal due to the presence of:

　1. *Low- to medium-voltage sharp waves, maximum in the right posterior temporal electrode during drowsiness and light sleep*
　2. *Increased slow-wave activity over the right mid- to posterior temporal area seen during both wakefulness and sleep.*

No other asymmetries or epileptiform activity was noted.

Note that this portion of the report could have described "a discharge maximum in P8, with delta waves maximum in T8 and P8." Because some readers of the report may not be familiar with the official names of electrode positions and other technical EEG terminology, in this section of the report it is preferable to use plain English terminology such as "right posterior temporal" rather than "P8." An abnormality list gives the report reader an opportunity to get a quick picture of the EEG findings by scanning the list. In reality, many report recipients may lack the time, patience, or expertise to go back and read the technical description portion of the report that you have prepared. The goal is to write an interpretation paragraph that can stand alone and communicate the main findings of the EEG. This type of stand-alone interpretation paragraph could be a significant aid to a clinician who has just received a patient in transfer or for a second opinion evaluation who would like to quickly review the results of the patient's previous eight EEGs.

In both the description and interpretation paragraphs, the location and field of EEG events should be given with as much specificity as the tracing allows. For instance, if a spike has been found in the F8 electrode, it is not sufficient to describe it simply as a "right temporal spike"; after all, there are at least three right temporal electrodes (anterior, mid-, and posterior temporal, not to mention such special electrode positions such as T2 or FT10 that also record the temporal lobe). In practice, a spike in the right anterior temporal area and a spike in the right midtemporal area may have significantly different clinical implications regarding the types of epilepsy they are associated with (e.g., lesional temporal lobe epilepsy versus rolandic epilepsy).

CLINICAL CORRELATION

The paragraph on clinical correlation is probably the most useful to the referring physician, yet it may be the most difficult to write, partly because many EEG findings are nonspecific (i.e., the patient's EEG findings usually do not by themselves establish a specific diagnosis). Therefore, writing this paragraph is not as simple as stating "Finding A is present, which implies that the patient has Diagnosis B." Also, writing a good Clinical Correlation paragraph requires both a good knowledge of clinical neurophysiology (i.e., EEG reading) but also of epilepsy. Because EEG abnormalities are not usually absolutely diagnostic of a particular disorder, when encountering a particular EEG abnormality in a patient we often want to communicate whether this raises or lowers the chances of a particular disorder. The challenge of writing this paragraph lies in neither understating nor overstating the specificity of the clinical implications of whatever findings are present. Thus, the clinical correlation paragraph must be worded with care. For example, it is well known that the presence of spikes in the EEG is not associated with a diagnosis of epilepsy 100% of the time. Some individuals may go through life with spikes in the EEG, possibly never knowing that they have them, and never experience a single seizure. Therefore, a spike in the EEG does not establish the diagnosis of a seizure disorder. Nevertheless, the presence of spikes in the EEG makes it considerably more likely that a person has epilepsy compared to another person who does not have such spikes. The report should, therefore, communicate this concept of "increased risk" or "an association" rather than appear to be diagnosing epilepsy:

Spikes seen in the right anterior temporal area suggest the possibility of a decreased seizure threshold in that area. Slowing over the right hemisphere suggests the possibility of an anatomical or functional (e.g., post-seizure) change in that region.

These sentences make it clear that the epileptiform abnormality seen in the EEG increases the chances that the patient has a seizure disorder or epilepsy arising from that area, but does not establish the diagnosis. The slowing over the right hemisphere could have a number of possible causes, such as stroke, tumor, infection, or the recent occurrence of a focal seizure from that hemisphere (post-ictal slowing) among others. The same type of thinking can be used when writing a clinical correlation for a normal EEG. Thus, when narrowing the clinical correlation discussion in an EEG report, in the spirit of the saying sometimes attributed to Albert Einstein that a theory should be "as simple as possible, but no simpler," EEG clinical correlations should be as precise as possible, but no more precise.

Some electroencephalographers choose to signal to the referring clinician that a normal EEG tracing does not exclude the diagnosis of epilepsy. Although such warnings can be useful, the necessity of including such reminders can be argued. For instance, blood testing laboratories do not find it necessary to say that a normal blood count does not exclude the possibility of an infection or leukemia. Whether or not to include such warnings is a matter of style that each reader can decide upon. Likewise, the routine addition of the phrase "clinical correlation is recommended" should be avoided as there is no situation in which an EEG result does not require clinical correlation. This phraseology should be reserved for the occasional situation in which the implications of the EEG findings depend in a special way on the clinical backdrop against which they have occurred, in which case the specifics of that issue should be discussed in the clinical correlation section.

The electroencephalographer must resist the temptation to suggest further diagnostic studies in the report. For instance, in the earlier example, the combination of spikes in the right anterior temporal area associated with slowing over the hemisphere does suggest the possibility of a fixed right hemispheric lesion. The findings are potentially consistent with the patient having a right temporal lobe tumor (among many other diagnoses). Why not suggest in the report that the patient undergo magnetic resonance imaging (MRI) of the brain? Because the electroencephalographer often does not know the patient firsthand, it may not be known that the patient had neuroimaging four months earlier, perhaps at a different hospital. In such a case, a suggestion that an MRI be obtained may be confusing. Is the electroencephalographer saying that the MRI should be repeated? Decisions about obtaining neuroimaging are best made by the clinician who knows all of the elements of the patient's story, one of which is the EEG report you are preparing. Similarly, the EEG report should not suggest that specific medications be used. The patient may have already been on a suggested medication in the past or could even be allergic to a suggested medication. Again, medication decisions should only be made by the treating physician who knows the whole story, not just based on the appearance of the EEG.

Some have suggested that the complexity level of the interpretation and clinical correlation sections of the EEG report should be written with the expertise level of the ordering provider in mind. Although this may seem to be a thoughtful approach, in many cases the ordering provider will not be the only one to review the EEG report and it is impossible to know at the time the report is prepared just who all of the future readers of the report will be. Keeping this in mind, ideally the style of the clinical correlation should be readable by a non-neurologist.

WHAT IS AN ABNORMAL EEG FINDING?

At first this question may seem too obvious to even pose, but it is worth thinking about what it means to label an EEG "normal" or "abnormal." In particular, what does the word "abnormal" mean? As an initial thought, one might feel that a finding not routinely encountered in normal EEGs, which is to say uncommon or rarely seen, should be considered abnormal. This would be a poor definition for many reasons. Is a person who is 6 feet 10 inches (208 cm) tall abnormal? No, that person may just be very tall, even though you may not be used to encountering people of that stature every day on the street. In certain localities, individuals who have red hair might be quite rare. Nevertheless, having red hair is not abnormal. The rarity of a given finding does necessarily indicate that it is abnormal. Rather, for the purposes of EEG interpretation, a good operational definition is that a finding should be considered abnormal if it is *associated with* pathology (disease or disability).

Consider the following hypothetical example: you have been reading EEGs for several years and have noticed a handful of patients with an atypical finding for which you have invented the term "x-wave." Because x-waves look so unusual and so few patients have them, you are inclined to consider them abnormal. What threshold should be used to make a

definite assertion of abnormality? You decide to conduct the following study: you look back through all of your lab's EEGs and collect 100 patients with x-waves and 100 patients of the same age who do not have x-waves (controls). You then compare the two groups, looking to see whether one group has more epilepsy (or any other pathologic condition) than the other. You find that the rate of epilepsy is 1% in both groups. No other disorder is more common in the x-wave group compared to the group without x-waves. Therefore, even though at first these x-waves *did not look right* to you, you finally conclude that x-waves represent a normal variant. (Publishing the results of your study could be a considerable aid to other electroencephalographers in the future!) Even though x-waves are rarely seen, it is incorrect to call them abnormal because they are not associated with an increased rate of pathology or disease. If, however, individuals with x-waves are found to have more seizures, or intellectual disability, or brain tumors than the 100 control patients who lack them, then the fact of any of these associations would be excellent additions to the clinical correlation section of the reports you and others prepare for patients who have these fictitious x-waves in the EEG.

In the real world, it is surprising how difficult it can be to perform this seemingly simple hypothetical study. Although it may not be particularly difficult to amass a good number of patients with one EEG finding or another in a busy EEG laboratory, the real challenge lies in assembling a "normal" comparison (control) group. Almost everyone referred to your EEG lab has been sent there for a reason, some worrisome symptom or suspicion of some disorder, so your laboratory patients cannot be considered "normal" as a group. Instead, the fact of their referral for an EEG study has enriched the persons recorded in your EEG lab for "disease." In practice, it is logistically very difficult to obtain the recordings of 100 "normal" 50-year-olds or 100 "normal" schoolchildren. How does one choose 100 normal patients and then induce them to come to the EEG laboratory for a study? If 100 patients are invited and 50 refuse, are the remaining 50 still a "random" group, or may there be a difference between refusers and non-refusers? How does one ethically handle the eventual occurrence of EEG abnormalities discovered in the so-called *normal group*—individuals who have no clinical indication for having an EEG and no neurologist, but have volunteered to help with your research study?

The example of the hypothetical "x-wave" serves as a cautionary tale. It reminds us that even if an EEG tracing "does not look right" to us, we should not jump to the conclusion that it is abnormal. Properly, if abnormal, whatever "does not look right" and is indeed not right should be categorizable as a known abnormality type. After it is categorized, the type of pathology that has been associated with that abnormality type based on past research studies can be cited in the Clinical Correlation section. If something does not look right in the EEG but it is not possible to categorize it as a known abnormality type, one must hesitate before calling it abnormal. The finding can still be described in the report, noting that it is unusual, but of "uncertain clinical significance."

The histories of several of the known "normal variants" (see Chapter 11) have followed this course. Initially, because they "looked abnormal" and were only seen occasionally in the lab, but were recorded in individuals with epilepsy (because most people referred for EEG recordings are persons with epilepsy), they were presumed to be abnormal. Only later was it recognized that certain findings were also present with a similar frequency in the normal population, leading them to be reclassified as normal variants.

THE THRESHOLD FOR "ABNORMAL" AND ITS IMPLICATIONS

In the course of interpreting EEGs, from time to time the question arises as to whether a wave is sharp enough or an asymmetry asymmetrical enough to label abnormal. For instance, several waves are seen in the EEG, but it is not definitely clear to you that they are sharp enough to be labeled as sharp waves or spikes. After a lot of thought, you still cannot definitely decide either way, and you estimate that the chances are 50-50 that the discharges represent an epileptiform abnormality. To boil it down to the basic question, what should you do if you are just not sure one way or the other? Is it best to err on the side of calling the wave (and, therefore, the EEG) normal or calling it abnormal? If an erroneous assessment is made in either direction, what would be the potential impact of each type of judgment, each of which could represent a different type of error with different potential consequences?

Imagine the following hypothetical story behind the patient described above with the 50-50 spike. Although the EEG reader may not know it, the EEG was obtained because the patient had an episode of loss of consciousness. The referring physician is undecided as to whether the patient has had a syncopal event (a simple fainting spell) or an epileptic seizure. Obviously, both types of error are undesirable, but what would the consequences be of either type of reading error in this patient's EEG: calling a normal wave a spike versus missing true spikes and calling the EEG normal?

First, consider the scenario in which the patient does not have epilepsy and the discharge is not really an epileptic spike, but you make the error of reporting that an epileptic spike is present. The referring physician reads your report and comes to the (erroneous) conclusion that the patient has epilepsy and considers starting an antiseizure medication. The patient is labeled as having a seizure disorder and cannot drive for a period of time according to local law. Some individuals who lose the right to drive may also be unable to get to their job and become unemployed as a result. In this scenario, the patient is now considered to have a potentially chronic disease where none exists and may be unnecessarily receiving antiseizure medications. Perhaps the referring physician should realize that the finding of a spike in the EEG does not necessarily compel the diagnosis of epilepsy. Unfortunately, the report of epileptiform findings in the EEG may carry more weight than it should, among both specialists and non-specialists.

In the second scenario, the patient does have epilepsy but you make the error of calling the EEG normal. In this situation, however, the "opposite" sequence of the events does not necessarily occur. This is partly because it is better known that individuals with epilepsy may still, from time to time (and occasionally repeatedly), have a normal EEG. The referring physician cannot exclude the diagnosis of seizure simply because of your report of a normal EEG. In reality, this patient does have a seizure disorder and your reading error may, at the very least, delay the diagnosis of epilepsy and incur any of the disadvantages to the patient consequent to that delay. If the patient does, in fact, have epilepsy, additional spells will probably occur providing additional descriptions of the event that may be more clearly suggestive of seizure. There will also be additional opportunities to recheck the EEG. One may argue that this type of error could delay the ordering of neuroimaging that could reveal an important finding, such as a tumor, leaving the patient inappropriately untreated. In fact, if a tumor (or some other serious pathology) is present, additional symptoms or spells will probably occur, eventually prompting the ordering of neuroimaging studies or other testing, though perhaps in a less timely fashion.

So, which type of error is worse, "overcalling" or "undercalling" the spike? In the scenario just described, the "overcalling reader" encountering 100 patients with a 50-50 spike could be responsible for giving 50 patients an erroneous diagnosis of epilepsy. That erroneous diagnosis could be carried just for a period of time, but also possibly life-long. The "undercalling reader" could be responsible for *delaying* a true diagnosis of epilepsy in 50 people. Although neither type of error is desirable, most would say that the first scenario in which 50 patients are given a diagnosis that they do not have is the less desirable outcome. Physicians are generally charged with alleviating disease, but in this scenario the physician has effectively given to these patients a disease they do not have, possibly relegating them to unnecessary long-term therapy and other possible negative consequences. In the second scenario, the diagnosis of a seizure disorder and its underlying cause may be missed or delayed. Although this is not desirable, if disease is present, it will likely declare itself again at some time in the future. If it never does, then perhaps no harm has been done. In summary, the type of error in which abnormalities are "undercalled" is usually the lesser of two evils: it is generally worse to erroneously label a patient with a disease he or she does not have than to delay the diagnosis of epilepsy in a patient. Part of this effect stems from the fact that clinicians are more likely to know that a normal EEG does not absolutely exclude the diagnosis of epilepsy. Conversely, it is more difficult for clinicians to receive the report of an epileptiform abnormality in the EEG and resist making the diagnosis of epilepsy.

For this reason, it is recommended that readers lean to the conservative side in making judgments about EEG findings that are not entirely clear. While giving an EEG tracing a normal interpretation, the electroencephalographer also has the option of including a comment in the EEG that reflects the difficulty of the decision.

Several waveforms seen in the right occipital electrode exhibit sharp contours at times, but probably fall within the range of normal. Although these do not clearly represent an example of sharp waves, the question could be further investigated by obtaining a repeat study, if clinically indicated.

Although the reader should be able to categorize the large majority of EEG tracings as normal or abnormal, in the case of unclear findings the reader may wish to communicate to the referring physician that "a repeat study may provide additional useful information, if clinically indicated." This kind of wording and the phrase "if clinically indicated" are chosen so as not to appear to compel the referring clinician to obtain a repeat study if one is not necessary when the patient's overall picture is considered.

THE CONCEPT OF INDEPENDENT OBSERVATIONS

Imagine that you are reading an EEG and you have a brief suspicion that there is slowing over the right hemisphere. By the time you get to the end of the EEG, however, you have not convinced yourself that the asymmetry was really there and you have decided to read out the EEG as normal. Before preparing the final report, however, by chance you come across the patient's MRI report (or maybe you even purposefully looked it up) which describes a stroke in the right hemisphere. Should you reverse your decision and rewrite your report so that it describes slowing in the right hemisphere? After all, the patient does have a stroke there! You begin to worry, how could there not be slowing if there is a stroke there? The answer is that you should not change your opinion of what the tracing shows based on the patient's clinical history. Often, clinicians refer patients for additional studies to confirm the importance of other findings and to see whether they "line up" with one another. In this case, it is possible that the referring physician has reviewed the MRI scan but doubts the presence of the stroke, thinking that the MRI was interpreted incorrectly. By ordering the EEG, the referring clinician was seeking an independent corroboration of the MRI finding. The purpose of the current EEG interpretation is not simply to echo the finding of what was found on a previous study. The ordering physician certainly has not referred the patient for EEG just to hear a repetition of the findings in the MRI report. Instead, to be useful, the results of your EEG interpretation should represent an independent observation.

To avoid the temptation of this type of error, many electroencephalographers do not read the patient's history before their initial review of the tracing. This is good practice, but is a matter of style and varies among readers. It also increases the sense of satisfaction the reader gets in picking up subtle right hemispheric slowing and then learning of the correctly situated stroke only after a definite conclusion of right-sided slowing has been reached. If the reader is already aware that the patient has a stroke on the right side before looking at the first page of the EEG, it may be psychologically difficult for some not to "see" slowing over the right hemisphere. This idea is captured by the unattributed humorous pseudo-aphorism: "I never would have seen it if I hadn't believed it with my own eyes." The search for slowing over the hemisphere "where it's supposed to be" may absorb so much mental energy that other abnormalities may be missed because of the distraction. The best time to review the patient's history is after the EEG has been read, at least for the first time, and a preliminary conclusion has been reached. After the initial reading, it is not "dishonest" to review the record again in light of the patient's history to make sure that something has not been missed. If the interpretation is changed at this point in the process, the reader fully realizes that the finding was not evident to him or her without the additional clue of knowing the patient's history and a higher standard of feeling convinced of the abnormality should be used.

SUGGESTED READING

Tatum WO, Olga S, Ochoa JG, Clary HM, Cheek J, Drislane F, Tsuchida TN: American Clinical Neurophysiology Society Guideline 7: Guidelines for EEG Reporting, *J Clin Neurophysiol* 33(4):328–332, 2016.

9

The Abnormal EEG

When discussing the abnormal EEG, it is worthwhile to start by asking what, specifically, we mean when we say "abnormal." The term can be used in many ways in many contexts, but when stating that an EEG is abnormal, we are implying that it has findings known to be associated with a pathologic or disease state. As discussed in Chapter 8, "The Structure and Philosophy of the EEG Report," this distinction is designed to prevent the interpreter from calling an EEG abnormal simply because it includes a finding that "looks unusual" or is uncommon, because findings that are uncommon still may not be abnormal.

When deciding which types of studies should be labeled *abnormal*, it is useful to consider the referring physician's purpose in ordering a diagnostic EEG. Ideally, based on the patient's clinical picture, the clinician has formed a list of possible diagnoses, also called the *differential diagnosis*, which might explain the patient's findings. If the results of an EEG have the potential to raise or lower the likelihood that one or more entities on the differential diagnosis list is the correct diagnosis, then the test may be indicated. However, if an EEG is not likely to sway opinion toward or away from any of the diagnoses on the list, then the test is much less likely to be useful, and perhaps should not be obtained. It is usually not a good idea to obtain an EEG just "to see what it looks like" without a specific question in mind that the EEG could potentially answer. Likewise, patients do not necessarily require a "yearly EEG" unless that EEG will be used for decision-making. Such decision-making could be as simple as confirming the working diagnosis if it is not completely clear, or helping to decide whether or not to discontinue medications, among other things. A related concept is that an EEG is indicated if there is some likelihood that the result will affect the patient's treatment. When reporting abnormalities on an EEG, ideally this can be done in a way that can impact the differential diagnosis. Simply reporting that the EEG looks "odd" or "unusual" will not likely be helpful to the referring physician. Rather, an EEG should only be considered abnormal if it contains a finding that has some association with a disease or an abnormal state.

The majority of EEG abnormalities do not specifically lead to a single diagnosis. Only a small minority of EEG abnormalities are associated with a short enough list of disease entities that they can be considered specific or pathognomonic for one diagnosis or another. The majority of EEG findings are diagnostically nonspecific and are associated with a list of disease states that may be lengthy and diverse such that no specific diagnosis can be made based on the EEG result alone. An example of a dramatically abnormal but nonspecific EEG abnormality is generalized delta slowing, a finding that is associated with so many types of abnormal states (e.g., coma, post-seizure state, meningitis, anesthesia) that the clinical implications of the finding can only be stated in the broadest terms in the EEG report. The utility of the EEG comes in combining the EEG result with the patient's history and other findings to narrow the differential diagnosis.

The referring physician is usually in the best position to put the EEG findings together with the clinical story to arrive at a clinical conclusion. Without the clinical history, the EEG is a considerably less powerful tool. Even when a clinical history has been submitted with the EEG request, the reader of the EEG should hesitate before suggesting specific clinical diagnoses. The submitted history may be incomplete and often lacks details such as the physical examination or certain laboratory or imaging findings. When reading the brief history that has been submitted with the EEG, the electroencephalographer usually cannot know whether that history is complete. For these reasons, the EEG reader should resist the temptation to make specific diagnoses based on the EEG results. Rather, a list of diagnoses that have been associated with the observed abnormalities, a sort of "EEG differential diagnosis," should be given at the end of the report, if feasible. The discussion given in the final clinical interpretation section of the report should take into account the clinical history provided, but the EEG differential diagnosis offered should not necessarily be limited by that history. After giving the broader EEG differential diagnosis, the reader may choose to close by making a more specific comment that takes the submitted history into account, such as, "the finding of left hemispheric slowing is consistent with the patient's reported diagnosis of left hemispheric stroke."

EEG abnormalities can be categorized in a variety of ways. Abnormalities may fall into the categories of (1) abnormal expressions of normally occurring rhythms (e.g., asymmetries or absence of normal rhythms), (2) inherently abnormal rhythms (e.g., "slow" delta and theta rhythms in an adult who is awake), (3) certain repetitive or periodic patterns (e.g., burst-suppression patterns or PLEDs/LPDs), (4) epileptiform abnormalities (spikes, sharp waves, etc.), and (5) abnormal "super-architecture" (e.g., abnormal sleep state cycling). These various abnormality types are discussed in the following sections. The first two abnormality families, abnormalities of normal rhythms and abnormal rhythms, are discussed by frequency range, starting with slow activity. Basic epileptiform abnormalities are discussed in this chapter. Various epilepsy syndromes and the EEG findings associated with them are discussed further in Chapter 10, "The EEG in Epilepsy."

ABNORMALITIES OF SLOW-WAVE (DELTA AND THETA) ACTIVITY

Descriptive Parameters for Slow Waves

Slow-wave abnormalities can be defined in multiple domains. The most obvious descriptor of a slow wave is its location. A slow wave may occur focally, such as in the left anterior temporal area or the right occipital area. Slowing may occur in broader regions, such as in the right posterior quadrant, in "anterior brain regions," or over a whole hemisphere (see Figures 9.1 and 9.2). Such regional slowing can be considered a subset of focal slowing. Finally, slowing may also be diffuse or generalized.

Slow waves may be rhythmic or irregular (nonrhythmic). When there is a tendency to rhythmicity but the waves cannot be considered truly rhythmic, the intermediate term *semirhythmic* may be used (see Figure 9.3). Slow waves can

be of varying amplitude. If slowing is only observed in a certain sleep stage, such as wakefulness or drowsiness, this fact should be described. Slow waves may occur intermittently (in brief runs or bursts) or continuously (in long, continuous runs with few pauses). These different parameters are worth remembering and should usually be included in the written description of slow-wave activity.

Parameter	Examples
Frequency:	Theta activity or 6–7 Hz activity
Rhythmicity:	Irregular versus semirhythmic versus rhythmic
Amplitude:	High voltage versus low voltage
Sleep Stage Specificity:	Seen in wakefulness versus drowsiness versus sleep
Continuity:	Intermittent versus continuous
Localization:	Focal versus regional versus generalized

The parameters can be remembered using the mnemonic FRASCL. Certain combinations of these parameters can define specific, well-described slow-wave abnormalities. For instance, a slow wave that is frontal, in the delta range,

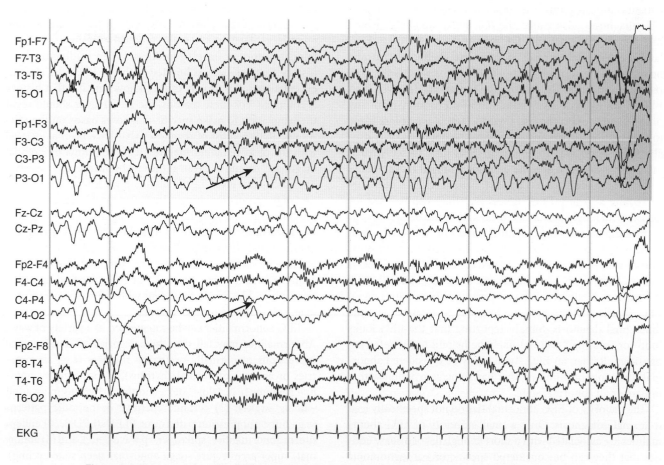

Figure 9.1 This page of waking EEG shows slowing in both the delta and theta ranges occurring predominantly over the left hemisphere. Compare the left hemisphere channels (shaded) to the right hemisphere (bottom eight channels, unshaded). Delta and theta waves are more plentiful and of higher voltage over the left. The difference is especially prominent comparing the left (top arrow) and right (bottom arrow) parasagittal areas.

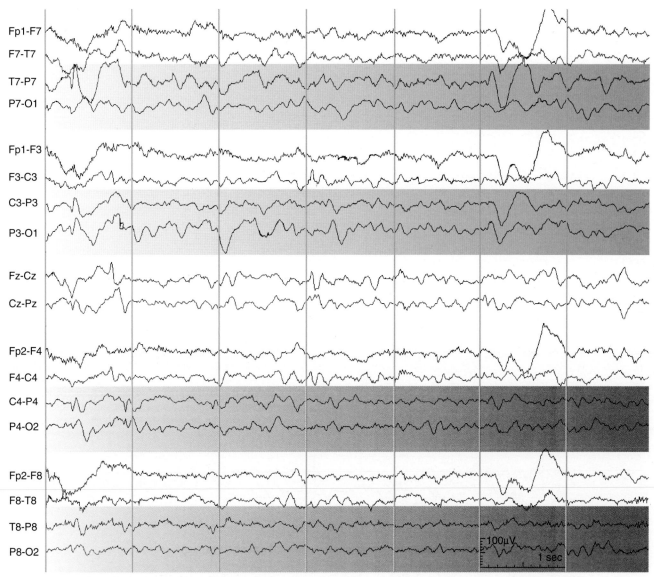

Figure 9.2 A mild but abnormal increase in slowing is seen in the left posterior quadrant (red rectangles) compared with the right posterior quadrant (gray rectangles) during drowsiness. The reader with a sharp eye will also catch low voltage spikes particularly in the posterior quadrants, left more than right, in the first second of the recording.

occurs intermittently, is rhythmic, and is seen during wakefulness has been given the specific and well-known name *FIRDA* (frontal intermittent rhythmic delta activity), discussed further later in the chapter. Although the term *slow wave* already implies that the waves are in the delta or theta range, the description of slow waves may be further refined by stating any narrower frequency range they may belong to. If waves have a distinctive morphology, a description of the shape may be added.

Focal Slowing

Focal slow waves are the classic sign of a lesion in the cerebral hemispheres. Before the era of modern neuroimaging, the electroencephalogram was an important tool for the localization of cerebral tumors. Today the magnetic resonance imaging (MRI) scanner has moved to the forefront

in localizing tumors, but the EEG may still play an important role in identifying certain types of focal lesions that may or may not be obvious on neuroimaging. The EEG has the advantage over imaging studies of identifying areas of electrical abnormality that may be "nonanatomical," that is, functional abnormalities of the brain that may not be visible on an MRI or computed tomographic (CT) scans. Examples of "nonanatomical" slowing may include postictal slowing (see Figure 9.4), slowing from trauma that has not caused an MRI lesion (Figure 9.5), or even migraine (discussed below).

Focal slow waves may mark an area of previous, rather than acute, injury. Brain lesions that cause focal slowing in the absence of epileptiform activity may not necessarily be prone to seizures. Figures 9.6 and 9.7 show a left temporal slow wave abnormality; the perinatally acquired lesion causing the slow wave is shown in Figure 9.8.

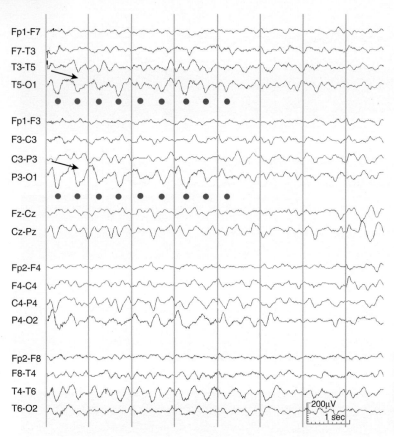

Figure 9.3 Although not perfectly rhythmic, the slow waves seen in the left occipital (O1) channels (arrows) are not completely irregular (dots). Some of the unpredictability of the appearance of these slow waves is caused by intermixing with other rhythms. Waves of this intermediate degree of rhythmicity can be termed semirhythmic.

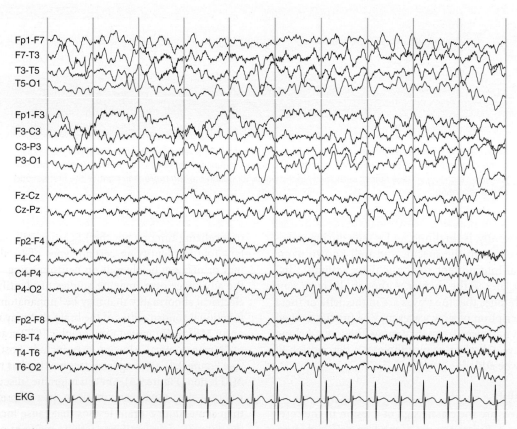

Figure 9.4 Significant slowing is evident in the top eight EEG channels (left hemisphere) compared with the bottom eight EEG channels (right hemisphere). The fact that this slowing represented a postictal change after a seizure was confirmed by demonstrating clearance of the slowing on a repeat EEG 2 months later. Depending on the nature of the patient and the intensity and duration of the seizure, postictal slowing may last from several seconds to as long as 4 weeks.

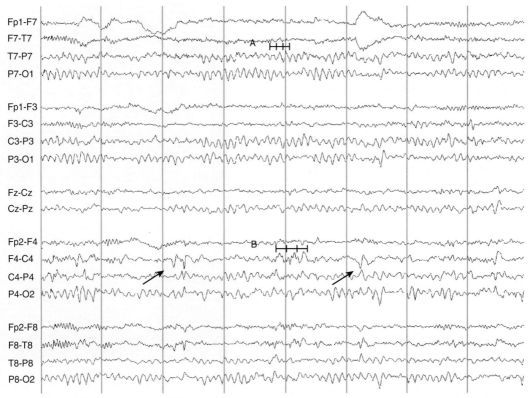

Figure 9.5 Slowing and sharp waves are seen over the right hemisphere in this patient following a brain contusion. Note the sharp waves (arrows) over the right hemisphere. Normal alpha range activity with short wavelengths (A scale) is seen on the left compared with slower, theta range activity with correspondingly longer wavelengths (B scale) on the right.

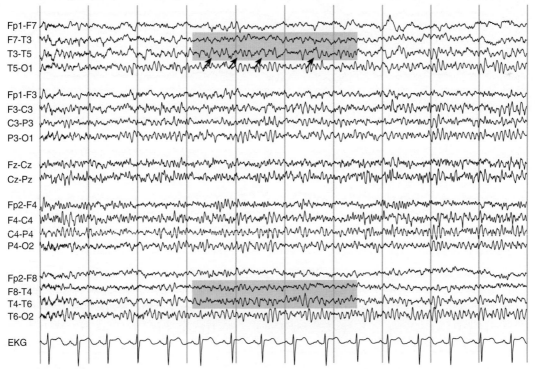

Figure 9.6 Close comparison of the temporal areas (shaded) shows an asymmetry of slow activity with increased theta waves on the left as a result of an old perinatal injury to the left temporal lobe tip in a 17-year-old girl. The arrows indicate individual theta waves in the left temporal area. The patient's scan is shown in Figure 9.8. The lesion resulted in complex partial seizures.

Figure 9.9 shows a subtle right occipital slow wave brought on by hyperventilation. If asymmetric slowing is only seen during hyperventilation, especially when the asymmetry is relatively mild as seen in this example, it is less likely to be associated with pathology than spontaneously occurring slow-wave asymmetries. Slow-wave asymmetries that alternate sides, whether spontaneous or elicited by hyperventilation, are much less likely to be clinically significant. To be convincing, slow waves should be confirmed in a referential montage.

Focal slow-wave abnormalities have generally been associated with deeper lesions located at the level of the deep white matter (as opposed to more superficial gray matter lesions), although exceptions to this rule occur. As discussed below, more superficial abnormalities of cerebral cortex are classically associated with decreases in beta activity.

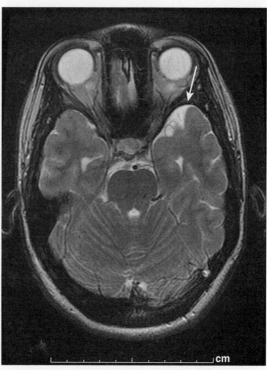

Figure 9.8 This is the T2-weighted magnetic resonance imaging (MRI) scan of the patient whose EEG is shown in the previous two figures. In this MRI sequence, the cerebrospinal fluid appears white. Note the loss of volume in the left temporal pole (arrow), which is responsible for the EEG asymmetry noted in the previous figures.

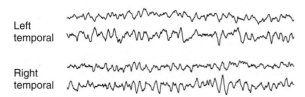

Left temporal

Right temporal

Figure 9.7 Close-up views of the left and right temporal channels taken from the shaded areas of the previous figure are shown. Note the mixture of slow waves with wider bases (wavelengths) in the top channels compared with the faster alpha rhythms with narrower bases in the bottom channels.

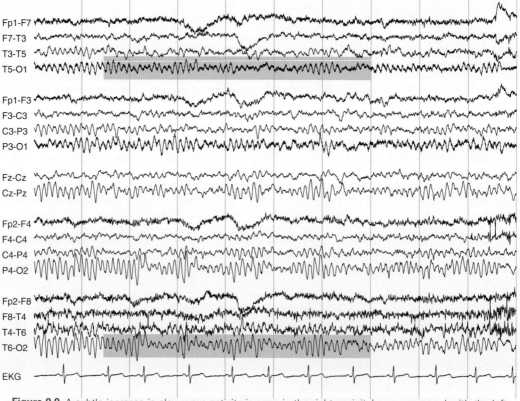

Figure 9.9 A subtle increase in slow-wave activity is seen in the right occipital area compared with the left (compare shaded areas). The posterior rhythm appears against a flat baseline in the T5-O1 channel (upper shaded area), but the posterior rhythm rides up and down on a low voltage wave in the T6-O2 channel (lower shaded area). The same comparison can be made between the P3-O1 and P4-O2 channels.

Intermittent Rhythmic Delta Activity

Frontal Intermittent Rhythmic Delta Activity and Occipital Intermittent Rhythmic Delta Activity

The term intermittent rhythmic delta activity (IRDA) refers to rhythmic delta activity occurring in brief bursts, usually lasting no longer than several seconds, typically located either frontally or occipitally (Figure 9.10). In some examples, the bursts can be more generalized (Figure 9.11) and occasionally they can be asymmetrical. IRDA is a pattern typically seen during wakefulness or mild drowsiness and is usually associated with processes of mild to moderate severity. Keeping in mind that the patient generally must attain some level of wakefulness to manifest frontal (FIRDA) or occipital IRDA (OIRDA), these patterns would not be expected in patients whose recordings are restricted to more deeply sedated or comatose states. Rather, they are most often seen in the outpatient laboratory. IRDA should be distinguished from more continuous rhythmic delta activity (RDA), discussed in Chapter 12, "EEG Patterns in Stupor and Coma."

One important feature of FIRDA and OIRDA is that these abnormal patterns do not suggest a specific localization. Surprisingly, the tendency for IRDA to occur either frontally or occipitally is not dictated by an anterior or posterior location of the patient's abnormality but rather by the patient's age. Up to approximately 10 years of age, IRDA, when present, tends to occur in the occipital areas. By the early teenage years and thereafter, IRDA tends to occur frontally. It is important to correctly identify an example of rhythmic slowing as IRDA to avoid being trapped into inappropriately using IRDA as a "falsely localizing sign." As stated above, FIRDA is not particularly associated with frontal lesions and OIRDA is not particularly associated with occipital lesions; either can be associated with anterior or posterior (or diffuse) brain abnormalities. Indeed, the location of the IRDA tells us more about the age of the patient than the location of the lesion.

It is interesting to note that the predilection of the hyperventilation response for the occipital area in children and for the frontal area in adults parallels this age dependence of FIRDA and OIRDA. In older patients, the hyperventilation response may mimic the appearance of FIRDA, and in younger patients it mimics OIRDA, which is to say that younger children tend to manifest the rhythmic high voltage slowing of hyperventilation in the occipital areas. Therefore, the localization of the hyperventilation response tracks with the localization of FIRDA and OIRDA by age.

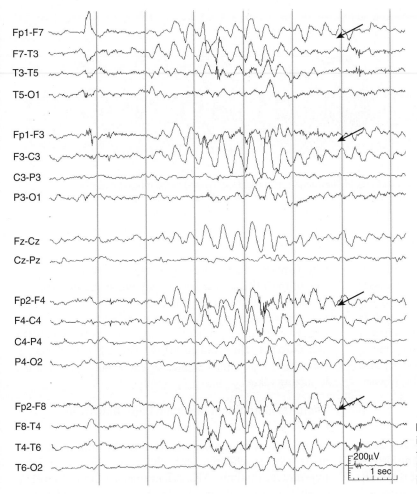

Figure 9.10 Frontal intermittent rhythmic delta activity (FIRDA) consists of rhythmic runs of delta activity in the frontal areas of varying duration (arrows). Although FIRDA appears frontally, the finding does not necessarily imply a frontal pathology (see text).

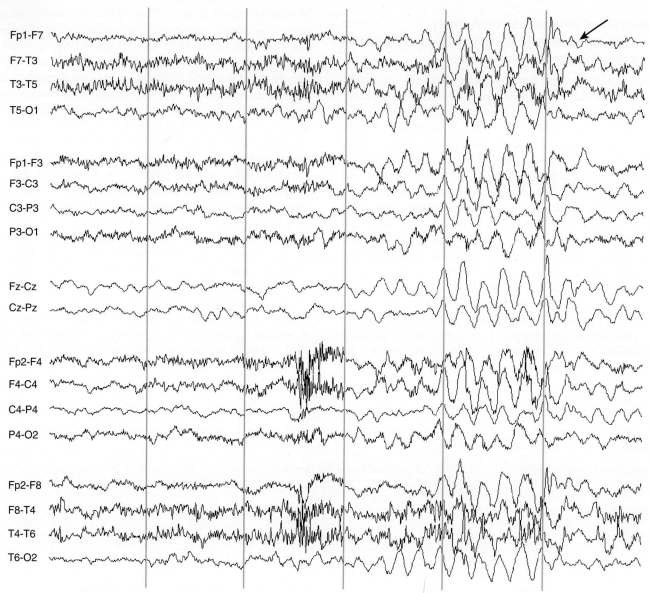

Figure 9.11 Compared with Figure 9.10, this burst of intermittent rhythmic slow (arrow) has a more diffuse (rather than frontal) distribution. It is seen equally well in the anterior and posterior channels. A small frontal spike-wave discharge is seen in the Fp1-F7 and Fp2-F8 channels at the end of the slow wave burst.

FIRDA and OIRDA are etiologically nonspecific, and can be caused by a variety of toxic, metabolic, and other processes that affect the central nervous system. Their presence signals some type of cerebral disturbance, focal or diffuse, and its nonspecific and nonlocalizing nature should be mentioned in the clinical conclusion of the report. One partial exception to this rule is the association of OIRDA with childhood absence epilepsy, discussed below and in Chapter 10, "The EEG in Epilepsy."

Temporal Intermittent Rhythmic Delta Activity

Temporal IRDA (TIRDA, or LRDA in the ACNS 2021 Terminology) should be considered separately from FIRDA and OIRDA. The presence of intermittent trains of rhythmic delta activity over either temporal lobe has been associated with temporal lobe epilepsy (Figure 9.12). Furthermore, the side of the TIRDA, which is usually unilateral and does not necessarily display sharp features, indicates the side of the lesion if one is present. This localizing property of TIRDA distinguishes it from the other two major types of IRDA (FIRDA and OIRDA). Thus, unlike FIRDA and OIRDA, TIRDA is considered a potentially epileptogenic abnormality and has localizing value.

Occipital Intermittent Rhythmic Delta Activity in Childhood Absence Epilepsy

A specific type of occipital intermittent rhythmic delta activity is seen in children with childhood absence epilepsy. Intermittent rhythmic 3 Hz delta activity, a form of OIRDA, can be seen in what can be either brief or prolonged runs in

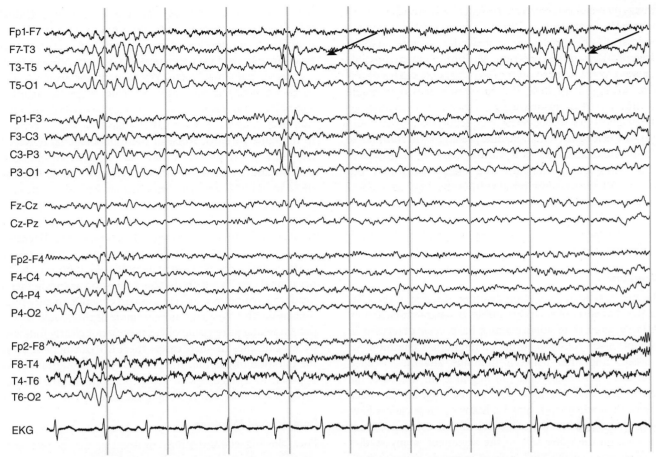

Figure 9.12 Temporal intermittent rhythmic delta activity (TIRDA) is seen in a patient with temporal lobe epilepsy. This rhythmic delta activity is seen best in the left temporal area (arrows), although the left parasagittal area is involved as well. In this example, some of the theta waves are sharply contoured, which is not a necessary feature for the identification of TIRDA.

the occipital areas in children who have childhood absence epilepsy (CAE). This type of rhythmic delta activity distinguishes itself from typical examples of OIRDA in that the runs can be quite prolonged, lasting many seconds. It is not seen in all cases of CAE, but can be a useful corroborative diagnostic finding. Knowing that OIRDA is seen in CAE can help distinguish this kind of delta activity from the slowing seen in encephalopathic states, which is to say that when OIRDA is seen in the context of known CAE, an additional explanation for the slowing need not be sought.

Generalized or Diffuse Slowing

In general, theta and delta rhythms are not expected in the waking adult EEG. In younger patients, however, theta waves may be seen in the normal waking EEG. The range of normal posterior rhythms in childhood may serve as a useful reminder that theta frequencies are commonplace in the EEG of the awake child (see Table 2.2 in Chapter 2, "Visual Analysis of the EEG"). For instance, in individuals young enough that a posterior rhythm of 7 Hz is considered normal, other 7 Hz rhythms may also be seen elsewhere in the normal waking EEG.

The determination that an adult EEG is abnormal simply because theta waves are present is made more difficult by the fact that it is normal for theta waves to appear with drowsiness. Therefore, in one way or another, the electroencephalographer must establish that a patient is not simply drowsy at the time that theta waves are seen in order to label them abnormal. Interpreting an EEG as abnormal on the basis of the presence of theta waves that are, in reality, related to drowsiness would constitute a significant error in interpretation. Indications that a patient is probably awake would include the presence of a posterior rhythm, temporalis or frontalis muscle artifact, eyeblink artifact, patient movements, or conversation. The alert technologist can document (or force) alertness by having the patient count or perform some other task to exclude drowsiness as an explanation for observed slow-wave activity.

The list of pathologic states that can cause diffuse slow-wave activity is long and includes almost any abnormal state that can cause a diffuse cerebral disturbance. The most common causes are postictal (post-seizure) states, post-anoxic states, diffuse traumatic injuries, infectious or inflammatory processes of the nervous system, toxic states related to drugs (recreational or pharmacologically-induced) or other metabolic derangements (hepatic, renal, etc.), and a large number of other processes that have the potential to affect large portions of the cerebrum. Most of the many possible causes of coma are also on the list of possible causes of diffuse slowing in the EEG. For this reason, it is not feasible for the electroencephalographer to give a specific differential diagnosis for this pattern in the report because it would just be too lengthy. Often the interpretation will summarize the possible etiologies as a "diffuse cerebral disturbance" or a "diffuse encephalopathy." The interpretation may also specifically discuss any clinical entities that have been questioned in the clinical history. EEG patterns in coma, many of which consist of slow-wave patterns, are discussed in more detail in Chapter 12, "Electroencephalographic Patterns in Stupor and Coma."

Migraine

Because it is such a common disorder, the role of the EEG in the diagnosis of migraine merits a separate discussion. A large number of abnormalities have been described in patients with common forms of migraine ("common" or "classic" migraine) between migraine attacks, so-called *interictal EEG abnormalities in migraine* (in this case, the terms *ictus* and *interictal* refer to the migrainous attack rather than an epileptic attack). Many of these claims have been challenged because of the lack of well-controlled studies and, on the other side of the argument, many studies have shown that the EEG in most migraine patients, both during and between attacks, is normal. One confounding factor is the high frequency of migraine in the general population, which increases the chance that an individual who has any particular EEG abnormality may also incidentally have migraine. Some authors have claimed that focal slowing, and even epileptiform activity, are seen with increased frequency interictally in migraine patients. The "high-frequency photic response" (the ability to maintain a photic driving response at particularly high flash stimulation frequencies, e.g., above 30 Hz) has also been described in migraine patients. None of these phenomena, however, has been clearly proven to have an incidence in migraine patients above that seen in the general population. Because there are no EEG abnormalities that have proven to be useful in helping to diagnose uncomplicated migraine patients between attacks, EEG is not recommended as part of the routine evaluation of migraine patients and the diagnosis of migraine is best made clinically using standard diagnostic criteria. The EEG may be indicated, however, in the occasional case in which there is a question as to whether a headache symptom may represent an epileptic seizure phenomenon. The most common example of this would be the patient with a pure visual phenomenon not clearly followed by a headache. In such cases, the EEG can help address the question of whether the phenomenon is migrainous as opposed to a seizure with visual phenomena (the former being much more common than the latter).

Complicated Migraine

Focal slowing, either rhythmic or irregular, may be seen during the course of complicated migraine attacks, making EEG a useful confirmatory study in this disorder if obtained during the attack. Figure 9.13 shows an example of high-voltage

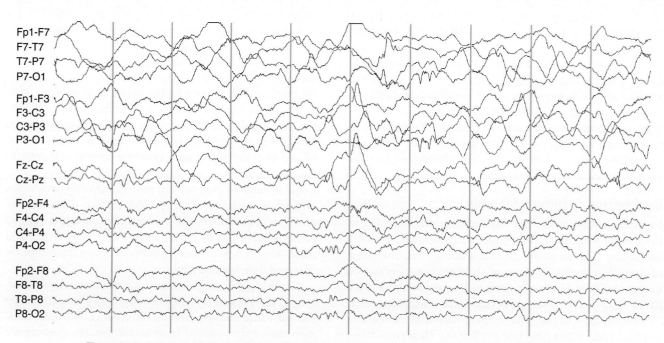

Figure 9.13 A 12-year-old girl recorded during an episode of hemiplegic migraine. Note the high voltage slowing over the left hemisphere (top eight channels) compared with the relatively more normal-appearing activity over the right hemisphere (bottom eight channels).

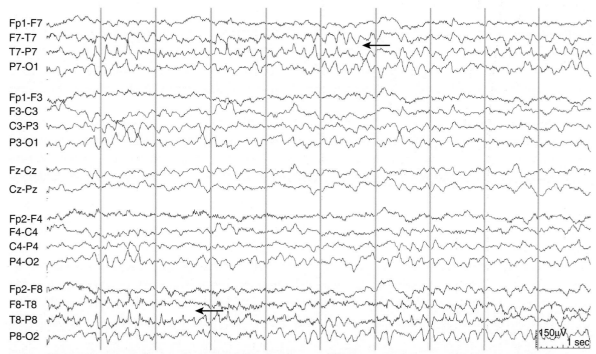

Figure 9.14 Sharp theta waves are seen in each temporal area (arrows). Note the varying degree of sharpness with some waves in the series appearing sharper and others appearing more rounded. This particular example of sharp theta waves may also represent an example of "wicket spikes," a normal variant (see Chapter 11, "Normal Variants in the EEG").

irregular slowing over the left hemisphere during an attack of hemiplegic migraine (a rare type of complicated migraine) in a 12-year-old girl. Confusional migraine, another rare type of complicated migraine that occurs predominantly in children, may cause bilateral slowing in the EEG during the attack. In some cases, migraine with visual aura can cause slowing during an attack, particularly in the posterior quadrants, although in many cases the EEG is not particularly remarkable even during attacks with visual symptoms.

In summary, EEG abnormalities, usually in the form of slowing, can be recorded in some patients during migraine attacks (particularly during complex migraine attacks). Whether certain other abnormalities are characteristic of the EEG between attacks in migraine patients remains an unsettled question. In the current environment of available neuroimaging, EEG does not play a major role in the diagnosis of migraine, which is best made based on clinical criteria.

"Sharp Slow"

At times, a hybrid between sharp waves and delta or theta waves is seen consisting of sharply contoured slow waves. An example of these slow waves with sharpened peaks is shown in Figure 9.14. The informal term for this type of wave is "sharp slow." Whether such sharply-contoured slow waves represent a true epileptiform abnormality or simply a variant of slow waves is unclear; some may be truly epileptiform and some may not. A variety of claims have been made regarding the significance of sharply-contoured slow waves, including their association with vascular abnormalities such as small strokes, although none of these associations has been definitely proven.

Abnormalities of Alpha Activity

Alpha range frequencies make their most dramatic appearance in the EEG in the form of the posterior rhythm. Asymmetries of the posterior rhythm are common, and certain asymmetries are even expected. For instance, the posterior rhythm is usually of higher voltage over the right, nondominant hemisphere (Figure 9.15). It may come as a surprise to learn that complete absence of the posterior rhythm may occur in a minority of otherwise normal individuals. It is also true that the posterior rhythm may be absent in individuals with brain injuries or other abnormalities, but in such cases the EEG usually shows other abnormal features. Therefore, an EEG whose *only* remarkable feature is absence of the posterior rhythm should be considered normal. Asymmetries of the posterior rhythm are discussed in more detail in Chapter 2, "Visual Analysis of the EEG."

In some patients, alpha rhythms take up much of the posterior quadrants of the EEG during wakefulness. This occurs either when the field of the posterior rhythm extends far forward or when the posterior rhythm blends with mu rhythms, a normal variant rhythm seen in the central areas that may also be in the alpha range. Mu rhythms are discussed in more detail in Chapter 11, "Normal Variants in the EEG." The specific entity of "alpha coma" is discussed in Chapter 12, "EEG Patterns in Stupor and Coma."

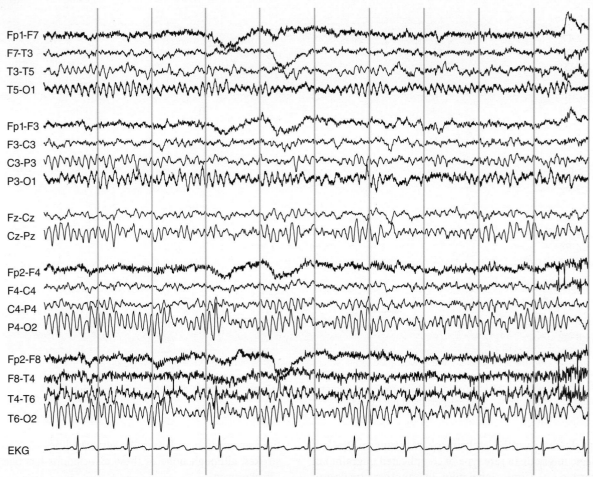

Figure 9.15 This EEG shows the typical asymmetry of the posterior rhythm. Higher voltages are seen in the right occipital area (P4-O2 and T6-O2 channels) compared with the left (T5-O1 and P3-O1 channels).

ABNORMALITIES OF BETA ACTIVITY OR "FAST ACTIVITY"

Excess Fast Activity

Unusually high voltage or plentiful beta activity is the most frequently encountered abnormality of fast activity in the EEG. By far, the most common explanation for excess fast activity in the waking EEG is pharmacologic effect. Benzodiazepines (such as diazepam, lorazepam, clobazam, and clonazepam) and barbiturates (such as phenobarbital and pentobarbital) are the most common causes of increased fast activity in the EEG, although other categories of medication may cause this effect less frequently. Because these two classes of drugs are frequently used in both the acute and chronic management of seizures, it is common to see increased fast activity as a pharmacologic effect in the EEG. Drug-related increases in beta activity are usually diffuse but may also be frontally predominant (Figures 9.16 and 9.17). A transient period of increased beta activity may be seen as a normal finding in many patients at onset of drowsiness and light sleep and usually subsides with deepening Stage II sleep.

Whether excess fast activity in the EEG as a drug effect should be considered an abnormal finding is, to some extent, a question of semantics. According to the definition used in this text—that a finding is abnormal only if it is associated with a pathologic or disease state—excess fast activity caused by drug administration would not represent a true abnormality because simply having received phenobarbital or diazepam should not be considered, in itself, a disease state. (A normal volunteer receiving these medications would manifest an increase in fast activity in the absence of a pathologic state.) If it is the only finding in the EEG, many readers note the presence of increased fast activity in the interpretation without calling the tracing abnormal.

A relatively rare cause of dramatically increased fast activity in the EEG is significant cerebral dysgenesis (e.g., lissencephaly); such abnormalities are associated with significant intellectual disability. In such cases, increased fast activity is not the only abnormality seen and other abnormal features would be noted, including a lack of normal EEG architecture. Often the beta activity seen in such cases is of a slower frequency than is seen in normal individuals.

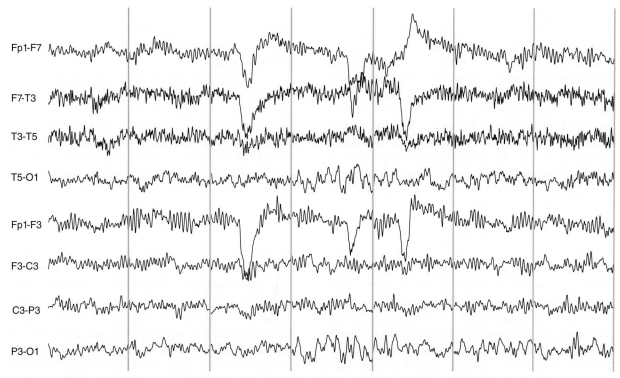

Figure 9.16 A large amount of beta activity is distributed across all channels in a patient on benzodiazepines. Scanning for low-voltage spike activity is made more challenging by the large amount of fast activity.

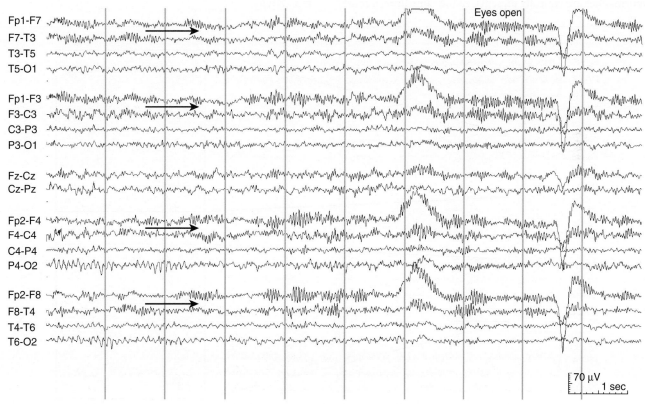

Figure 9.17 The amount of fast activity in this patient has been markedly increased by the administration of lorazepam. In this example, the fast activity is most prominent in the anterior quadrants (arrows).

It is not uncommon to see increased fast activity in an otherwise normal EEG without apparent explanation. This should not become a major problem for the electroencephalographer. Often the submitted medication list is incomplete or perhaps there is a scenario where barbiturates have been administered previously and subsequently discontinued but may not yet have been cleared from the bloodstream. Because the EEG reader is usually not in a position to carry out the detective work of seeing if the patient has taken a medication that was not in the medication list, it is acceptable to simply comment that "increased fast activity is usually a pharmacologic effect" and leave it up to the referring provider as to whether to pursue the matter further.

"Slowed" or Absent Fast Activity

Cortical fast activity recorded during wakefulness is usually within the range of 18 to 30 Hz. A reduction in the frequency of the fast activity may represent an abnormality. "Slow" (or perhaps better, "slowed") fast activity is most commonly encountered in cases of diffuse cortical injury, as may be seen after an anoxic episode. In other cases, a decreased frequency of fast activity may represent the pharmacologic effect of certain sedative or anesthetic medications, such as those used for pharmacologic induction of coma.

A relative absence of fast activity in the EEG may also represent an abnormality. Absent fast activity may be seen in the setting of severe, diffuse cortical injuries (in which case, other abnormalities are typically present). At the same time, it must be appreciated that some patients have less fast activity in the EEG than others, and apparently decreased amounts of fast activity in the waking EEG may represent a normal variant in some individuals.

In assessing the amount of fast activity in an EEG, the reader should not be led astray by the situation of a tracing that has been displayed with low amplifier gains. Tracings with large amounts of high-voltage slow activity are typically displayed with low amplifier gains so that adjacent channels will not collide and cross. At these lower gains, the lower voltage fast activity, although present in normal amounts, may not be visible in the display. This effect is discussed in more detail in Chapter 2, "Visual Analysis of the EEG," and illustrated in Figure 2.24.

Asymmetry of Beta Activity

A true asymmetry in fast activity between brain regions is an important abnormality. Fast waves are believed to be generated at the level of cerebral cortex, reflecting the activity of cortical circuits nearer the scalp surface (rather than activity arising from deeper levels, such as the deep white matter). Thus, asymmetry of fast activity can be an important marker of cortical damage (Figure 9.18). Most often, the region with lower voltage fast activity marks the area of abnormality; in the region of a cortical stroke, it is expected that beta activity will be reduced. Much more rarely, cases are seen in which an area of abnormal cortex is associated with higher voltage fast activity.

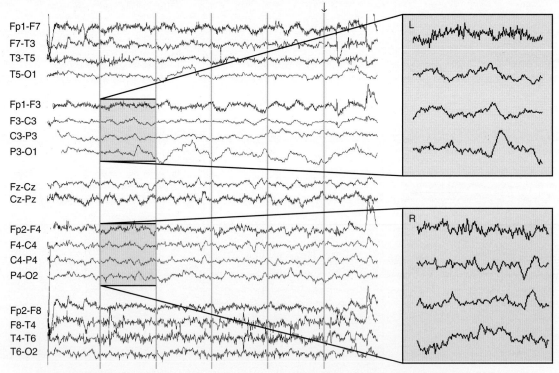

Figure 9.18 The waking EEG of this patient who has suffered a left middle cerebral artery infarct shows decreased fast activity over the area of the stroke. The close-ups emphasize the lower voltage of fast activity over the left parasagittal area compared with the right, especially in the bottom three lines of each as they do not include muscle artifact. This asymmetry of fast activity is relatively subtle and would be easy to miss without a systematic comparison of the left versus the right sides by individual frequency bands.

ASYMMETRIC RHYTHMIC ACTIVITY

In cases in which not just a single frequency range but all frequency bands of electrical activity are depressed in a certain area, the shorthand term *decreased rhythmic activity* can be used to denote a decrease in activity of all frequencies (Figure 9.19). There are many possible causes for decreased rhythmic activity in a particular region, and care should be taken not to suggest a list of possible causes that is too narrow because even noncerebral causes are on the list of possibilities.

When rhythmic activity is decreased over a discrete area, an anatomical injury such as loss of brain parenchyma (e.g., a stroke or encephalomalacia) is an initial consideration. This makes sense because less brain tissue would be expected to generate less in the way of brain waves. However, it is best to consider the various anatomical spaces between the mass of neurons creating brain wave activity and the recording electrode in order to organize a differential diagnosis of such voltage asymmetries. This would include broadly the intraparenchymal space (the brain tissue itself), the extra-axial space (including the space between the brain and the skull: subarachnoid, subdural, and epidural spaces), the skull itself, and the extracranial space (the scalp and the space under the outer periosteum of the skull bone, for example the space where cephalhematomas accumulate). Fluid collections in the subarachnoid, subdural, or epidural spaces, which may consist of blood, pus, cerebrospinal fluid, or proteinaceous fluid collections, may cause an attenuation of recorded voltages. Individuals with large but asymmetrical subgaleal hemorrhages (bleeding into the scalp) or other scalp swelling such as a caput succedaneum (a type of scalp swelling seen in the newborn soon after delivery) or cephalhematoma (a collection of blood under the periosteum of the outer skull bone as mentioned above, seen most commonly in newborns after delivery) may cause dramatic voltage asymmetries even in the absence of cerebral abnormalities. It would be undesirable to make the error of reporting an EEG with a voltage asymmetry in a patient who has been in a car accident as indicating a brain injury in the

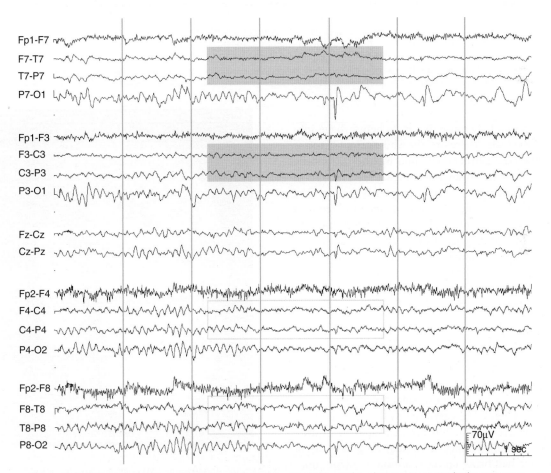

Figure 9.19 This patient, who has experienced a left hemispheric stroke, shows a more marked asymmetry of rhythmic activity (i.e., for waves in multiple frequency ranges) in the highlighted areas. Whereas in the previous figure the asymmetry was mostly restricted to fast frequencies, in this example all frequencies are relatively diminished over the left central and temporal areas (shaded rectangles), giving them a relatively flat appearance. Compare with the right central and temporal areas (unshaded rectangles). It is also wise to confirm such voltage asymmetries in a referential montage. Incidental note is made of left occipital-maximum spike-wave discharges in the last 3 seconds of the page.

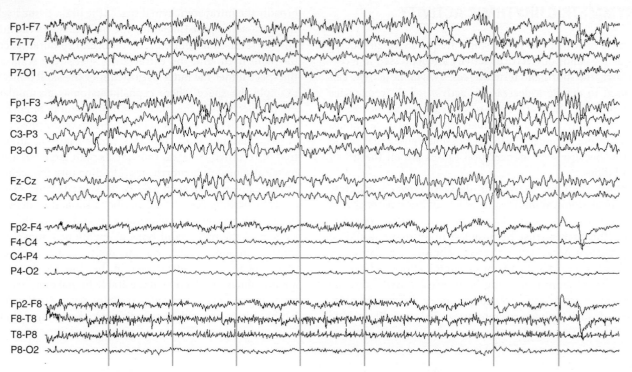

Figure 9.20 The most dramatic examples of voltage asymmetry can be seen in patients who have undergone surgical hemispherectomy. Note that all apparent rhythmic activity over the right hemisphere can either be ascribed to artifact or to projection of voltages from the left hemisphere (e.g., low-voltage alpha frequencies seen in F4-C4 and C4-P4). The patient's magnetic resonance imaging scan is shown in the next figure.

left hemisphere simply because of a large hemorrhage into the left side of the scalp. Therefore, the whole gamut of intra-axial and extra-axial/extracranial abnormalities should be considered in the case of an EEG tracing with a voltage asymmetry that includes multiple frequency bands. The report may include a clinical correlation such as "reduced voltages seen over the left hemisphere could reflect injury to brain tissue in that hemisphere from a variety of causes, or an extra-axial or extra-cranial fluid collection." Figures 9.20 and 9.21 show a dramatic asymmetry of rhythmic activity as an aftereffect of surgical removal of the right hemisphere for refractory epilepsy.

ASYMMETRIES OF SLEEP ELEMENTS

In the case of asymmetric sleep spindles or vertex waves, the magnitude and persistence of the asymmetry are important in deciding whether or not to label the asymmetry as abnormal (Figure 9.22). Mild asymmetries in the amplitude of sleep spindles are occasionally seen and may be of little consequence. Spindle voltage asymmetries greater than one third to one half bring up the question of a true functional brain asymmetry (Figure 9.23). In certain patients, occasional asymmetry of vertex waves is seen and may not be significant; mild or nonpersisting shifts of vertex wave maxima to the left or right may not be clinically important. More persistent or dramatic asymmetries in the appearance of spindles or vertex waves may, however, reflect an

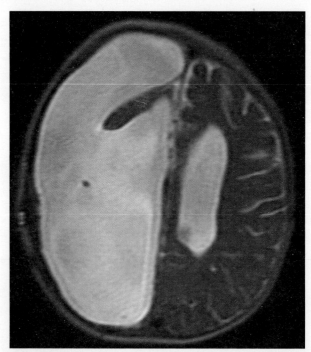

Figure 9.21 The magnetic resonance imaging scan of a patient who has undergone right hemispherectomy for intractable epilepsy is shown. A small tongue of disconnected frontal brain tissue remains. The patient's EEG is shown in the previous figure. Of note, complete removal of a hemisphere for large hemispheric dysplasias (e.g., hemimegalencephaly) as was done previously in this patient has fallen out of favor. Surgical disconnection of the abnormal hemisphere (leaving the hemisphere in place) is now the favored treatment because of its lower complication rate.

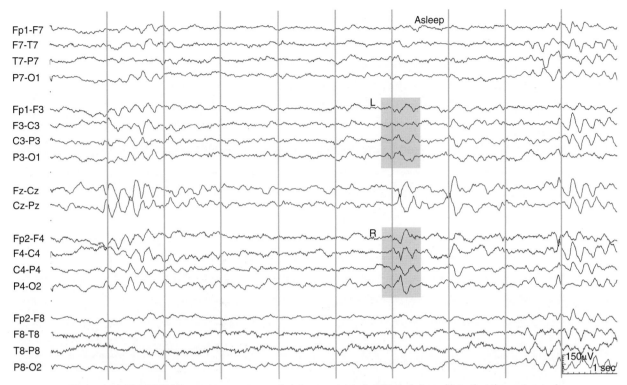

Figure 9.22 This EEG shows an asymmetry of vertex waves during Stage I sleep. Note that the vertex wave is well seen in the midline and in the right central area (shaded area marked "R") but not well seen in the left central area (shaded area marked "L"). Such asymmetries are only considered to be potentially clinically significant if they are persistent.

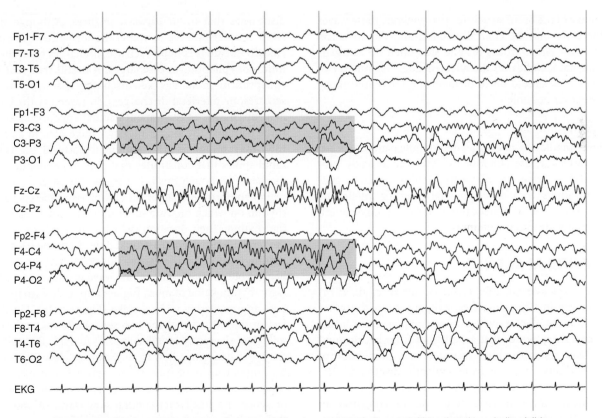

Figure 9.23 Persistent asymmetry of sleep spindles is considered abnormal. Note that the spindle visible in the right central region (lower shaded area) and the midline can barely be seen during this interval in the left central region (upper shaded area). As a further confirmation of the presence of an abnormal asymmetry, note the decreased amount of delta activity in the T3–T5 and T5–O1 channels compared to T4–T6 and T6–O2.

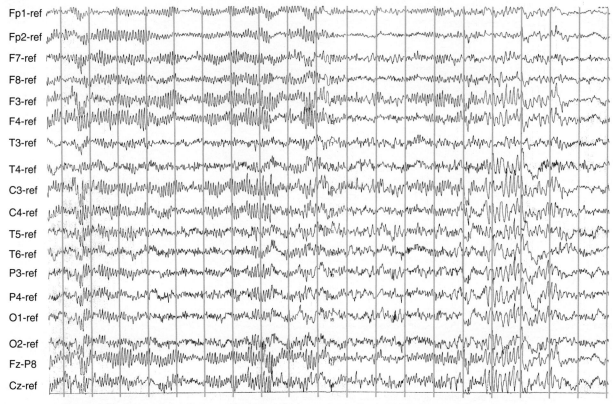

Figure 9.24 An example of extreme spindles is shown in a referential "alternating" montage. Note that spindle voltages are highest in the C3 and C4, F3 and F4, and Fz and Cz electrodes, as expected.

asymmetry of the brain structures that generate these waves and therefore may be clinically significant. For instance, persons with large strokes on one side often do not generate normal spindles on the affected side. Asymmetry of sleep elements should be confirmed in a referential montage whenever possible.

Extreme Spindles

"Extreme spindles" is an exaggerated spindle pattern in sleep and represents a rare abnormality. These abnormally prolonged and persistent spindles have been described in children and adults with developmental delay or intellectual disability (Figure 9.24). Rarely, this abnormal spindle pattern may even intrude into wakefulness.

EPILEPTIFORM ACTIVITY

In the 1974 glossary of EEG terms (Chatrian et al., 1974) and similarly in later glossaries, epileptiform activity has been defined as "distinctive waves or complexes, including spikes and sharp waves that are distinct from background activity and resemble those recorded in a proportion of human subjects suffering from epileptic disorders." The word epileptiform itself suggests that these are waves that appear in the "form" of epilepsy but do not constitute an example of epilepsy (i.e., epileptic seizures) themselves. By definition, epileptiform activity refers to abnormal

discharges that occur *between* seizures. Although it may seem counterintuitive to some, the formal definition specifically excludes epileptic seizure discharges from the definition of epileptiform discharges. It is still true that many epileptiform discharges (i.e., discharges that occur between seizures, or interictal discharges) do resemble the component discharges of the patient's actual epileptic seizures in some patients. The single interictal spike seen in a patient's EEG may resemble the component parts of the train of rapid spikes that constitutes that patient's epileptic seizure discharge, although this is not always the case.

Epileptiform discharges should interrupt the background rhythm on which they are superimposed rather than fit into the rhythm. Their duration (which is to say their width on the screen or wavelength) should differ from the background rhythm from which they arise. This portion of the definition helps avoid the possibility of one wave in a train of a physiologic rhythm being of much higher amplitude than its neighbors and appearing to be a spike (Figure 9.25). Finally, the fact of the existence of the two separate terms, *spike* versus *spike-and-slow-wave complex*, appears to imply that spikes are not associated with a slow wave. However, close inspection of the large majority of epileptiform spikes (as compared with apparent spikes that are actually artifact) will disclose the presence of a small after-coming slow wave, an observation that can help confirm that an apparent spike represents a true epileptiform discharge.

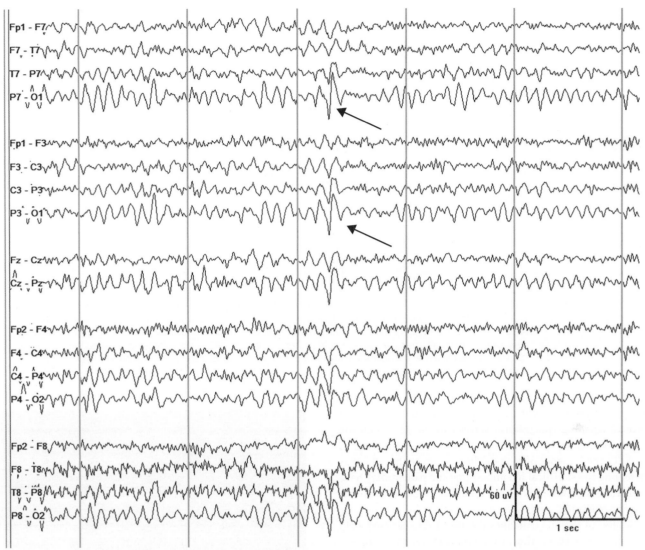

Figure 9.25 A spike-like wave is seen to stand out in the occipital region (arrows), somewhat sharper than its neighbors, and catches the eye. This is not an example of an epileptic spike, however. This higher voltage wave fits into the surrounding rhythm rather than interrupting it. Note that it appears "in rhythm" with the five preceding waves. This is an example of a single wave in the posterior rhythm that happens to be of higher voltage than its neighbors. Remembering that even a mathematically perfect sine wave appears to have sharper peaks and troughs than lower voltage sine waves of the same frequency, the higher amplitude of this individual wave lends to its sharper appearance.

Occasionally, it may be difficult to distinguish interictal activity from electrographic seizure activity (discussed in more detail in Chapter 10, "The EEG in Epilepsy"). The electroencephalographer must always be conscious of the distinction between discharges that take place during the seizure or "ictus," referred to as ictal activity, and activity that takes place between seizures, or interictal activity. It is presumed that ictal discharges (seizures) have more negative consequences to the patient compared to interictal discharges. Whether or not and in what situations interictal discharges can contribute to (rather than be an indicator of) brain dysfunction is a matter of current and lively debate. Antiseizure medications may be necessary and effective in the treatment of ictal events, but those same medications may have little effect on interictal

discharges. In fact, trial infusions of antiseizure medications are occasionally necessary to help distinguish ictal patterns from interictal patterns. The idea here is that antiseizure medications may halt seizure discharges, but are less likely to affect interictal patterns.

The definition of epileptiform activity has been extended by some to include specific types of paroxysmal bursts of slow-wave activity, reasoning that these bursts are an indicator of a decreased seizure threshold in such patients (see the discussions of OIRDA associated with childhood absence and TIRDA earlier in this chapter), even though these bursts do not include sharp forms. Again, this is a question of semantics.

Keeping in mind that approximately 1% of asymptomatic adults and 3% to 4% of asymptomatic children will have

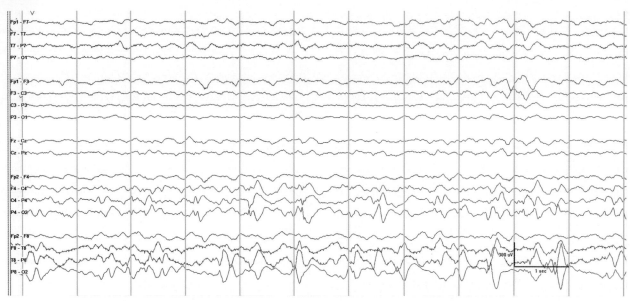

Figure 9.26 The waking EEG with eyes open of a 16-year-old boy after surgical resection of a large right posterior quadrant tumor during early childhood, subsequently treated with radiation. Frequent independent sharp waves are seen independently in P4 and T8 that occur against the backdrop of background slowing over the right hemisphere, especially over the involved right posterior quadrant. The lower voltage slow waves in the delta and theta range seen over the opposite (left) hemisphere are also abnormal in an awake teenager. The patient's MRI scan is shown in the next figure.

epileptiform activity in the EEG, it is important to avoid the error of equating epileptiform activity in the EEG with the diagnosis of epilepsy. Unless an actual seizure is observed in the EEG, the presence of such discharges can be thought of as increasing the statistical likelihood that the patient may have seizures, but certainly does not establish a diagnosis of epilepsy by itself.

Several of the abnormalities discussed thus far may help localize a brain lesion. These would include areas of decreased fast activity (often associated with more superficial, cortical lesions), decreased rhythmic activity (lesions with multiple levels of tissue loss), increased slow wave activity (classically deep white matter lesions), and focal epileptiform activity. The EEG in Figure 9.26 is markedly abnormal and shows abnormalities concentrated in the right posterior quadrant associated with the brain abnormalities show in Figure 9.27.

Electrographic Versus Electroclinical Seizures

By definition, a seizure is an event during which a clinical change in the patient is accompanied by a characteristic abnormal change in brain waves. The clinical change may either be outwardly observable by those surrounding the patient or the change may be experienced subjectively by the patient. The outward clinical change may be as dramatically obvious as generalized tonic-clonic seizure activity, or more subtle such as a mild slumping of the shoulders, slowed responsiveness, or a pause in an ongoing activity. Internally experienced seizure manifestations, such as olfactory hallucinations or the psychic experience of fear, may be invisible to outside observers. Because most of a patient's seizure events are unlikely to occur while they happen to be recording on

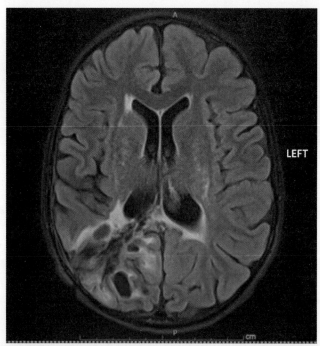

Figure 9.27 MRI scan (FLAIR sequence) of the patient whose EEG was shown in the previous figure. There is a dramatic abnormality in the right posterior quadrant that includes gliosis (scarring) and encephalomalacia (tissue loss). Mild generalized volume loss is also noted.

EEG, the brain wave portion of the definition implies a presumed change in the EEG at the time of the clinical event had the patient been recorded by an appropriate technique at the time.

The question may arise as to how to classify an apparent EEG seizure discharge that is not accompanied by a known clinical change in the patient. When a clear EEG seizure discharge is seen in the record but there is no outwardly observable clinical change in the patient, the term *electrographic seizure* is used. To distinguish these electrographic seizures from seizures with a clinical component, the term *electroclinical seizure* can be used to denote a seizure that is both seen on EEG and a clinical change has been observed in or reported by the patient. Imagine a patient who has 10 similar seizure discharges recorded in the EEG. Five are recorded during wakefulness and are associated with behavioral arrest (therefore representing clear electroclinical seizures), and the other five are identical discharges recorded during sleep, a state during which behavioral arrest cannot be observed. The electroencephalographer may then correctly report that five electroclinical seizures and five electrographic seizures were recorded during the study, keeping in mind the distinctions between the two terms as described below.

Whether a seizure is truly "electrographic" as opposed to "electroclinical" can sometimes resemble a philosophical question. How does one deal with the electrographic seizure discharge during sleep as described in the preceding paragraph or in a child too young to describe experience? One might argue that if you awakened the sleeping patient immediately during the seizure discharge for quick testing you might detect decreased responsiveness as compared to waking the patient up at other times when a seizure discharge was not in progress in the EEG. Similarly, what can one say about one electrical seizure discharge that was previously seen to interrupt an ongoing activity, but another seizure discharge that occurs while the patient is not in the midst of an activity during which behavioral arrest could potentially be observed. In such a case, had the patient been speaking or carrying out an activity, perhaps a behavioral arrest or slowed response time would have been observed. Finally, how should one classify a seizure that would otherwise have produced a clinical convulsion if not for administered pharmacologic paralytic agents in the ICU? Often such questions regarding individual events may not be answerable and the convention is to label any seizure discharge as an electrographic seizure if no behavioral or experiential change can be ascertained. If appropriate, the limitations of the specific situation can be discussed in the report.

In some patients, it can be difficult or even impossible to determine whether a run of discharges represents an interictal discharge or an electrographic seizure discharge. This is a particular problem in patients with slow

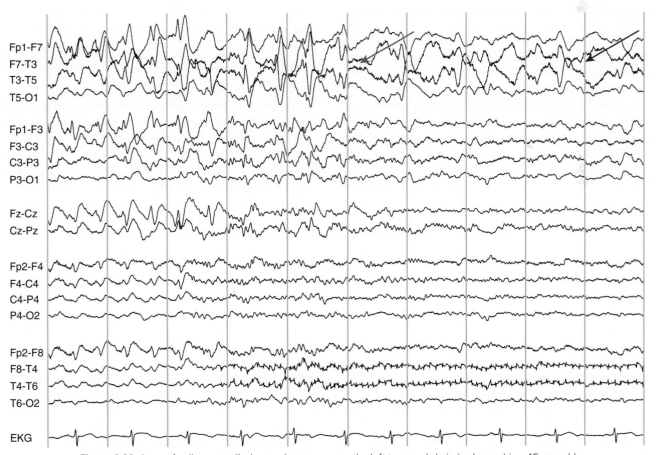

Figure 9.28 A run of spike-wave discharges is seen across the left temporal chain (red arrow) in a 15-year-old girl with focal seizures with impaired awareness. The sharp slow waves seen at the end of the page (gray arrow) suggest a hybrid between slow waves and sharp waves, sharing the characteristics of both.

spike-wave discharges in which the interictal (slow spike-wave complexes without clinical change) and electroclinical discharges (slow spike-wave complexes associated with an atypical absence seizure) can look quite similar. At least in the critical care setting, guidelines have been proposed (see discussion of the Salzburg criteria and the ACNS 2021 guidelines in Chapter 12, "EEG Patterns in Stupor and Coma") to aid in making the distinction between ictal and interictal activity.

Limitations to the Localization Value of Interictal Epileptiform Activity

Descriptions and definitions of epileptiform spikes, sharp waves, and spike-wave discharges are given in Chapter 3, "Introduction to Commonly Used Terms in Electroencephalography." Because the large majority of epileptic patients do not happen to experience an actual epileptic seizure during routine recording in the EEG laboratory, it is the interictal epileptiform discharges that are the main tool in further defining an individual's specific epilepsy diagnosis in most cases (Figure 9.28).

Interictal discharges can be valuable in localizing the epileptogenic zone in epileptic patients, but there are instances where their localization value may be limited. Certain cerebral regions are particularly difficult to localize using scalp recordings. Some types of discharge may even be "falsely localizing," implying a scalp localization that is actually different from the true cerebral source. This is especially true of discharges that arise from areas of cortex that are not adjacent to the scalp, such as the interhemispheric fissure, orbital surfaces, the mesial temporal lobe, the basal surfaces of the occipital and frontal lobes, and insular cortex.

To give just one curious example of this phenomenon, consider a discharge that might arise from an epileptic focus deep in the interhemispheric fissure on the mesial surface of the *left* frontal lobe near the foot area of the motor strip (Figure 9.29). Recall that the motor strip begins on the lateral convexity of the brain just above the Sylvian fissure with representations for the larynx and face, and moving up the central sulcus toward the vertex, the hand and hip are represented. Continuing over the crest of the frontal lobe into the interhemispheric fissure, the leg and foot areas are represented deeper on the mesial surface of the frontal lobe (as it gets closer to the cingulate gyrus and the corpus callosum). Considering a discharge from the left frontal lobe foot area (which is closest to the overlying C3 electrode), by the time the dipole of this discharge reaches the recording scalp electrodes, because of its orientation it may be picked up better by the contralateral scalp electrode, C4 rather than C3 (right central electrode rather than the left central electrode)! For this reason, it can be difficult to localize/lateralize discharges in the interhemispheric fissure based on scalp recordings alone with confidence.

A second potential problem is that the location of an epileptiform discharge, even if well ascertained, may not always indicate the seizure onset zone. Interictal discharges often arise from the seizure focus, but this is not true 100% of the time. Keep in mind that some individuals with interictal

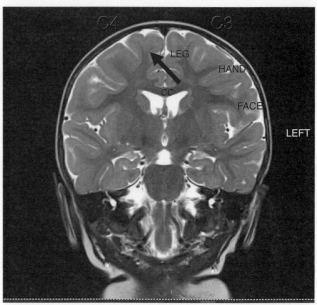

Figure 9.29 The red arrow in this figure depicts a spike focus arising from the mesial surface of the left hemisphere where the leg motor area is usually located. Note the labeled locations of the "FACE," "HAND," and "LEG" areas of the motor strip as well as the locations of the C4 (right central) and C3 (left central) scalp electrodes. The spike in question originates from the tail of the red arrow (left mesial frontal lobe surface which is on the right side of the image) and projects toward the scalp in the direction of the arrowhead. While it may initially seem counterintuitive, spikes arising from this left-sided location may be better detected by the contralateral right central scalp electrode. Of course, a spike that has a maximum amplitude in C4 may, indeed, arise from the right hemisphere from the area directly under the right central electrode. Alternatively, this could represent a false localization, as the dipole of such interhemispheric foci may be better detected by the electrode opposite to the side of the spike's origin.

discharges may never have a seizure, which implies that at least some interictal discharges never give rise to seizure activity (and therefore could not possibly localize a seizure focus). Conversely, there are some patients with seizures who never have interictal discharges. Acknowledging these two situations, if it is possible for an area of the brain to generate interictal discharges but never originate a seizure and another area may generate seizures but be interictally quiet, it is easy to imagine a circumstance in which an interictal discharge could occasionally "point to the wrong place" in some patients with seizures. Continuing on this line of thought, some individuals may have two separate foci of epileptiform activity, although seizures may only arise from one of those regions. In such a patient, the location of one of the discharges could then be thought of as indicating an incorrect localization of the seizure focus. It is not hard to imagine how this could happen. Imagine a person who has experienced a patchy injury to the brain, perhaps from trauma or infection. Two areas are damaged, one in such a way that it generates abnormal epileptiform discharges but, by chance, does not generate actual seizures. The second area is damaged in such a way that it generates both epileptiform activity and seizures. In such a patient, only one of the spike localizations is pertinent to the correct localization of the seizure onset zone. Therefore, a spike localization often, but not always, corresponds to the area of seizure onset. Other factors such as the history, imaging results, and seizure semiology should be used to confirm localization. These examples remind us to inject a level of humility regarding the level of confidence we have when reporting the localization of seizure foci based on interictal EEG findings.

A secondary use for localizing epileptiform activity, apart from locating seizure-onset zones, is to localize different types of lesions in the brain. In the past, electroencephalography was among the most useful tools for localizing brain tumors, but modern neuroimaging has supplanted electroencephalography as a primary tumor localization tool. Still, despite the primacy of MRI in imaging tumors, epileptiform activity in the EEG may sometimes give the first clue to the presence of a tumor, as occurred in the patient discussed in the paragraph that follows on secondary bilateral synchrony.

Secondary Bilateral Synchrony

Secondary bilateral synchrony refers to the phenomenon of generalized discharges arising from a unilateral/focal cortical lesion. Typically we think of focal discharges in the EEG as associated with focal lesions and generalized discharges as associated with generalized processes or generalized epilepsies. Apparent generalized discharges in the EEG are not always associated with truly generalized seizure onsets, however. Occasionally, a unilateral focal lesion can originate a discharge that spreads rapidly and synchronously across both hemispheres. Such discharges, although arising from a single focus, may spread throughout the brain so rapidly that they are virtually indistinguishable from a primary generalized discharge. Figure 9.30 shows an example of an apparent generalized spike-wave discharge. Figures 9.31 through 9.33 are taken from other pages of the same patient's EEG and give clues to the phenomenon of secondary bilateral synchrony. The patient's causative lesion is shown in Figure 9.34.

Because of this phenomenon, it is good practice to consider the possibility that *any* generalized discharge might possibly be an example of secondary bilateral synchrony and to look for clues to the latter. One such clue is voltage asymmetry of the discharge—the discharge may be of persistently higher voltage over one hemisphere as compared with the other. An even more compelling finding is a consistent "lead-in" of the discharge from one hemisphere, the hallmark finding of secondary bilateral synchrony. In these cases, the discharge is seen to originate from one hemisphere followed by rapid generalization. Indeed, if this patient had had a relatively shorter EEG recording period and only the discharges in the first three of the four figures had been observed, there would have been little cause to suspect that these apparently generalized discharges were caused by a focal lesion.

There is a flip side to the process of examining all generalized discharges for a "lead-in." Because close analysis of even genuine generalized discharges may disclose an apparent onset that starts briefly ahead on one side compared to the other (which is to say that even true generalized discharges are often not *absolutely* synchronous), the most compelling "lead-ins" are those of 2 seconds or more duration that always occur persistently on the same side. In some patients, it is not uncommon for true generalized discharges to alternate the apparent side of onset with brief "lead-ins" seen in one hemisphere and then the other. When the side of the lead-in alternates, this makes the chance that the generalized appearance of the discharge is due to secondary bilateral synchrony much less likely.

The criteria for a definite diagnosis of secondary bilateral synchrony are fairly strict and include a definite "lead-in" of the discharge from one side, a possible voltage asymmetry, or possible focal interictal epileptiform activity seen at other times in the record arising from the same side as the lead-in. The threshold for questioning that a generalized discharge is truly generalized (i.e., suspecting the diagnosis of secondary bilateral synchrony) is considerably lower. At times, focal lesions may cause discharges to generalize so rapidly

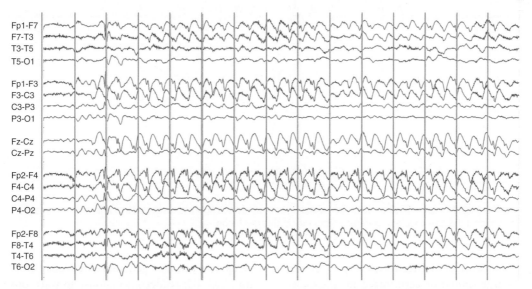

Figure 9.30 An apparent generalized, frontal-predominant spike-wave discharge is seen with no definite indicators to the contrary; no significant asymmetries or "lead-in" is seen. In fact, the discharge shown in this figure was triggered by a tumor in the right temporal lobe. The following figures show additional pages taken from the same EEG that do have clearer clues as to the discharge's focal onset.

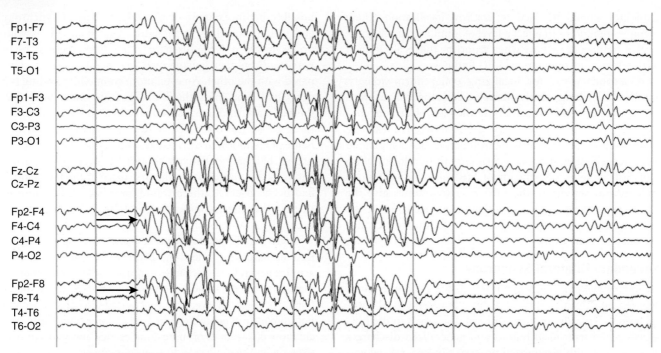

Figure 9.31 During this burst taken from a different page of the same EEG shown in the previous figure, higher spike-wave voltages are seen on the right side (arrows) compared with the left. There is also a probable "lead-in" in the right frontal area (arrows). Although slight voltage asymmetries may occur in truly generalized discharges, the presence of a voltage asymmetry should bring up the question of secondary bilateral synchrony.

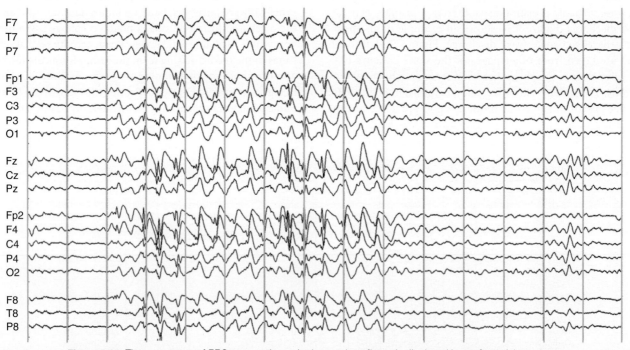

Figure 9.32 The same page of EEG as was shown in the previous figure is displayed in a referential montage, confirming the presence of a voltage asymmetry in this discharge.

that a lead-in is not identifiable. Therefore, every apparently generalized discharge should be scrutinized for the possibility that it has a hidden focal onset, even if not meeting strict criteria for secondary bilateral synchrony. When other signs of a primary generalized epilepsy are not present in the EEG, the reader may choose to warn of the possibility of a focal onset, even when generalized spike-wave or other generalized discharges are seen. This would be particularly

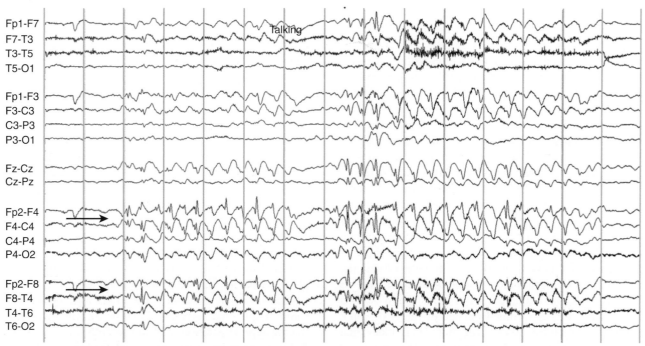

Figure 9.33 Another page of EEG is taken from the same tracing as shown in the previous three figures. This example of the patient's generalized spike-wave discharge now shows a clear and prolonged lead-in from the right hemisphere (arrows). An asymmetrical lead-in, especially if of longer duration, is one of the most convincing clues to the presence of secondary bilateral synchrony.

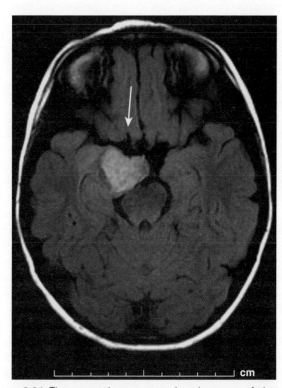

Figure 9.34 The magnetic resonance imaging scan of the child whose EEG is depicted in the previous four figures demonstrates the causative lesion. A glioma enlarging the tip of the right temporal pole (arrow) is seen on this fluid-attenuated inversion recovery (FLAIR) image. This unilateral lesion was responsible for generating a discharge that, at times, was indistinguishable from generalized spike wave.

true if an apparently generalized discharge was also associated with, for example, a spike focus or focal slowing in the EEG. If appropriate, the clinical correlation paragraph can include wording to the effect that "the generalized discharges present in this EEG are potentially consistent with a primary generalized epilepsy, although the possibility of a focal onset with rapid secondary generalization cannot be completely excluded."

PERIODIC PATTERNS

The term *periodic pattern* refers to the presence of a periodic waveform in the EEG. It is to be distinguished from abnormal *rhythmic* waveforms. The term *periodic* implies repetitive recurrence of the waveform with an approximately fixed interval between the waveforms. Moreover, to be called a *periodic pattern*, some amount of the background EEG activity should be seen between each waveform. This should be compared with rhythmic patterns, a term that implies a more fixed, shorter, and regular interval with no intervening background activity between waveforms. Sinusoidal waves or runs of rhythmic spike-wave complexes are examples of rhythmic activity that are easy to envision—no background activity intervenes between each waveform. (Note that *periodic patterns* may occur with a particular rhythm, and therefore rhythmically, but the criterion of intervening background activity between waves is the best way to distinguish them from abnormal rhythmic activity according to this definition.)

Since the publication of the first edition of this text, a new set of terms has been proposed for use in the interpretation and description of critical care EEG: American Clinical Neurophysiology Society's *Standardized Critical Care EEG Terminology*: 2021 version. This new terminology was specifically created for use with EEG tracings recorded in the ICU. Although much of this revision of critical care terminology is likely to become widely accepted, the new classification replaces some time-honored EEG terms, such as *PLEDs*, which will almost certainly remain in common use alongside the newer terms, and are included below. An additional consideration is that some of these periodic patterns may be observed outside of the critical care setting. Because this new proposed EEG terminology was specifically designed for critical care recordings, one might reasonably suppose that it does not necessarily apply to patterns recorded outside the ICU. On the other hand, the idea that one set of terminology would be used for patterns seen in the ICU but a different set of terms would be used for identical patterns recorded outside of the ICU would be unreasonably burdensome. Therefore, it is likely that many of the elements of the new terminology proposed for critical care EEG will eventually migrate into descriptions for all EEGs. The bulk of the 2021 ACNS terminology is described in Chapter 12, "EEG Patterns in Stupor and Coma." Because periodic patterns are also observed in outpatients, some of these concepts will be introduced here.

A particularly useful and simple classification system for periodic EEG patterns was described by Brenner and Schaul (1990) and will almost certainly be supplanted by the new system. The older system is described here because the two different classification systems were designed with different goals in mind. The new 2021 system strives for uniformity in the terms used to describe different EEG patterns so that two different laboratories far apart might classify the same pattern or waveform the same way. Thus, excellent interrater reliability is one of the main goals of the ACNS terminology, which should allow research studies on different EEG patterns to be more easily compared between centers. The older system, which is retained in this edition because it may still be conceptually useful to readers, looked to simplicity but also strived to associate different types of periodic patterns with different diagnoses, which was not a primary goal of the newer ACNS classification. Thus, unlike the ACNS terminology, the goal of this classification is to create groupings of periodic patterns according to their specific attributes and associate them with the different diagnostic groups that may have caused the patterns.

In the older system (described below), a periodic pattern is classified according to whether it occurs over a single hemisphere or both hemispheres (unilateral vs. bilateral), whether it occurs over both hemispheres in a synchronous or asynchronous (bilaterally independent) fashion, and whether the intervals between waves are less than or greater than 4 seconds (short interval vs. long interval). In practice, combinations of these three parameters result in four categories of patterns: (1) periodic lateralized epileptiform discharges (PLEDs), (2) bilateral periodic lateralized epileptiform discharges (BiPLEDs), (3) periodic short interval diffuse discharges (PSIDDs), and (4) periodic long interval diffuse discharges (PLIDDs) (See Tables 9.1 and 9.2.)

PLEDs or LPDs (ACNS 2021)

Of the periodic patterns, the best known is PLEDs (Figure 9.35). Of the four letters in this abbreviation, the "L" for lateralized is the most useful to keep in mind. The word lateralized is used in place of the word focal, reflecting the fact that, rather than being confined to a small focal area, the field of a PLED typically spreads across a whole hemisphere. If an apparent periodic discharge is focal rather than lateralized, the diagnosis of PLEDs should be questioned.

PLED waveforms, apart from being lateralized to a single hemisphere, may be simple, complex, or polymorphic. Typically, though not always, the PLED waveform contains sharp or spike-like features. PLEDs occur repetitively in the tracing approximately every 1 to 4 seconds. In general, when PLEDs are present, they are present for the entirety of the tracing; they do not tend to appear and disappear within a single recording. If a periodic waveform is seen only intermittently, the diagnosis of PLEDs should be questioned.

Etiologies associated with PLEDs include a list of acute and subacute processes with stroke, infection, and tumor at the top of the list. Classically, the finding of PLEDs has a particularly well-known association with herpes simplex virus (HSV) encephalitis (although the finding is not pathognomonic). In HSV encephalitis, PLEDs may either be unilateral or bilateral but independent (BiPLEDs, discussed in the next subsection).

Occasionally, the distinction between PLEDs and seizure activity can be difficult. For instance, when PLEDs are associated with contralateral jerking movements of the body, the diagnosis of epilepsia partialis continua (EPC) is suggested. Unless there is such a contralateral motor response in association with the discharges, the electrical patterns associated with EPC can be indistinguishable from PLEDs. In general, however, PLEDs are not considered to represent an electrographic seizure discharge but rather an interictal pattern. This is borne out by the fact that PLEDs are usually resistant to treatment with antiseizure medications. Rare exceptions to this concept are seen in the form of confusional states associated with PLEDs that have cleared with the administration of antiseizure medications.

PLEDs may be seen less commonly after a prolonged seizure discharge, so-called *postictal PLEDs*. After the clinical seizure has ceased, periodic afterdischarges identical to PLEDs may be seen over a single hemisphere, eventually burning out with time. Except in unusual cases, PLEDs are a temporary phenomenon and do clear with the passage of time. PLEDS in an ICU recording would be classified as LPDs (lateralized periodic discharges) in the 2021 ACNS system.

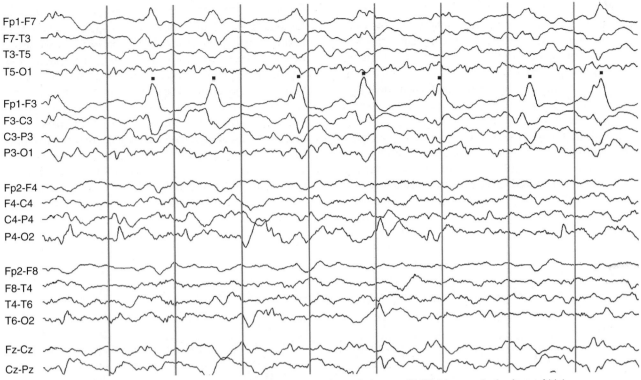

Figure 9.35 An example of periodic lateralized epileptiform discharges (PLEDs) is seen in the form of high-voltage, repetitive complexes over the left side (dots). The discharges have a fairly broad, hemispheric field. At times, the waveform seems sharp and at other times it appears more rounded. This duality is characteristic of PLEDs, which may or may not manifest obviously sharp features.

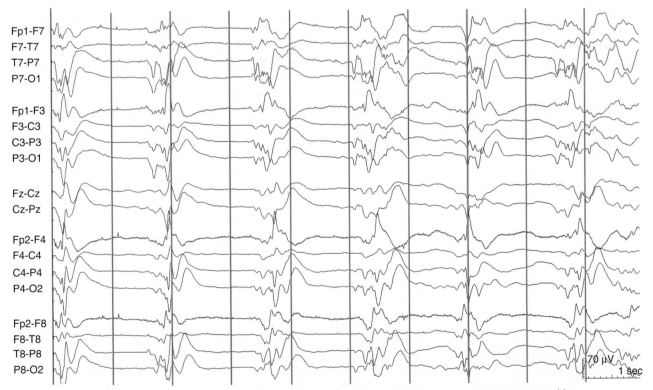

Figure 9.36 Periodic short-interval diffuse discharges (PSIDDs or GPDs) are characterized by a repetitive discharge that occurs synchronously over both hemispheres with a relatively short interdischarge interval (approximately 1.5 seconds in this example). In this patient, the diffuse discharges have a complex but similar morphology.

BiPLEDs or BIPDs (ACNS 2021)

PLEDs that occur over both hemispheres in the same record but in an asynchronous or independent fashion are termed bilateral periodic lateralized epileptiform discharges (BiPLEDs). The possible causes of BiPLEDs is similar to the causes of PLEDs but favor those processes that are more likely to be bilateral. Therefore, a tumor or a discrete, focal stroke, both of which tend to be unilateral processes, are not common causes of BiPLEDs, but anoxic encephalopathy (the equivalent of bilateral, diffuse strokes) is a more common cause. As mentioned earlier, BiPLEDs are particularly characteristic of HSV encephalitis which is usually a bilateral process. BiPLEDS would be classified as BIPDs (bilateral independent periodic discharges) according to the 2021 ACNS system.

PSIDDs or GPDs (ACNS 2021)

Periodic short interval diffuse discharges (PSIDDs) are periodically occurring waveforms that may consist of sharp waves, spikes, spike-wave discharges, or triphasic waves. As the name implies, the field is spread diffusely over the brain and the interdischarge interval is 4 seconds or less (Figure 9.36). The most common clinical association of PSIDDs is anoxic encephalopathy. Each discharge may or may not be associated with a body jerk (myoclonus). In general, the presence of PSIDDs in anoxic encephalopathy suggests a poor neurologic prognosis. PSIDDs may also occur as a seizure phenomenon (see the section on nonconvulsive status epilepticus later in the chapter). PSIDDs are classified as GPDs according to the 2021 ACNS system.

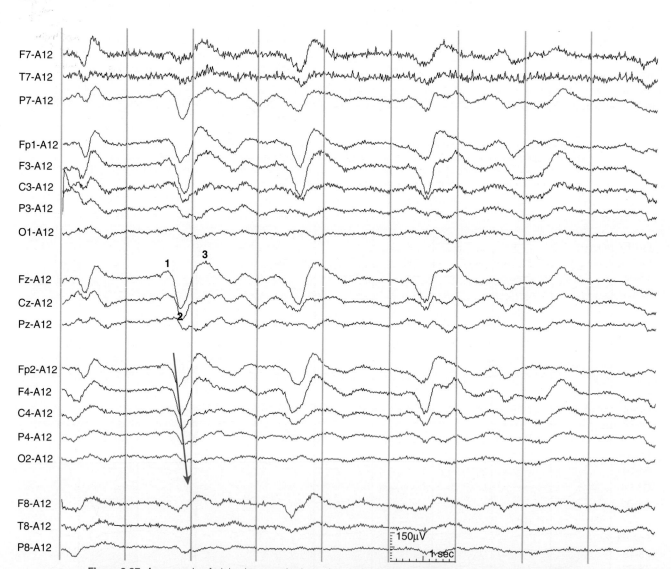

Figure 9.37 An example of triphasic waves is shown in a patient with hepatic failure. The waves are displayed in a referential montage using a reference that consists of the average of both earlobes, A1 and A2. The three separate phases of the triphasic waves ("up-down-up") are labeled "1," "2," and "3," respectively. The characteristic time shift often seen with triphasic waves is highlighted by the red arrow. Note that the trough of the wave begins earlier in the frontal area and is delayed by several milliseconds in each successively more posterior channel. Although a classic feature of triphasic waves, this back-to-front delay is not seen in all cases of triphasic waves.

Triphasic Waves

Triphasic waves may be considered a subset of PSIDDs. Triphasic waves are medium- to high-voltage complexes with a characteristic triphasic pattern, often with a sequence of negative–positive–negative deflections, repeating at rate of 1.5 to 2.5 Hz (Figure 9.37). The first phase of the deflection has been said to resemble a blunted spike and the whole complex may resemble a blunted spike-wave discharge, although usually the initial deflection is too rounded for the complex to be considered a true spike-wave discharge. Triphasic waves usually occur diffusely and symmetrically, often with a frontal predominance. The most frequent and best known clinical association is with hepatic encephalopathy or hepatic coma, but other metabolic derangements (such as renal failure) may also be associated with triphasic waves. In fact, a wider range of causes of encephalopathy, even including certain structural abnormalities, may also be associated with triphasic waves so the finding is not necessarily pathognomonic for metabolic encephalopathy. Triphasic waves may also show the unusual manifestation of an anterior-to-posterior time lag in which the wave is seen frontally up to 200 ms before it is seen posteriorly.

Extreme Delta Brushes

Extreme delta brushes (EDBs) is a distinctive EEG pattern that was first described relatively recently in patients with anti-NMDA receptor encephalitis, an autoimmune encephalitis. Since then, it has also been recognized in Febrile infection-related epilepsy syndrome (FIRES). The term *delta brush* has been borrowed from the characteristic beta-delta complex that is seen in premature babies and which it resembles, but to which it may have no physiologic relationship whatsoever (Figure 9.38). Anti-NMDA receptor encephalitis affects younger patients, including children, and is seen more commonly in women than men. A tumor triggers the causative autoimmune response in some patients and must be excluded, with ovarian teratoma being the most common type. Patients with this autoimmune encephalitis typically have cognitive and behavioral deterioration in addition to sleep abnormalities. There is often a movement disorder that includes both abnormal orofacial and limb movements. Even with prompt treatment, recovery can be slow and incomplete. In FIRES, the patient (the large majority being children) develops refractory status epilepticus without other clear cause 1 day to 2 weeks following a fever. The status epilepticus is highly refractory and may last days. Many therapies in addition to antiseizure medications for the status epilepticus have been tried, including immunotherapy and the ketogenic diet, though the best therapy has yet to be established. Survivors of the acute phase of refractory status epilepticus may enter a chronic phase of sporadic seizures, usually without regaining their baseline level of function. EDBs have been reported in both disorders.

Nonconvulsive Status Epilepticus

Generalized nonconvulsive status epilepticus (NCSE) may also technically fulfill the criteria for PSIDDs or GPDs in that this pattern may consist of repetitive, diffuse sharp discharges (Figure 9.39). Both the EEG appearance and the clinical context may aid in distinguishing between NCSE and other causes of PSIDDs/GPDs, although at times the distinction is difficult. Because NCSE is an epileptic seizure pattern, its presence requires a different treatment approach aimed at terminating the seizure activity, usually with aggressive use of antiseizure medications.

Creutzfeldt-Jakob Disease

Creutzfeldt-Jakob disease (CJD) is a rare disorder that consists of a progressive dementia characteristically associated with repetitive myoclonus. The disease may be transmitted by unique infectious particles called *prions*. CJD is often associated with the finding of PSIDDs in the form of sharp wave complexes, often with triphasic morphology (Figure 9.40). The myoclonus typically associated with this disease may occur synchronously with the PSIDDs. The findings of PSIDDs and myoclonus alone cannot establish the diagnosis of CJD. Rather, the distinctive clinical picture of CJD should be considered supported by finding this characteristic pattern in the EEG.

PLIDDs or GPDs (ACNS 2021)

Periodic long-interval diffuse discharges, or PLIDDs, refer to repetitive waveforms that are separated by intervals of four to 20 seconds' duration. PLIDDs are the hallmark finding of subacute sclerosing panencephalitis (SSPE), a very rare disorder related to a slow measles infection of the central nervous system. Measles immunization has almost completely wiped out this disease in many parts of the world, although a low rate of SSPE persists even in the immunized population; a possible relationship between the slow virus infection and the vaccine is unclear. This fatal disorder begins with mental status changes and behavioral deterioration followed by dementia and myoclonic seizures that correlate with the periodic discharges. Over weeks or months, the disorder inexorably progresses to a vegetative state and death. The presence of such discharges in the appropriate clinical context is considered highly characteristic of SSPE. PLIDDs would also be classified as GPDs under the 2021 ACNS system, which does not distinguish between GPDs with short and long intervals.

Burst suppression patterns related to anoxia or drugs (including pharmacologic agents used in the intensive care unit) may fall into the category of either PSIDDs or PLIDDs (Figure 9.41) because the interval between bursts in burst suppression may be both less than or greater than 4 seconds in duration. Burst suppression patterns are discussed in more detail in Chapter 12, "EEG Patterns in Stupor and Coma."

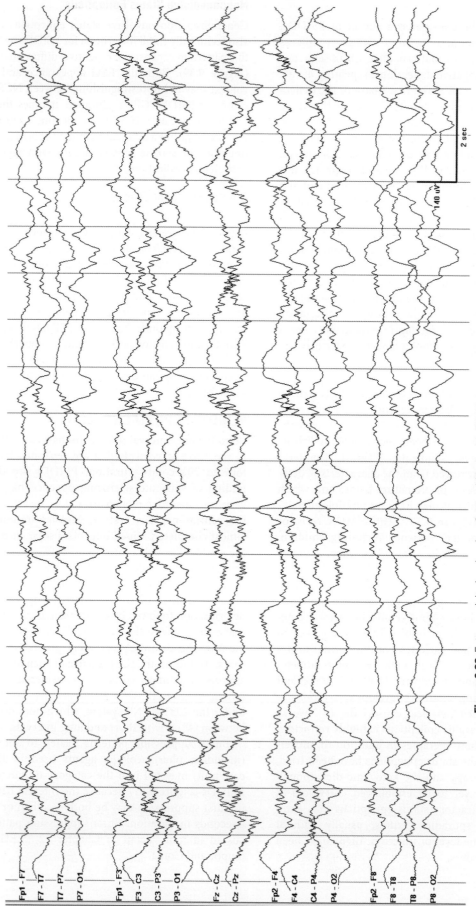

Figure 9.38 Extreme delta brushes in a 6-year-old boy with FIRES. The patient had no previous past medical history and presented in super-refractory status epilepticus after a 6-day course of headache and fever. Note the superimposition of fast activity on the delta waves that resemble the delta brushes seen in premature infants.

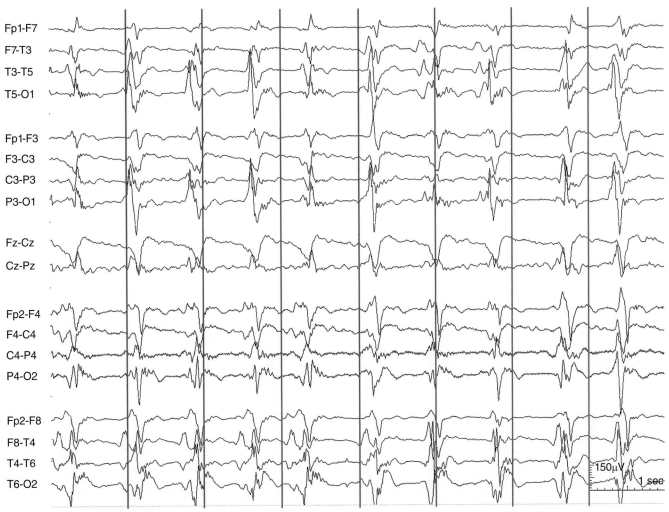

Figure 9.39 During the episode of nonconvulsive status epilepticus shown in this figure, this 19-month-old girl was motionless and unresponsive. This seizure pattern was eventually terminated with anticonvulsant medications.

TABLE 9.1   Periodic Patterns Seen in Both the Inpatient and Outpatient Setting

	Short Interval (0.5–4 sec)	Long Interval (4–30 sec)
Unilateral	Periodic lateralized epileptiform discharges (PLEDs)	—
Bilateral asynchronous	Bilateral periodic lateralized epileptiform discharges (BiPLEDs)	—
Bilateral synchronous	Periodic short-interval diffuse discharges (PSIDDs)	Periodic long-interval diffuse discharges (PLIDDs)

ABNORMAL SLEEP STRUCTURE

Abnormalities of sleep structure fall into a variety of categories, including sleep disorders that are beyond the scope of this text. Abnormal sleep structure, including the absence of normal sleep elements or the abnormal ordering of sleep staging, may be the result of an abnormal central nervous system, a disease process, or a pharmacologic effect. For instance, instead of proceeding in an orderly fashion through the stages of slow wave sleep when falling asleep, patients with narcolepsy may manifest very short sleep latency and immediate transition to REM sleep at sleep-onset (sleep-onset REM). This phenomenon is best demonstrated on a multiple sleep latency test (MSLT), a sleep study that is specifically designed to detect it.

Occasionally, patients are seen who lack the expected synchrony seen in normally occurring sleep elements. This type of abnormality has been associated with agenesis of the

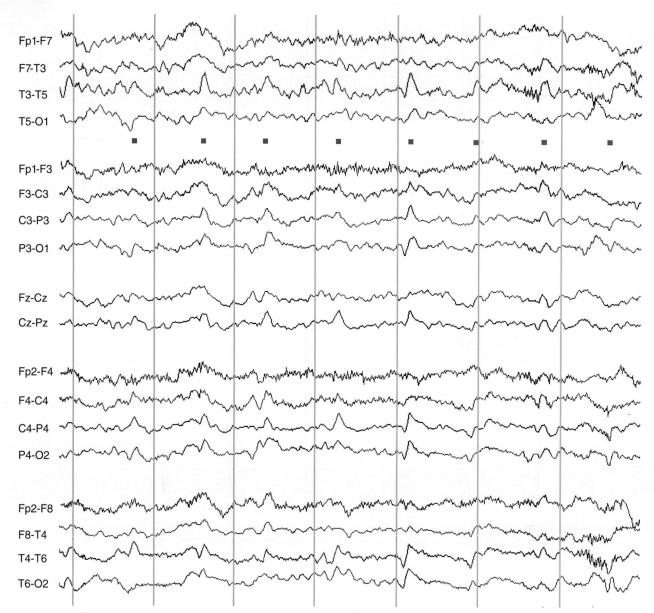

Figure 9.40 Periodic short interval diffuse discharges (PSIDDs or GPDs) ranging from 30 to 50 μV are seen in a patient with Creutzfeld-Jakob disease (dots). Note that the field of the discharge is diffuse, although this patient's variant of the disorder is posteriorly predominant. (Image courtesy of Dr. Edward Bromfield and Dr. Barbara Dworetsky.)

TABLE 9.2	Clinical Features of Periodic Patterns		
Characteristic	**PLEDS or BiPLEDS**	**PSIDDS**	**PLIDDS**
Etiology	Varied; most often vascular or tumor (PLEDs) CNS Infection, anoxia (BiPLEDS)	Metabolic (e.g., hepatic encephalopathy), anoxia, CJD, toxic, NCSE	SSPE, toxic (anesthetics), anoxia
Seizures	Common	Rare	Rare
Myoclonus	Rare	Common	Common

PLEDs = periodic lateralized epileptiform discharges; BiPLEDS = bilateral periodic lateralized epileptiform discharges; PSIDDS = periodic short-interval diffuse discharges; PLIDDS = periodic long-interval diffuse discharges; CJD = Creutzfeld-Jakob Disease; NCSE = nonconvulsive status epilepticus; SSPE = subacute sclerosing panencephalitis. Brenner RP, Schaul N. Periodic EEG patterns: classification, clinical correlation, and pathophysiology. *J Clin Neurophysiol* 7:249–267, 1990.

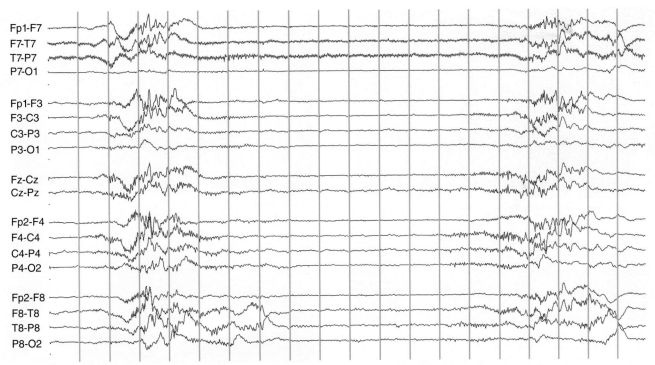

Figure 9.41 This burst-suppression pattern consists of 2- to 3-second bursts of mixed activity that includes sharp elements, separated by several seconds of diffuse suppression. Technically, this example could fall into the older category of periodic long interval diffuse discharges because of the long interburst interval, but the term *burst-suppression* is much more commonly used for this type of pattern.

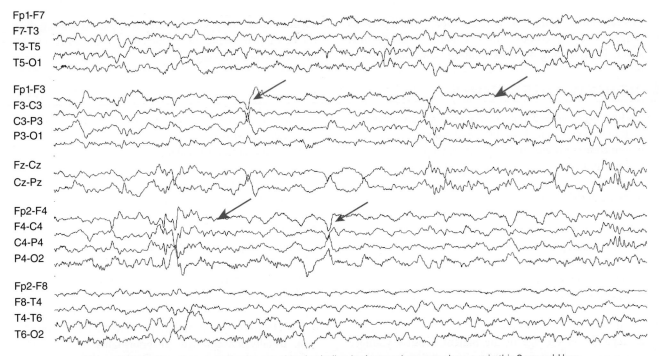

Figure 9.42 Both vertex waves (gray arrows) and spindles (red arrows) are asynchronous in this 3-year-old boy with agenesis of the corpus callosum. Although it seems logical that vertex waves and spindles might not be synchronous in individuals who lack a corpus callosum, some patients with agenesis of the corpus callosum still do manifest vertex wave and spindle synchrony. Likewise, the presence of spindle and vertex wave asynchrony does not always indicate absence of the corpus callosum.

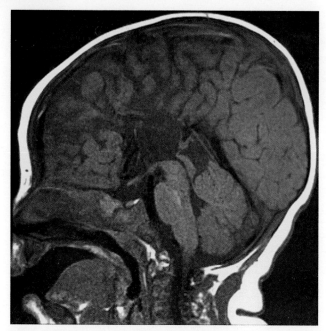

Figure 9.43 The magnetic resonance imaging (MRI) scan of the patient whose EEG was shown in the previous figure demonstrates absence of the corpus callosum. The next figure shows the MRI of an individual with an intact corpus callosum for comparison.

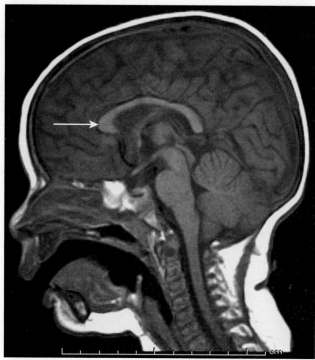

Figure 9.44 A magnetic resonance imaging scan of an individual with an intact corpus callosum is shown for comparison to the previous figure. The arrow indicates the lighter-colored horseshoe-shaped corpus callosum cut in cross-section. The corpus callosum is the large bundle of neurons that joins the two hemispheres. This structure is absent in the previous figure.

corpus callosum (Figures 9.42 through 9.44). Not all patients with agenesis of the corpus callosum manifest this finding, however. Representing an early stage in EEG maturation, asynchronous sleep spindles are an expected finding during the first 2 years of life, after which sleep spindles are expected to occur synchronously.

REVIEW QUESTIONS

1. An EEG is considered abnormal if it has features that are
   a. found in less than 3% of the population.
   b. not commonly encountered in normal subjects.
   c. known to be associated with pathologic or disease states.
   d. None of the above

2. A specific diagnosis one may expect to make with EEG is
   a. hepatic encephalopathy.
   b. active absence seizure disorder.
   c. herpes simplex encephalitis.
   d. hypoglycemia.

3. The definition of slow waves
   a. depends on the age of the patient because younger patients tend to have lower frequency EEG waves compared to adults.
   b. includes a requirement that the waves be of sufficient amplitude.
   c. cannot be applied to waves seen during sleep.
   d. refers to any wave with a wavelength longer than 0.125 seconds.

4. Focal slow wave abnormalities in the EEG have been associated with
   a. lesions at the cortical level.
   b. lesions at the deep white matter level.
   c. lesions in the thalamus.
   d. lesions of the brain stem.

5. Epileptic spikes
   a. should interrupt the underlying rhythm.
   b. should have a wavelength less than 70 msec.
   c. almost always have an aftercoming slow wave.
   d. All of the above

6. FIRDA (frontal intermittent rhythmic delta activity)
   a. usually denotes a frontal abnormality.
   b. cannot be depended on to localize a lesion.
   c. is a common but nonspecific pattern seen in coma.
   d. is not always in the delta range.

7. When a focal area of the EEG lacks beta activity,
   a. a lesion at the cortical level is suspected.
   b. a lesion in the deep white matter is suspected.

c. the pattern is often brought on my barbiturates or benzodiazepines.

d. it is usually the result of failing to set the correct amplifier sensitivity.

8. Regarding the role of the EEG in the diagnosis of migraine,
   a. it has been eliminated by the advent of MRI technology.
   b. it is not indicated in the routine evaluation of migraine.
   c. it is not expected to show a change during a migrainous attack.
   d. it is confined to the diagnosis of confusional migraine.

9. Secondary bilateral synchrony should be suspected when a patient's EEG manifests apparent generalized spike-wave discharges, but
   a. other focal abnormalities are found in one hemisphere.
   b. there are persistent "lead-ins" of the discharge from one side.
   c. the discharge is of higher amplitude over one hemisphere.
   d. All of the above.

ANSWERS

1. ANSWER: **C**. The fact that an EEG finding is uncommonly encountered in normal subjects or only occurs in a few percent of the population does not, in and of itself, qualify it as abnormal. Several normal variants have been identified in the EEG (see Chapter 11, "Normal Variants in the EEG") that are not common but are not associated with disease or pathologic states, which is the best definition of abnormality.

2. ANSWER: **B**. It is not common that the EEG alone can make a specific diagnosis, but the diagnosis of an active absence seizure disorder can, indeed, be established by EEG if such seizures are successfully recorded. Although the finding of triphasic waves is often associated with hepatic encephalopathy, it is not diagnostic of that disorder. Likewise, HSV encephalitis can be suggested by the presence of PLEDs or BiPLEDs, but these findings are still nonspecific and there are other possible causes of these EEG findings. There is no pathognomonic EEG finding associated with hypoglycemia.

3. ANSWER: **D**. Although younger patients do manifest more EEG activity in the slow-wave range, the definition of slow waves is not dependent on patient age, wave amplitude, or sleep state. Slow waves are defined as waves in the delta and theta range, which means that they must have a frequency below 8 Hz. Because an 8 Hz wave has a wavelength of 125 msec, by definition all slow waves have a wavelength longer than 125 msec.

4. ANSWER: **B**. Slow waves have been classically associated with abnormalities at the level of the deep white matter, though with exceptions, rather than with the other anatomical structures mentioned here.

5. ANSWER: **D**. By definition, epileptiform activity, including spikes, should interrupt the underlying rhythm. The formal definition of a spike (versus a sharp wave) is that the base of a spike should be 70 msec or less. If examined closely, almost all epileptic spikes will be associated with an aftercoming slow wave.

6. ANSWER: **B**. Although a frontal phenomenon, FIRDA does not necessarily denote a frontal lesion. FIRDA usually is seen in wakefulness or drowsiness and is not typically found in sleep or in comatose states. By definition, FIRDA should be in the delta range because it is a subset of intermittent rhythmic delta activity.

7. ANSWER: **A**. Fast activity is believed to be generated by cortical circuits and injuries at the cortical level are particularly associated with a loss of beta (fast) activity. Lesions at the level of the deep white matter are more often associated with focal slow wave abnormalities. Barbiturates and benzodiazepines tend to increase beta activity, but diffusely. Using amplifier gains that are too low may make it difficult to appreciate beta activity, but should not cause the appearance of a focal loss of beta activity.

8. ANSWER: **B**. MRI technology only plays a secondary role in the diagnosis of migraine (that of excluding lesional headache) as the MRI of a migraine patient is expected to be normal. Although not a consistent finding, the EEG sometimes shows focal slowing during complicated migraine attacks, including confusional migraine. In the evaluation of migraine, EEG is perhaps most useful in the minority of patients in whom it is difficult to distinguish between a migraine attack and a seizure.

9. ANSWER: **D**. All of the findings listed above increase the possibility that apparently generalized spike-wave discharges are caused by an underlying focal abnormality that is causing secondary bilateral synchrony and, therefore, mimicking a truly generalized spike-wave discharge.

SUGGESTED READINGS

Blume WT, Pillay N: Electrographic and clinical correlates of secondary bilateral synchrony, *Epilepsia* 26:636–641, 1985.

Brenner RP, Schaul N: Periodic EEG patterns: classification, clinical correlation, and pathophysiology, *J Clin Neurophysiol* 7:249–267, 1990.

Chatrian GE, Bergamini L, Dondey M: A glossary of terms most commonly used by clinical electroencephalographers, *Electroencephalogr Clin Neurophysiol* 37:538–553, 1974.

Gloor P, Kalaby O, Girard N: The electroencephalogram in diffuse encephalopathies: electroencephalographic correlates of gray and white matter lesions, *Brain* 91:779–802, 1968.

Hirsch LJ, et al: American Clinical Neurophysiology Society's Standardized Critical Care EEG Terminology: 2021 Version, *J Clin Neurophysiol* 38:1–29, 2021.

Kane N, Acharya J, Benickzy S, Caboclo L, Finnigan S, Kaplan PW, Shibasaki H, Pressler R, van Putten MJAM: A revised glossary of terms most commonly used by clinical electroencephalographers and updated proposal for the report format of the EEG findings. Revision 2017, *Clin Neurophysiol Pract* 2:170–185, 2017 Aug 4.

10

The EEG in Epilepsy

There are many indications for EEG testing, but the most common reason that an EEG is obtained is to assist in the diagnosis of seizures and epilepsy. Although the patient's history is still the cornerstone of the diagnostic process, in some cases the results of the EEG can make an equal or even greater contribution to the diagnosis of seizures, especially when some elements of the history are unclear. The EEG is a particularly powerful tool in helping to classify seizure types. Previous chapters in this book were written from the point of view of various EEG findings, discussing their potential clinical implications, including possible associations with epilepsy. This chapter provides a review of selected seizure types and epilepsy syndromes and discusses the EEG findings most commonly associated with each.

SEIZURES VERSUS EPILEPSY

There is considerable overlap between the concepts of seizures and epilepsy, but they are distinct concepts. In general, persons are said to have epilepsy if they have a persistent tendency to experiencing unprovoked seizures. Note the importance of the concept of provoked seizures versus unprovoked (spontaneous) seizures. An example of a provoked seizure would be a seizure episode occurring in a diabetic person who injects too much insulin causing a hypoglycemic seizure. Febrile seizures in young children are also considered provoked seizures. Seizures occurring in newborns immediately after birth asphyxia are also considered provoked seizures. If that baby grows up and continues to have seizures after the acute phase of the injury, then those seizures would be considered unprovoked. Likewise, seizures occurring in close proximity to a stroke or head trauma may be considered provoked seizures, but those occurring in the convalescent period would be considered unprovoked. The idea is that the seizure that occurs immediately after a head trauma may have been provoked by a temporary perturbation from the acute injury, which is not expected to persist. Late posttraumatic seizures, however, occur in the healed or healing state and are more likely to signal a longer-lasting tendency to spontaneous seizures. The concept of the epileptic brain implies that there is some pathologic process in the CNS that is predisposing to recurrent, unprovoked seizures. How, then, best to define epilepsy?

The longstanding working definition of epilepsy has been quite simple: a person who has experienced two or more unprovoked seizures can be said to have epilepsy. A key strength of this definition is how easy it is to apply—one can simply count the number of unprovoked seizures a person has had and if it is two or more, that person can be diagnosed with epilepsy. The thinking behind requiring two seizures for this definition is that the chances of having a second seizure after presenting with a first seizure is approximately 50%, but after a second seizure the chance of having additional seizures rises considerably.

This working definition of epilepsy was reconsidered by a committee of the International League Against Epilepsy (ILAE), which approached the question of how to classify individuals who present with only a first seizure episode, but whose clinical information implies a higher risk for repeat episodes, similar to the elevated risk for the group that has already had two seizures. As an example, if a 15-year-old woman experiences a first recognized prolonged staring spell with unresponsiveness and the EEG shows generalized spike-wave discharges and a photoparoxysmal response, the diagnosis of juvenile absence epilepsy is highly likely and the risk for recurrent seizures if the patient is left untreated is high. According to the new paradigm, that person, even though she has only had a single known seizure, can be diagnosed with epilepsy as the clinician has ascertained through history and testing that she likely has an epilepsy syndrome and will have a long-term tendency two recurrent seizures. The definition of epilepsy from the 2014 ILAE publication from Fisher et al. extends the original definition and includes any of the following conditions:

1) At least two unprovoked (or reflex) seizures occurring > 24 hours apart, or
2) One unprovoked (or reflex) seizure and a probability of further seizures similar to the general recurrence risk (at least 60%) after two unprovoked seizures, occurring over the next 10 years, or
3) Diagnosis of an epilepsy syndrome.

Note that fulfilling the diagnosis of epilepsy in a patient according to these parameters is not the same as deciding that treatment with medications is necessary. Although a positive diagnosis of epilepsy often runs in parallel with the decision to treat, there are occasions where a diagnosis of epilepsy can formally be made but the patient and physician decide to defer treatment for a variety of reasons.

SEIZURE TYPES AND SEIZURE SYNDROMES

Seizure Types

The distinction between seizure types and seizure syndromes (or epilepsy syndromes) is central to both the practice of clinical epileptology and clinical electroencephalography. It is worthwhile to consider the distinction between the two and how the diagnosis of each is made.

The concept of seizure type refers to the classification of an individual seizure event. To define a key term, a seizure's *semiology* includes the patient's appearance during the seizure combined with the patient's own subjective description (if able to give one) of what the experience of the seizure was like. Thus, the semiology is what happens during the seizure from the patient's and observers' point of view—essentially what the seizure looks like and feels like. In theory, a seizure type can be determined by simply knowing the seizure's semiology and the appearance of a simultaneous EEG recording, without necessarily having access to additional background history. Thus, a seizure type can usually be assigned based on an electroencephalographer's interpretation of the video EEG of a seizure event without knowing further background information.

The following hypothetical example illustrates how the two key features of semiology and EEG recording are used: a patient experiences an event that starts with a subjective report of a feeling of fear. Next, observers report that the patient begins to stare and is unresponsive, followed by rhythmic jerking of the left arm. Simultaneously, an EEG is recorded that shows a rhythmic discharge starting in the right temporal lobe and evolving to include much of the right hemisphere over a brief period of time (Figure 10.1A, B, and C). The combination of a psychic aura reported by the patient, staring, the specific motor phenomena reported by observers, and observation of an EEG seizure discharge that starts in the right temporal lobe all establish the diagnosis of a specific seizure type: focal seizure with impaired awareness arising from the right temporal lobe. Note that the age and previous history of the patient are not of primary importance in diagnosing seizure type; rather, the behaviors observed during the episode and any recordings made at the time of the event are the essential elements in defining seizure type. We can assign the seizure type "focal seizure with impaired awareness arising from the right temporal lobe," or more casually "right temporal lobe seizure," without knowing whether the seizures are occurring in a broader context of possible posttraumatic epilepsy, or perhaps temporal lobe epilepsy with mesial temporal sclerosis. Of course, often the seizure type can be diagnosed without the aid of a simultaneous EEG recording, which often is not available. In most cases the seizure type can be established based mostly on the seizure semiology, sometimes supplemented by confirmatory information from interictal EEG recordings. This contrasts with the approach to diagnosing seizure syndromes, described next.

Seizure Syndromes

To discern a patient's seizure syndrome, it is useful to know the patient's age, history, neurodevelopmental or cognitive status, and the seizure types he or she has experienced. For instance, a 28-year-old man with normal intellect and neurologic examination and a history of generalized convulsions and morning myoclonic jerks since the early teenage years

likely has the diagnosis of the seizure syndrome known as juvenile myoclonic epilepsy. In this example, this patient's seizure syndrome includes two *seizure types*: myoclonic seizures and generalized tonic-clonic seizures. Typically, the diagnosis of these seizure types can be confirmed by patient and observer descriptions of the seizure semiologies. Less often, simultaneous video/EEG recording of the individual seizure events could be confirmatory of the seizure types (though the latter is usually not necessary). The diagnosis of the seizure syndrome of juvenile myoclonic epilepsy, however, is best established by knowing the age at onset of the seizures, the seizure types the patient has, and additional pertinent history. Consider that, if this patient happened to have a grand mal seizure while on video EEG, an electroencephalographer would be able to correctly assign the seizure type—generalized tonic-clonic seizure—but would not be able to establish that the patient's seizure syndrome was juvenile myoclonic epilepsy without knowing the surrounding historical information.

CLASSIFICATION OF SEIZURE TYPES

The most frequently used series of classifications of seizure types was initially established by a committee of the ILAE in 1981 and has subsequently undergone a set of revisions. The most recent revision of the ILAE classification of seizure types at the time of this writing was published in 2017. Of the philosophical shifts represented in this latest classification, perhaps the most interesting is an emphasis on choosing to use terminology more understandable to the general public. Thus, opaque terms such as *complex partial seizure* and *dyscognitive seizure* have been discarded in favor of the somewhat cumbersome but more readily understandable *focal seizure with impaired awareness*.

This chapter primarily discusses the most recent 2017 terminology system. As with most new classification systems, it may not be the case that the medical community will adopt all of the proposed changes in their entirety. It is also useful to ask why a term that may have been in use for decades has been changed in a new classification. Keep in mind that most of the nomenclature changes have not necessarily been driven by any new scientific understanding of seizure types. This is to say that we did not discover that, under closer analysis, partial seizures are really focal seizures and then change their name—the name change does not reflect any new understanding of what focal seizures are. In the majority of cases, names have been changed because they are hoped to be more accurate or understandable. Some changes have been made to highlight details of seizures that have long been known, but were felt to deserve more emphasis. Readers may ask themselves if they are always obliged to use the newest nomenclature just because it is the latest one proposed and endorsed by a committee representing a highly respected organization. After all, based on recent historical patterns, many of the terms in these classifications have been proposed but then later rejected and replaced over the past 20 years. This question can be debated and reasonable people will have different opinions. Because

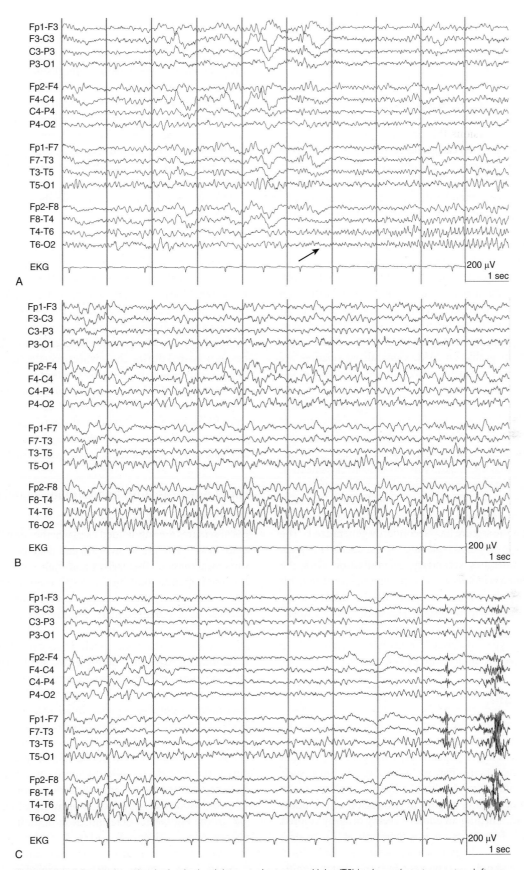

Figure 10.1 A focal seizure beginning in the right posterior temporal lobe (T6) is shown (montage setup: left para-sagittal chain over right parasagittal chain, left temporal chain over right temporal chain). The arrow indicates the location of seizure onset, which consists of a low-voltage, fast rhythm initially confined to the bottom two channels (compare with homologous channels on the left: T3-T5 and T5-O1). This fast rhythm then spreads through the right temporal chain, subsequently involving the right parasagittal chain as well. As is characteristic of many seizures, the discharge slows in frequency and increases in voltage throughout its course before abruptly coming to an end.

new classifications rarely completely sweep away the use of the previous terminology, both the older and newer terms are discussed below so the reader can gain familiarity with both the old and new terms.

FOCAL VERSUS GENERALIZED

Similar to previous versions, this classification divides seizures into focal and generalized categories according to the *onset* of the seizure, adding a smaller "unknown onset" category. This initial step in categorization, determining whether the seizure onset is focal versus generalized, is the most important step in seizure classification. Whether or not a seizure is focal as opposed to generalized will have a strong impact on determining its cause, but also which medications might be most effective in suppressing it, and also help assess its prognosis. In brief, focal seizures are more likely to be associated with focal anatomical abnormalities, the type that would show up on imaging studies. If imaging is normal in a case of focal seizures, sometimes we suspect that there is still a focal anatomical abnormality but that it may be present on a microscopic basis and not imageable on MRI. Generalized seizures are more likely to have a genetic cause and are typically associated with normal neuroimaging.

When a seizure is classified as focal versus generalized, this always refers to its onset. A focal seizure that rapidly spreads to both hemispheres and quickly resembles a generalized seizure is still classified as focal because it is the onset that matters. In fact, one major change in this most recent classification is to use the term *generalized* exclusively to refer to a seizure's onset. When a seizure spreads from a focal location to both hemispheres, the traditional expression for this sequence has been to say that the seizure has "secondarily generalized." The new terminology proposes replacing the concept of the focal seizure that undergoes secondary generalization with the term *focal to bilateral tonic-clonic*, reserving the term *generalized* for seizures whose *onsets* are generalized and *bilateral* for patterns of diffuse/bilateral *spread*. The strengths and weaknesses of this approach are discussed further below. Each category of seizure type is described briefly in this section, along with its characteristic clinical and EEG findings.

FOCAL SEIZURES

Because a seizure can arise from nearly any location on the cortical surface, the range of potential seizure manifestations is quite varied and depends on what part of the brain is involved. Focal seizures may include motor findings (such as jerking or stiffening of a limb), sensory findings (such as a sensation of tingling or pain over a region of the body, hearing a sound, smelling an odor, or seeing brightly colored shapes), psychic features (such as a sensation of fear or déjà vu), or autonomic findings (such as sweating, palpitations, or salivation). It should also be kept in mind that a significant portion of the cortical surface is functionally relatively silent. When a seizure discharge starts in one of these "silent" cortical areas, it is possible for the discharge to occur on the

cortical surface in a clinically silent fashion. Frequently, a seizure discharge may begin in one of these "silent" areas and subsequently spread to a less silent area, such as the motor strip, by which time obvious clinical signs may appear such as clonic jerking of an extremity. Thus, when a patient manifests clonic jerking, we can infer that the seizure discharge has involved the motor strip, but this is not a guarantee that the seizure discharge originated in the motor strip—the seizure discharge may have started elsewhere and spread to the motor strip. Figures 10.2 and 10.3 show examples of how two focal-onset seizures propagated.

On a historical note, as mentioned above, the original term used for focal seizure was *partial seizure*, and you will still hear that term from time to time. The current classification has favored the term *focal* because it was felt that some were understanding the term *partial seizure* to mean that the event was not a true or "complete" seizure. *Focal* was also preferred because it was felt that the term clearly referred to the anatomical localization of the seizure, while the term *partial* was more ambiguous with regard to what particular feature of the seizure was partial.

Focal seizures are further classified as to whether awareness is impaired during the seizures, whether its onset is motor as opposed to non-motor, and whether it becomes bilateral in distribution. Each of these attributes can then be further described. These three attributes are not meant to be hierarchical, which is to say that one attribute does not come first and determine what the possibilities are for the next—each attribute can be independently assessed for each seizure.

Focal Seizures with and without Impaired Awareness

Focal seizures are subdivided as to whether or not they impair awareness. There are many ways and degrees to which a person's awareness of themselves and their environment might become impaired, but there is no absolutely straightforward way to assess awareness during a seizure with complete confidence. As a practical matter, awareness is often assessed by the patient's responsiveness, an attribute that is distinct from awareness but with which it has considerable overlap. Imagining an example where the two attributes diverge, the current definition of impaired awareness specifically excludes individuals who are completely aware of their surroundings but cannot respond to outside stimuli because they are immobilized by the seizure and therefore cannot signal that they are aware. In theory, patients' awareness during a seizure can be assessed by asking if they were aware of what was going on during the episode, though this approach would tend to misclassify patients who are amnesic for (cannot remember) the seizure episode but happened to be aware while it was ongoing. In the end, strict determination of awareness is usually not crucial for patient care, and we do the best we can with the observations of the seizure that have been made in each case.

Some focal seizures may be associated with completely retained awareness, such as a focal seizure with clonic spasms of the face or hand—the patient may remain completely alert and aware during such a seizure. The majority of focal

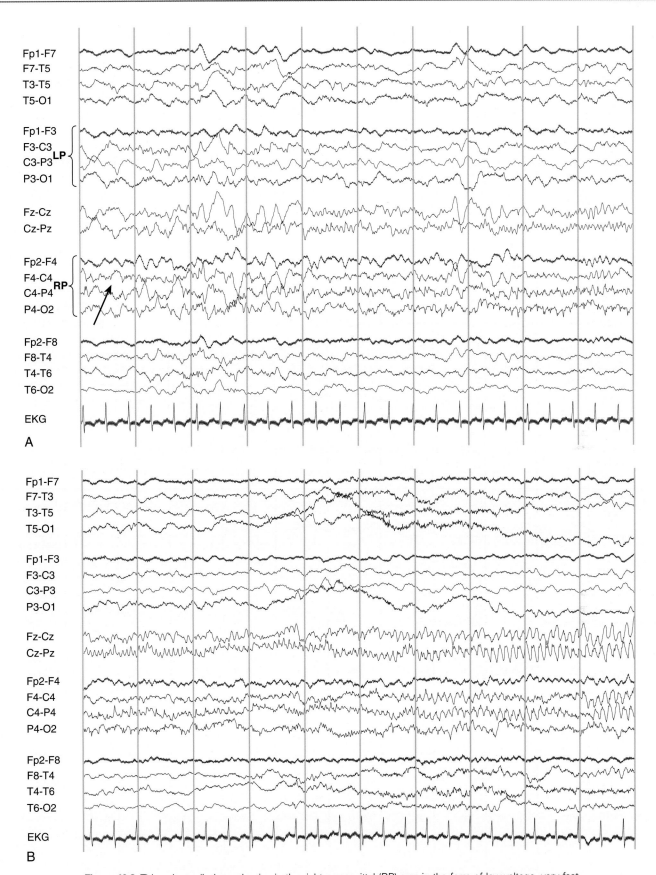

Figure 10.2 This seizure discharge begins in the right parasagittal (RP) area in the form of low-voltage, very fast activity (arrow) and spreads quickly to the midline electrodes (see Fz-Cz and Cz-Pz channels). The EEG seizure onset is detected by noting the first asymmetry between the right parasagittal and left parasagittal chains (labeled RP and LP)—compare the asymmetry of low-voltage fast activity in C4 compared to C3, most obvious in the third and fourth seconds after the arrow. The discharge then becomes most prominent and well formed in the midline channels (Fz-Cz and Cz-Pz) and then spreads to involves the right parasagittal area, with the field eventually spreading to the right temporal chain before termination. The seizure is then followed by postictal slowing.

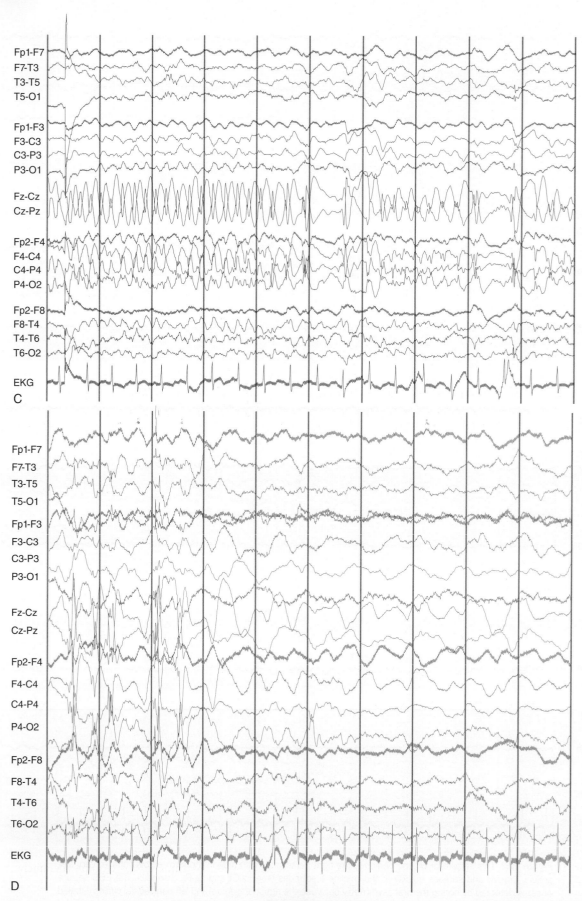

Figure 10.2, cont'd

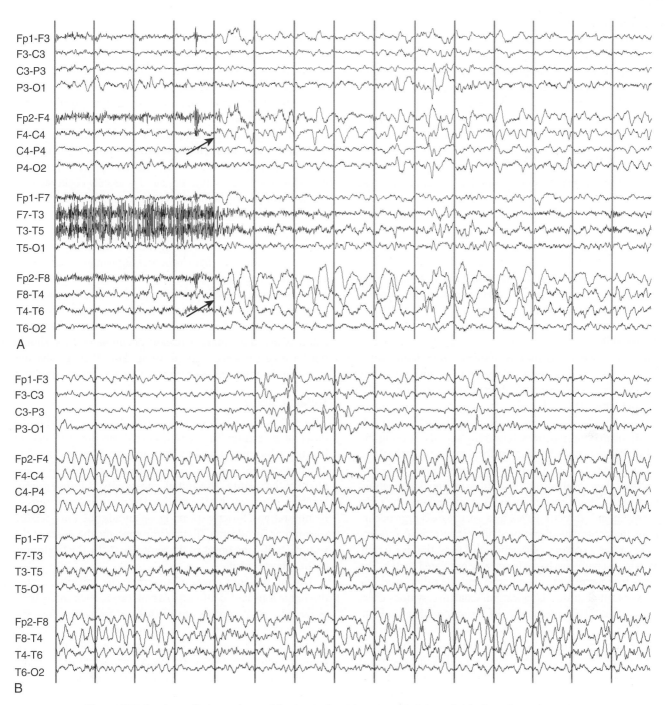

Figure 10.3 A seizure discharge (arrows) begins in the right temporal chain and right frontal area (montage setup: left parasagittal chain over right parasagittal chain, left temporal chain over right temporal chain). Initially, the seizure waveforms consist of higher voltage sharp forms, but as this seizure spreads to involve the whole of the right hemisphere, it attains a more rounded or sinusoidal morphology. This is an example of a discharge in which the frequency initially accelerates, and then decelerates before termination (final termination not shown).

seizures, however, are associated with diminished responsiveness/awareness and are properly classified as focal seizures with impaired awareness. Indeed, it is only during a minority of focal seizures that complete responsiveness is maintained—focal aware seizures. During focal seizures with impaired awareness, the patient often appears awake but may be staring or unresponsive (or only partially responsive) to stimulation. Only rarely does a patient appear to completely lose consciousness during focal seizures, though examples definitely occur.

According to previous classifications, focal aware seizures were termed *simple partial seizures* and focal seizures with impaired awareness *complex partial seizures* (CPS). In an intermediate version of the classification, the CPS term was changed to *dyscognitive* seizures, a clumsy term that was disliked by many and not easily understood by the lay public (and perhaps by some practitioners as well). Although the term *dyscognitive* came and went over a period of several years, the CPS term was in use for decades and, because of that and the fact that it forms an easy-to-use acronym, the term's usage may persist for a period of time.

Motor and Non-Motor Onsets

Focal seizures are classified as to whether the initial or most prominent feature includes a motor component. For those with motor onset, specifically named subsets of focal seizures include automatisms, atonic, clonic, epileptic spasms, hyperkinetic, myoclonic, and tonic. For non-motor onsets, primary descriptors include autonomic, behavioral arrest, cognitive, emotional, and sensory. In general, these descriptors are self-explanatory. Among these focal seizure subsets, the automatisms subset merits further discussion.

Automatisms

In the context of epilepsy, the term *automatisms* refers to automatic rather than consciously planned movements that occur during seizures. Examples include repetitive fumbling of the hands or picking at clothing, slow mechanical chewing movements, lip-smacking movements, running the fingers through the hair, or making repetitive humming sounds. Among the focal attributes that are listed in the focal seizure classification, focal seizures with automatisms may be qualitatively different from the other focal seizure attributes in the classification. When a focal clonic seizure includes clonic jerking, the jerking movement is directly driven by a seizure discharge occurring in the contralateral motor strip. When a focal sensory seizure causes a sensory experience, this sensation is directly caused by a seizure discharge in sensory or related cortex. The same is true for psychic phenomena and the other focal seizure types listed in the classification. Controversy does exist, however, around the mechanism of the automatisms, which, in contrast, may not be directly driven by a seizure discharge.

Although there is still a school of thought that some automatisms may be directly driven by a difficult-to-record seizure discharge, automatisms may occur by an entirely different mechanism—they may represent a release phenomenon rather than a direct seizure manifestation. The idea here is that certain automatic programs exist in the brain but are routinely suppressed by normally functioning cortex. When normal cortical function is disrupted by being engulfed with a seizure discharge, these automatic programs can be released from their usual state of being suppressed and start to play out repetitively. Note that, if this is the case, the observed automatic behavior does not necessarily arise from the seizing cortex, but rather from another area that has been released from the normal suppression of that program, possibly at some distance from the seizure focus.

Here is a list of observations that would support the view that automatisms are not directly generated by a focal seizure discharge. Automatisms have been observed both during the ictal period *and* the postictal period of seizures. Automatisms can occur during absence seizures and are more likely to be seen when the absence episodes become more lengthy. It does not seem likely that the automatisms that occur during the generalized discharges of absence episodes could be commanded by a small subpart of the cortex specific to that automatic behavior during a generalized discharge. When it occurs during a focal seizure, the fumbling hand automatism is not seen contralateral to the seizing temporal lobe as would be expected if it were directly driving the automatic fumbling behavior. Rather, the fumbling hand is usually observed *ipsilateral* to the seizing hemisphere, suggesting that an automatic program in the non-seizing hemisphere has become unsuppressed and is running the automatic motor program. Thus, automatisms are not necessarily directly driven by a seizure discharge in the way that clonic jerking would be driven by repetitive spikes in the EEG. Unfortunately, listing automatisms as a focal seizure type among other focal seizure attributes that are direct seizure manifestations may cause some confusion. This is of more than academic interest because, if automatisms do represent release phenomena, they should not be used for seizure localization. Also, their persistence also would not be a reliable sign that a seizure is continuing.

Epileptic Auras

An epileptic aura is a subjective sensation that heralds the onset of a seizure. The sensations can be diverse, such as hearing a buzzing sound in the ears, experiencing déjà vu, or having a feeling of nausea immediately preceding the next phase of the seizure. This initial, comparatively minor semiological feature may then be followed by more dramatic seizure manifestations. Strictly speaking, an aura is not a pre-seizure warning or "prodrome." Rather, it represents the onset of the seizure itself—the onset of the aura is actually the beginning of the seizure event.

During the aura phase of a seizure, the epileptic seizure discharge is usually confined to a small area, often in the temporal lobe. As it spreads out of that out from that area, the seizure's manifestations may become more dramatic. Because the aura itself should properly be considered the onset of the clinical seizure, true epileptic auras, even when they do not evolve, can be counted as a seizure and in certain instances can represent the seizure in its entirety.

RECORDABLE EEG PATTERNS ASSOCIATED WITH FOCAL SEIZURES

In contrast to generalized seizures, focal seizures are distinguished by EEG patterns that involve only subsets of the brain. Although most epileptic seizures can be recorded using standard scalp electrodes, in some cases a seizure discharge may occur in a cortical area that is not readily accessible to recording with conventional electrodes. These include such areas as the mesial surfaces of the frontal, parietal, and occipital lobes, the orbitofrontal surface of the frontal lobe, and the basal occipital and temporal lobes, and the mesial surface of

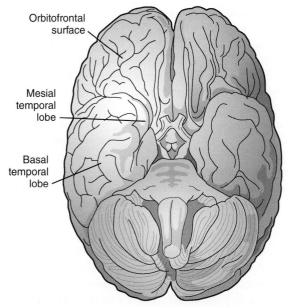

Figure 10.4 The basal surfaces of the brain are at some distance from the scalp and difficult to record well using routine techniques. The orbitofrontal surface of the brain lies on the floor of the anterior cranial fossa, above the eyes (orbits). The basal temporal lobe lies on the bone of the middle cranial fossa, and the mesial temporal lobe, including the amygdala and hippocampus, also lies at some distance from the scalp electrodes.

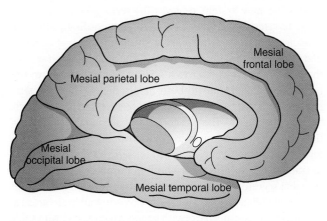

Figure 10.5 A section through the sagittal midline of the brain shows the mesial surfaces of the frontal, parietal, occipital, and temporal lobes, which can be difficult to record.

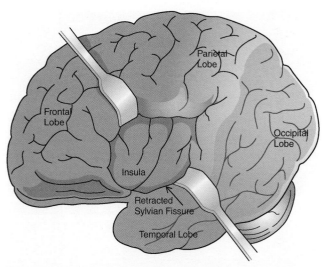

Figure 10.6 The insula (literally "island") represents an infolding of cerebral cortex covered by the lips (opercula) of the Sylvian fissure. The frontal and temporal opercula are retracted to reveal this hidden area of cortex.

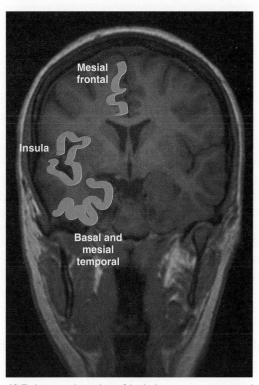

Figure 10.7 A coronal section of brain is seen on a magnetic resonance imaging scan. The mesial frontal lobe, insula, and basal and mesial temporal lobes are highlighted.

the temporal lobe, and the insula, among others (Figures 10.4 through 10.8). Therefore, most, but not all focal seizures are well recorded at the scalp. For these reasons, a negative EEG recording cannot, in and of itself, exclude the diagnosis of an epileptic seizure. In these occasional cases of definite epileptic seizure with negative scalp recordings, other factors must be taken into account to make the correct diagnosis, such as the specific features of the patient event and the history. In cases of focal epileptic seizures associated with a negative EEG, the seizure definition implies that there is some theoretical electrode placement that could record the seizure discharge, even if that placement location would have to be deep within

the brain. In fact, such depth recordings are possible and the technique is introduced in Chapter 14.

The EEG patterns associated with focal seizures usually consist of a rhythmic, sharp discharge over the affected area (e.g., spikes or spike-wave discharges) as shown in the previous figures. However, different appearances are possible. Especially when seizure sources are located deeper in the brain and at some distance from the recording electrode, the

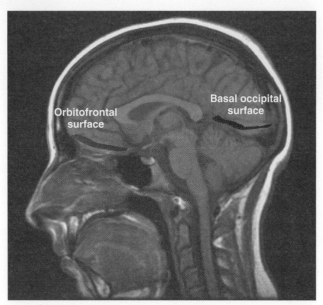

Figure 10.8 The basal frontal and occipital lobes are highlighted on a sagittal MRI scan. The gyri of the mesial surface of the cerebral hemisphere (frontal, parietal, and occipital) are also visible.

seizure may only appear as a rhythmic focal slowing in the theta or delta range over the involved area without obvious sharp features when recorded from the scalp. In the case of focal seizures, the epileptic discharge is usually unilateral. Although a unilateral focal seizure discharge may spread incrementally through the initially involved hemisphere, at such time as the discharge might cross to the opposite hemisphere, both hemispheres become completely engulfed with seizure activity; there is no incremental spread through the opposite hemisphere. This process has been referred to as secondary generalization, but the newer classification favors the term *focal to bilateral tonic-clonic*. An important exception to this rule is the example of temporal lobe seizures in which the seizure discharge may spread from one temporal lobe to the other without simultaneous involvement of the remainder of the hemispheres (Figure 10.9).

Focal Seizures with Secondary Generalization or "Focal to Bilateral Tonic-Clonic"

As described earlier, a seizure discharge may start focally and subsequently spread to involve all brain areas (generalize). This flow of the discharge from a subset of cerebral cortex to all of cerebral cortex is reflected both by the spread of the recorded discharge from a subset of EEG channels to all EEG channels and also by the evolution of the patient's seizure behavior from a focal manifestation to involvement of the whole body. This classic progression was first described by the English neurologist John Hughlings Jackson in 1863 and is referred to as a "Jacksonian march." He described examples of seizures that could begin with clonic contractions in the right hand and arm and subsequently spread to include the right face and leg. Thereafter, the seizure could spread to

the opposite side of the body so that bilaterally synchronous clonic activity of the whole body is seen. This clinical progression is mirrored electrographically by an evolution of the discharge from a small area in the left hemisphere which might include the hand area of the motor strip, to the whole of the left hemisphere and then, finally, to involvement of both hemispheres (Figure 10.10).

Focal seizures that secondarily generalize (or become bilateral) are classified among the focal seizures rather than the generalized seizures for diagnostic reasons. Focal seizures that do not generalize and focal seizures that do secondarily generalize have the same list of possible causes. In comparison, the list of causes of (primary) generalized seizures, i.e., seizure that *start* in all brain areas at once, is distinctly different from the list of causes of focal-onset seizures. In short, focal seizures are often caused by focal lesions in the brain (e.g., acquired lesions or dysplasias), while seizures that begin with a generalized pattern are often caused by a genetic predisposition to generalized seizure volleys. Whether or not a focal seizure secondarily generalizes usually has little to do with the etiology of the seizure.

Although the expression *secondary generalization of focal seizures* has been used for decades, a new terminology for this concept has been proposed in the 2017 ILAE classification of seizure types. The previous term, *partial onset with secondary generalization*, has been replaced by *focal to bilateral tonic-clonic*. The new system reserves the term *generalized* exclusively to refer to the onset of a seizure. According to the new classification, if a seizure *starts* in all brain areas, it is classified as generalized, much as before. The new system now uses the term *bilateral* to refer to a seizure that has started in one hemisphere but *spreads* to both hemispheres. Thus, the term *bilateral* is meant to be reserved for a seizure that propagates to both hemispheres—the old concept of secondary generalization. It is not clear, however, what advantages using the new term *bilateral* has over *generalized* for seizures that have spread to (rather than originated in) both hemispheres. If it were the case that secondarily generalized seizures were *less generalized*, but merely bilateral (i.e., not really involving all brain areas as much as their counterparts with generalized *onsets*), this could bolster the motivation for the change, but that claim is not made. Because "generalized" indicates a process occurring all over the brain and "bilateral" merely means present to some degree on both sides, the change in terms would seem to imply that primary generalized seizures are more all-encompassing in the brain and those that originate in one hemisphere and spread secondarily ("bilateral"), are less all-encompassing, but that is not the case. It has long been known that both seizures with generalized onset and those that have spread to both hemispheres after onset may have asymmetries and preponderances in some brain areas over others, but that is not the point that the new classification is making.

Another quirk of this new terminology is that the only term offered in the new classification for a seizure that has spread from one to both hemispheres is "focal to bilateral tonic-clonic" which would seem to imply that all secondarily propagated seizures are tonic-clonic, which is not the case.

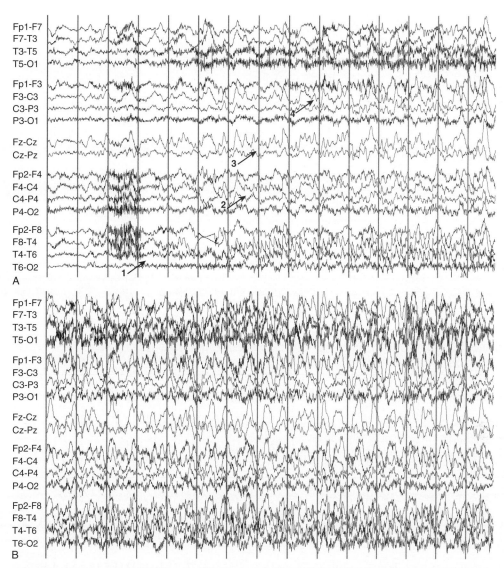

Figure 10.9 The beginning of the low-voltage sharp seizure discharge that is evident on the second half of the first page can be traced back to (1) in the right midtemporal area where the muscle artifact stops—this is the first point at which activity in the right temporal area clearly differs from the left temporal area (compare T4 to T3). After 3 seconds, the discharge spreads to the right parasagittal area (2) and then quickly to the midline (3). After 2 more seconds, the discharge has become bilateral and can be seen in the left parasagittal area (4). The sharp waves may be present simultaneously in the left temporal chain as well but would be difficult to discern because of the muscle and motion artifact in that area. As it nears its end, the seizure discharge increases in voltage and slows in frequency. The increased muscle and motion artifact is not unexpected as the clinical manifestation of seizures often includes muscle tensing and patient movement.

The classification does not make clear whether it means to allow terms such as *focal to bilateral tonic* or *focal to bilateral clonic* if that happens to be the pattern of the seizure. Because it is the only term for seizures that become bilateral, does the classification expect a pure tonic seizure that becomes bilateral to be called *focal to bilateral tonic-clonic*, even when there is clearly no clonic component? Finally, there are seizure types that can become bilateral, but are clearly not generalized, such as the bilateral temporal lobe seizures described above. The new classification seems to indirectly imply that all seizures that transition from focal to bilateral become secondarily generalized (according to the original meaning of the term), which is not the case

with bilateral temporal seizures. Thus, it remains to be seen whether the new proposed terminology regarding seizures that spread to both hemispheres will completely supplant the old terminology.

GENERALIZED SEIZURES

The classification of generalized seizures is now divided into motor and non-motor groups. The motor group includes tonic-clonic, clonic, tonic, myoclonic, myoclonic-tonic-clonic, myoclonic atonic, atonic seizures, and epileptic spasms. The non-motor generalized seizures essentially consist of the different types of absence and absence-related

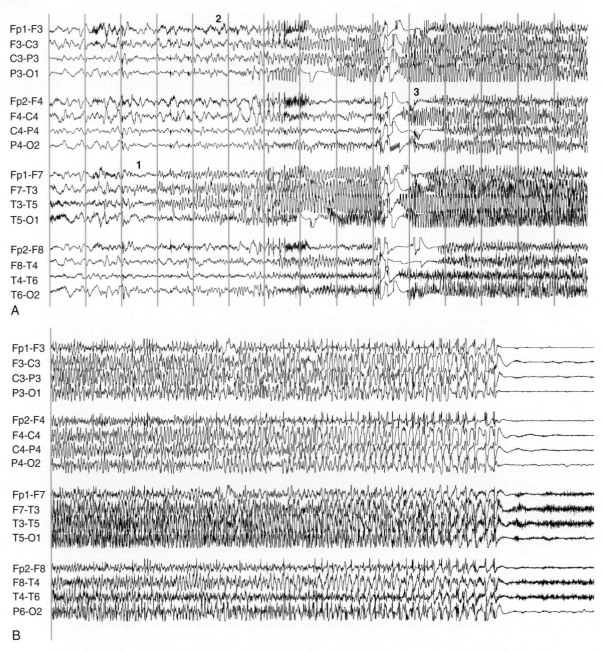

Figures 10.10 A seizure in a child with severe myoclonic epilepsy of infancy (SMEI, or Dravet syndrome) is shown that begins in the left temporal chain (1) and quickly spreads to the left parasagittal chain (2). After a brief period of amplifier blocking (possibly related to patient movement), the discharge becomes bilateral (3). Although SMEI is related to the generalized epilepsies, this patient had similar focal seizure onsets arising from the opposite (right) side at other times. Also, note the left parasagittal/right parasagittal, left temporal/right temporal setup of this montage.

seizures: typical, atypical, and myoclonic absences and eyelid myoclonia. Even though all of these seizure types fall into the category of generalized seizures, their manifestations differ widely and are described below.

Generalized Tonic-Clonic Seizures

The generalized tonic-clonic seizure (GTC) is the prototypical generalized motor seizure. The term refers specifically to the

sequence of whole-body tonic stiffening, followed by clonic jerking. Unfortunately, this term is often used indiscriminately to refer to any generalized convulsion, a use which is technically incorrect; properly, the term generalized tonic-clonic seizure should be reserved exclusively for the sequence of whole-body tonic stiffening followed by whole body clonic jerking. This distinction can be important, as some clinical events that mimic seizures, such as convulsive syncope (nonepileptic stiffening or jerking body movements that may occur with syncope/fainting) do not tend to manifest this specific sequence. The sequence of tonic body stiffening followed by clonic jerking, compared with other possible sequences of movements, is highly suggestive of an epileptic seizure and should be duly noted when observers give this description. Unfortunately, the new classification of seizure types may be indirectly blurring this important distinction as it is explicitly attempting to replace the term *grand mal seizure*, which refers to generalized convulsions in a generic sense, with the term *GTC*, which indirectly implies that all grand mal seizures are GTCs, which is definitely not the case.

The term *grand mal seizure* is sometimes used synonymously with GTC, but is somewhat less precise, which can be an advantage in some circumstances. The GTC term implies a generalized onset. If a patient has a major motor seizure but the onset is not confirmed, referring to the episode as a grand mal seizure is noncommittal as to its onset and, therefore, avoids the false precision that using the GTC term might communicate in such a circumstance. It also does not necessarily imply that the observer reported the progression from tonic stiffening to clonic jerking that the GTC term indicates. The term *grand mal seizure* is juxtaposed against another older term, *petit mal seizure*, which used to be a synonym for absence seizure, but has fallen out of favor.

The EEG correlate of the GTC seizure often begins with an abrupt onset of generalized rapid spikes that then slow in frequency over the course of the event. As the firing frequency of the spikes slows, the spikes may begin to manifest a clearer spike-wave morphology. From the clinical perspective, rapid spikes are often associated with tonic stiffening. Typically, during the course of the seizure, the firing rate of the rapid spikes gradually slows on EEG. At a certain point in the seizure, the firing rate of the spikes slows to a point that allows each spike or spike-wave discharge to generate its own separate clonic jerk (Figure 10.11) rather than a continuous tonic muscle contraction. This is the reason that the progression from tonic stiffening to clonic jerking is so common in generalized epileptic seizures. Over the course of a GTC seizure, the clonic jerking is seen to slow in frequency and eventually cease as the discharge blends into a slow-wave pattern: "postictal slowing," or even postictal flattening. Less commonly, a clonic-tonic-clonic seizure may occur in which clonic jerking speeds up and melds into tonic stiffening, followed by the usual progression back to clonic jerking. As expected, the EEG correlate of this type of seizure often consists of spike-wave discharges that speed up to become rapid spikes, and then slow down again (Figure 10.12).

Clonic Seizures

Clonic seizures are characterized by repetitive clonic jerks. These clonic jerks can occur in nearly any skeletal muscle group in the body depending on the location of the discharge in the motor strip. Clonic jerking from seizure activity tends to have a rhythmic quality. Because each clonic jerk is driven by an EEG discharge, a simultaneous spike or spike-wave discharge is expected in the EEG just before each clonic jerk, the frequency of the EEG discharges matching the frequency of the jerks. The jerks can fire up to approximately four times per second and tend to slow down during their course before the seizure terminates. Because clonic jerking is typically driven by discharges from the area of the motor strip, it is uncommon for scalp EEG electrodes to fail to record them, especially if they involve the face or hand. Pure clonic seizures are especially common in newborns.

Tonic Seizures

Tonic seizures cause tonic stiffening of a limb, several limbs, or the whole body. When the whole body is involved with a generalized tonic seizure, tonic stiffening in extension is most common; however, tonic stiffening with flexion of the hips, knees, arms, or back may also be seen. Especially with generalized tonic seizures, tonic contraction of the diaphragm may occur resulting in a forced inhalation or a grunting/moaning sound, which sounds unnatural and unlike typical moaning (the same sound may be heard during the tonic phase of GTC seizures). Most often, the EEG correlate of tonic seizures is a spray of rapid spikes in the affected area, often with an initial frequency between 10 and 25 Hz, which subsequently slows, similar to the onset of GTC seizures as described above. Other EEG correlates may also be seen, including an abrupt desynchronization (flattening) of the EEG. When such flattening occurs, there is often a suggestion of low voltage rapid spikes superimposed on the flattened pattern though these are not always identifiable (Figure 10.13). Therefore, although most ictal patterns are dramatic and show higher-voltage, repetitive discharges, the electroencephalographer must also be alert to abrupt flattening of the EEG (an electrodecrement) as a possible EEG seizure correlate. Other patterns are less common.

Myoclonic Seizures

Myoclonic seizures consist of a lightning-like or shock-like contraction of the muscles driven by an epileptic discharge. Thus, appearance of a myoclonic seizure is similar to the appearance of a brief electric shock. Myoclonus may consist of a single jerk or a quick series of jerks that occur in a burst, either rhythmic or nonrhythmic. Epileptic myoclonus may manifest as a muscle jerk in nearly any part of the body, although the most common location for epileptic myoclonus is the upper shoulder girdle, as is seen in the syndrome of juvenile myoclonic epilepsy. In such cases, the myoclonus usually consists of a quick series of abduction jerks at the shoulders. During the series of jerks, there may be a tendency for slight net abduction of the upper arms away from the body with each jerk. The most common EEG manifestation of epileptic myoclonus is a high-voltage polyspike-wave discharge, which may occur singly or in brief, repetitive bursts (Figures 10.14 and 10.15).

Because myoclonic seizures and clonic seizures both generate body jerks, the definitions of both sound similar. Epileptic myoclonus is more of a lightning-like jerk and, when repetitive, occurs in a brief non-rhythmic sputtering burst lasting approximately one second. The jerks generated

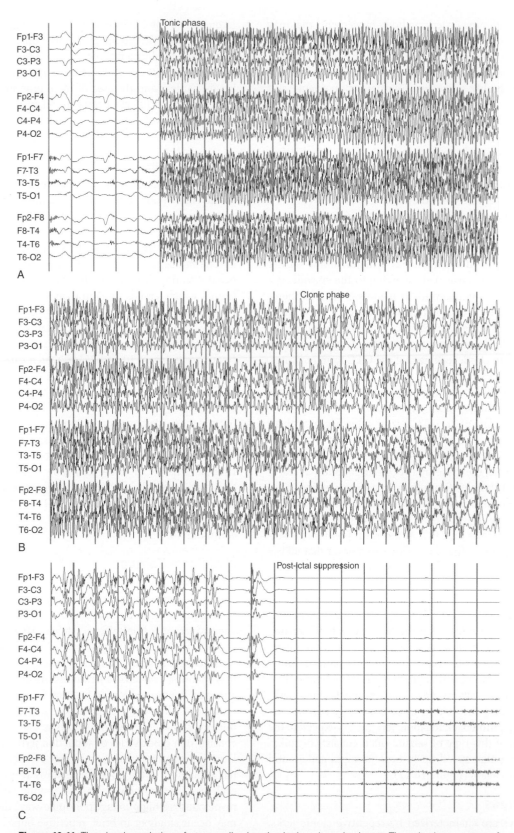

Figure 10.11 The classic evolution of a generalized tonic-clonic seizure is shown. There is abrupt onset of generalized rapid spikes at the start of the tonic phase. As the firing frequency of the spikes decreases the individual spikes become far enough apart from one another that each spike can generate a separate clonic jerk, representing the clonic phase of the seizure. In this case, there is a period of postictal suppression after cessation of the seizure discharge. After seconds or minutes, generalized slow-wave activity may appear eventually blending into the EEG background. The slowing can last from minutes to days depending on the duration of the seizure and the nature of the patient, so-called *post-ictal slowing*.

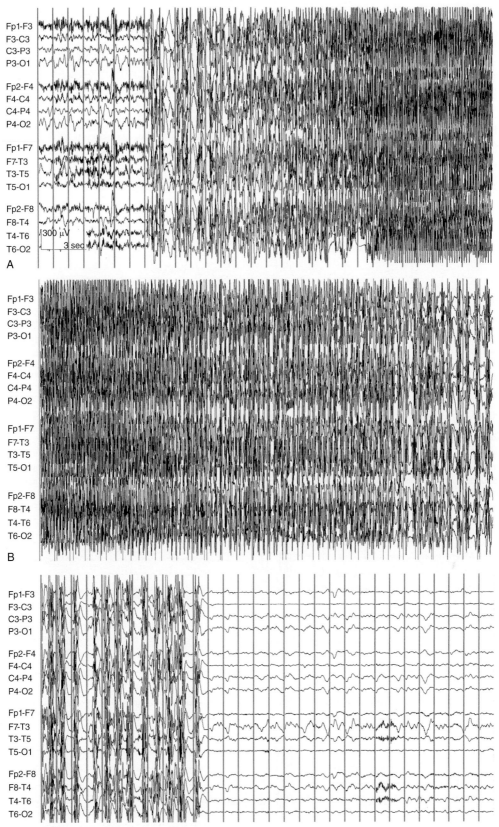

Figure 10.12 A clonic-tonic-clonic seizure discharge is shown. Note that, in comparison to the previous example, the initial rapid spikes appear in brief bursts (seconds 8–10 of panel A) each associated with a clonic jerk. After a few seconds, the rapid spikes consolidate and their firing frequency increases, corresponding to the tonic phase of the seizure. The seizure discharge then follows a pattern similar to that of the tonic-clonic seizure shown earlier, with slowing of the spike frequency associated with the next clonic phase EEG the seizure. Postictal slowing is seen after this seizure discharge.

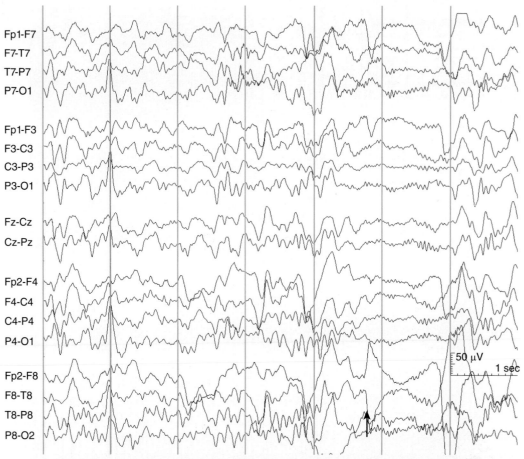

Figure 10.13 Electrodecremental seizure patterns consist of an abrupt flattening of the EEG, usually only lasting a few seconds. In some examples, low-voltage rapid spikes can be seen during the decrement (arrow), but in other cases spikes cannot be identified.

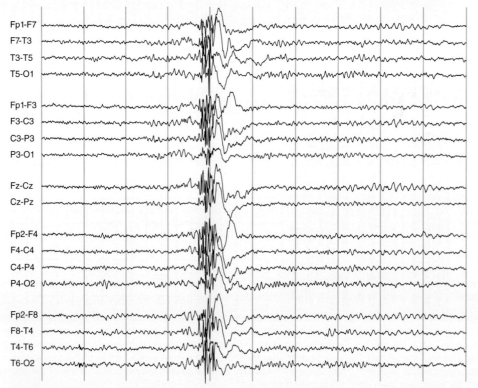

Figure 10.14 This 15-year-old girl was referred for tremor. The movements in question actually represented epileptic myoclonus driven by the high-voltage polyspike-wave discharge shown.

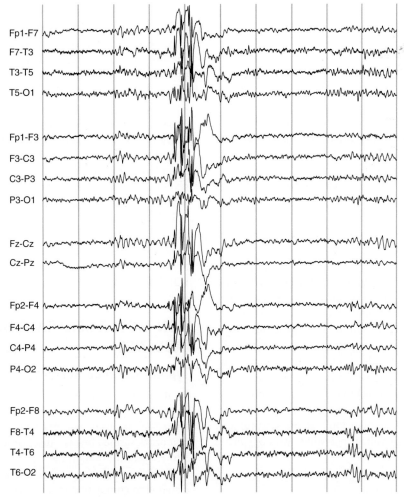

Figure 10.15 Myoclonic jerks often occur in quick succession. In this teenage patient, this quickly repetitive series of polyspike-wave discharges caused a series of quick abduction jerks at the shoulders.

by clonic seizures are more rhythmic and separated by longer intervals.

It is important to keep in mind that not all myoclonus is epileptic. Nonepileptic myoclonus may originate in the central nervous system at levels below cerebral cortex, including the subcortical areas, brainstem, and even the spinal cord (segmental myoclonus). The question of whether an instance of myoclonus is epileptic myoclonus is best confirmed by demonstrating the presence of a concomitant EEG discharge driving the movement. No EEG discharge would be expected to precede nonepileptic myoclonus. Sleep myoclonus is a common physiologic phenomenon that is nonepileptic. In fact, because sleep myoclonus may trigger a subarousal in the sleeping patient, it may be accompanied by a K-complex, a normal burst occurring in Stage II sleep often triggered by a sound or other outside stimulus. Epileptic myoclonus can usually be easily distinguished from sleep myoclonus in that, with epileptic myoclonus, the EEG burst precedes and drives the myoclonic jerk. In the case of sleep myoclonus, the jerk comes first and any change in the EEG, such as a K-complex, closely follows it.

Myoclonic-Tonic-Clonic Seizures

The myoclonic-tonic-clonic seizure type has long been clinically recognized but is a new element of the 2017 classification. This seizure type is specifically seen in the juvenile myoclonic epilepsy syndrome. In this syndrome, the GTC episodes are often (but not always) heralded by a series of the patient's myoclonic jerks. The jerks are immediately followed by a progression, beginning with whole body tonic stiffening, that is similar to a GTC. An interesting clinical layer to this progression is its relation to the general rule that, during a seizure with generalized or bilateral motor activity, consciousness is not preserved. For that reason, patients who experience a GTC are not able to describe the tonic stiffening or the clonic jerking they experience. When a patient self-describes bilateral motor activity at seizure onset, this raises a strong suspicion that the event is nonepileptic. An exception to this rule is the series of myoclonic jerks that might initiate a myoclonic-tonic-clonic seizure. Because patients do have preserved consciousness during the phase of myoclonic jerks, they are often able to self-describe that portion of the seizure, though they would not be conscious of the tonic-clonic portion of the event.

Myoclonic-Atonic Seizures

The myoclonic-atonic seizure is the hallmark seizure of myoclonic-atonic epilepsy (MAE). This seizure type and the syndrome were previously referred to as myoclonic-astatic seizures and myoclonic-astatic epilepsy (or Doose Syndrome). As the name implies, myoclonic-atonic seizures are atonic seizures that begin with myoclonic activity. The term *astatic* specifically indicates the failure to maintain the erect position (standing), which is to say a seizure that can cause a fall. An atonic seizure is a seizure associated with a loss of muscle tone, which, of course, can also cause a fall, so atonic seizures can be seen as a subset of astatic seizures. The term *astatic* had the nice advantage of not requiring the user of the term to know whether all of the patient's muscles became atonic during an event. This is made more complicated by the fact that, during some types of seizures, muscle electrodes show that some muscle groups lose tone while some stiffen, still resulting in a fall. Although the falling seizures of MAE are generally associated with a loss of muscle tone, it may not be the case that all muscles become atonic and, indeed, some patients may even fall from the initial myoclonic portion of the seizure. Thus, and somewhat ironically, the lack of precision of the previous *astatic seizure* terminology did have some advantages over the newer myoclonic-atonic term. Myoclonic-atonic seizures are usually associated with high-voltage polyspike-wave or spike-wave discharges on EEG.

Atonic Seizures

As the name implies, atonic seizures consist of a loss of tone, usually of the truncal muscles. In its mildest form, an atonic seizure may simply cause a subtle slumping of the shoulders. More frequently, an atonic seizure may manifest as a head-drop spell in which the patient's head slumps forward. The most dramatic version of an atonic seizure is the drop attack in which the patient collapses to the ground, possibly resulting in injury. There are many possible EEG correlates to atonic seizures, including slow spike-wave discharges, EEG desynchronization (flattening), or polyspikes, sometimes followed by flattening.

Epileptic Spasms

The term *epileptic spasms* has replaced the original term *infantile spasms* in some settings to avoid the awkwardness of using the term *infantile* for a patient who might have this seizure type persist well after infancy. In fact, the new classification still approves of the use of the original term *infantile spasms* term when the seizure is occurring during infancy. Epileptic spasms can be thought of as a special subset of tonic seizures. Most commonly, the patient has a brief tonic stiffening of the body, with arm abduction and some neck flexion, held for about one second. Variations from this classic appearance do occur, including spasms in extension or with mixed flexion and extension. So-called *hemispasms* involve half of the body and are strongly suggestive that a focal lesion is causative. Although some muscle groups undergo tonic stiffening during epileptic spasms, others may simultaneously become atonic. Occasionally, the appearance of the epileptic spasms can be quite subtle, with only very mild slackening of proximal tone or a subtle upgaze—such mild manifestations may be seen in the partially treated state. Epileptic spasms characteristically occur in clusters, often after the patient awakens from sleep, though neither this timing nor occurrence in clusters is mandatory for the diagnosis of this seizure type. When occurring in clusters, the patient may have an individual spasm every 10 to 20 seconds over a period of several minutes. Epileptic (infantile) spasms are quite distinct from myoclonic seizures, which consist of an extremely brief or lightning-like jerk. In contrast, the change in body position caused by infantile spasms is sustained for a brief period of time. Infantile spasms are the hallmark seizure type of West Syndrome. West Syndrome and the EEG patterns associated with infantile spasms are discussed later.

NON-MOTOR GENERALIZED SEIZURES (ABSENCE)

Typical Absence Seizures

In its purest form, the sole clinical manifestation of the absence seizure is a pure stare, though typical absence seizures seldom occur without some of the additional features that are described below. Absence seizures typically last from 3 to 15 seconds, though there is no strict upper or lower limit to their duration. Absence seizures are characteristically associated with complete unawareness of the environment. From a practical point of view, defining a possible minimum duration of an absence seizure is limited by the ability of observers or the patient to document unawareness or unresponsiveness for very brief periods of time. For instance, in practice, it would be very difficult to document lack of awareness during a discharge that lasts only one second. Although most absence seizures are brief, they can be of any duration, and examples of very prolonged absence seizures, including absence status epilepticus, may occur.

To distinguish them from atypical absence seizures (described below), the term typical absence seizure may be used, but when no modifier is used, typical absence is assumed. Typical absence seizures are characterized by abrupt onset and termination of the spells. In the past, some have used the term *absence* to denote any seizure associated with staring (even including focal seizures with impaired awareness). In modern usage, the term *absence seizure* refers to staring seizures associated with generalized spike-wave discharges as described below—focal seizures with impaired awareness that cause staring are excluded.

A simple typical absence seizure consists of staring alone, but such examples of completely bland staring with no other accompaniments are rare. In fact, subtle, rhythmic clonic movements of the eyelids occur with the majority of typical absence seizures (each blink occurring in synchrony with a generalized spike-wave discharge seen on EEG); pure staring with no additional signs is uncommon. The eyes may also drift upwards during the episodes, and sometimes upward and a bit off to the side. Less frequent additions are clonic or myoclonic movements of the face or upper body, which also occur in synchrony with the spike-wave discharges. Review of video recordings of absence seizures can show a subtle slackening of facial muscle tone during the episodes. Mild changes in body tone during typical absence are much less common. Because some type of accompaniment is expected during absence seizure episodes, these seizures should not look like persons who simply have a fixed gaze because they are deep in thought.

As a rule, patients are usually completely unaware of the environment during absence seizures, though an occasional patient reports partial awareness including the ability to hear or see during the discharges. In the majority of cases, after an absence seizure, patients themselves are unaware that the episode has even occurred, the only potential clue being the subjective feeling that something has been missed in the observed sequence of events.

Although 3 Hz generalized spike-wave discharges are the hallmark EEG accompaniment of the typical absence seizure, the occurrence of such discharges is not a guarantee that an absence seizures has occurred. A fraction of patients may have EEG patterns that are indistinguishable from the 3 Hz generalized spike-wave discharges that occur during clinical absence but may have no discernible change in awareness at all during the discharges. For instance, these individuals may be able to continue a conversation or typing on a keyboard

without pause during the discharges which then, by definition, would not represent a clinical seizure (the definition of a clinical seizure requiring that an objective or a subjective change occur in the patient at the time of the abnormal EEG discharge). Realizing that this phenomenon exists, the electroencephalographer must resist the impulse to assume that all 3 Hz generalized spike-wave discharges represent absence seizures. Even "classic" 3 Hz generalized spike-wave discharges may occur as an interictal abnormality. Strictly speaking, the diagnosis of clinical absence seizures requires some observable or reported change during the discharge.

EEG

The most frequent EEG correlate to typical absence seizures is the "classic" 3 Hz generalized spike-wave discharge (Figure 10.16). When these discharges are analyzed closely, the maximum voltage of the spike component of the spike-wave complexes is most commonly seen in the superior frontal electrodes (F3 and F4). Less often, the spike maximum is seen in the occipital area, and even less frequently in other locations.

Although the term 3 Hz generalized spike wave is well known and implies a consistent frequency, observed firing frequencies are not necessarily as consistent as the term implies. Often, the first few discharges fire at a frequency slightly faster than 3 Hz. After onset of the discharge, the firing frequency typically slows, often to 2.5 Hz and sometimes to 2 Hz before terminating (Figure 10.17). One of the most characteristic attributes of the typical absence seizure is the abrupt onset

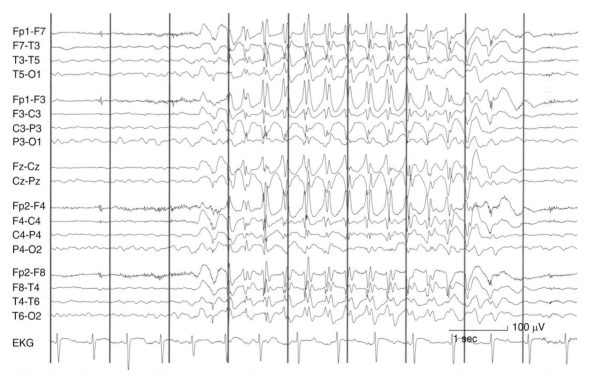

Figure 10.16 This 3 Hz generalized spike-wave discharge shows the abrupt onset and termination that is characteristic of absence seizures. Note the frontal maximum of the waveforms and also that, on closer examination, what we casually refer to as generalized spike-wave discharges actually are polyspike-wave discharges.

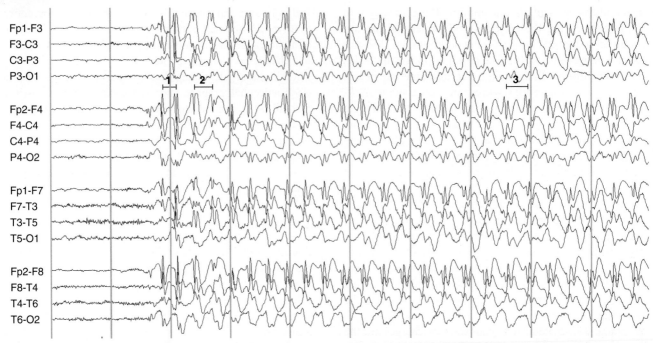

Figure 10.17 Although the discharge associated with this typical absence seizure is classified as 3 Hz generalized spike-wave, note that the discharge's firing frequency still evolves throughout its course. The first wavelength measured suggests a firing rate just above 4 Hz but (1), 1 second later at the time of the second measured wavelength, the firing rate has dropped to 3 Hz (2). Later in the discharge, the third measured wavelength implies a firing frequency of 2.5 Hz (3).

and termination of the discharge. The classic 3 Hz generalized spike-wave discharge tends to abruptly interrupt a normal background and has a clear time of onset and a fairly well demarcated termination. After termination, the EEG returns to the previous background after a few seconds or less.

Finally, close examination of most examples of "classic generalized 3 Hz spike-wave" often shows that the discharges often have multiple phases and are actually polyspike-wave discharges. Therefore, the reader should be aware that in the case of "classic 3 Hz generalized spike-wave discharges," the discharges may not be strictly generalized (they often show an F3/F4 maximum), they may not fire consistently at 3 Hz, and the discharges themselves may not actually be spike-wave discharges, but rather polyspike-wave discharges!

Atypical Absence Seizures

As with typical absence seizures, the core clinical features of atypical absence seizures are staring and unresponsiveness. Atypical absence seizures differ, however, in that onset and termination of the episodes, both clinically and electrographically, are less clear, and the associated spike-wave firing rates are slower. In addition, atypical absence seizures tend to occur in individuals with intellectual disability, whereas typical absence seizures are most often seen in subjects who are cognitively normal. Changes in tone are more common during atypical absence seizures, with slumping of the head, shoulders, and sometimes the whole torso seen during some examples.

EEG

The EEG hallmark of atypical absence seizures is the slow spike-wave discharge. Slow spike-wave discharges differ from "classic" 3 Hz generalized spike-wave discharges in two important respects: slow spike-wave discharges, as their name implies, fire at a slower rate, usually 2.5 Hz or less at onset (Figure 10.18). Slow spike-wave discharges also lack the clear-cut onset and termination characteristic of typical absence seizure discharges—slow spike-wave discharges tend to drift in and out. Finally, whereas slow spike-wave discharges may be generalized, asymmetries, both between the left and the right hemispheres and the anterior and posterior head regions, are more common. There is no single characteristic location for the discharge maximum for the slow spike-wave discharges associated with atypical absence seizures and the location of the voltage maximum may differ even within the same patient at different times. Atypical absence seizures often occur against the backdrop of an otherwise abnormal EEG, which may include scattered epileptiform activity or a slowed background.

From the point of view of seeing slow spike-wave discharges on the EEG, while these may be associated with atypical absence seizures, this is often not the case. Although slow spike-wave discharges are expected as the EEG correlate of atypical absence seizures, the converse is often not true: most slow spike-wave discharges are *not* associated with clinical atypical absence seizures. In practice, slow spike-wave discharges are often seen as interictal abnormalities in the EEG.

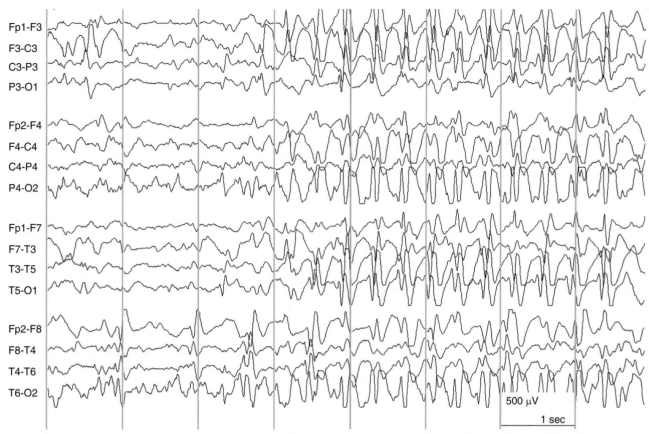

Figure 10.18 Slow spike-wave discharges are seen in a young man with mixed seizures. Note the slowed firing rate of the train of spike-wave discharges on the second half of the page and the scattered, single discharges in multiple locations seen on the first half of the page.

The simple observation of slow spike-wave discharges in the EEG is no guarantee that the patient is actually experiencing an atypical absence seizure, although the finding does raise suspicion that the patient could have this seizure type. When this pattern is seen, the concurrent observation of associated staring or some form of decreased responsiveness or change in tone is necessary to establish the diagnosis of an electro-clinical seizure.

Eyelid Myoclonia

Eyelid myoclonia represents a very distinctive seizure type, best known for its appearance in the syndrome of Eyelid Myoclonia with Absence (EMA), also known as Jeavons syndrome. The eyelid myoclonia consist of a very fast fluttering or jerking movement of the eyelids. What makes the movement unusual is that sometimes it is associated with an absence seizure and sometimes not. Therefore, unlike the rhythmic clonic eye-blinking that occurs with typical absence seizures that is clearly driven by generalized spike-wave discharges, eyelid myoclonia can occur both with and without spike-wave discharges, which implies that the eyelid movements are not directly driven by epileptic discharges. This is also consistent with the observation that the very fast and irregular frequency of the eyelid fluttering seen in eyelid

myoclonia would not be in synchrony with the slower-paced spike-wave discharges that can be seen in these patients.

The myoclonia typically begin with eye closure and Jeavons noted that this phenomenon of eye-closure-triggered myoclonia does not occur in the dark, implying that it is a photosensitive phenomenon rather than simply related to physical closure of the eyelids. This is a childhood-onset syndrome and patients may manifest absence seizures both with and without the eyelid myoclonia. GTC seizures occasionally occur. Although eyelid myoclonia is highly characteristic of EMA/Jeavons syndrome, the phenomenon may also be occasionally encountered outside of the syndrome.

Unknown Onset

In some cases the onset of a seizure cannot be ascertained. A straightforward example of this is the generalized tonic-clonic seizure where the beginning of the seizure is not observed. It may have begun focally on one side of the body, or it may have had a bilateral onset, but if there are no reports of how it started, the onset is unknown. Later, it is possible that the onset will be ascertained, perhaps with a subsequent seizure seen to begin on one side, the EEG showing a clear unilateral focus, or the MRI showing a clear epileptogenic lesion, which would then allow the onset to be classified as focal. The classification makes clear that the term *unknown* does not apply to the situation where it is unknown that an event was a seizure, but only to an epileptic seizure with unknown onset.

There are also a few potential seizure types that do not easily fit into the foregoing focal versus generalized dichotomy. These would include seizure semiologies such as swimming or bicycling movements, apneas, or roving eye movements. In fact, it is unclear whether many of these behaviors necessarily represent direct epileptic phenomena. As previously discussed, some of these behaviors may represent automatic movements (automatisms) rather than seizure activity directly driven by an epileptic seizure discharge. The nature of such events therefore remains to be clarified. Infantile spasms (or epileptic spasms) also represent a seizure type that is not easily classified. Epileptic spasms are usually associated with a generalized EEG discharge but it is well known that in some cases, focal lesions may also cause what seem to be generalized epileptic spasms and, once the lesion in these cases is surgically resected, the spasms may be cured (see the later section on West syndrome).

Neonatal Seizures

Although the classification paradigm for neonatal seizures generally parallels the classification presented here for other age groups, there are some differences. A discussion of the classification of neonatal seizures can be found in Chapter 13, "The Electroencephalogram of the Newborn."

CLASSIFICATION OF EPILEPSY SYNDROMES

Epilepsy syndromes are defined by the "big picture" of the patient's seizure disorder. This may include the type or types of seizures experienced, age of onset, neurologic status (abnormal neurologic status before or after seizure onset), progression, cognitive status, family history, physical examination, and EEG patterns seen. In some cases, genetic testing may suggest a specific syndromic diagnosis. Identification of a particular seizure syndrome will often suggest possible treatments and a specific prognosis. The importance of correct identification of a seizure syndrome is evident when you consider that for certain seizure syndromes, specific medications are known to be quite effective and certain other medications may actually be known to make the seizures worse. Select seizure syndromes are discussed below, generally in order of age of onset.

Developmental and Epileptic Encephalopathies (DEE)

The central concept of epileptic encephalopathy is that the patient's seizures themselves contribute to cognitive decline. To consider a counterexample, before effective treatment was available, some individuals with childhood absence epilepsy would have dozens of absence seizures per day and could continue to have the seizures over a period of years or even decades, yet they did not experience a fundamental cognitive decline. By contrast, in individuals with disorders in the epileptic encephalopathy group, the epileptic process itself is

felt to contribute to the intellectual decline. Unfortunately, this conceptualization of epileptic encephalopathy is not as simple as this. The definition might lead one to believe that, if one succeeded in eliminating the seizures completely in an individual with an epileptic encephalopathy (a theoretical goal that unfortunately is not usually practicably achievable), cognitive status might become normal or at least improve significantly. Recognizing that many of the epileptic encephalopathies are caused by genetic syndromes that may have severe developmental consequences even in the minority of cases where seizures are absent, the term *epileptic encephalopathy* was expanded to *developmental and epileptic encephalopathy* or DEE—acknowledging the fact that in many of these syndromes the disability may be caused both by the ongoing epileptic activity and the underlying developmental disorder.

Epileptic Syndromes of Early Infancy Associated with a Burst-Suppression Pattern

Early myoclonic epilepsy (EME) and early infantile epileptic encephalopathy (EIEE) are the two major catastrophic epilepsies of early infancy. Although these two syndromes have much in common, it appears that they represent two distinct entities, albeit with considerable overlap.

Early Myoclonic Encephalopathy

Infants with EME present soon after birth with both fragmentary and massive myoclonic seizures. In some cases, mothers report that they felt the seizure movements before delivery. Other seizure types also occur. The magnetic resonance imaging (MRI) scan at birth is almost always normal, and a large fraction of these babies are eventually found to have a specific metabolic disorder, nonketotic hyperglycinemia (NKH). Those babies with EME who do not prove to have NKH may have other inborn errors of metabolism, and an ever-lengthening list of genetic abnormalities has more recently been associated with EME. Babies with EME tend to have anatomically normal brains at birth by MRI, and there is usually no history of a previous neurological injury. Babies with EME go on to have complete developmental failure and the seizures tend to be refractory to treatment. Later in the course, tonic seizures may occur as well. The EEG shows an unremitting burst-suppression pattern that may continue unabated through childhood (Figure 10.19).

Early Infantile Epileptic Encephalopathy

EIEE, also known as *Ohtahara syndrome*, initially was thought to be a "lesional" epilepsy syndrome that, in contrast to EME, was often associated with an abnormal MRI scan. More recently, several genetic etiologies have been established for EIEE as well. Thus, the EIEE phenotype is now understood to be caused by both structural lesions in the brain and genetic abnormalities. Tonic spasms are the hallmark seizure type, and are more prominent in EIEE compared with EME. Erratic myoclonus does not tend to occur. MRI abnormalities associated with this syndrome can include cerebral malformations, or cerebral injuries as may occur in babies with hypoxic-ischemic encephalopathy. Therefore, EIEE often occurs as

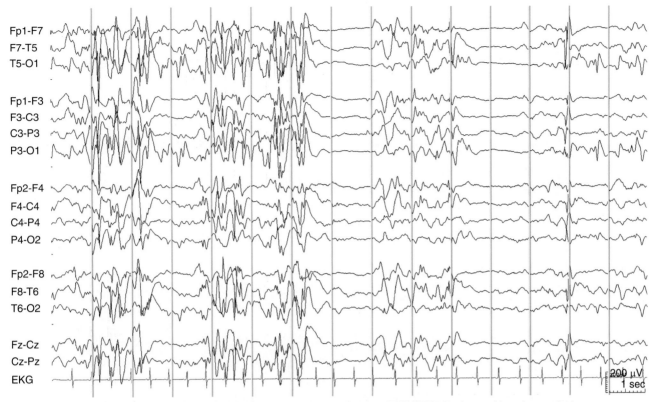

Figure 10.19 A dramatic burst-suppression pattern is seen in the EEG of this newborn with early myoclonic epilepsy (EME). No sleep cycling occurred in this recording, and every page of the record showed the same burst-suppression pattern. In patients with EME, this discontinuous pattern may persist for years.

an epileptic syndrome that is symptomatic of a preexisting abnormality, be it a cerebral malformation or some type of brain injury. In other cases the MRI is normal and there is a genetic underpinning. EIEE is more likely to evolve to West syndrome or the Lennox-Gastaut syndrome.

Like EME, EIEE is typically associated with a burst-suppression pattern on EEG. The EEG patterns of EIEE and EME are not easily distinguished without the benefit of the clinical history (Figure 10.20), though mild differences have been proposed. The amplitude of the interburst periods may be more suppressed in EME, and the burst-suppression pattern more often occurs independent of sleep state. In EIEE, there is more of a tendency for the burst-suppression pattern to occur more prominently in sleep compared to wakefulness. The burst-suppression pattern of EIEE is more likely to evolve into other EEG background patterns later in life, compared with the EME burst-suppression pattern, which may persist indefinitely.

Therefore, despite the many aspects they share in common (similar EEG pattern, intractable seizures, poor prognosis), EIEE distinguishes itself from EME in that in EIEE some cases are caused by an acquired lesion or cerebral malformation. In contrast, children with EME are believed to have the disorder on a genetic or biochemical basis rather than from a postnatal or acquired event. In EME, MRI brain anatomy is typically normal. Although the prognosis is poor

in both disorders, it can be somewhat better in EIEE compared to EME.

The Concept of the Age-Dependent Epileptic Encephalopathies

EIEE is considered one of the age-dependent epileptic encephalopathies. The idea is that there is a different characteristic epileptic response of the brain to injury depending on the age of the patient. For instance, when the brain expresses its reaction to an injury in the neonatal period, the response may present as the EIEE syndrome as described here. When the epileptic response to an injury or abnormality begins later in infancy (typically after 3 months of age), the child may develop a pattern of infantile spasms or West syndrome (discussed later). The epileptic response to an injury that manifests after 3 years of age may present as the Lennox-Gastaut syndrome (also discussed later). Because different maturational states of the brain are only associated with certain syndromic patterns, West syndrome does not present in adults, and Lennox-Gastaut syndrome cannot present in early infancy. Presumably, because of the way the human brain matures, it cannot mount those types of seizure patterns at those ages.

Pyridoxine-Dependent Epilepsy

The syndrome of pyridoxine-dependent epilepsy is extremely rare in its pure form. In the classic presentation of this

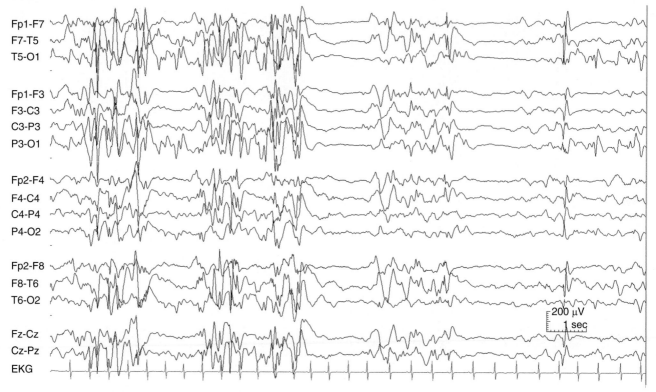

Figure 10.20 The burst-suppression pattern of a newborn patient with EIEE shown in this figure is essentially indistinguishable from the patterns seen in EME. In EIEE, however, eventual evolution to other patterns over months or years is not uncommon.

disorder, a newborn is found to have refractory seizures associated with a persistent burst-suppression pattern on EEG. Administration of pyridoxine, sometimes in high doses, abruptly breaks the abnormal EEG pattern and promptly terminates the seizure activity. Without continued supplementation with pyridoxine, the seizures will relapse. Because this is such an easily treatable form of what would otherwise be a catastrophic epilepsy, pyridoxine infusion is routinely carried out on newborns with seizures that potentially match the phenotype of this disorder (in particular, those having a burst-suppression pattern on EEG without other explanation). Variant presentations of pyridoxine-dependent epilepsy exist, even without a burst-suppression pattern on EEG, but are even less commonly encountered.

Benign Familial Neonatal Convulsions and Benign Neonatal Convulsions

Benign familial neonatal convulsions (BFNC) and benign neonatal convulsions are the two important benign seizure syndromes of the newborn. With the goal of eliminating the term *benign* from the classification of epilepsy syndromes, the terms *self-limited familial neonatal epilepsy* and *self-limited neonatal epilepsy* have been proposed to replace these names. The essence of both of these seizure syndromes is similar: seizures early in the newborn period in a previously well infant followed by a generally benign outcome. Although these two syndromes have significant similarities, they are discussed separately.

Benign Neonatal Convulsions

The syndrome of benign neonatal convulsions is also known to as "fifth day fits," a name that serves as a useful reminder that the fifth day of life is the most common age of onset for the seizures seen in this syndrome. To some extent, the diagnosis of benign neonatal convulsions must be made in retrospect because a benign long-term course is a key feature of the syndrome. Still, the diagnosis can be strongly suspected when there is a typical presentation of convulsions occurring in a newborn who appears normal at birth and who may have already been uneventfully discharged home from the hospital. (This is in distinction to the typical story of babies with neonatal seizures presenting soon after delivery, sometimes after an asphyxial event, whose seizure presentation would prevent early discharge from the hospital.) The seizures begin in the first week of life, with the most common age of incidence being the fifth day of life; 90% of babies present between the fourth and sixth days of life. The seizures tend to alternate sides and generally subside by the second month or earlier, followed by continued normal development.

The family history for seizures is negative. There is no antecedent history of a difficult delivery or birth injury, and neuroimaging is normal. Apart from possible mild hypotonia, the interictal examination is normal. A search for central nervous system infection is negative and no electrolyte or other metabolic disturbances are found. The clinician is left with a story of an otherwise perfectly well newborn with unexplained onset of seizures in whom all testing is normal.

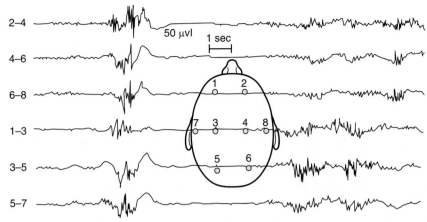

Figure 10.21 Théta pointu alternant, or alternating sharp theta, may be seen in each central area in both the syndromes of benign neonatal convulsions and benign familial neonatal convulsions. (Modified from Dehan M, Quillerou D, Navelet Y, et al. Convulsions in the fifth day of life: a new syndrome? Arch Fr Pediatr 1977;34:730–742).

In babies with benign neonatal convulsions, the EEG background pattern tends to be normal. A characteristic EEG finding has been described in such babies, termed théta pointu alternant. This is a pattern of sharpened theta waves occurring in brief runs, typically in each central area, and alternating sides (Figure 10.21). Although this pattern is said to occur in the majority of patients with this seizure syndrome, it may be difficult to identify, and its presence is not necessarily diagnostic of benign neonatal convulsions.

Whether or not benign neonatal convulsions represents a single, distinct syndrome has been questioned. From one point of view, it should not be a surprise that if you consider the entire group of all newborns with seizures and then separate out the subgroup that has a negative history and normal testing, that that group would have a more favorable outcome than newborns with seizures who have abnormal histories or testing. In fact, at least in some babies with benign neonatal convulsions the seizures may be caused by de novo changes in the genes that are known to cause the familial form of the syndrome (see below). There also does appear to be an incidence of later epilepsy in these infants that is higher than that of the unaffected population.

Benign Familial Neonatal Convulsions

The syndrome of benign (or self-limited) familial neonatal convulsions (BFNC) has many elements in common with the previously described syndrome of benign neonatal convulsions. As the name implies, however, in such babies there is a positive history of seizures in the newborn period in other family members. In this syndrome, the seizures may begin slightly earlier, typically on the second or third day of life, usually resolving by the second month. Moreso than in the case of benign neonatal convulsions, in BFNC an increased risk for later life epilepsy appears to have been more clearly demonstrated. Also, mild developmental problems may occur with a slightly increased frequency compared with the unaffected population. The majority of kindreds have an abnormality in the KCNQ2 gene,

and a smaller number in KCNQ3, both potassium-channel genes. Other genes also appear to be involved less frequently.

The typical seizure in BFNC is the clonic seizure, preceded by tonic stiffening and apnea in some (Hirsch et al., 1993). Most commonly the interictal EEG is normal; however, the théta pointu alternant pattern, as has been described in benign neonatal convulsions, has also been reported in some babies with this syndrome.

Febrile Seizures

Febrile seizures are seizures that occur with fever during childhood in the absence of CNS infection. There are mild variations in the age range that various groups have used to define febrile seizures of childhood, with ranges such as 3 months to 5 years and 1 month to 6 years being used. These stated age ranges are somewhat misleading in that it is uncommon for febrile seizures to *start* at the end of these age ranges; usually when a febrile seizure occurs after the age of 4 years, the child has already had previous episodes. The large majority of affected children have had the first febrile seizure by 3 years of age. According to the definition, the seizure should not have been caused by central nervous system infection, and children with previous unprovoked seizures are also excluded by the definition. In general, the fever should exceed 38.4°C (101°F), but this cutoff is flexible. The diagnosis of febrile seizures is usually made in a normal-appearing child with a normal central nervous system. Nevertheless, there is no reason that children with preexisting neurologic abnormalities should be any less prone to febrile seizures than their normal counterparts, leaving the underlying cause of the seizures more difficult to sort out in this group.

Although one may speak of a "febrile seizure syndrome," febrile seizures are not considered an example of an epilepsy syndrome. Epilepsy is defined as a tendency to recurrent, unprovoked seizures and because the presence of fever is considered a provocative factor, febrile seizures are not considered examples of epileptic (unprovoked) seizures.

Febrile seizures are common. They occur in 3% to 5% of all children and, in the large majority, disappear during childhood. Only 2% to 4% of children with febrile seizures are destined to have future seizures without fever (epilepsy). On the other hand, fever is known to be a common seizure-triggering factor for persons who do have epilepsy, and the question may arise as to whether an apparent febrile seizure episode might represent a first epileptic seizure that happened to be triggered by fever in a child who is destined to have epilepsy.

It is known that certain features of a febrile seizure episode increase the odds that a child will later develop epilepsy. A febrile seizure is termed a complex febrile seizure when one or more "complex" features are present. These complex features have been defined by epidemiologic studies that have found these factors to be associated with an increased risk for developing later afebrile seizures (epilepsy). They include seizure duration longer than 10 or 15 minutes, focal (as opposed to generalized) febrile seizures, or two or more febrile seizure episodes within a 24-hour period. The more of these "complex" features a child has, the higher the risk for developing later epilepsy. Still, the majority of children who have even more than one of these complex factors do not go on to develop later epilepsy. A preexisting abnormal neurological status at the time of seizure onset and a positive family history of epilepsy also independently increase the chance of later epilepsy in a child with febrile seizures (as they also would in children who do not have febrile seizures).

A relationship between febrile seizures and temporal lobe epilepsy has long been suspected. Case-control studies of individuals with temporal lobe epilepsy appear to show an increased incidence of a history of febrile seizures, particularly prolonged febrile seizures, in temporal lobe epilepsy patients compared with control subjects. These findings suggest the possibility that prolonged febrile seizures may cause hippocampal damage (hippocampal sclerosis) and predispose to later temporal lobe epilepsy. An alternative interpretation is that those children destined to have temporal lobe epilepsy later in life may automatically be more prone to prolonged febrile seizures in childhood and that the early febrile seizures may not have been the *cause* of the later epilepsy. Finally, there is some worry about ascertainment bias, that patients with temporal lobe epilepsy and their families are more likely to recall febrile seizure episodes from childhood compared to control patients who do not have epilepsy. Still, the association between prolonged febrile seizures and later temporal lobe epilepsy does appear to be fairly strong.

The Role of EEG in the Evaluation of Febrile Seizures

Despite the fact that EEG abnormalities may be seen in children with febrile seizures, the EEG has not proven to be a particularly useful tool in predicting which children with febrile seizures will go on to develop epilepsy. When an EEG is obtained, the most common epileptiform abnormality found in children with febrile seizures is generalized spike-wave discharges. This pattern is, of course, nonspecific in that it is also seen in the generalized epilepsies, but some feel it also may serve as a specific marker for a tendency to febrile seizures. It may come as a surprise that its

presence in the EEG of a child with febrile seizures has not been shown to predict an increased risk for later epilepsy. Increased slowing, especially in the posterior quadrants, may be expected within a few days of a febrile seizure. In general, because the EEG has not been found to be useful in predicting later epilepsy in children with febrile seizures, EEG testing is not routinely indicated in the evaluation of febrile seizures, including complex febrile seizures. Indeed, it is not clear what one would do with an abnormal EEG result after a febrile seizure. If generalized spike wave is found, the abnormality may simply represent a marker for febrile seizures as described above. Even if another type of EEG abnormality were found, the child still would not have a diagnosis of epilepsy and initiating treatment with antiseizure medications would not be appropriate. Except in exceptional cases, daily antiepileptic medications are not indicated in children with febrile seizures.

Infantile Spasms and West Syndrome

Although the terms infantile spasms and West syndrome are sometimes used interchangeably, infantile spasms is best used to refer to a seizure type (most often, but not exclusively seen as a part of West syndrome) and West syndrome to an epilepsy syndrome. Because infantile spasms can persist past infancy, the term *epileptic spasms* has also been introduced to refer to this seizure type, mostly to avoid the awkwardness of using the term *infantile* for a seizure type a person might have who is well past infancy. The term *West syndrome* denotes a syndrome consisting of the triad of infantile spasms, an EEG pattern of hypsarrhythmia, and neurodevelopmental abnormality in childhood. The original clinical description of this syndrome appears in a letter to *Lancet* by Dr. W. J. West in 1841, who first described this seizure syndrome in his own son, requesting advice on its treatment from the medical community. More recently, the term "Infantile Spasms Syndrome" has been proposed to replace West Syndrome.

The hallmark seizures of West syndrome are infantile spasms. Infantile spasms may occur as flexor spasms, extensor spasms, or mixed (asymmetrical) spasms. Flexor spasms are the most common form, consisting of a brief tonic contraction in flexion of the body on the hips, flexion of the head on the chest, and tensing of the shoulders and upper arms, sometimes in abduction. Because of the flexed position attained during the seizures, these episodes have also been referred to as "jackknife seizures" or "salaam seizures." The position is typically held for approximately one second, followed by relaxation. The individual spasms tend to occur in clusters; a series of repeat spasms may last several minutes, each separated by a brief interval. Less commonly, spasms can result in extensor rather than flexor posturing. The presence of asymmetrical spasms should always prompt a search for an underlying focal lesion. Other, milder variants of spasms can be seen, including relatively subtle bobbing of the head with upward eye deviation and milder shoulder movement. These milder expressions of spasms may also be seen in partially treated children. Because epileptic spasms are seen in both apparently generalized and focal forms, this seizure type defies easy categorization into one group or the other. Infantile spasms are occasionally erroneously classified as myoclonic seizures, but the episodes are not consistent with the lightning-like jolt that is the definition of myoclonus. Rather, the clinical spasm usually lasts approximately one second, too long to be classified as myoclonus.

The infantile spasms of West syndrome can be surprisingly difficult to diagnose. Because West syndrome is a rare disorder, many pediatricians and family practice providers have not personally encountered this seizure type in their clinical practice. The tensing up seen during infantile spasms can mimic gastrointestinal discomfort or episodes of colic. Often, the primary care physician does not have the opportunity to witness the seizures personally but must rely on a verbal description of flexing up of the knees followed by crying, a history that may not initially suggest seizures. Features of the history that increase the suspicion of infantile spasms include the short duration of the individual tensing movements, the tendency for the episodes to cluster, and the predilection for the clusters to occur in the period after awakening from sleep.

The spasms of West Syndrome usually begin between the ages of 3 and 18 months. Only rarely is onset of this seizure type seen outside of childhood. In many, the seizures resolve spontaneously but may be replaced later by other seizure types, such as focal seizures or the mixed seizures of the Lennox-Gastaut syndrome. Only a relatively small minority of patients are intellectually normal after developing infantile spasms and hypsarrhythmia.

EEG in the Diagnosis of Infantile Spasms and West Syndrome

Because West syndrome has distinctive ictal and interictal EEG signatures, electroencephalography is a fundamental tool in the diagnosis of infantile spasms and West syndrome. EEG helps establish the diagnosis of infantile spasms, either by identifying the characteristic interictal pattern of West syndrome (i.e., hypsarrhythmia) or by recording the spasms and demonstrating an ictal discharge during the events. EEG may also be used to monitor the success of treatment.

The EEG term *hypsarrhythmia* is derived from the Greek meaning "high" or "lofty" rhythm. In fact, some of the highest voltages measured in electroencephalography are seen in babies with hypsarrhythmia. Compared with adult EEGs in which voltages typically do not exceed $200\,\mu V$, hypsarrhythmia EEGs may exceed $1\,mV$ $(1,000\,\mu V)$. The essential features of the hypsarrhythmic pattern are high voltage and chaos. In this context, chaos refers to the opposite of synchrony or predictability. A completely chaotic EEG pattern is a pattern in which different electrical events and rhythms are occurring in different brain regions at different times in an unsynchronized and seemingly unrelated fashion. In contrast, the generalized spike-wave discharge, although abnormal, represents a pattern with a very high degree of synchrony with all cortical areas acting in unison. In the chaotic hypsarrhythmia pattern, rapid spikes, high-voltage slow waves, and other abnormalities may occur in scattered locations at different times and in a seemingly random fashion (Figure 10.22). Intermediate states between synchrony and complete chaos are also seen (Figure 10.23).

Activation by sleep is an important feature of the hypsarrhythmia pattern. In fact, in some individuals the waking tracing can be relatively normal with the EEG only blossoming into the highly abnormal hypsarrhythmia pattern after the patient falls asleep (Figure 10.24).

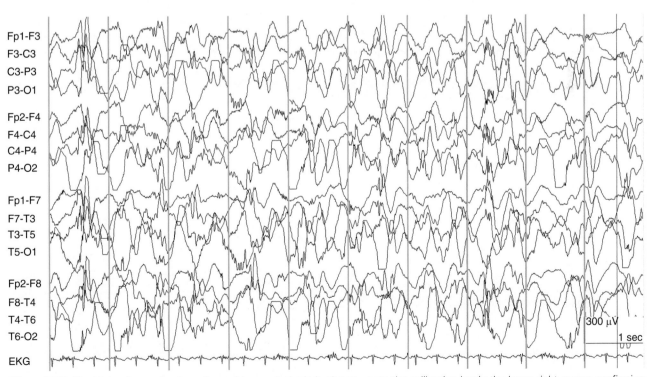

Figure 10.22 The high-voltage, chaotic pattern of hypsarrhythmia is shown—note the calibration bar in the lower right corner, confirming the high-voltage pattern. "Random delta" activity and scattered spikes are seen, occurring both singly and in brief runs in a chaotic fashion.

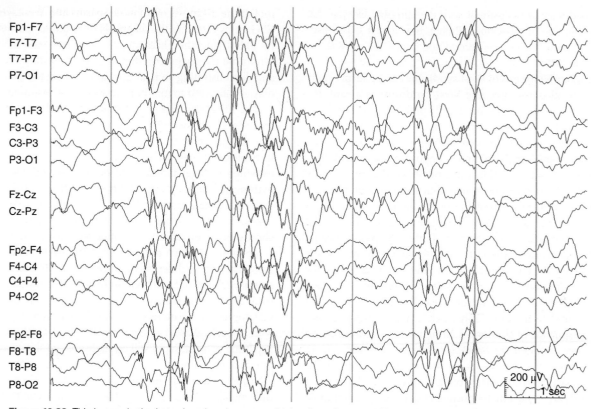

Figure 10.23 This hypsarrhythmia tracing also shows very high-voltage bursts and intermixed spikes. The pattern is somewhat less chaotic than the previous figure as the bursts show more bilateral synchrony. In the fifth second of the tracing, sleep spindles can be identified.

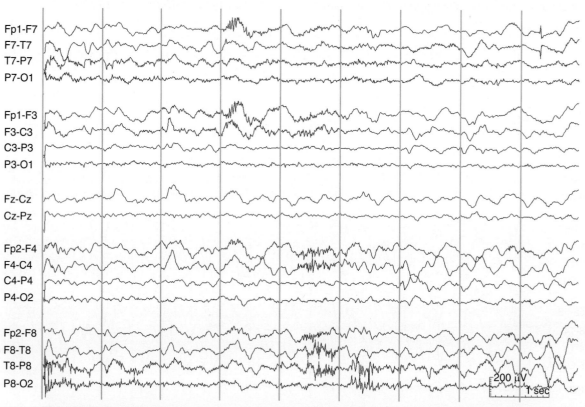

Figure 10.24 The EEG of the same patient whose hypsarrhythmia pattern was shown in Figure 10.21 is seen during wakefulness. While awake, almost all evidence of the hypsarrhythmia has cleared. The EEG diagnosis of hypsarrhythmia would almost certainly have been missed if this infant had not been recorded during sleep.

It can be challenging to describe the intensity of a hypsarrhythmia pattern in words. The hypsarrhythmia scoring system designed by Jeavons and Bower (1961; Table 10.1) is a useful reminder of the various parameters of chaos and high voltage that are scrutinized during analysis of the hypsarrhythmic EEG. Note that the main factors are degree of chaos, magnitude of voltage, amount of bursting, number of locations of focal spiking, and presence of asynchronous delta activity. This scoring system is not in common use today but is presented here because its parameters reflect a well-thought-out picture of the features of hypsarrhythmia. Other scoring systems have been proposed more recently, but none yet has gained general acceptance as the standard.

EEG Recording of Infantile Spasm Events

Recording a hypsarrhythmia pattern is usually adequate to confirm the diagnosis of West syndrome in an infant with a history suggestive of infantile spasms. Because the seizures occur so frequently, often with multiple clusters per day that may show linkage to the sleep-wake cycle, it is often possible to record the seizures themselves on EEG. In centers with adequate resources, infants may have prolonged or overnight recordings to directly establish the diagnosis by demonstrating the seizures on EEG and video. The ictal pattern associated with infantile spasms can vary, but most often it is seen as a "complex" or "poorly-organized" slow wave of moderate or high voltage and approximately one second's duration followed by very low-voltage rapid spikes. The slow-wave portion of the discharge is termed complex here because the phase of the wave is often flipped up and down in different channels in a way that defies a single, accurate localization. Because the infant is tensing up during the seizure and the rapid spikes, if present, are of low voltage, muscle artifact may obliterate some of the low-voltage rapid spiking activity in some recordings. At times the ictal correlate may only consist of a slow wave followed by a brief, relative flattening of the background pattern. In other examples, the slow wave is not evident and only a simple flattening is seen (Figures 10.25 and 10.26). Additional "EMG electrodes" (EEG electrodes placed over muscles to record electrical muscle activity associated with muscle contractions) can be placed on shoulder or neck muscles to record the distinctive diamond-shaped muscle burst that occurs with the spasm. Because it always takes some amount of time for the cerebral discharge to propagate from cortex to the body and cause the spasm, there should always be some time latency between the onset of the poorly-organized slow wave and the muscle burst associated with the spasm. If a muscle burst is seen in the EEG at the exact same time as or even before the slow wave deflection, the slow wave deflection may represent motion artifact rather than an epileptic discharge. This is an important point because tensing movements that are non-epileptic will show the muscle burst and motion artifact (which may also resemble a poorly-organized slow wave) at the very same time. With true epileptic spasms, the high-voltage slow wave should *precede* the body movement (which it is causing) by approximately 100 milliseconds or more.

Because the hypsarrhythmia pattern is an interictal pattern (i.e., seen between seizures), the electrographic seizure pattern of infantile spasms may interrupt the high-voltage, chaotic hypsarrhythmic pattern resulting in a relative flattening in the EEG at the time of the seizures (Figure 10.27). This type of transition from high-voltage background to low-voltage seizure pattern contrasts with the more common occurrence of non-spasm seizure discharges that often attain a higher voltage than the background from which they arise.

Modified Hypsarrhythmia

The term modified hypsarrhythmia has been used for EEG patterns that share many of the characteristics of full-blown hypsarrhythmia but do not meet the chaos or voltage criteria that would qualify as a fully hypsarrhythmic pattern. Some have attempted to create a classification of modified hypsarrhythmias; however, such classifications are cumbersome as there are so many ways that an EEG pattern can be similar to (but not quite a classic example of) frank hypsarrhythmia. Rather than simply using the nonspecific term *modified hypsarrhythmia* as if it referred to a specific entity, it is more useful to describe exactly what variations are seen from the classic pattern.

One common variation of hypsarrhythmia is presence of the pattern only during sleep. In these patients, the waking EEG pattern is not particularly remarkable but may show a few epileptiform discharges (Figure 10.24). As the child falls asleep, the pattern blossoms into the typical high-voltage, chaotic pattern. The hypsarrhythmia pattern may also be suppressed during rapid eye movement (REM) sleep. For these reasons, it is mandatory that a portion of the recording be obtained in slow-wave sleep before excluding the presence of hypsarrhythmia. Another less common but noteworthy variant of hypsarrhythmia is hemi-hypsarrhythmia. In hemi-hypsarrhythmia, the hypsarrhythmia pattern is essentially confined to a single hemisphere. When present, this pattern should prompt a search for a focal lesion.

West Syndrome as an Age-Dependent Epileptic Encephalopathy

Because onset of the combination of hypsarrhythmia and spasms in West syndrome is only seen during a specific age range, West syndrome is considered one of the age-dependent epileptic encephalopathies. As discussed earlier, the idea behind the concept of the age-dependent encephalopathies is that the brain mounts a characteristic pattern of response to the abnormal or injured state based on the age of the individual. EME and EIEE (Ohtahara syndrome) are the earliest age-dependent patterns and are seen in very early infancy, at ages before West syndrome typically presents. Lennox-Gastaut syndrome, described later, is an age-dependent encephalopathy seen in later childhood and adulthood and may appear after the resolution of West syndrome in some cases.

Benign (Self-Limited) Focal Epilepsies of Childhood

The benign focal epilepsies of childhood are a group of seizure disorders associated with normal neurodevelopmental status, normal neuroimaging, a favorable long-term outcome,

TABLE 10.1   Hypsarrhythmia Scoring System (Jeavons and Bower)

GRADE	
Grade 1: 12 points	Complete chaos with total asynchrony, no organized discharges, and no normal background activity.
Grade 2: 8 points	Chaos, with some discernible synchronous bursts. The bursts are of chaotic makeup, and the episodic nature can only be seen by reducing the gain.
Grade 3: 6 points	Mainly chaotic, but with more bilaterally synchronous activity than in Grade 2.
Grade 4: 4 points	Bursts of chaotic makeup, some bilaterally synchronous discharges and a little normal background activity.
Grade 5: 3 points	Discharges mainly bilaterally synchronous, but some showing a chaotic makeup. Some normal activity.
Grade 6: 1 point	Bilaterally synchronous epileptic discharges (centrencephalic). No chaos. Normal background activity.
Grade 7: 1 point	Focal epileptic discharges. No chaos. Normal background activity.
Grade 8: 1 point	Nonspecific abnormality.
Grade 9: 0 points	Normal.
Voltage: 0–4 points	
100–200 µV	1 point
200–400 µV	2 points
>500 µV	4 points
Bursts of Very Chaotic Makeup containing delta waves from 0.75 to 3 Hz, with spikes of varying site and amplitude:	2 points
Bursts of Slow or Rapid Spikes appearing simultaneously in all regions:	2 points
Focal Spikes 0–4 points	
1 point each for:	
Left	1 point
Right	1 point
Anterior	1 point
Posterior	1 point
Completely Random Spikes	4 points
Completely Random Delta	2 points
Normal Background Activity	−1 point
HYPSARRHYTHMIA	13–30 points
MODIFIED HYPSARRHYTHMIA	9–12 points
EPILEPTIC (CENTRENCEPHALIC)	2–8 points
NORMAL OR NONSPECIFIC	0 or 1 point

Adapted from Jeavons P, Bower B: The natural history of infantile spasms. *Arch Dis Childhood* 36:17–22, 1961.

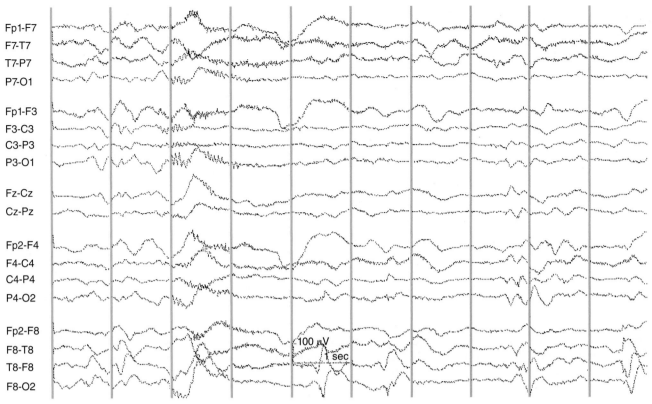

Figure 10.25 The rapid spikes seen in the third second of this tracing are associated with an infantile spasm. In some examples, the large slow wave at the onset of the seizure is more prominent. This seizure pattern could be easy to miss if this tracing were scanned too quickly. An abrupt suppression of voltage, often with superimposed rapid spikes, is the key finding in the infantile spasm seizure pattern. This pattern must be distinguished from simple arousals, which are also associated with an abrupt reduction in voltage.

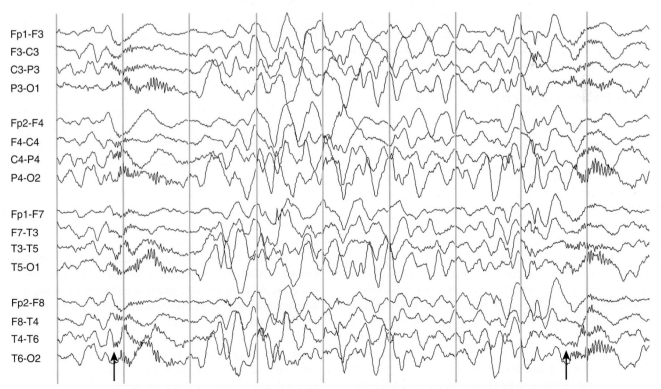

Figure 10.26 Two separate runs of rapid spikes associated with infantile spasms are seen (arrows) against the backdrop of a hypsarrhythmic EEG. This page was recorded in the middle of a cluster of spasms.

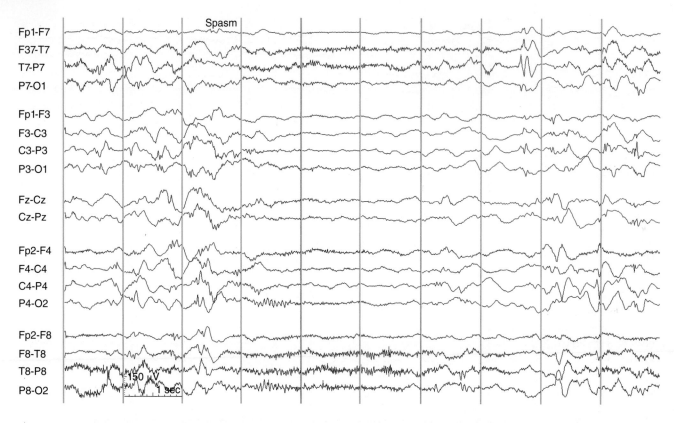

Figure 10.27 The initial clue to the occurrence of this infantile spasm is the abrupt flattening of the previous hypsarrhythmic pattern. Closer analysis shows two seconds of diffuse, rapid spikes. Although the rapid spikes are helpful in ascertaining the seizure pattern of infantile spasms, they are not always visible.

and a specific age range of occurrence. This is a group of disorders that are believed to be genetically based and are often associated with distinctive EEG patterns. It has recently been proposed that the term *benign* be replaced by *self-limited* in the official nomenclature for these epilepsy syndromes (discussed further below), so both terms will likely persist and both are used interchangeably in this text.

In contrast to the large number of focal epilepsies that are caused by one or more distinct cortical lesions such as an area of injury or dysplasia, the self-limited focal epilepsies of childhood (SeLFEs in the new nomenclature) are considered non-lesional; no causative abnormalities are seen either on imaging or on pathologic examination. In the benign focal epilepsy syndromes, bilateral independent seizure onsets and bilateral independent EEG abnormalities are commonplace. This type of symmetrically bilateral presentation would not be expected in a lesional epilepsy presenting in a typically developing child because such a pattern would imply the presence of symmetrical cortical lesions in both hemispheres, a relatively unlikely occurrence in an otherwise neurodevelopmentally normal child. For this reason, when bilateral focal or even multifocal discharges are seen during childhood in the right clinical setting, particularly in a child with a normal neurodevelopmental status, the diagnosis of a benign focal epilepsy of childhood should be considered.

The two most common forms of benign or self-limited focal epilepsy of childhood are benign childhood epilepsy with centrotemporal spikes (BCECTS; also known as benign rolandic epilepsy, and as more recently proposed, self-limited epilepsy with centrotemporal spikes or SeLECTS) and benign childhood epilepsy with occipital paroxysms (BCEOP, but as more recently proposed, self-limited occipital epilepsy of childhood). These two benign focal epilepsy syndromes are now discussed in more detail.

Benign Rolandic Epilepsy or Benign Childhood Epilepsy with Centrotemporal Spikes, or Self-Limited Epilepsy with Centrotemporal Spikes

Benign rolandic epilepsy (or Benign Childhood Epilepsy with Centrotemporal Spikes, abbreviated BCECTS but pronounced "*bects*") is one of the most common forms of childhood epilepsy. The term rolandic epilepsy is based on the most frequent localization of the EEG spikes in this syndrome to the region of the rolandic sulcus (Figure 10.28). By linguistic coincidence, the initial description of the syndrome was made by a Bavarian physician, Martinus Rulandus, and for that reason some favored the term *Rulandic seizures*, which is quite similar to the more commonly used term, rolandic seizures. Several other synonyms for this seizure type exist, including sylvian seizures, based on the localization of the discharges to the area around the Sylvian fissure. The EEG spikes of benign rolandic epilepsy are usually centered around the central (C3 and C4) and/or midtemporal (T7 and T8) electrodes, hence the term *centrotemporal spikes*. In the most recent epilepsy classification, which seems to place

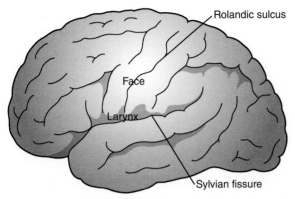

Figure 10.28 A lateral view of the left cerebral hemisphere shows the location of the rolandic (central) sulcus and the Sylvian fissure. The cortical areas for the larynx and face, which are near the Sylvian fissure, are shown.

a high value on pronounceable acronyms, the term *self-limited* is favored over *benign*, and it has been proposed to rename the syndrome *Self-Limited Epilepsy with Centrotemporal Spikes* and abbreviate it as SeLECTS. The committee explained that the term *benign* was replaced because this epilepsy type is associated with a somewhat higher rate of school, attentional, and occasionally language problems compared to unaffected children. Because, when they occur, these problems generally remit as the child grows out of this epilepsy syndrome, the syndrome can still be considered benign in the large majority of cases. In any case, both old and new nomenclatures are still in common use.

The Two Seizure Types of BCECTS (SeLECTS)

Two specific seizure types may occur in this seizure syndrome. The first is a focal seizure primarily involving the face, either with hemifacial clonic spasms or a pulling of the face to one side. Because the cortical representation of the larynx lies near the face area at the most inferior portion of the motor strip, the seizures also typically include speech arrest and the child may experience a choking sensation. Children who are old enough to do so often describe a sensory change inside the mouth or on the inside of the cheek at the onset of the seizure, presumably caused by the seizure discharge's involvement of the adjacent postcentral gyrus (face sensory area).

The focal seizures of rolandic epilepsy tend to occur in the early morning. The classic description is of a child who walks into her parents' room in the early morning with hemifacial clonic contractions, drooling, and unable to speak. Although the most characteristic time for these seizures to occur is in the early morning hours, the next most common time for children to experience these focal seizure episodes is soon after falling asleep. Less often, the focal seizures occur later in the day when the child is out and about, but this is the exception rather than the rule. Thus, the seizures only occasionally occur during school hours. When these spells occur during wakefulness, the children are usually fully aware of the seizure, even if they cannot respond during the event. More rarely the focal seizures in BCECTS may be associated with impaired awareness.

The second type of seizure associated with benign rolandic epilepsy is a grand mal convulsion that almost always occurs out of sleep, either during the night or less often during daytime naps. This means that if a child has a grand mal convulsion that begins out of wakefulness, the diagnosis of rolandic epilepsy is unlikely. Therefore, the focal seizures of BCECTS usually occur during wakefulness, most often in the morning, but more rarely can occur any time of day, and they also can occur out of sleep. The grand mal seizures of BCECTS occur during sleep with only very rare exceptions.

Age Range in BCECTS (SeLECTS)

Most rolandic seizures occur between the ages of 6 and 13 years and it is rare to see the seizures persist past 13 years of age in this syndrome. Of all seizure types and seizure syndromes, the seizures of benign rolandic epilepsy are the type that most reliably disappears with age (i.e., is "self-limited") and the only type for which the physician can more or less guarantee the patients and families that the seizures will "go away." Loiseau et al. (1988) were able to locate 168 of the 267 patients who were over age 20 years who they had earlier treated for rolandic epilepsy. Of these, 165 of the 168 were seizure-free; of the three with recurrences, two had only had a single additional seizure. The three cases of 168 who had experienced later seizures represents a prevalence rate that is not dramatically different from the rate of epilepsy seen in the general population.

EEG Findings in BCECTS (SeLECTS)

The EEG pattern seen in BCECTS is distinctive and this seizure syndrome is one of the few that has been named after its EEG finding. Typically, high-voltage spike-wave discharges are seen in the centrotemporal areas (C3/T7 and C4/T8). In a given patient, the discharge maximum may classically be seen in the central electrode, the midtemporal electrode, or it may be shared between the two (Figure 10.29). During wakefulness, the discharges may occur independently on each side; in sleep, the discharges often become bilaterally synchronous. It is particularly reassuring to find centrotemporal discharges over both sides of the brain when making the diagnosis of rolandic epilepsy, but in some patients the discharges are only recorded over a single hemisphere, a pattern that is still consistent with the diagnosis of BCECTS. In fact, such patients with unilateral discharges may have unilateral discharges seen only over the opposite hemisphere on the next recording. This ability of the discharges to switch sides or appear on both sides confirms the idea that benign rolandic epilepsy is not a lesional epilepsy but rather represents a genetic disorder. To say that a symmetrical, bilateral independent pattern is caused by a lesional epilepsy would imply that the patient has two separate lesions in the same brain location but on opposite sides, an unlikely occurrence, especially in an otherwise normally developing child.

Although, by far, centrotemporal spikes are the most common finding in benign rolandic epilepsy, other spike localizations may be seen less frequently. The most common alternate spike locations are the centroparietal areas (C3/P3 and C4/P4), the parietal areas (P3 and P4), and the central and parietal midline (Cz and Pz electrodes; Figure 10.30). Occipital discharges

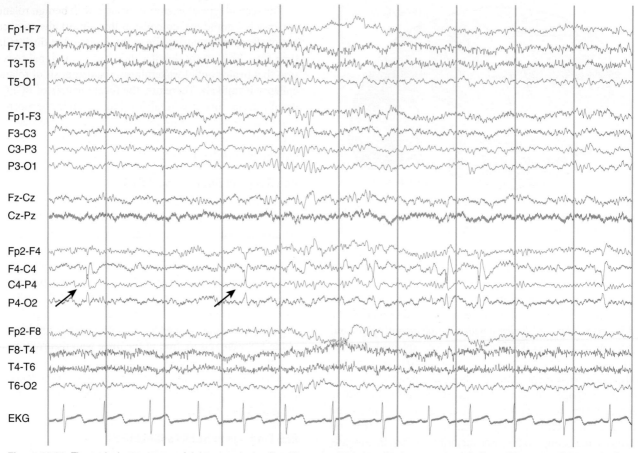

Figure 10.29 The typical appearance of right central rolandic spike-wave discharges is shown; two are indicated by arrows followed by four additional examples. These discharges are highly localized to the C4 electrode, but in other cases the discharge may be maximum in the midtemporal electrode, or the maximum may be shared between the two positions.

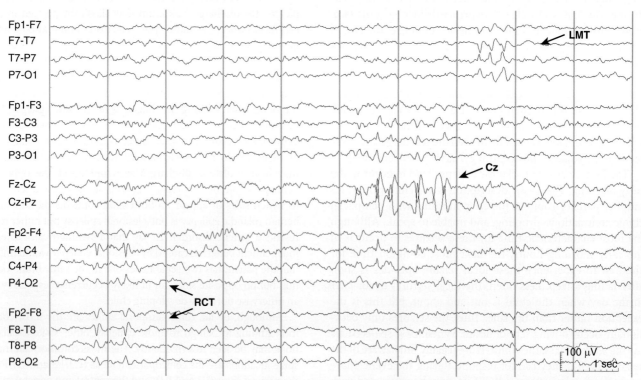

Figure 10.30 In addition to the more "standard" spike localizations in the right centrotemporal (RCT) and left midtemporal (LMT) areas, this 12-year-old boy also has spike-wave discharges in the central midline (Cz), a less common spike location for this syndrome.

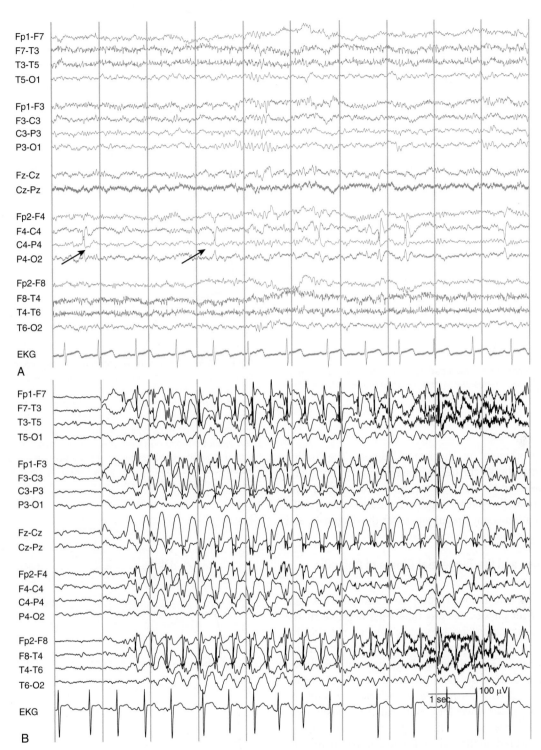

Figure 10.31 The first page (A) shows right central spike-wave complexes (arrows) in a patient with rolandic epilepsy. The second page (B) is recorded later in the same patient at sleep onset showing a run of generalized spike-wave discharges. Despite the apparent focal nature of rolandic epilepsy, many benign rolandic epilepsy patients manifest generalized spike-wave in the EEG at some point in their course. Despite the propensity to these generalized discharges, rolandic epilepsy patients rarely manifest frank absence seizures.

are known to occur with increased frequency along with the centrotemporal spikes of rolandic epilepsy. Certain spike localizations, such as the anterior temporal areas (F7 and F8), are not expected in BCECTS. Interestingly but somewhat unexpectedly, generalized spike-wave discharges frequently are also seen to

coexist with centrotemporal spikes in the EEGs of patients with BCECTS (Figure 10.31). This does not mean that absence seizures are expected in the BCECTS syndrome, however.

The centrotemporal spikes of rolandic epilepsy have a distinctive topography, referred to interchangeably as a

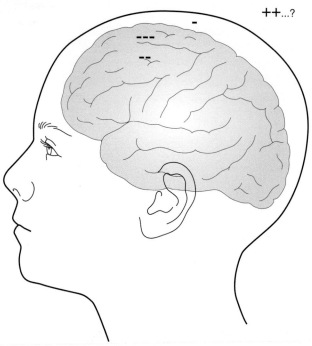

Figure 10.32 When a spike recorded from the scalp surface consists of pure negativities (minus signs), the question arises: where is the (unrecorded) counterbalancing positivity?

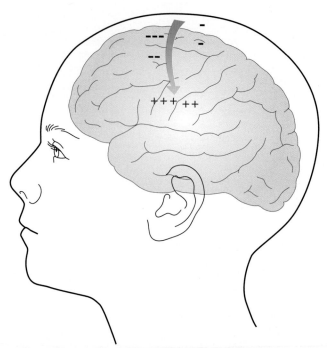

Figure 10.33 When pure negativities are recorded from the scalp surface, the "missing" positivities are presumed to lie at a location deeper in the brain. This implies the presence of a dipole that is oriented more or less parallel to one of the axes emanating from the brain's center—a so-called *radial orientation*. The "hidden" positivities are shown in lighter color, indicating that they are more deeply located and cannot be recorded from the scalp surface. The large majority of scalp-recorded epileptic spikes are oriented as radial dipoles, with a negativity recorded on the scalp and a simultaneous unrecorded positivity deeper in the brain.

"tangentially oriented" or "horizontal" dipole. The finding of a horizontal dipole further increases the certainty that a centrotemporal spike found in the EEG is associated with the benign rolandic epilepsy syndrome, though this specific dipole orientation is not a requirement for the diagnosis, and is only seen in about half of such cases.

Spike Dipoles and the Tangential Dipole of Rolandic Epilepsy

Considering the orientation of the dipole of any spike, it is clear from the laws of physics that any time a net negative charge is measured, there must be a counterbalancing net positive charge in some other location (Figure 10.32). In the practice of conventional EEG recording, the large majority of epileptic spikes manifest a negativity measured on the scalp, but no concurrent scalp positivity is measured. In such cases, it would be reasonable to wonder where the counterbalancing positivity is for the negativity measured on the scalp. When purely negative spikes are measured on the scalp, it is inferred that there must be an unmeasured positivity somewhere deep to the scalp. The simultaneous coexistence of a scalp negativity and a deep positivity implies a radially oriented dipole, by far the most common orientation of epileptic spikes (Figure 10.33).

In contrast, the dipole of the centrotemporal spikes of BCECTS often is not oriented in the direction of the more common radial dipoles just described, but rather manifests a tangential dipole. At the same time that a negativity is measured in the centrotemporal electrodes, a simultaneous positivity is measured in the anterior scalp electrodes (Figure 10.34). The simultaneous recording of a negativity in the

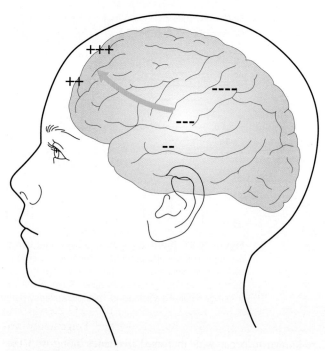

Figure 10.34 The classic discharge of benign rolandic epilepsy consists of a negativity recorded from the centrotemporal area and simultaneous positivities recorded from the anterior brain areas. This configuration of polarities suggests the presence of a dipole oriented tangent to the scalp as shown.

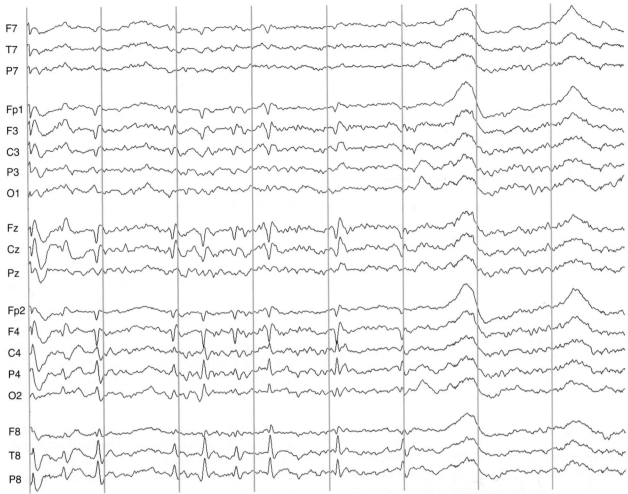

Figure 10.35 This EEG is recorded in a referential montage using the nose as the reference electrode. Negativities manifest as upgoing waves and the positivities as downgoing waves. The primary (highest voltage) negativity is seen in T8 with secondary negativities in P4 and P8. A still smaller amount of negativity is picked up by the O2 electrode. What distinguishes this discharge from most scalp-recorded spikes is the positive deflections recorded by the anterior electrodes: Fp2, F4, Fz, Cz, and Fp1 and F3. The simultaneous recording of a negative charge in one scalp location and a positive charge in another scalp location constitutes a tangential or "horizontal" dipole. The next figure shows a schematic representation of this dipole as viewed on the scalp from above.

centrotemporal area and a positivity in the frontal area implies an electrical dipole oriented *tangent* to the scalp, pointing from the centrotemporal area where the negative end of the dipole is to the frontal areas where the positive end is (Figures 10.35 and 10.36). Thus, with the more commonly occurring radial dipoles, a negativity is measured on the scalp, and a positivity is inferred deep to the scalp. Discharges manifesting a tangential or horizontal dipole manifest a scalp-to-scalp dipole, with a negativity in one scalp area and a visibly measured positivity in another scalp area.

Note that in this discussion and in the EEG literature in general, the terms horizontal dipole and tangentially oriented dipole are used interchangeably. Although both terms are commonly accepted, the latter is technically preferable because the dipole being described is always tangent to the scalp, no matter what the patient's head position. As patients move their heads, a tangential dipole will not always remain

parallel to the horizon as the word *horizontal* implies. Still, the term *horizontal dipole* remains in common usage.

Pitfalls in the Identification of the Tangential Dipole

The successful identification of a tangentially oriented dipole in the setting of rolandic epilepsy relies on the ability to detect the spike's simultaneous frontal positivity. As it happens, this pattern is most easily demonstrated using referential montages. In referential montages with a well-chosen (i.e., neutral) reference, the primary centrotemporal spike is seen as an upgoing (negative with respect to the reference) deflection in the centrotemporal area, and the anterior positivity is seen as a simultaneous downgoing (positive) deflection in the frontal areas. As it happens, the pattern of the horizontal dipole (specifically, demonstration of the frontal positivity) is more difficult to appreciate in bipolar montages. In fact, even when a significant horizontal dipole is present, it often cannot

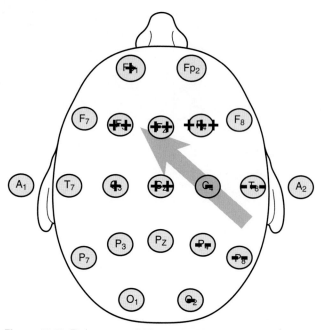

Figure 10.36 The net negativities and positivities recorded in the EEG trace from the previous figure are shown schematically on the scalp. The presence of a peak negativity in the right midtemporal area and area of net positivity in the anterior electrodes suggests a dipole tangent to the scalp as depicted by the dipole arrow.

be easily appreciated in a bipolar montage (Figure 10.37). In only a small minority of cases can a horizontal dipole be easily seen in a bipolar montage by way of an anterior positive phase reversal (Figure 10.38). For that reason, a referential montage must be examined before the presence of a horizontal dipole can be excluded. Because a horizontal dipole provides important confirmatory information regarding a possible diagnosis of rolandic epilepsy, the presence or absence of this distinctive dipole orientation should always be sought when a discharge is seen in this location. The absence of a horizontal dipole does not, however, exclude the diagnosis of rolandic epilepsy because such a dipole is not demonstrable in approximately half of all cases.

As noted earlier, the horizontal dipole of the rolandic discharge is best demonstrated on referential montages. The choice of reference in this setting deserves special attention. The search for the positive component of the rolandic discharge entails identification of downgoing ("positive") deflections in the frontal and contralateral channels. Consider, however, the situation in which the reference chosen for a referential montage is inadvertently contaminated with the active discharge. This issue arises most problematically when an earlobe reference (A1 or A2) is used. The example of a contaminated earlobe reference is easy to visualize, in particular because the earlobe is so close to the centrotemporal area. First, we examine the example of a non-rolandic discharge (that does not manifest a horizontal dipole) that is maximally negative in the left midtemporal electrode (T7). Recall that it is not uncommon for the nearby earlobe electrode (A1) to pick up a fair amount of the electrical activity

occurring in T7. If the A1 electrode is used as the reference electrode, A1 will partially record the negative event coming from the nearby centrotemporal area. When A1 is used as a reference electrode (for instance in an Fp1-A1 derivation), the voltage measured in A1 is subtracted from the frontal electrodes that, in this example, are truly neutral, and the subtraction of the A1 reference signal will result in downgoing deflections in the channels corresponding to those neutral electrodes. The appearance of these downgoing waves is quite similar to the usual appearance of a true horizontal dipole, with negativities (upward deflections) in the centrotemporal area and positivities (downward deflections) in the anterior electrodes. In fact, in this type of case in which the reference is contaminated with the active discharge, downward deflections will also be present in the channels of the other neutral electrodes that use A1 as a reference as well (Figures 10.39 through 10.41).

This type of error can be avoided first by choosing a reference that is distant from the active discharge and therefore inactive. When it occurs, this type of error can be detected by noting the distribution of downward deflections in *all* of the neutral electrodes' channels (rather than just the frontal channels) as is seen in Figure 10.41, thereby identifying those deflections as contamination of the reference rather than true positive events in anterior regions. The same type of error can be made when an average reference electrode is used if the centrotemporal discharge is so large that it is visible in the average. The general problem of misinterpretation of discharge topographies based on contaminated reference electrodes is discussed in Chapter 4, "Electroencephalographic Localization."

Rolandic EEG Trait

Almost all children with benign rolandic epilepsy manifest rolandic discharges during the course of their seizure disorder. Interestingly, it has long been known that the siblings of children with rolandic epilepsy may also manifest rolandic discharges in the EEG, even when those siblings do not have the seizure disorder. Therefore, the tendency to manifest rolandic discharges in the EEG appears to be a heritable trait, and only a subset of all children who have rolandic discharges in the EEG actually have rolandic epilepsy. The finding of rolandic discharges in the EEG in the absence of the seizure disorder is referred to as rolandic EEG trait. It may come as a surprise to learn that rolandic EEG trait is much more common than rolandic epilepsy itself. Some estimate that of all children in the general population with rolandic discharges in the EEG, as many as 90% only have rolandic EEG trait and do not actually have the epilepsy syndrome, that is, they never experience the seizures of rolandic epilepsy. Others estimate this percentage to be even higher. This fact has important ramifications in EEG interpretation. Rolandic EEG trait has such a high frequency in the population that the mere observation of rolandic discharges in the EEG should not automatically lead to the diagnosis of a seizure disorder or even of rolandic epilepsy, without careful consideration of the clinical history.

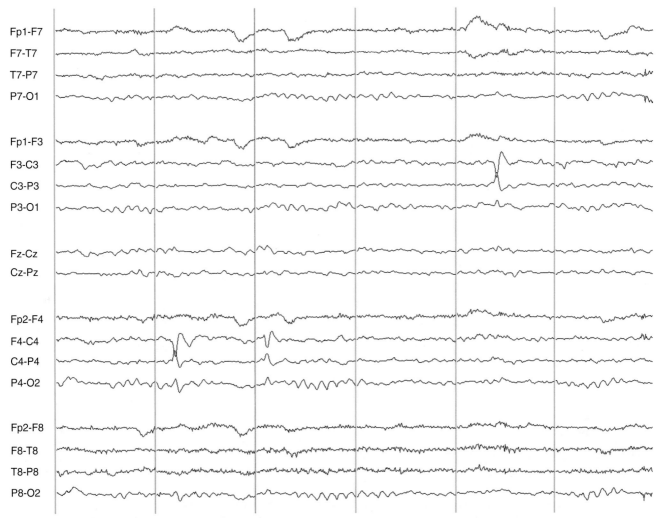

Figure 10.37 Even when centrotemporal discharges have a true horizontal dipole, the dipole orientation is often not easily detectable in bipolar montages. For instance, the horizontal dipole of these independent C3 and C4 discharges cannot be discerned from this tracing (compare to Figure 10.37).

Because of the relatively high frequency of rolandic EEG trait in the population, the presence of centrotemporal spikes in the EEG often represents an incidental finding. Consider the scenario of an 11-year-old boy with an episode of loss of consciousness in science class. An EEG is obtained that shows typical rolandic discharges with a horizontal dipole. In reality, the likelihood that this child's episode was an epileptic seizure are not increased by the abnormal finding in the EEG. As discussed earlier, the BCECTS syndrome consists either of focal seizures out of wakefulness or grand mal convulsions arising out of sleep. Because this child lost consciousness from the awake state, this event is not likely to have represented a focal seizure and, if it had represented an example of a grand mal convulsion, it does not fit with the rolandic epilepsy syndrome because it occurred out of wakefulness. Even though the EEG findings are formally considered abnormal, the finding of rolandic discharges does not match the clinical picture of the event. It is quite possible that this episode represented an example of syncope (further questioning might reveal that

the child was dissecting a frog!), despite the abnormal EEG finding. Because such a high proportion of individuals with rolandic discharges do not have epilepsy, the clinician should always confirm that the event history is consistent with the seizure types seen in the BCECTS syndrome before arriving at the diagnosis of epilepsy in this group of children, and the EEG reader should confirm that the EEG report does not imply a definite diagnosis of rolandic epilepsy.

Another way to look at this problem is to consider the difference in the rate of epilepsy between two groups of children who are found to have rolandic discharges. One is a group of children with rolandic discharges who have been referred to an EEG laboratory because of a possible seizure event—this is the scenario that EEG readers are most often dealing with. The other is a group of children whose rolandic discharges have been identified during a hypothetical school-based research study in which all children in the school of a certain age group, regardless of their medical history, are recorded on EEG. In the case of the school study, the large majority of children

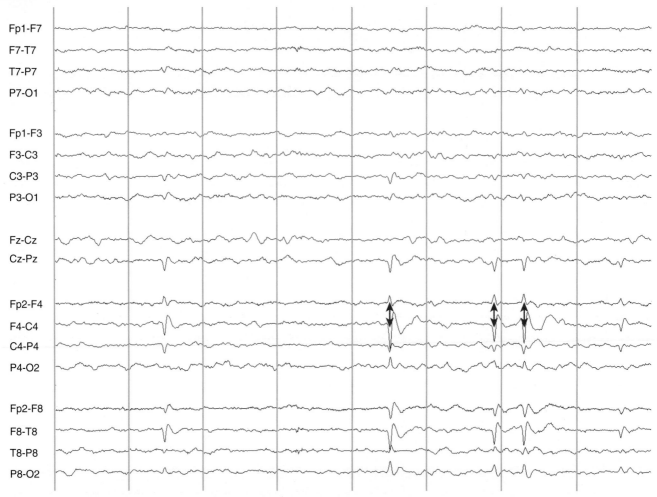

Figure 10.38 A right centrotemporal discharge is seen in a bipolar montage. The presence of an anteriorly oriented horizontal dipole is indicated by the positive phase reversals anterior to the peak negativities (arrows). In fact, this appearance represents the exception to the rule—even when present, horizontal dipoles usually cannot be so easily appreciated in bipolar montages. The presence of a horizontal dipole can only be excluded with certainty by examining an appropriate referential montage.

with rolandic discharges in the EEG will not have epilepsy. However, in the laboratory-referred group the patient group is significantly enriched for epilepsy because the majority have been referred for seizures or seizure-like events. For this reason, if you are sitting in an EEG lab, it appears that most children with rolandic spikes do, indeed, have rolandic epilepsy. Nevertheless, some children are referred for EEG evaluation in whom suspicion that a particular clinical event was a seizure is low, and the odds of having epilepsy in this group, despite the presence of rolandic discharges, may be closer to the group from the hypothetical school-based study example than the laboratory-referred group. In such cases, the mere presence of rolandic discharges should not compel a diagnosis of epilepsy. This is an excellent example of the maxim that "an abnormal EEG does not make the diagnosis of epilepsy." A properly written EEG report should somehow reflect this fact by describing rolandic discharges as potentially consistent with both rolandic epilepsy and rolandic EEG trait.

When reporting spikes in centrotemporal locations in children in the appropriate age range, it is not enough to simply report their location and let the reader surmise that

these might be rolandic spikes. If the morphology, location, and other EEG findings (or better, the absence of other abnormal findings) make the discharges you are reporting consistent with rolandic spikes, it is best to explicitly state this in your report and not leave the reader guessing. In such cases, it may be useful to simply write that "these centrotemporal discharges may represent an example of rolandic spikes." This may tip off the referring provider to a possibility that may not have been considered, for instance that a single nocturnal grand mal seizure in a 12-year-old boy may have been a rolandic seizure. As mentioned above, the presence of a tangential dipole is not mandatory for centrotemporal discharges to be in the rolandic category, nor must the spikes be bilateral. On the other hand, there may be a finding in the EEG that makes it much less likely that a centrotemporal spike is a rolandic spike, such as a slow background or other findings, and you may wish to communicate your thought process regarding the entirety of the EEG picture this to the ordering provider.

Because the presence of a tangential dipole is a strong factor in support of a centrotemporal spike being a rolandic

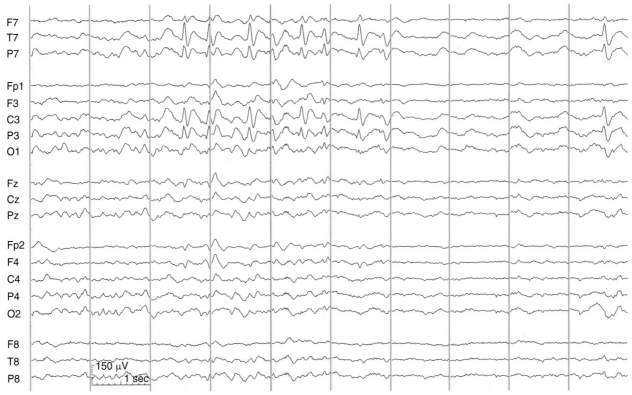

Figure 10.39 This left centrotemporal discharge, maximum in the T7 and C3 electrodes and recorded in a referential montage using the nose as the reference electrode, does not manifest an obvious horizontal dipole. Note that all of the principal deflections are upgoing implying that only negative charges are present on the scalp, with only the smallest hint of positivity in Fz, Fp2, and F4 (compare with Figure 10.34).

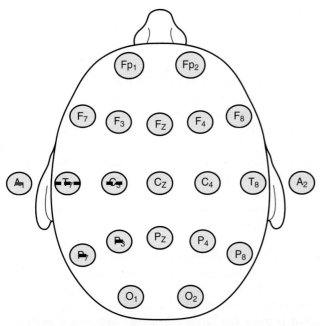

Figure 10.40 A schematic is shown of the purely negative discharge seen in the previous figure (Figure 10.38). Only negativities are recorded on the scalp implying that a positivity must be present deep to the scalp. Note the small amount of negativity overflows the left earlobe.

spike, sophisticated providers will be wondering if one was present. For that reason, when a centrotemporal spike is seen without a tangential dipole, this should be explicitly stated.

Otherwise, you will leave the referring provider wondering whether there was such a dipole or whether you simply neglected to check for it or describe it.

Benign Childhood Epilepsy with Occipital Paroxysms (BCEOP)

Two types of benign or self-limited occipital epilepsy syndromes have been recognized, a more common, early-onset variety (also referred to as Panayiotopoulos type) and a late-onset variety (referred to as Gastaut type). BCEOP is the second most common self-limited epilepsy category after BCECTS. There is a more recent proposal by the ILAE to rename the early onset version of BCEOP to *Self-limited Epilepsy with Autonomic Seizures (SeLEAS)* and the late-onset version to *Childhood Occipital Visual Epilepsy (COVE)*. Thus, multiple names for each of these syndromes will be in circulation.

Early-Onset Benign Childhood Epilepsy with Occipital Paroxysms (BCEOP)—Panayiotopoulos Type (or SeLEAS)

In the early onset form of childhood occipital epilepsy, seizures typically begin between the ages of 3 and 6 years. The seizures of this syndrome are distinctive and autonomic symptoms are prominent. The majority of seizures occur at night. The episodes tend to be lengthy, often lasting 20 minutes or more with pallor, sweating, irritability, nausea and vomiting, and prolonged eye deviation. In some cases, there is further progression to convulsions (either hemiclonic or bilateral clonic). Even taking into

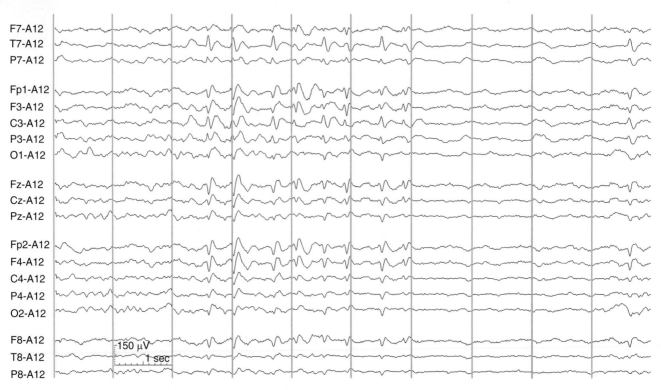

Figure 10.41 A left midtemporal (T7) rolandic discharge is recorded with suboptimal technique, giving the false impression of a horizontal dipole. The reference electrode used in this recording is an average of the earlobe electrodes, A1 and A2 (labeled as A12). Because A1 is adjacent to T7, it also detects the negativity from the left midtemporal area. When this negativity is subtracted from neutral electrodes, a downgoing deflection results. Note that electrodes in areas that are presumably completely neutral (e.g., the right occipital area, O2) still manifest the downgoing deflection, which represents contamination of the reference rather than a true positivity in that location. Another way of saying this is that the downward deflection in the O2-A12 channel reflects activity in the A12 reference rather than the O2 electrode. Compare this appearance to the true horizontal dipole shown in Figure 10.34 in which, because it was recorded with an appropriate reference electrode, uninvolved electrodes appear correctly as neutral.

account the fact that the ability to report visual manifestations may be limited in children in this younger age group, visual phenomena are felt to be rare. Because of the nausea and vomiting, in some cases the episodes are mistaken for migraine attacks. Approximately two thirds of children manifest occipital spikes or occipital paroxysms (discussed later). In the early-onset version of this syndrome, seizures tend to be infrequent with some children experiencing only one or two seizure episodes throughout the syndrome's entire course. The seizures tend to remit within a few years of presentation. The small number of lifetime seizures in some cases and tendency toward natural remission reduce the necessity of treating with antiseizure medications. The proposed renaming of this seizure syndrome as SeLEAS is meant to emphasize that many of the features of the seizures are autonomic, though the new terminology unfortunately drops the term *occipital*, which served as a reminder of the classic EEG finding of this syndrome and its heritage as an occipital epilepsy.

Late-Onset Benign Childhood Epilepsy with Occipital Paroxysms (BCEOP)—Gastaut type (or COVE)

The late-onset version of childhood occipital epilepsy is felt to be considerably (five-fold) less common than the early- onset

version. The mean age of onset in the late-onset form is 8 years, compared with 5 years for the early onset form. In the late-onset form, seizures are much more frequent and tend to occur in the daytime. Unlike the early-onset form, visual phenomena are highly characteristic of the seizures in the late-onset form, consisting of elementary (or more rarely complex) visual hallucinations. Blindness may occur as either an ictal phenomenon or a postictal phenomenon. Headache and, more rarely, nausea and vomiting can be associated seizure symptoms.

EEG Findings in Childhood Occipital Epilepsy

Both the early and late forms of occipital epilepsy may show the classically described pattern of occipital spikes that suppress with eye opening, the so-called *fixation-off* effect (so-called because the spikes "turn off" with visual fixation). In fact, any maneuver that interrupts visual fixation, such as shutting off room lights, can prompt the appearance of occipital spike activity. Although fixation-off occipital spiking is the classic EEG finding of the benign occipital epilepsies, it is not uniformly seen in these syndromes; estimates vary, but occipital spikes are only seen in approximately two thirds of children with benign childhood occipital epilepsy. In the remaining third, spikes may be seen in extraoccipital

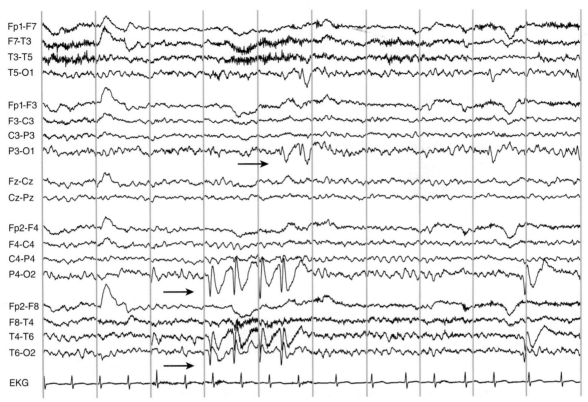

Figure 10.42 A paroxysm of occipital spikes is seen in the right occipital area (black arrows). Independent but lower voltage occipital spikes are seen in the left occipital area (lighter arrow). The paroxysmal bursting pattern seen here is consistent with that seen in the BCEOP (benign childhood epilepsy with occipital paroxysms) although the spikes are often bilaterally synchronous in those syndromes. Fixation-off spiking as may be seen in BCEOP is not demonstrated in this figure.

locations or the EEG may even be normal, making the diagnosis considerably more challenging. Although some children may have the classic finding of paroxysms of occipital spikes, in others the spikes may occur singly. The spikes are often bilateral, but in some they may be unilateral (see Figure 10.42). The yield of finding EEG abnormalities is increased by obtaining sleep. Although it is the classic EEG finding of the childhood occipital epilepsy syndromes, fixation-off occipital spikes may also occasionally be seen in other types of occipital epilepsy outside of the benign group described here; the presence of fixation-off occipital spikes does not guarantee the presence of a benign occipital epilepsy syndrome.

More recently, a specific pattern of spike-wave discharges has been associated with the early onset variant with a broad field spanning the occipital and frontal areas. These occipitofrontal discharges show a downward deflection in the occipital channels and an upward deflection in the frontopolar channels in AP bipolar montages suggesting negativities in the frontal and occipital areas and a broad relative positivity in between (Figure 10.43).

Especially in the early-onset version of the syndrome, spikes may be seen in extraoccipital locations, including the centrotemporal areas. Like in BCECTS, generalized spike-wave discharges may also be seen in the childhood occipital epilepsy syndromes. The not infrequent co-occurrence of

occipital spike-wave discharges and centrotemporal spike-wave discharges suggests the possibility of a link between BCECTS and BCEOP. The concept of benign childhood seizure susceptibility syndrome has been proposed to encompass the group of children who manifest a tendency toward the benign focal epilepsies, including children with benign rolandic epilepsy, rolandic EEG trait, benign childhood epilepsy with occipital paroxysms, and other less well defined benign focal epilepsies of childhood. Further delineation of the genetics of this group of disorders may help clarify whether the construct of a benign childhood seizure susceptibility syndrome is valid. The early and the late-onset versions of the syndromes are compared in Table 10.2.

Autosomal Dominant Nocturnal Frontal Lobe Epilepsy

Autosomal dominant nocturnal frontal lobe epilepsy (ADNFLE) is an unusual epilepsy syndrome that may have onset as early as infancy but as late as adulthood, although onset in the childhood years is typical. The seizures can be difficult to diagnose because they manifest as violent, uncoordinated thrashing occurring out of light sleep ("hypermotor seizures" or more recently "hyperkinetic seizures"). The spells are often mistaken for nightmares or other parasomnias, for

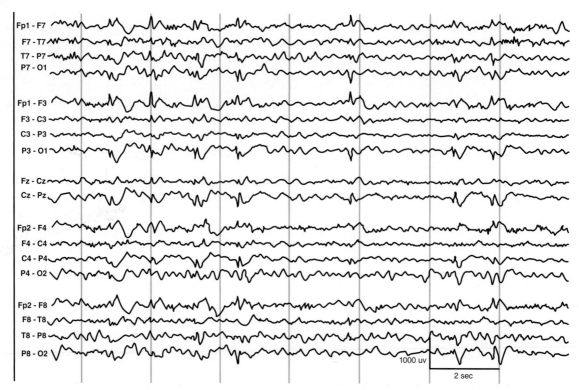

Figure 10.43 This image shows a specific variant of the typical occipital discharges seen in the benign occipital epilepsies of childhood. Note the downgoing waves seen in the posterior channels and the upgoing waves seen in the anterior channels in this AP bipolar montage. A review of this discharge in referential montages shows that this distinctive pattern was caused by a primary occipital negativity, as expected, and a smaller frontal negativity, with an intervening positivity marked by the evident broad "positive phase reversal" that is seen with this discharge. Note that an overly hasty review of this pattern could allow it to be mistaken for a generalized spike-wave discharge because of the apparent broad field of the spike across the head.

TABLE 10.2 Childhood Epilepsy with Occipital Paroxysms Subtypes		
	Early-Onset—Panayiotopoulos type or SeLEAS	Late-Onset—Gastaut type or COVE
Population Frequency	More common	Less common
Mean Age of Onset	5 years	8 years
Seizure Duration	Lengthy	Brief
Number of Lifetime Seizures	Few	Many
Timing of Seizures	Most at night	Most during day
Typical Seizure Semiology	Sweating, pallor, irritability, eye deviation, vomiting, culminating in convulsion (visual phenomena rare)	Pure visual phenomena without loss of consciousness
Long-Term Course	Early remission	Inconsistent remission during childhood, later course unclear

a movement disorder, or sometimes for a psychiatric disturbance. Distinguishing between the seizures of ADNFLE and nocturnal movement disorders such as paroxysmal nocturnal dystonia can be difficult in some cases, and controversy persists regarding the exact demarcation between these two syndromes. In a minority of cases, heterozygous genetic abnormalities have been identified in the neuronal nicotinic acetylcholine receptor and more rarely in other genes.

EEG Findings in ADNFLE

The EEG findings in ADNFLE are variable; typically the interictal EEG is normal. When the interictal EEG is abnormal, anterior focal epileptiform discharges may be seen. Ictal EEG recordings can be difficult to interpret because they are often obscured by motion artifact associated with the ictal hypermotor behaviors. An intracranial electrode recording of an ADNFLE seizure has been made that demonstrated onset from the left operculoinsular cortex (Picard et al., 2000).

Genetic Generalized Epilepsies

The genetic generalized epilepsies are a group of generalized epilepsy syndromes characterized by generalized seizures and generalized spike-wave discharges in the EEG. The question of exactly how broad or restrictive the boundaries for this group of syndromes should be has still not been settled. It is useful to consider the three terms that have historically been used, sometimes interchangeably, for the conceptualization of these syndromes: *idiopathic* generalized epilepsies, *primary* generalized epilepsies, and *genetic* generalized epilepsies.

Considering the strict meaning of each of these three adjectives, idiopathic, meaning of unknown or uncertain cause (idios, Greek, "unto itself"), is probably the weakest choice. It implies that, with the current state of research, science has not yet found a particular cause or explanation for the epilepsy. Of course, today's idiopathic disorder may no longer be idiopathic tomorrow once the cause might have been discovered, and the successive identification of the cause of various other genetic epilepsies has been occurring before our eyes. Considering the strict meaning of the term, at such time as the genetic cause of all these epilepsy syndromes is discovered, this term would immediately become obsolete. As it currently stands, the genetic causes of this group of common epilepsies have been surprisingly elusive, so the term *idiopathic* still has some standing, at least for now.

The term *primary* implies that a disorder is not caused by another medical condition. For instance, individuals with high blood pressure in whom all investigations for the cause are found to be negative are said to have primary hypertension. The hypertension is not secondary to some other condition—the person simply has it. The term *primary generalized epilepsy* was also naturally juxtaposed against the older term *secondary generalized epilepsy*, which implied a generalized epilepsy that was caused by (i.e., secondary to) another disorder, a concept no longer in use.

The meaning of the term *genetic generalized epilepsy* is straightforward, and clearly all three of these terms should potentially refer to a group of epilepsy syndromes that would have considerable overlap, which they do, because almost all primary or idiopathic syndromes would be expected to have a genetic basis.

How did the new classification choose among these terms? To some degree the choices seem somewhat arbitrary. Of the three, the term *primary generalized epilepsy* has been discarded from the most recent classification. The new classification recognizes the importance of a core group of four of the genetic generalized epilepsy syndromes. Notwithstanding the disadvantages of the term *idiopathic* discussed above but recognizing the term's historical precedent, it has chosen the term *idiopathic generalized epilepsies* for these four syndromes: childhood absence epilepsy, juvenile absence epilepsy, juvenile myoclonic epilepsy, and epilepsy with generalized tonic-clonic seizures alone. A wider group of *genetic generalized epilepsies* includes this core group and adds myoclonic-atonic epilepsy (Doose syndrome), epilepsy with eyelid myoclonia (Jeavons syndrome), epilepsy with myoclonic absences, and myoclonic epilepsy in infancy. Generalized epilepsy with febrile seizures plus (GEFS+) may also be included in this group in individuals who have this syndrome but do not have focal seizures (which occasionally do occur in this syndrome). Therefore, *idiopathic generalized epilepsies* is now the proposed term for the core group of generalized epilepsies and represent a subset of the genetic generalized epilepsies.

Idiopathic Generalized Epilepsies

The idiopathic generalized epilepsies occur in individuals with otherwise normal neurologic and cognitive status: childhood absence epilepsy, juvenile absence epilepsy, juvenile myoclonic epilepsy, and epilepsy with tonic-clonic seizures alone. Although many patients with these syndromes conform to their classic presentations and timeframes for age of onset, in occasional patients these syndromes may appear to blend into one another. For instance, some individuals with absence seizures in childhood may go on to develop a picture consistent with juvenile myoclonic epilepsy, blurring the border between juvenile myoclonic epilepsy and childhood absence epilepsy, suggesting the possibility that some of these syndromes with different names may represent varying presentations of the same genotype. Also, the generally held belief that these syndromes have no cognitive or behavioral impact has more recently been questioned and subtle effects may be present in some patients.

The genetics and pathogenesis of the idiopathic generalized epilepsies is just beginning to unfold. At least some of the generalized epilepsies have been demonstrated to be caused by sodium-, chloride-, or calcium-ion channel disorders ("channelopathies") and others by errors in synaptic receptors such as gamma-aminobutyric acid (GABA) receptors. As the genetics of these syndromes is further elucidated, many additional subtypes and biochemical errors will doubtlessly be identified. At the current time, the large majority of individuals with idiopathic generalized epilepsy do not have an identified genetic cause, which is to say that genetic testing is largely not yet available to confirm the diagnosis of these disorders.

Some previous terminology for this group of disorders focused on the generalized spike-wave mechanism. The terms primary corticoreticular epilepsy and centrencephalic epilepsy are older terms that reflect the basic susceptibility in these patients to the occurrence of thalamocortical volleys that are the generalized spike-wave discharges characteristic of these syndromes. The same biochemical abnormality that allows for generalized spike-wave discharges to cause absence seizures is also presumed to be responsible for the more rapid discharges associated with generalized tonic-clonic seizures and the brief polyspike discharges that drive epileptic myoclonus in some patients, as described earlier.

Childhood Absence Epilepsy

Childhood absence epilepsy (CAE) usually has its onset between 4 and 8 years of age. The main seizure type of CAE is the typical absence seizure, described earlier, consisting of brief periods of staring with subtle clonic eye blinking and unawareness of the environment. Children with untreated CAE may have frequent absence seizures, often more than 100 per day. A large fraction of children with CAE grow out of the tendency to absence seizures during the teenage years, and in approximately 90% of CAE patients the absence seizures have cleared by the age of 20 years. Patients and families should be made aware, however, of the lifelong increased risk for GTC seizures, estimated to be around 40%, even in previous CAE patients in whom the absence seizures have remitted during childhood. In a minority of CAE patients, GTC seizures occur during childhood while the absence seizures are still active.

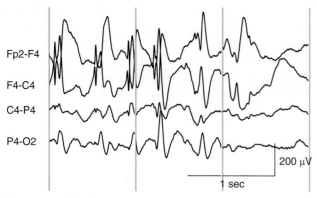

Fp2-F4

F4-C4

C4-P4

P4-O2

200 μV

1 sec

Figure 10.44 This close-up of a discharge associated with an absence seizure shows the multiphasic morphology of the spike component of the discharge. In fact, close analysis of many discharges casually referred to as "generalized spike wave" actually shows that these represent generalized polyspike-wave discharges.

Both ethosuximide and valproic acid have a high success rate in CAE, although ethosuximide is only active against the absence seizures. Lamotrigine is a second line medication.

EEG Findings in CAE

Confirmation of the diagnosis of absence seizures hinges on EEG demonstration of 3 Hz generalized spike-wave discharges with simultaneous staring/decreased responsiveness. Well-trained EEG technologists are adept at testing the child's responsiveness during 3 Hz generalized spike-wave volleys that occur during EEG recordings, usually by speaking a string of words during the discharge and asking the child to repeat the words back after the volley is over. In this way, awareness during the spell can be assessed. Although absence seizures are classically associated with "3 Hz generalized spike-wave discharges," close examination of the discharges often reveals polyspike-wave morphology in most cases. The presence of spike-wave versus polyspike-wave morphology at the same frequency does not have a diagnostic or prognostic impact in children with CAE (Figure 10.44). OIRDA (occipital intermittent rhythmic delta activity) may also be seen in children with absence epilepsy.

The diagnosis of absence seizures can be definitively established by recording the seizures in the EEG laboratory, something that is usually not difficult to do in the untreated child given how frequently the seizures occur. In addition to the 3 Hz spike-wave discharges that are associated with clinical seizures, patients often also have generalized spike-wave fragments that are not clearly associated with clinical change. In sleep, brief, generalized polyspike-wave discharges may also appear. Most commonly, generalized spike-wave discharges show a voltage maximum in a band across the frontal region, including the F3, F4, and Fz (superior and midline frontal) electrodes with flanking maxima in the adjacent F7 and F8 (anterior temporal) electrodes.

Hyperventilation

Hyperventilation is an effective tool for demonstrating absence seizures. Hyperventilation is carried out during most conventional EEG recordings when it can be feasibly performed, depending on the patient's age, cognitive level, degree of cooperation, and absence of medical contraindications. The patient is asked to overbreathe for 3 to 4 minutes. It can be helpful to have younger children blow a pinwheel. In children who do not have epilepsy, hyperventilation typically causes high-voltage hypersynchronous slowing, often dramatic, thought to be a consequence of the cerebral vasoconstriction associated with the lowered CO_2 levels caused by hyperventilation. Such dramatic hyperventilation responses are less common in adults (Figure 10.45). In children who do have a tendency to generalized spike-wave discharges, the discharges are often provoked by the hyperventilation technique. Among children with active absence seizures, hyperventilation will elicit an absence spell in approximately 80%. In some children, the absence seizures provoked by hyperventilation are more prolonged than those that occur spontaneously. At times, hyperventilation elicits high-voltage slowing with some definite spike-wave discharges mixed in (Figure 10.46), but no clinical seizure.

It is not uncommon for patients to become fatigued and to appear to lose alertness from the effort of hyperventilation and the malaise it may cause. It is important to be able to distinguish the "dreamy look" or lack of alertness brought on by the fatigue and discomfort of the hyperventilation exercise from actual clinical absence seizures. Certain clues can help distinguish between the two scenarios. First, during a true absence seizure, the patient almost always halts the hyperventilation effort with a noticeable change in the pace of respirations. Second, if the patient is asked to hold the arms outstretched during hyperventilation, a mild but distinct slumping of the arms is seen at the time of absence seizures. This is easiest to observe when the patient hyperventilates in the seated position. Finally, the ability to repeat words spoken during an absence seizure is reduced or absent.

In CAE, generalized spike-wave discharges are often also seen in drowsiness as the patient passes into light sleep. Because responsiveness is impossible to evaluate in a patient who is falling asleep, whether these discharges should be considered electrographic seizures or electroclinical seizures remains an open question.

Patients and families who are aware that hyperventilation provokes absence seizures during the EEG often ask whether exercise that causes heavy breathing should be avoided. In fact, exercise is not expected to provoke absence seizure because of the physiologic differences between voluntary hyperventilation and hyperpnea during exercise. During exercise, CO_2 accumulates as a metabolic waste product, and the blood CO_2 rises. The body responds to this increased CO_2 level by increasing minute ventilation in an effort to bring CO_2 levels back down to normal. During strenuous exercise with rapid breathing, the CO_2 level does not typically dip significantly below normal. In contrast, the patient who hyperventilates in the EEG laboratory presumably starts with a normal CO_2 level at baseline, and the hyperventilation effort brings the level significantly below normal, potentially provoking an absence seizure if the patient is prone to them.

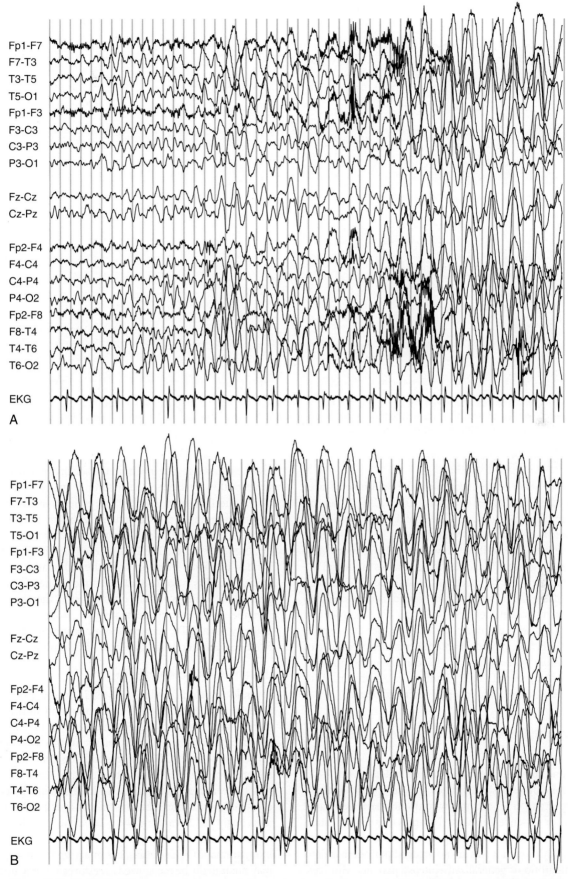

Figure 10.45 (A–B) The EEG response to hyperventilation can be dramatic. Factors associated with higher voltage hyperventilation responses include greater effort, younger patient age, and lower blood glucose levels. As long as no epileptiform (spike) activity is present, very high-voltage hyperventilation responses should not be considered abnormal. Also note that, while the hyperventilation response's amplitude dramatically increases and decreases, the frequency of the hypersynchrony remains fixed.

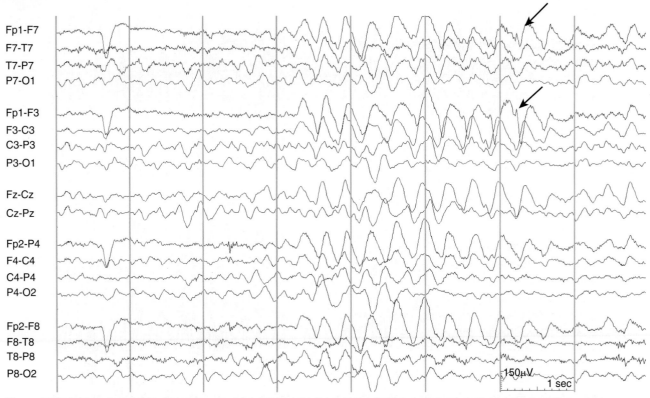

Figure 10.46 Definite spikes intermixed with a hyperventilation response are considered abnormal. A transient is most likely to represent a true epileptic spike (rather than an artifact) when it is time-locked to the slow wave. Peaking or sharpening of the high-voltage slow waves themselves during hyperventilation is less likely to be abnormal.

Juvenile Absence Epilepsy

Although they share much in common, the syndrome of juvenile absence epilepsy (JAE) is distinct from CAE in several ways, beginning with a later age of onset of the absence seizures in JAE. There is an important overlap between JAE and juvenile myoclonic epilepsy (described below) in that JAE patients may also experience generalized tonic-clonic seizures (although the JME diagnosis cannot be made in the absence of myoclonic seizures). In the JAE syndrome, the absence seizures tend to be less frequent, sometimes only occurring once or twice per week compared with the dozens of episodes per day seen in untreated CAE. The individual absence episodes tend to be of longer duration, with spells up to 20 seconds long not uncommon in the JAE group. The EEG findings in JAE are similar to those of juvenile myoclonic epilepsy, described below.

Epilepsy with Generalized Tonic-Clonic Seizures Alone

As the name implies, the syndrome of epilepsy with GTC seizures alone describes individuals with idiopathic generalized epilepsy and GTC seizures who do not have associated myoclonic or absence seizures. The previous classification described a syndrome of Epilepsy with GTC Seizures on Awakening. Although it was acknowledged that there is definitely a subgroup of generalized epilepsy patients who have their GTC seizures exclusively on awakening, it was not felt that there was a clear distinction apart from the timing of their seizures between these patients and patients with

identical findings, but in whom the seizures occurred at other times of the day. Hence, the syndrome was renamed. There is also a question as to whether this epilepsy syndrome simply represents a subset of JME patients who only experience GTC seizures and who do not happen to have myoclonic seizures or absence seizures. The EEG findings in this syndrome are similar to those found in the other idiopathic generalized epilepsies. This is to say that the three of the four idiopathic generalized epilepsies that occur during the teenage years, juvenile myoclonic epilepsy, juvenile absence epilepsy, and epilepsy with GTC seizures alone, cannot be distinguished from one another based solely on EEG findings.

Juvenile Myoclonic Epilepsy

Juvenile myoclonic epilepsy (JME) is an epilepsy with onset in the second decade of life, most commonly during the early teenage years, and is a classic example of an idiopathic generalized epilepsy. The hallmark seizure of this syndrome is the myoclonic seizure; GTC seizures and, less commonly, absence seizures occur as well. Any subset of these three seizure types may be seen in an individual with JME, though, by definition, myoclonic jerks should be present. On average, the myoclonic jerks begin at 12 years and the GTC seizures begin at 13 years of age. Because the onset of myoclonic jerks may precede the more dramatic GTC seizures, in some patients these quick jerks may not initially be recognized as seizures and not attract medical attention. Some patients only seek medical attention once a GTC seizure has occurred. For this reason, when younger patients present with generalized seizures, the clinician should

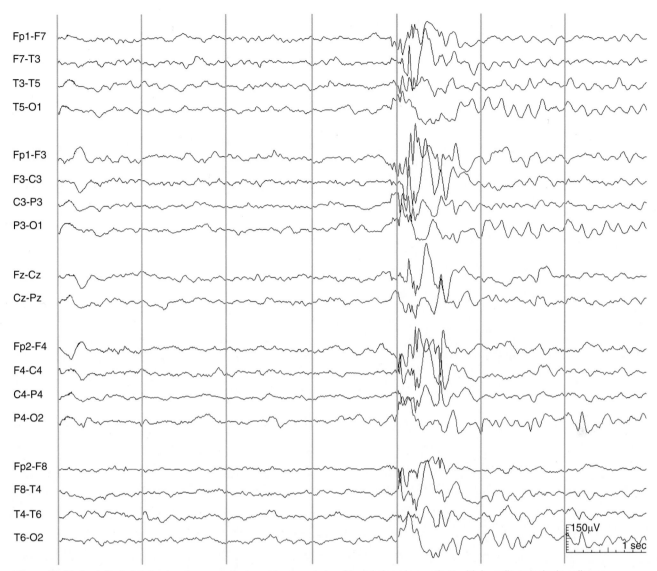

Figure 10.47 A relatively brief polyspike-wave discharge is seen during Stage I sleep in a patient with juvenile myoclonic epilepsy.

specifically ask the patient about the presence of myoclonic jerks even if that history has not been volunteered. In those patients in whom the diagnosis of JME is made based solely on the presence of myoclonic jerks before the occurrence of a GTC seizure, effective antiseizure therapy may prevent the patient from ever experiencing GTC seizures.

The myoclonic seizures in JME characteristically consist of quick abduction jerks of the upper arms. The jerks have a predilection for the morning hours, and the patient may describe events such as involuntarily flinging a glass of orange juice into the wall because of the jerks. Consciousness appears to be preserved during these very brief episodes. Occasionally, a succession of myoclonic jerks can culminate in a GTC. This is one of the rare scenarios in which individuals appear to report observing the onset of a GTC seizure in themselves. They may remember the initial series of myoclonic jerks but they should not be able to recall the ensuing GTC seizure; an observer may have a difficult time determining when the myoclonic jerks stopped and the GTC seizure began. This seizure sequence is described by the newly classified myoclonic-tonic-clonic seizure.

The clearance of myoclonic seizures can be used as a barometer of the effectiveness of drug therapy in JME patients. Approximately one quarter of patients with JME will also manifest absence seizures, which tend to be less frequent but of longer duration than the absence episodes that occur in the context of CAE (when present, similar to the pattern described earlier in JAE). Valproic acid is the drug of choice in JME, with a high success rate, but it must be used with caution in women of childbearing age because of its teratogenic potential. In terms of its ability to completely clear the seizures, lamotrigine is a second choice in JME (although in a minority of cases it may exacerbate the myoclonic jerks), and levetiracetam is less effective.

EEG Findings in JME and Related Disorders

The classic EEG findings in JME are fast spike-wave discharges, high-voltage polyspikes in sleep, and less frequently a photoparoxysmal response. The polyspikes may be either brief or more lengthy, well organized or poorly organized (Figures 10.47 and 10.48). Fast spike wave refers to 4 to 5 Hz

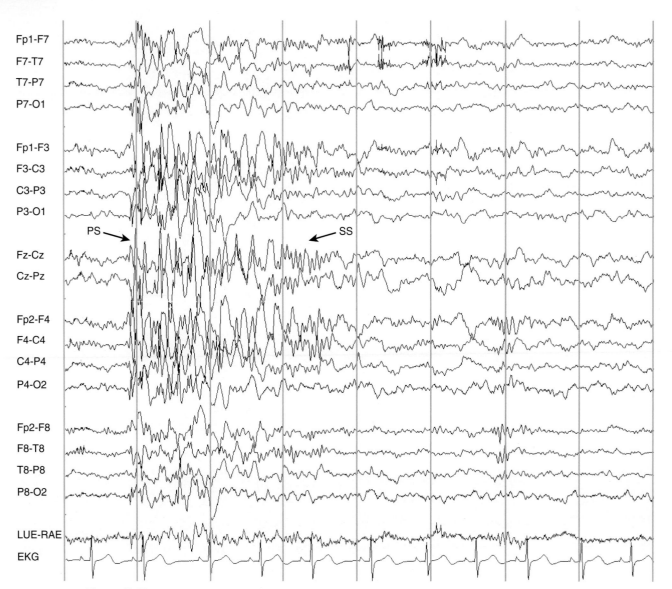

Figure 10.48 More prolonged polyspikes may be seen in patients with primary generalized epilepsy. This polyspike discharge (PS) merges with a sleep spindle (SS). The polyspike portion of the discharge can be distinguished from the spindle on the basis of the respective wave frequencies (14 Hz in the case of the sleep spindle).

generalized spike-wave discharges that resemble classic 3 Hz generalized spike-wave discharges except for their faster firing rate (Figure 10.49). A minority of patients may also exhibit a photoparoxysmal response: spike-wave discharges that are triggered by strobe light stimulation (discussed later). The epileptiform findings of JME are activated both by hyperventilation and by slow-wave sleep; during REM sleep, the discharges are relatively suppressed. A normal background is expected. Unless caused by a recent seizure, the presence of abnormal slowing calls the diagnosis of an idiopathic generalized epilepsy into question. Some patients with JME may have a normal EEG study, but abnormalities are usually discovered with repeated studies. The diagnostic yield of the EEG in JME can be increased by the use of hyperventilation and strobe activation techniques. Recording sleep, which may be facilitated by sleep-depriving the patient before the study, also increases diagnostic yield.

At times, patients with JME may appear to manifest focal discharges. This occurs when asymmetric or fragmentary versions of the generalized discharges appear in the tracing (Figures 10.50 and 10.51). When spike asymmetries are seen in a presumed primary generalized epilepsy patient, the apparent focal discharges should not occur consistently on one side but should appear to be somewhat evenly distributed on both sides. Focal spike-wave discharges that represent fragments of generalized spike-wave discharges should occur at the same locations as the patient's generalized spike-wave discharge maxima, most commonly the superior frontal electrodes, F3 and F4. Therefore, apparently focal discharges that are present at the same maximum points as the generalized spike-wave discharges are still potentially consistent with an idiopathic generalized epilepsy, especially when those apparent focal discharges appear on both sides—in which case they should not be reported as separate focal abnormalities.

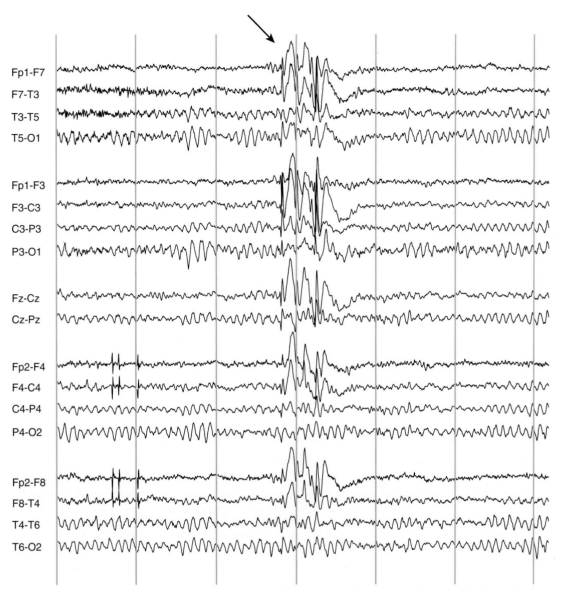

Figure 10.49 A brief, generalized fast spike-wave discharge is seen firing at approximately 4 Hz. Fast spike wave is particularly characteristic of the juvenile myoclonic epilepsy and juvenile absence epilepsy syndromes. The spike-like discharges seen in the first second of the tracing in the Fp2-F4, F4-C4, Fp2-F8, and F8-T4 channels represent artifact.

Persistent, mild asymmetries of spike-wave voltage can be seen from time to time in some patients with truly generalized discharges. Persistent lead-in of the spike wave discharges from one hemisphere, however, is not expected and may signal that a focal lesion is triggering the apparently generalized discharges, so-called secondary bilateral synchrony. A photoparoxysmal response is seen in about a third of patients, described below.

Strobe Stimulation and the Photoparoxysmal Response

Strobe stimulation, or intermittent photic stimulation, is one of two routine activation procedures (in addition to hyperventilation) carried out during most EEGs performed in the EEG laboratory. During the photic stimulation procedure, a strobe light is flashed in front of the patient at varying

frequencies, usually between 1 and 35 Hz, for 5 to 10 seconds at each frequency, separated by pauses of similar length. The EEG is then analyzed for a photic driving response (a normal finding) and a photoparoxysmal response (an abnormal finding).

Visual Evoked Potentials versus the Photic Driving Response

A visual evoked potential is a mainly positive-polarity wave seen in the occipital area approximately 100 msec after a visual stimulus such as a flash or a reversing pattern is shown to the patient. The individual wave produced by a single flash may be difficult to sort out from the background activity, so when formal visual evoked potentials are being performed, special averaging techniques are carried out with repeated flashes to define where this wave is in terms of its timing after the flash and what its morphology is. The

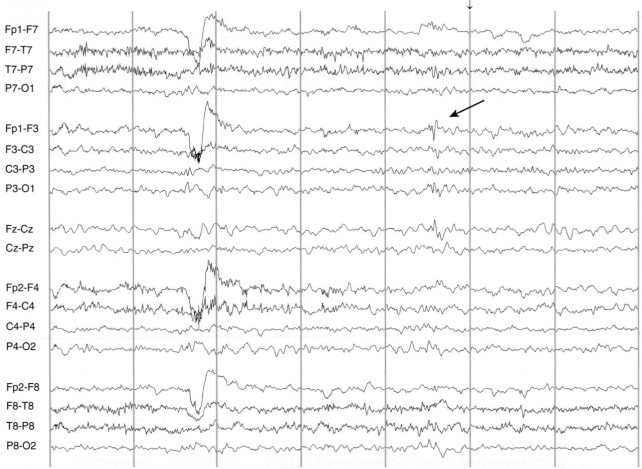

Figure 10.50 A single apparent focal spike-wave discharge is seen (arrow), maximum in the left superior frontal area. When seen as an isolated event, this spike-wave complex suggests a focal discharge. When seen in the context of the generalized spike-wave discharges seen elsewhere in the tracing of this patient with absence epilepsy, it is recognized as a fragment of a generalized discharge without focal significance (see Figure 10.48).

photic driving response consists of a train of these occipital waves or potentials driven by repetitive strobe flashes. Each individual wave of the driving response can then be considered an individual visual evoked potential, though no averaging technique is used for strobe stimulation during an EEG—the train is identified by the EEG reader visually. The photic driving response differs from visual evoked potentials in that it measures the ability of the occipital lobe to "follow" strobe flashes at varying frequencies with repetitive responses (Figure 10.52). The strobe may be able to entrain occipital waves at low flash frequencies, but the driving response may "drop out" at higher flash frequencies. Occasionally, the driving response is seen at a subharmonic of the strobe frequency, usually half the strobe frequency (Figure 10.53). The ability to produce driving at very high strobe frequencies, the high frequency photic response or H response has been reported to be associated with migraine and certain other clinical states, although the usefulness of this sign has been questioned.

A photic driving response can usually be observed in a calm, cooperative subject, but absence of an identifiable driving response is not considered abnormal. Amplitude asymmetries in the driving response may be seen in normal individuals. Because each occipital lobe responds to photic stimulation from the opposite visual hemifield, some observed asymmetries may be related to asymmetric retinal stimulation from off-center strobe placement or eye- or head-turning by the patient. Although it is true that structural asymmetries of brain may cause an asymmetry of the photic driving response, many neurologically normal individuals may have an inherently asymmetrical driving response. Therefore, isolated asymmetries of the photic driving against the backdrop of an otherwise normal EEG are not considered abnormal.

High-Amplitude Photic Response

Certain rare disorders have been associated with an unusually high-amplitude photic driving response, particularly at low strobe frequencies. Such high-voltage driving responses are probably the equivalent of abnormally high-voltage visual evoked potentials. The high-amplitude photic response has been described in the early stages of the late infantile form of neuronal ceroid lipofuscinosis (Jansky-Bielschowsky

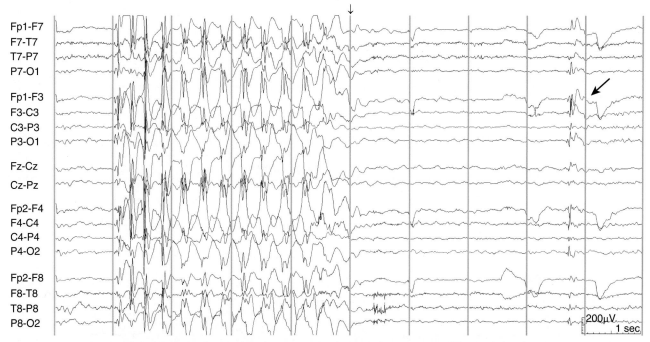

Figure 10.51 A high-voltage generalized spike-wave discharge is seen on a different page of the same patient's EEG that was shown in the previous figure. Of note, later in this page, a spike-wave discharge is seen (arrow), again representing a fragment of the generalized discharge. When several such fragmentary discharges are seen, approximately the same number would be expected on the left as on the right.

disease) as well as the juvenile form (Batten's disease)—neurodegenerative diseases of infancy and childhood associated with myoclonic seizures and progressive visual loss. Later in the course of these diseases, the photic response is completely lost, possibly because of ongoing retinal degeneration. A high-amplitude photic response may also occasionally be present in other neurodegenerative conditions.

The Photoparoxysmal Response

The phenomenon of intermittent photic stimulation eliciting generalized spike-wave discharges is referred to as the photoparoxysmal response (PPR; see Figure 10.52). Strobe stimulation can provoke a range of epileptiform activity in the EEG. Different features of the response are felt to increase or decrease the chances that the elicited activity is abnormal (i.e., associated with seizure disorders). When they occur, generalized or frontal-predominant spike-wave discharges are felt to be more abnormal than posterior spike-wave discharges. Higher voltage discharges are felt to be more abnormal than lower voltage discharges. Finally, spike-wave discharges that outlast the strobe stimulus are more likely significant compared to those that end immediately with the stimulus. Some of these guidelines, especially the distinction between posterior responses and responses in other locations, are designed to distinguish atypically exuberant (but non-epileptic) driving responses from true epileptiform bursts.

In patients with seizures, the PPR is most often seen in the idiopathic generalized epilepsies such as JME and JAE. When present, the PPR is most commonly seen during the adolescent and teenage years and tends to become less prominent with age. The presence of a PPR is not synonymous with photosensitive epilepsy, however. Photosensitive epilepsy most accurately refers to the situation in which the patient's seizures (as opposed to spike-wave discharges on the EEG) are triggered by flashing lights (Figure 10.54). Examples of light stimuli encountered during daily life that may elicit a seizure in a patient with photosensitive epilepsy include flashing strobe lights, driving down a sun-dappled street, or flashing lights from video screens. Patients with photosensitive epilepsy often do manifest a PPR on the EEG. However, of all patients with a PPR on the EEG (such as JME patients), most do not have a history of light-induced seizures among their naturally occurring episodes. The distinction between photosensitive epilepsy and a PPR is highlighted by the intriguing fact that, while it is not uncommon to record a PPR in the EEG lab, it is quite rare for strobe stimulation in the EEG lab to elicit an actual GTC seizure.

An intermediate situation may be seen in which each strobe flash generates a frontal-predominant spike-wave discharge and an epileptic myoclonic jerk. This phenomenon is referred to as a *photoconvulsive response*. When seen, the photoconvulsive response usually occurs in patients with idiopathic generalized epilepsy and the PPR triggered by the strobe flashes often outlasts the stimulus.

The *photomyoclonic response* is likely a non-epileptic phenomenon in which each strobe flash generates a (non-epileptic) muscle jerk in the patient, possibly related to a startle response. The EEG can be difficult to interpret as each body jerk can produce an artifact in the EEG that can be difficult to distinguish from polyspike-wave discharges. In such cases, the jerks should not outlast the strobe stimulus. The photomyoclonic response is not particularly associated with epilepsy and is

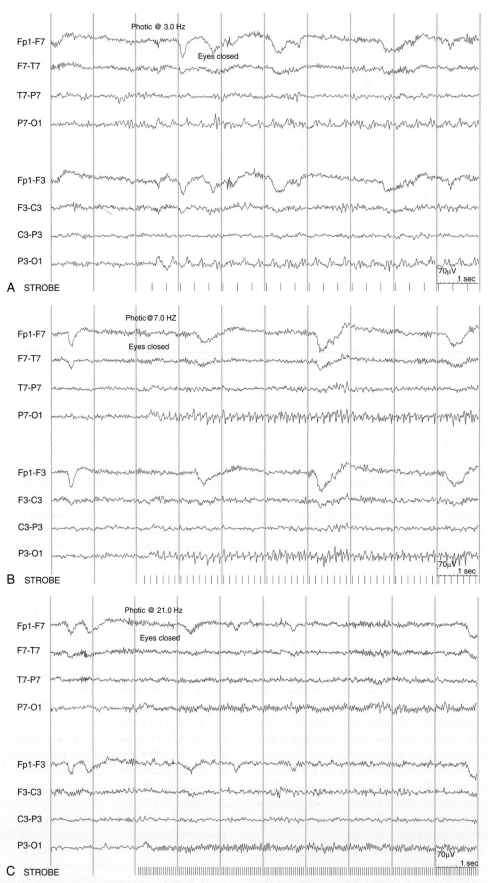

Figure 10.52 The strobe flashes of photic stimulation are denoted by each vertical line in the bottom strobe channel. A photic driving response can be seen in the occipital channels (P7-O1 and P3-O1) in the form of low-voltage, repetitive rhythmic waves that closely follow the strobe flashes. A similar response was also seen in the right occipital area but is not shown.

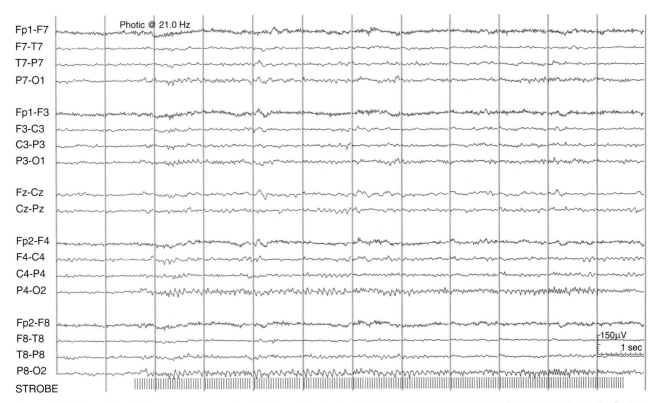

Figure 10.53 The photic driving response occasionally follows the strobe at a subharmonic (half) frequency. In this example, strobe flashes at 21 Hz generate a 10.5 Hz driving response.

more likely to occur in patients with a heightened level of anxiety at the time of the recording.

In support of the genetic nature of the PPR phenomenon, it may also be seen as an EEG trait in the unaffected siblings of patients with primary generalized epilepsy. A PPR is only rarely encountered in patients with focal epilepsies.

Generalized Epilepsy with Febrile Seizures "Plus": GEFS+

The GEFS+ syndrome is a familial genetic syndrome in which the different family members affected with the syndrome may have widely varying clinical presentations. Indeed, perhaps the most remarkable aspect of the GEFS+ syndrome is that the same single gene mutation can cause such a wide array of seizure types and seizure syndromes in different members of the same kindred. Individuals with the same GEFS+ mutation may manifest several combinations of (usually) generalized seizure types including febrile seizures, absence seizures, myoclonic seizures, generalized tonic-clonic seizures, and in the most severe phenotype, seizures indistinguishable from those that occur in myoclonic-atonic epilepsy (Doose syndrome, discussed later). In the general population, febrile seizures typically subside by the age of 6 years or earlier. Individuals with the GEFS+ syndrome may have febrile seizures that continue past this age, hence the term febrile seizures "plus." At the time of this writing, more than seven specific genetic mutations associated with the sodium channel, GABA receptor, and other errors have been identified that

can cause the various phenotypes of the GEFS+ syndrome in different families (and additional putative genetic loci have been identified). In a single family, multiple carriers of a given mutation may have strikingly different phenotypes.

It is surprising to see that a single gene mutation can cause seizure syndromes as apparently disparate as a febrile seizure syndrome and the syndrome of myoclonic-atonic seizures. At the same time, some obligate carriers of the GEFS+ mutation are asymptomatic. It is hypothesized that the dramatic variation seen in the clinical expression in carriers of the same mutation is related to other modifying genes in affected individuals. Patients with this syndrome may also manifest seizure disorders that are indistinguishable from JME, CAE, or epilepsy with GTC alone. Surprisingly, occasional individuals with this genotype may also manifest focal seizures. EEG findings in individuals with GEFS+ generally resemble the EEG patterns expected in the particular seizure syndrome the patient manifests as described earlier—there is no GEFS+-specific EEG pattern.

OTHER MYOCLONIC EPILEPSY SYNDROMES

Lennox-Gastaut Syndrome

Lennox-Gastaut syndrome (LGS) consists of the triad of mixed seizure types, a slow spike-wave pattern on EEG, and cognitive dysfunction beginning in early childhood. Seizure types seen in LGS include atypical absence seizures, atonic seizures, tonic seizures (occurring particularly during sleep),

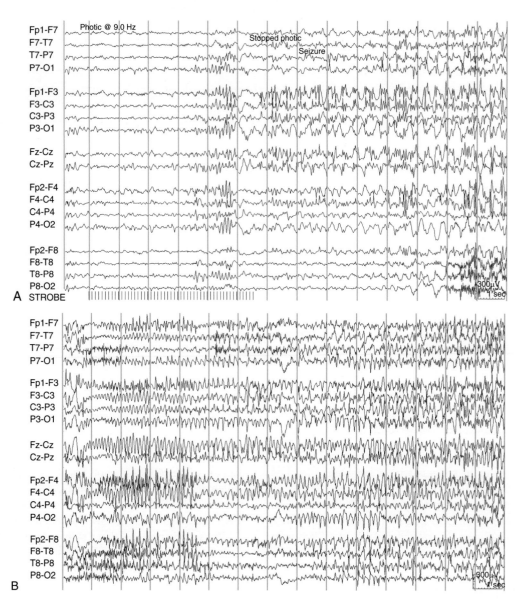

Figure 10.54 A generalized seizure is elicited by strobe stimulation. The phenomenon of an actual clinical seizure triggered by strobe flashes represents a true photosensitive epilepsy. Fortunately, this is an uncommon occurrence in the EEG lab. In contrast, many patients with a photoparoxysmal response as seen in Figure 10.75 may never actually have a clinical seizure triggered by flashing lights. Indeed, the photoparoxysmal response illustrated in that figure represented an EEG finding, but not a seizure.

and myoclonic seizures. Although some authors have classified LGS as a myoclonic epilepsy, myoclonic seizures are not an obligatory part of the syndrome. Previously LGS has also been classified as a *symptomatic generalized epilepsy*, a term and concept no longer favored. The idea was that the generalized (or bilateral, in terms of the newer conceptualization) seizures seen in LGS were symptomatic of some disorder that was already present. Although LGS includes many seizure patterns that resemble generalized seizures, in many patients the EEG also shows significant focal or multifocal abnormalities and seizures of clearly focal onset may occur among the mixed seizures of LGS. Therefore, LGS is no longer considered a member of the group of generalized epilepsies.

The seizures of LGS are often refractory to treatment. In most, cognitive problems are already evident at the time of

onset of the LGS syndrome, although a minority of children have an apparent normal neurodevelopmental status at the time the seizures start and subsequently lose ground as the seizures continue. In some patients, the LGS begins against the backdrop of a previously recognized encephalopathy, such as a pre-existing history of stroke, meningitis, cerebral dysgenesis, cerebral palsy, or West syndrome. In others with LGS, the syndrome appears to occur *de novo*.

Seizure Types and EEG Findings in Lennox-Gastaut Syndrome

Patients with LGS have a mixture of seizure types. The atypical absence seizures of LGS are associated with a simultaneous slow spike-wave pattern on the EEG that usually has a diffuse distribution. With atypical absence, neither the outwardly

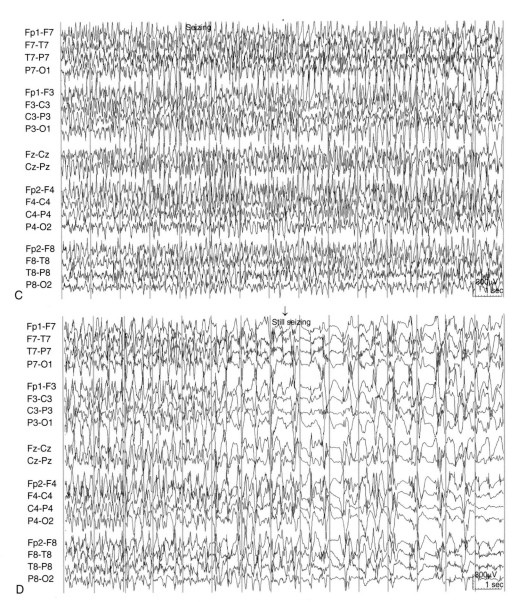

Figure 10.54, cont'd

apparent staring spell nor the slow spike-wave pattern seen on EEG necessarily shows a sharply demarcated onset or termination. This is in contrast to the case with typical absence seizures, where onset and termination are fairly abrupt. Making the situation yet more complicated, slow spike-wave discharges are also frequently seen as an interictal abnormality in LGS. This is to say that, when a run of slow spike-wave discharges is seen on the EEG, it is generally not possible for the reader to know whether the discharges represent an electroclinical seizure or an interictal abnormality without concurrent evidence of loss of awareness or responsiveness in the patient. In LGS patients, the slow spike-wave discharge that cause a seizure and the slow spike-wave that occurs between clinical seizures can look the same.

The atonic seizures in LGS may occur in their mildest form as a brief bobbing of the head or slumping of the shoulders. More severe versions may occur, such as dramatic "head drops" in which the face may fall forward and hit a table in front of the patient. The most severe version is the drop attack in which the patient falls to the ground. Patients with "drop seizures" may need to wear a helmet for head protection. Multiple EEG correlates are seen to for drop seizures or atonic seizures (discussed earlier). Tonic seizures may occur at any time of the day, but the tonic seizures of LGS occur most characteristically during sleep and are typically associated with brief runs of generalized rapid spikes (Figure 10.55). In fact, the tonic seizure out of sleep is considered the hallmark seizure type of LGS.

Not all seizures that cause a head drop or a fall necessarily belong to the category of atonic seizures as seizures with tonic or myoclonic components may also culminate in a fall. Careful studies with the use of EMG electrodes have documented that many such "drop seizures," instead of being caused by a loss of tone, are actually associated

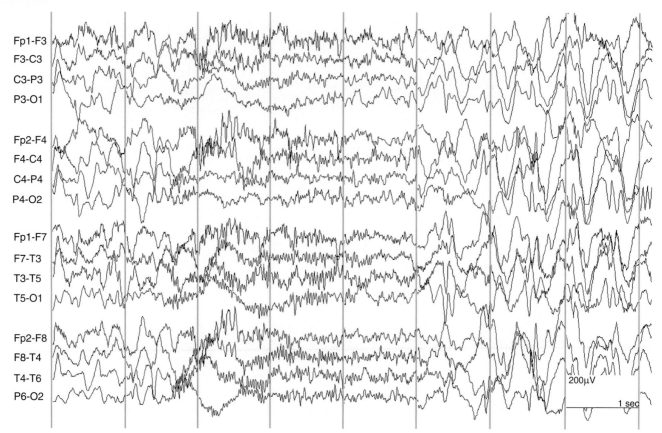

Figure 10.55 A tonic seizure occurs in sleep in a patient with the Lennox-Gastaut syndrome. The background pattern of slow spike-wave discharges is interrupted by a brief train of generalized rapid spikes associated with whole body tonic stiffening. The fact that this is more than just an interictal EEG abnormality but rather a clinical seizure is supported by the appearance of the muscle artifact superimposed on the rapid spikes.

with an initial tonic muscle contraction. Some prefer the more general term astatic seizure for such episodes (literally meaning the loss of the ability to stand—astasia), which can properly be used for any seizure type in which loss of posture is the primary feature. This term had the advantage of not implying that its user knew for certain whether various muscle groups had undergone tonic or atonic changes during the seizure.

The typical interictal EEG in LGS includes generalized and/or focal slow spike-wave or polyspike-wave discharges (at 1–2.5 Hz) that are sometimes activated by sleep, a slow background, and brief bursts of rapid spikes in sleep. Many patients also manifest multifocal spikes or sharp waves.

Myoclonic-Atonic Epilepsy or Doose Syndrome

In 1970, Doose et al. described an epilepsy syndrome with myoclonic seizures and falling spells that appeared to be distinct from LGS. Whereas children with LGS usually appeared to have a symptomatic epilepsy, those with this new syndrome had no clear etiology for their seizures but did have a strong family history of epilepsy. Therefore, a genetic etiology was suspected. In previous classifications, this syndrome was referred to as myoclonic-astatic epilepsy.

The most characteristic seizure type seen in myoclonic-atonic epilepsy is the myoclonic-atonic seizure, which consists of one or more brief myoclonic jerks followed by a loss of posture, often culminating in a fall. There is brief loss of consciousness during the attacks followed by quick recovery. Seizure onset is usually between 1½ and 5 years of age. A variety of other generalized seizure types also may occur including GTC seizures, absence seizures, and tonic seizures. Response to treatment and prognosis vary widely in this group, with some patients nicely responsive to treatment but others who are refractory to therapy and who have a downhill developmental course.

EEG Findings in Myoclonic-Atonic Epilepsy

The EEG may be normal at onset. Often, the background shows slowing in the 4 to 7 Hz range, although the posterior dominant rhythm often is in the normal range. In sleep, slow spike-wave discharges can be seen, although this finding is not as prominent as in LGS. Slow spike-wave discharges are not expected during wakefulness. Both the myoclonic and myoclonic-atonic seizures are typically accompanied by a brief burst of 2 to 4 Hz generalized spike-wave or polyspike-wave discharges, often one to three discharges in quick succession.

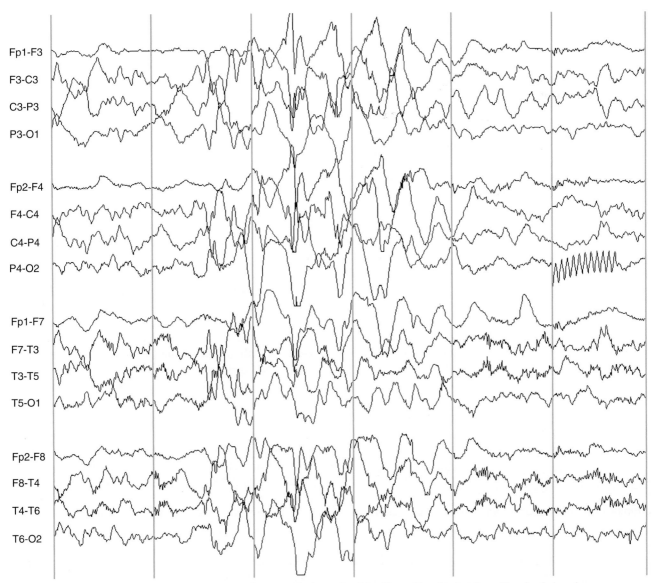

Figure 10.56 A brief, generalized spike-wave discharge is elicited by patting this toddler with reflex-induced myoclonic epilepsy on the back. The artifact in the P4-O2 channel on the last second of the page is an event marker made by the child's caretakers at the time of the clinical event.

Myoclonic Epilepsy in Infancy

Myoclonic epilepsy in infancy (previously referred to as benign myoclonic epilepsy of infancy) is a syndrome consisting mainly of myoclonic seizures typically presenting between the ages of 1 and 5 years in an otherwise normal child. The ictal EEG shows a brief series of generalized polyspikes driving rapidly repetitive myoclonic jerks which are usually relatively mild and occur only a few times a day. The myoclonic seizures are usually responsive to valproic acid. The syndrome usually remits spontaneously during childhood, but later learning and developmental difficulties may occur with a higher frequency in affected individuals compared with the general population. Strobe stimulation may elicit the jerks in a subset of infants. Because of the occasional occurrence of generalized tonic-clonic seizures in children with this syndrome, myoclonic epilepsy in infancy may exist on a continuum with other primary generalized epilepsy syndromes.

Reflex-Induced Myoclonic Epilepsy

Reflex-induced myoclonic epilepsy may represent a subset of myoclonic epilepsy in infancy in which the myoclonic jerks are elicited by sound or touch. In certain infants, auditory or tactile stimulation such as a loud sound, brushing the cheek, or patting the back may elicit a train of spike-wave discharges associated with a brief run of rapid myoclonic jerks (see Figure 10.56). Reflex-induced myoclonic epilepsy, too, is generally expected to remit during childhood.

Severe Myoclonic Epilepsy of Infancy (Dravet Syndrome)

Severe myoclonic epilepsy of infancy (SMEI) is a childhood-onset epilepsy that is refractory to treatment. Because it is believed that the ongoing neurological deterioration seen in this syndrome may be caused by the occurrence of the seizures themselves, it is also considered one of the developmental epileptic encephalopathies. The typical presentation begins with repeated prolonged febrile seizures during the first year of life. Afebrile seizures then become more prominent, which may be either generalized or focal. Despite the original name of the syndrome (SMEI), the presence of myoclonic seizures is not invariable. For that reason, the eponym Dravet syndrome is increasingly used. Despite its relationship to the generalized epilepsies, focal seizures that can arise from either hemisphere are frequent, often with secondary generalization as was seen in Figure 10.10. Tonic seizures are uncommon.

The majority of cases of SMEI are caused by mutations in the SCN1A gene, the same gene that has been implicated in some GEFS+ kindreds and that may cause the variety of epilepsy syndrome presentations seen in that syndrome. Borderline versions of SMEI are seen, suggesting that the syndrome may lie on the severe end of the spectrum of primary generalized epilepsies. Other genes have been implicated in individuals with a Dravet syndrome phenotype in a minority of cases.

Early in the course, the EEG may be normal. Later, high-voltage spike-wave and polyspike-wave complexes appear, sometimes generalized but in some examples surprisingly focal and concentrated over one hemisphere (Figure 10.57). The discharges are activated by sleep and may manifest photosensitivity. The EEG pattern in SMEI is variable and not highly characteristic. The association of the seizures with fever, especially early on, is a useful diagnostic feature.

Epilepsy with Continuous Spike Wave of Slow Sleep and the Landau-Kleffner Syndrome

Epilepsy with Continuous Spike Wave of Slow Sleep

Continuous spike wave of slow sleep (CSWS) is a relatively rare epileptic encephalopathy associated with neuropsychological impairment and a variety of possible seizure types, both generalized and focal. It shares many clinical features with Landau-Kleffner syndrome, described next. CSWS is associated with a distinctive EEG pattern during slow-wave sleep termed electrical status epilepticus of sleep (ESES). The term CSWS is used to refer to the clinical syndrome, while ESES refers specifically to the EEG pattern. The ESES pattern consists of continuous, rhythmic 1.5 to 2.5 Hz spike-wave discharges, often with a diffuse field but occasionally unilateral, that appear in non-REM sleep. The essence of this sleep-activated EEG pattern is the appearance of spike-wave discharges so rhythmic that they could potentially be mistaken for an electrographic seizure (Figure 10.58). Despite the name of the syndrome, which might seem to imply that the pattern should only be present during the sleep stages with slow waves, Stages III and IV (or N3), the ESES pattern appears with onset of Stage I or early in Stage II sleep. Therefore, ESES is essentially seen in the non-REM sleep stages. It is not necessary to insist on recording Stage III and IV sleep to exclude the presence of the ESES pattern—indications of the ESES pattern should be recognized by onset of Stage II sleep if it is to be present. In REM sleep, the continuity of the ESES discharges is significantly disrupted. Scattered, focal discharges may be seen in REM sleep, similar in density to what is seen during wakefulness.

The patterns of clinical seizures seen in this syndrome range from rare or no seizures to seizures that occur several times per week. A wide variety of seizure types is seen, including nocturnal seizures, either hemiclonic or apparent generalized tonic-clonic, typical absence seizures or, more rarely, atypical absences that may also be associated with falls. Tonic seizures as are seen in LGS generally do not occur. Although epilepsy with CSWS is generally considered an idiopathic syndrome with no causative lesion expected on the MRI, in some children, a clinical picture otherwise similar to idiopathic CSWS may be seen as a symptomatic syndrome related to preexisting lesional abnormalities. The question of whether the classification should separate such symptomatic cases from the main CSWS group has yet to be resolved.

By what may seem to be an arbitrary definition based on the earliest descriptions, the ESES pattern should be visible during 85% or more of non-REM sleep. The term electrical status epilepticus reminds us that the pattern should have sufficient rhythmicity and continuity as to mimic a seizure discharge. The term ESES should not apply to patterns in which there may be a very high density of interictal activity during sleep but without the rhythmicity seen in seizure discharges. When making the diagnosis of ESES, the reader should have the impression that the discharge is so rhythmic that it could actually represent electrical seizure activity but that its duration, lack of evolution, and disappearance in REM sleep and on awakening make this unlikely. Whether other EEG patterns with a spike-wave density significantly below 85% or that manifest less rhythmicity and continuity should be included with ESES is controversial. In straightforward cases of ESES, it is visually obvious that the spike-wave pattern is present for 85% or more of the non-REM tracing and strict quantification of the percentage usually is not necessary. The 85% term was likely used in the original description descriptively to allow for the brief breaks in the highly rhythmic spike-wave pattern seen in classic ESES (and which may also be seen in other versions of electrographic status epilepticus). For that reason, it is usually unnecessary to make a formal count of the percentage of involved seconds in individuals who have classic ESES.

Some readers calculate and report a "spike-wave index," the percentage of one-second bins that include a spike-wave discharge, independent of their rhythmicity or resemblance to seizure activity. The clinical importance of changes in the spike-wave index has yet to be established. For instance, if a clinician changes a patient's medication dose and the spike-wave index changes from 52% to 40%, is the patient really any better? Although you may think that providing this type of information can't hurt, including this quantification in your report may represent false precision. The very act of including it in the EEG report may imply to referring providers that the reader believes that the number has an inherent value by which one might adjust the patient's treatment regimen, or that it has some correlation with the patient's well-being, which it may not. In fact, this type of change may simply represent natural variation, which can be considerable from study to study, even in the absence of a change in therapy or the patient.

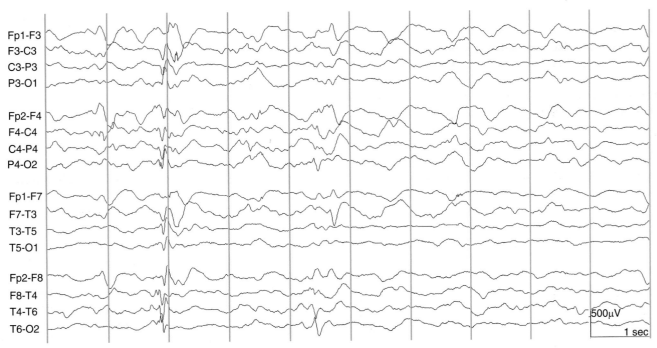

Figure 10.57 This child with severe myoclonic epilepsy of infancy (SMEI or Dravet syndrome) has both generalized and focal discharges. EEG findings vary widely among patients with SMEI.

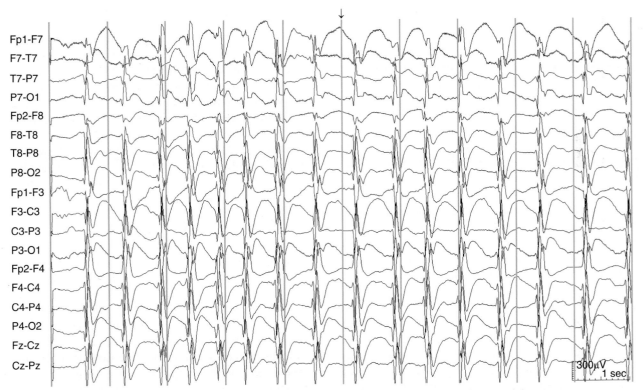

Figure 10.58 This highly rhythmic generalized discharge mimics a seizure discharge; however, it is present exclusively during non–rapid eye movement (REM) sleep and dissipates during REM sleep and on awakening. The ESES pattern consists not only of spikes activated by sleep but of a pattern so rhythmic and continuous that it could be mistaken for a seizure discharge, as is seen in this figure.

Another potential pitfall is to equate an EEG with a *spike-wave index* over 85% with ESES. Although it remains to be seen whether a spike-wave index of 85% versus 55% in two different patients tells us a lot about a difference between the two patients, the original 85% benchmark was only meant to refer to the density of rhythmic and entrained spike-wave discharges that resemble electrical status epilepticus, and not to a spike-wave index. Indeed, some children with benign rolandic epilepsy can develop very high spike-wave indices in sleep.

Epilepsy with CSWS is associated with a global cognitive impairment that may include the behavioral, language, and motor realms. A variety of patterns of cognitive deficits may be seen. The presence of the ESES pattern appears to be age-dependent, even in those who have organic lesions on imaging. The continuous spike-wave pattern tends to "burn out" by the early teenage years independent of treatment. In some individuals, the EEG may even normalize. In general, children with CSWS appear to fall into two groups. In some children, the MRI is normal and the disorder appears to be a genetic epilepsy, possibly with strong links to BCECTS because the initial presentation and EEG pattern as well as the tendency for the EEG pattern to remit spontaneously after childhood resemble that disorder. In the other group, the MRI is abnormal and may show cortical dysplasia or early strokes, often involving the thalamus or basal ganglia.

Long-term outcome may depend on a variety of factors, particularly the underlying etiology. Many children improve significantly after CSWS has run its course, although some amount of residual disability is the rule. The ESES pattern may be resistant to treatment; however, high-dose diazepam therapy can result in periods of remission and clinical improvement of varying duration in some (De Negri et al., 1995). ACTH or corticosteroids also may be effective.

Acquired Epileptic Aphasia or the Landau-Kleffner Syndrome

The Landau-Kleffner syndrome (LKS) or acquired epileptic aphasia is a childhood epilepsy syndrome that may exist in the middle of a spectrum that includes benign rolandic epilepsy on one end and epilepsy with CSWS on the other. In children with LKS, the language disturbance predominates. In contrast to the majority of language disturbances observed in childhood in which expressive language lags behind the ability to comprehend, in LKS difficulties with language comprehension are more prominent than expressive difficulties.

The most characteristic pattern is of a child who develops language normally and then acquires an aphasia pattern that is most pronounced in the receptive realm. Concurrently or soon after, an EEG abnormality is noted over one or both temporal lobes, strongly activated by sleep. Behavior and attention may also be adversely affected. Children with LKS may also have seizures, but these are usually sporadic and few in number. In rare instances, LKS may begin before significant language has developed, and the "acquired" nature of the syndrome may not be evident. Such children may appear to present as having pure language delay. How often LKS plays a role in the language

and behavioral regression seen in children with autism has been a matter of some debate. It does not appear that LKS explains more than a very small percentage of the larger population of children with autistic disorders.

The interictal EEG in LKS may show focal discharges, often in the centrotemporal areas or the posterior temporal/parietal areas and may also occasionally show generalized spike-wave discharges (Figure 10.59). In a minority, the discharges may have a frontal localization. In some, the waking EEG is normal. At some point in the disorder, not always at onset, bilateral generalized spike-wave activity is seen in a pattern consistent with ESES with more than 85% of the slow-wave sleep tracing involved with continuous spike-wave activity. This ESES pattern, when present, is essentially indistinguishable from the patterns that can be seen in epilepsy with CSWS, suggesting the possibility that LKS actually represents a subset of CSWS. In LKS, more unilateral or focal patterns of persistent spike-wave complexes are more common compared with the CSWS syndrome in which discharges tend to be more bilateral and diffuse. Clinically, deficits in LKS are more concentrated in the language sphere whereas the deficits seen in CSWS tend to be more global.

Because the discharges seen in LKS often show voltage maxima in the centrotemporal areas, a relationship between this syndrome and BCECTS has been proposed, although not yet proven. In fact, some children with benign rolandic epilepsy show so much sleep activation on the EEG that they may strongly resemble, at least from the EEG point of view, the EEG patterns seen in LKS. In children with LKS, initial EEGs are often interpreted as being consistent with BCECTS because of the presence of centrotemporal spikes. The fact that some children with BCECTS may manifest a developmental language abnormality also supports the possibility that the syndromes are related.

Although cases of an EEG pattern consistent with LKS have been reported after acquired brain lesions, in general, those with LKS have a normal MRI and, apart from the EEG, other diagnostic testing is normal. Thus far, a small minority of LKS presentations have been found to be associated with a genetic abnormality in the GRIN2A gene.

Angelman Syndrome

Angelman syndrome is a rare genetic disorder that has also been referred to as the "Happy Puppet Syndrome" because of the jerky, puppet-like movements and inappropriate laughter that marks some of the affected children's behavior, though some patients do not display either of these attributes. Most patients have moderate to severe intellectual disability and some can walk while others are wheelchair-bound. Many of the children have seizures that are resistant to treatment. The inheritance pattern of Angelman syndrome is distinctive, and shows a classic example of genetic imprinting. In most, the disorder is caused by an error in the UBE3A gene, located on the long arm of chromosome 15, when the abnormality is inherited from the mother. In neurons, the paternal copy of this gene is normally turned off so that proper function of the gene product is dependent on the maternal copy of the gene.

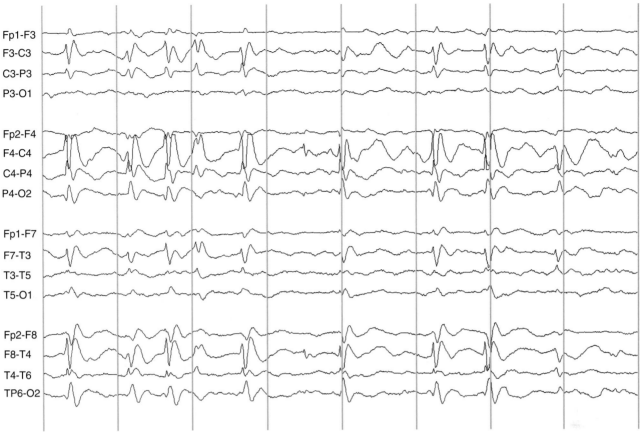

Figure 10.59 The EEG findings of Landau-Kleffner syndrome (LKS) are more widely variable than strict ESES patterns (an example of which was illustrated in the previous figure). The component discharges seen in LKS may resemble rolandic discharges and are typically activated by sleep. They may be seen over one or both hemispheres. Although the discharges shown here are semirhythmic, they would not be mistaken for continuous electrographic seizure activity. A sharp eye will capture a subtle left frontal positivity in F3.

(Individuals who inherit a mutated copy of the UBE3A gene paternally may manifest the Prader-Willi syndrome, known for profound early hypotonia and poor feeding but a later tendency to hyperphagia and obesity.)

Several EEG patterns have been described in Angelman syndrome, but the most characteristic pattern is of high-voltage 2 to 2.5 Hz rhythmic delta waves which are seen during both wakefulness and sleep. The delta waves variably manifest a spike component, in which case they resemble slow spike-wave discharges. In some patients, these waves can have a triphasic morphology (Figure 10.60).

Alpers Disease—POLG1 Disease

Alpers disease, also known as Alpers-Huttenlocher disease, should be suspected in a child who presents with a neurodegenerative disorder in the first years of life that combines seizures and progressive neurologic deterioration with liver failure. Convulsive status epilepticus at presentation is common and epilepsia partialis continua may be seen as well. The disorder is caused by a mutation in the POLG1 gene, the gene that codes for the polymerase gamma enzyme that is responsible for replication of mitochondrial DNA. In children with this disorder, the use of valproic acid may improve seizures but can precipitate worsened liver failure and should, therefore, be avoided. With discontinuation of the valproic acid, in some patients liver function may improve. Children with Alpers disease have been shown to have a distinctive finding in the EEG called *RHADS*: rhythmic high-amplitude delta with superimposed (poly)spikes (Figure 10.61). Recognition of this distinctive EEG pattern may suggest the possibility of a POLG1 abnormality in a child in whom the diagnosis has not yet been made.

FOCAL EPILEPSIES

Temporal Lobe Epilepsy

Temporal lobe epilepsy is the most common focal epilepsy. The seizure type most often associated with temporal lobe epilepsy is the focal seizure with impaired awareness. Focal seizures *without* impairment of awareness may also occur, such as those that consist only of a sense of déjà vu, a feeling of fear, olfactory sensations, etc., if they remain confined to the

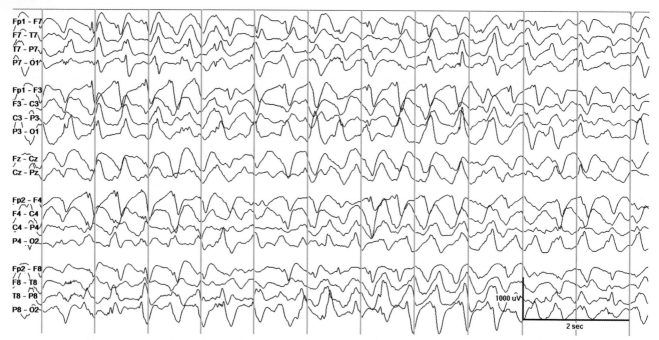

Figure 10.60 This is the EEG of a 3-year-old boy with Angelman syndrome while awake and interactive. Note that the fundamental background feature in this EEG is high-voltage, highly rhythmic 2 Hz delta activity. A frontal spike component is seen in a waxing and waning pattern. (Courtesy of Dr. Rachel Hirschberger).

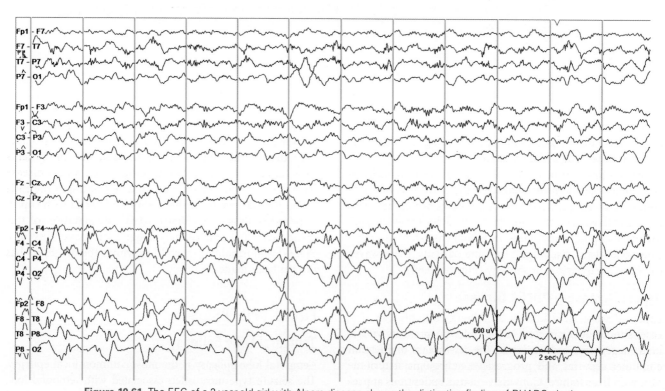

Figure 10.61 The EEG of a 2-year-old girl with Alpers disease shows the distinctive finding of RHADS: rhythmic high-amplitude delta with superimposed (poly)spikes. In this patient, the RHADS are unilateral, but they may be bilateral in some patients. RHADS typically show a posterior predominance. At other times in this patient's recording, the RHADS would accelerate and coalesce into convulsive seizures from time to time. (Courtesy of Drs. Coral Stredny and Agnieszka Kielian).

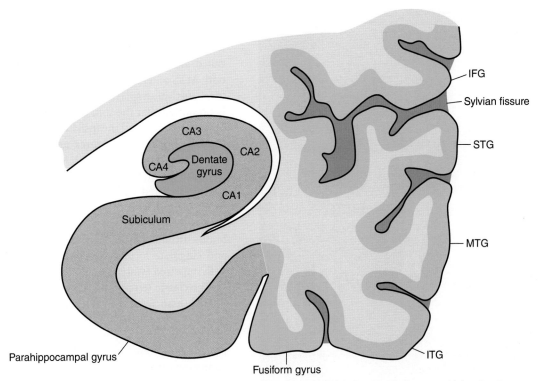

Figure 10.62 This image shows the relationship between the medial and neocortical temporal lobe structures in the coronal plane. The hippocampus is the most epileptogenic structure in the temporal lobe, and is labeled CA1 through CA4 in this figure to denote the four subsections of Ammon's horn of the hippocampus. The dentate gyrus is closely apposed to Ammon's horn and is considered part of the hippocampal formation. The fine ultrastructure of the hippocampus can often be appreciated on higher resolution MRI scans through this area (see next figure). The remainder of the surface of the temporal lobe has a six-layered neocortical structure. In counter-clockwise order, the gyri of temporal lobe neocortex are shown: The parahippocampal gyrus, fusiform gyrus, ITG = inferior temporal gyrus, MTG = middle temporal gyrus, and STG = superior temporal gyrus. The sylvian fissure, the major fissure on the lateral surface of the hemisphere that leads down to the insula, separates the temporal lobe from the inferior frontal gyrus (IFG) of the frontal lobe.

medial temporal lobe. Such seizures may not be detected on scalp EEG until such time as they might spread more widely.

Temporal lobe epilepsy can be anatomically categorized into two groups: medial temporal lobe epilepsy and neocortical temporal lobe epilepsy. In the temporal lobe, the hippocampus and closely associated dentate gyrus are medial structures that have an architecturally older, four-layered cortical architecture (also referred to as allocortex), shown in Figure 10.62. Despite being small and tucked away in the medial temporal lobe, the hippocampus is the most epileptogenic area of the brain and is a frequent location of seizure onset. As a shorthand, epilepsies whose seizure-onset zones are substantially in the medial temporal lobe and include the hippocampus are referred to as medial temporal lobe epilepsy.

The term *neocortex* refers to the highly organized six-layered cortex that is evolutionarily the newest part of the brain and found only in higher mammals. The large majority of the gyri and sulci of the brain consist of neocortex and this applies to the temporal lobe as well (excluding the hippocampus and its closely related structures as described above). The term *neocortical temporal lobe epilepsy* then implies that the seizure-onset zone for the epilepsy involves a cortical surface of the temporal lobe that is specifically not in the hippocampus or its closely related structures. For instance, a seizure may arise from the auditory area of the superior temporal gyrus producing unusual sound manifestations for the patient. This would be an example of a neocortical temporal lobe epilepsy that could further be specified as lateral temporal lobe epilepsy (because the superior temporal gyrus is on the lateral surface of the temporal lobe), a subset of the neocortical temporal lobe epilepsies. Note that lateral temporal lobe epilepsy is not necessarily everything in the temporal lobe that is not medial temporal lobe epilepsy because epilepsies may also arise from the basal temporal lobe.

The medial temporal lobe, especially the hippocampus, is a comparatively epileptogenic structure. Even though the large majority of the temporal lobe consists of neocortex, including the base and lateral surface of the temporal lobe, the majority of temporal lobe epilepsies are medial temporal lobe epilepsies and arise from the hippocampus.

The hallmark pathologic finding in medial temporal lobe epilepsy is mesial temporal sclerosis (MTS), also referred to as *hippocampal sclerosis*. On pathologic examination, this is seen as pyramidal cell loss in the hippocampus, which may occur in different zones of the Ammon's horn portion of

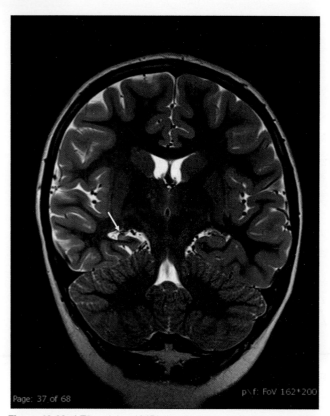

Page: 37 of 68   p\f: FoV 162*200

Figure 10.63 A T2-weighted MRI showing a coronal slice through the temporal lobes. The black arrow denotes a normal-appearing left hippocampal formation in which the "jelly roll" ultrastructure of the hippocampus can be appreciated. The white arrow shows an example of mesial temporal sclerosis in the right hippocampus: the right hippocampus is smaller, its architectural features are harder to see, and it shows increased T2-weighted signal (brightness) on this scan.

the hippocampus or the dentate gyrus with associated hardening (sclerosis) of the tissue. (Ammon's horn is written as *cornu ammonis* in Latin, explaining the nomenclature of CA1 through CA4 for the four subparts of Ammon's horn.) On MRI, the architecture of Ammon's horn and the dentate gyrus create the characteristic flattened jelly roll appearance of the hippocampus. On MRI, MTS is best seen on coronal slices of the temporal lobes when specific sequences tailored to the diagnosis of epilepsy are used. Findings suggestive of MTS on MRI include a smaller hippocampus, increased T2 signal in the hippocampus, and a loss of the ability to appreciate the details of the internal ("jelly roll") architecture of the hippocampus (Figure 10.63).

It is not entirely clear whether a patient develops MTS, which in turn causes seizures, or whether seizures occur which then causes MTS. For instance, a higher percentage of patients with MTS have a history of prolonged febrile seizures in childhood compared to individuals without MTS, which suggests a causative link. It is important to remember that the large majority of children with febrile seizures, even if prolonged, still do not develop MTS or temporal lobe epilepsy, suggesting there could be a genetic predisposition to developing MTS after febrile seizures in some patients. Current thought is that some initial event (possibly seizures,

an infection, or an initial ischemic injury) causes MTS, which can then later become a primary onset zone for seizures. This idea is also supported by the observation of cases with so-called *dual pathology*. In dual pathology, an individual has both MTS and another lesion causative of seizures, such as a focal cortical dysplasia or tumor, in the same hemisphere. It is presumed that the initial epileptogenicity of the dysplasia or tumor has caused the ipsilateral MTS, which later becomes capable of triggering seizures autonomously.

The term focal seizure with impaired awareness should not be equated with temporal lobe epilepsy. Most, but not all, seizures associated with the temporal lobe can be classified as focal seizures with impaired awareness. Focal seizures with impaired awareness can, however, arise from any lobe of the brain—frontal, parietal, and occipital foci (including insular and cingulate localizations) can all result in focal seizures with impaired awareness.

The classic temporal lobe seizure may begin with staring, possibly associated with automatisms such as fumbling movements of a hand, chewing, or lip-smacking automatic behaviors. If there is a seizure prodrome or aura, it may include psychic symptoms such as a feeling of fear or déjà vu, or hallucinations involving the senses of taste or smell. Here, the term prodrome is misleading because such psychic symptoms actually represent the beginning of the ictal discharge rather than a warning that one is to occur. Dystonic posturing of a hand, when it occurs, is typically seen contralateral to the seizure focus. Conversely, automatic behaviors in a hand such as fumbling or picking movements usually occur ipsilateral to the side of the seizure focus. It is likely the case that these automatic movements are not actually driven directly by the seizure discharge (in which case they would be expected to occur contralaterally) but rather occur as a release phenomenon. Temporal lobe seizure activity may spread to the ipsilateral motor cortex and include clonic or tonic movements of the contralateral side of the body, or the seizure may secondarily generalize and evolve to a bilateral convulsion.

EEG Findings in Temporal Lobe Epilepsy

Because most temporal lobe epilepsy originates in the anterior temporal lobe, the classic interictal EEG finding of temporal lobe epilepsy is the anterior temporal spike or sharp wave. An isolated spike in either the F7 or F8 or adjacent electrodes can aid significantly in localizing a seizure focus to the temporal lobe. Focal temporal discharges are often activated by sleep. An associated slow-wave abnormality may also be seen in the temporal lobe, either in the form of intermittent slow (temporal intermittent rhythmic delta activity, or TIRDA) or continuous slowing. The use of additional electrodes over the anterior temporal lobes, such as the T1 and T2 positions (or the similar FT9 and FT10 positions) can enhance the recording of discharges from the temporal lobes. Because the yield of invasive electrodes such as sphenoidal and nasopharyngeal electrodes is not significantly better than these additional surface temporal electrodes, the use of these invasive contacts has become much less common. Depending on their particular localization on the temporal lobe surface, interictal discharges from the temporal lobe may also appear in other nearby electrodes.

Temporal lobe seizures can be associated with focal discharges as described earlier, with spikes or sharp waves that manifest a broader field across the temporal lobe, or with discharges that are triggered by irritability in the temporal lobe but that spread quickly and express themselves across the whole of the involved hemisphere. In some cases, a focal temporal lobe abnormality can trigger an apparently generalized discharge (secondary bilateral synchrony) resulting in generalized spike-wave discharges with varying amounts of interhemispheric symmetry (see Chapter 9, "The Abnormal EEG," for a more detailed discussion of secondary bilateral synchrony).

Because the hippocampus and related structures are hidden away in the medial temporal lobe, relatively far from the scalp, it is not obvious how seizure activity in this area might express on scalp electrodes. After all, depending on its orientation, the dipole of a discharge from the hippocampus could point in a variety of possible directions, like a searchlight beam, and be picked up best by any of a number of surface electrodes. To determine when and how seizure activity in the medial temporal lobe would become recordable by surface EEG electrodes, ideally, one would want to record seizures simultaneously from two sources: from intracranial electrodes placed directly on the surfaces of the temporal lobe (as is done during the process of epilepsy surgery) comparing them to simultaneous recordings from scalp electrodes. This is the strategy Pacia and Ebersole used when they recorded temporal lobe seizures simultaneously from both subdural electrode grids placed on the surface of the brain and from scalp EEG electrodes. They described specific ictal patterns that may distinguish mesial temporal lobe seizures from neocortical seizures on scalp EEG. A preponderance of their "Type 1" patterns were seen in seizures of hippocampal origin and "Type 2" patterns were associated with seizures of neocortical temporal origin. Their Type 1 pattern began with a regular 5 to 9 Hz discharge, either seen best in the inferior temporal electrodes such as T1 and T2 or FT9 and FT10 (Type 1a) or instead in the vertex and parasagittal electrodes (Type 1b) at onset. This projection to the vertex was explained by seizure dipoles on the base of the temporal lobe projecting up to the vertex and parasagittal areas. These specific localizations were best appreciated in referential montages and the described pattern referred to the seizure onsets. Interestingly, the observed discharges did not appear on the scalp until the seizure discharge spread from the hippocampus to adjacent neocortical temporal structures. Type 2 patterns were more frequently associated with neocortical epilepsies. These discharges were distinguished by somewhat irregular 2 to 5 Hz patterns that later increased in frequency up to 7 Hz after several seconds (becoming similar in appearance to the Type 1a discharge), in some cases marking spread to the hippocampal electrodes on the subdural recordings. Type 3 discharges showed little on scalp EEG or perhaps some background slowing. As noted, when seizures remained confined to the hippocampus on the subdural recordings, they often were not seen on scalp EEG. These scalp EEG patterns were associated with the above-described anatomical locations on intracranial recordings in the majority, but not all, cases.

Other Lesional Epilepsies

Although the temporal lobe is the most common location for lesional epilepsies, lesions that cause focal-onset seizures can be located in any area of cerebral cortex, including deeper cortical areas. Lesions that cause localization-related epilepsies may be either congenital or acquired. Congenital lesions include cortical dysplasias and other malformations, including the hamartomas associated with tuberous sclerosis or pre- of perinatally acquired cortical scars. In childhood and adulthood, seizure foci may be created by a variety of processes including traumatic injury, vascular injury (including stroke and complications of vascular malformations), tumors, inflammation including infectious and autoimmune phenomena, and neurodegenerative processes.

The EEG signs of lesional epilepsy in non-temporal locations are analogous to those of temporal lobe epilepsy as described earlier. Focal spikes or sharp waves arising from the epileptogenic area are the most characteristic signs of a focal epilepsy. Associated slow wave abnormalities may also be present.

At times, the EEG reader may encounter what appear to be generalized spike-wave discharges in which the spike foci do not have a clear localization (Figure 10.64). Although this type of spike-wave discharge may appear to be generalized, the mechanism of onset could be either focal or generalized. This is possible because focal brain lesions can sometimes trigger discharges that spread so quickly that they resemble generalized discharges. In such cases, asymmetries in the discharge, lead-ins from one side, or other focal findings in the EEG may serve as a clue to the focal nature of the discharge's mechanism. When attempting to localize a discharge that has a broad field, it is the localization of the spike component of the discharge that is of greatest interest.

If you encounter an EEG that has apparent generalized spike-wave discharges but another clearly focal finding, it may be risky to conclude that the diffuse discharges do, indeed, arise by a truly generalized mechanism. Remember that, in a person who has apparent generalized discharges but also a focal slow wave in the EEG, stating that the patient may have a generalized mechanism of onset would imply that you think there are two independent processes going on. The generalized mechanism, as described earlier, represents a genetic tendency to generalized thalamocortical volleys (generalized spike-wave discharges). The focal slow wave would then have to be explained by a completely separate process. Although it is not impossible that a person with the generalized spike-wave discharges of a genetic generalized epilepsy could also have had an unrelated focal stroke or other focal lesion, we usually prefer the most parsimonious explanation for the set of observations we make—as a first step, we try to explain all of the findings by a single process. In this example, rapid generalization from the focus that may have also caused the slow wave may be the simpler and favored explanation.

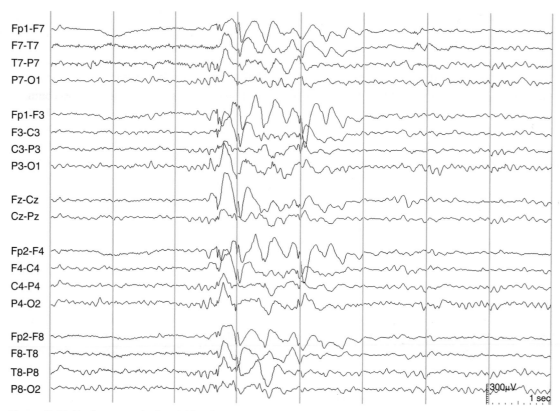

Figure 10.64 The burst seen in the middle of this page could be classified either as generalized spike wave with unclear spike localization or a burst of rhythmic slowing with intermixed spikes. These poorly organized spike-wave bursts could be generated by either a generalized or a focal mechanism.

Figures 10.65 through 10.68 show examples of focal discharges associated with lesional epilepsies in different locations. Depending on the location of the seizure focus, the semiology of focal seizures varies widely. The subjective and observed manifestations of seizures provide important supplemental localization information in addition to EEG data.

Multifocal Spikes

EEGs with multifocal spikes are usually found in patients with some degree of developmental delay or intellectual disability. Spikes or sharps waves are classified as multifocal when three or more independent localizations are seen, with at least one location in each hemisphere (see Figure 10.69). This finding is generally felt to be suggestive of an epileptic encephalopathy, a multifocal or diffuse epileptic process associated with a decreased seizure threshold and usually with a history of seizures. One important apparent exception to this rule is the patient with a benign developmental epilepsy, such as BCECTS. In addition to bilateral independent centrotemporal discharges, these patients may also manifest occipital discharges and, less frequently, discharges in other locations. Technically, these children have multifocal spikes, but they usually do not manifest clinical signs of a true epileptic encephalopathy and should be separated from the general group of patients with multifocal spikes. Thus, in a child with apparent multifocal spikes but with normal intellectual status, it is worth rethinking the EEG and asking whether the pattern could possibly be related to one of the benign/self-limited epilepsy syndromes of childhood.

Identification of Seizure Discharges

The large majority of seizure discharges are rhythmic discharges. The converse is not true: by far, most rhythmic discharges are not seizure discharges. How, then, to distinguish which rhythmic discharges are seizure discharges? The key features that mark a seizure discharge are a sudden change from the preceding background and gradual variations of the discharge in frequency and amplitude. Of the latter two parameters, the variation in frequency is most important. Typically, a seizure discharge will show a decrease or an increase in its firing rate (or both) throughout its course. Sometimes the change in rate is subtle enough that the spiking frequency must be formally counted (Figure 10.70). Occasionally a seizure discharge maintains an unvarying firing rate for a time (Figure 10.71), although a tailing-off of frequency may still be observable at the end of the discharge.

The most typical evolution of a seizure discharge is from lower voltage, faster activity to higher voltage, slower activity. This pattern may be seen in both generalized discharges, as

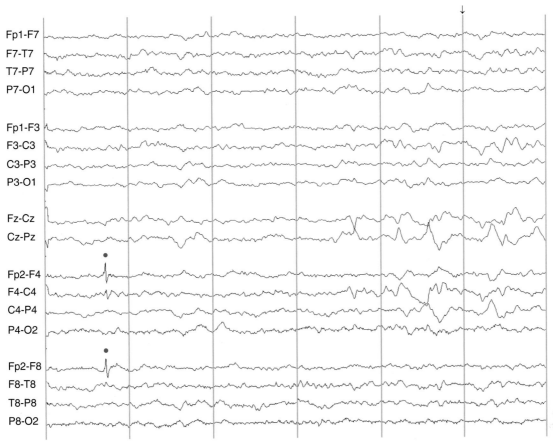

Figure 10.65 A right frontopolar spike-wave discharge seen in Stage I sleep (dots) is related to a focal lesion in the anterior right frontal lobe. This discharge is so focal that one might question whether it represents an artifact in the Fp2 electrode. If that were the case, one would not expect to see the small deflection in the F4-C4 channel, which implies that the F4 electrode is involved in the discharge as well and that this does not, therefore, represent a single-electrode artifact in Fp2.

was seen in Figure 10.11, and in focal discharges as is seen in Figure 10.72. Other patterns of frequency change are possible and are more likely to occur with lengthier discharges, including both accelerations and decelerations of the firing frequency. Occasional seizure discharges do not manifest this characteristic evolution in frequency and must be recognized by their sudden onset and their clear contrast from preceding background rhythms. When suspicion arises that a brief, non-evolving discharge may represent a seizure discharge, it is important to search for similar rhythms elsewhere in the tracing. For instance, if a run of suspicious, sudden onset 20 Hz beta activity is noted, but similar 20 Hz rhythms are identified elsewhere in the tracing with a haphazard pattern that drifts in and out, it is much less likely that the rhythm represents a seizure—this patient may simply have 20 Hz waves intermittently in the background. It is important not to mistake the waxing and waning in amplitude of an underlying background rhythm for an EEG seizure.

Wave amplitude typically shows some variation throughout a seizure discharge's evolution, but this sign alone is not reliable in distinguishing seizure from non-seizure activity.

Rhythmic waves that vary only in amplitude and not in frequency usually do not represent seizure activity. Well-known examples of waveforms that fit this description would include the posterior dominant rhythm and sleep spindles. Both of these familiar waveforms are well known to vary in amplitude (in fact, the term *spindle* refers to the increasing and decreasing amplitude of the waveform, similar to the pattern that spun yarn creates when collected on a wooden spindle) but not in frequency, and neither would be mistaken for seizure activity.

Arousal rhythms may sometimes resemble seizure discharges, partly because they can appear as an abrupt change from the previous sleep pattern. Abrupt change from the background is characteristic of seizure discharges, but is also characteristic of the process of awakening. A suddenly appearing high-voltage arousal rhythm usually maintains a consistent frequency that helps to distinguish it from a seizure discharge. The high-voltage hypersynchronous responses to hyperventilation and arousal patterns are both good examples of this phenomenon. These dramatic but benign wave patterns often show waxing and waning amplitudes but maintain

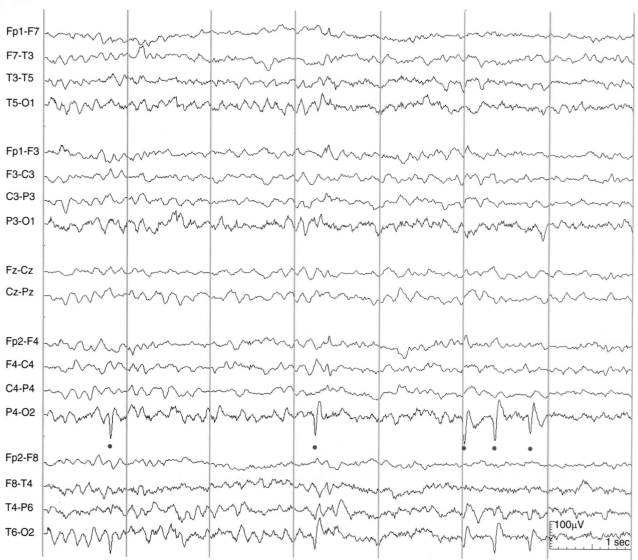

Figure 10.66 Focal right occipital spike-wave discharges (dots) are seen at the transition from wakefulness to drowsiness (note dropout of the posterior rhythm halfway through the page).

steady frequencies, helping to distinguish them from seizure discharges (Figure 10.73). Because arousal patterns can consist of an abrupt relative flattening of the EEG, it is important not to mistake these for electrodecremental seizures.

The component waves of a seizure discharge often, but not always, show epileptiform morphology. Commonly, seizures manifest as a spray of rapid spikes or spike-wave discharges. Nevertheless, some seizure discharges may have no sharp features, appearing as rounded, sinusoidal waves. In general, the closer the recording electrode is to the seizure, the more likely it is to manifest sharp features. Seizure discharges that show more rounded (as opposed to sharp) features are assumed to arise at a greater distance from the recording electrode.

During a focal seizure discharge, slow waves may appear in the adjacent or opposite hemisphere.

The foregoing discussion presupposes that the rhythmic waveform being analyzed in the EEG is true cerebral activity and not some type of artifact. As with the assessment of epileptiform activity, the first step in assessing a rhythmic waveform is to exclude artifact. Many types of rhythmic movements may occur in patients, creating an artifact that may mimic a seizure discharge. Repetitive movements from patting or chest physical therapy, toothbrushing, head scratching, and head rocking may all resemble seizure discharges (Figure 10.74), especially if no video is available. As with evaluation of epileptiform activity, a seizure discharge

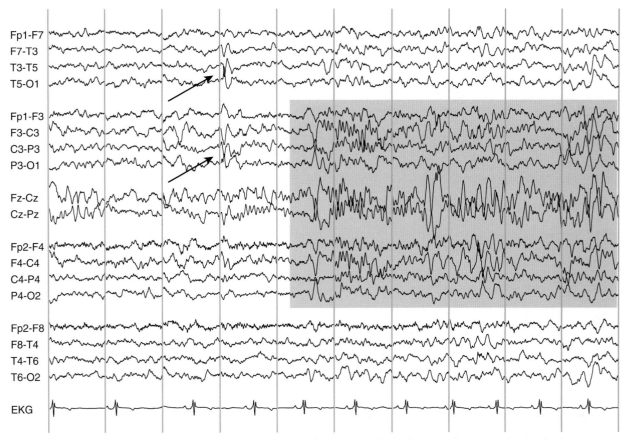

Figure 10.67 A focal spike-wave discharge is seen with a maximum in the left posterior temporal and parietal electrodes (T5 and P3) during Stage II sleep (arrows). Vertex waves and sleep spindles (red rectangle) are distinct from the temporoparietal discharge.

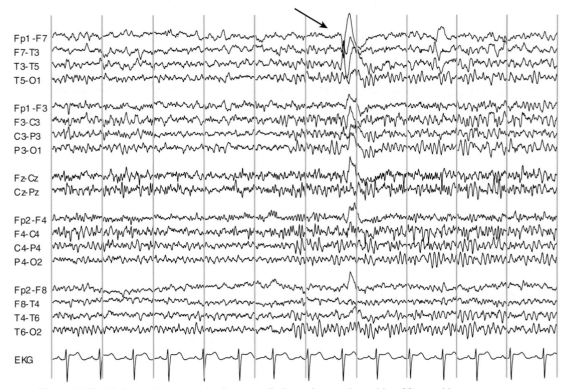

Figure 10.68 A left anterior temporal spike-wave discharge is seen (arrow) in a 22-year-old woman with temporal lobe epilepsy.

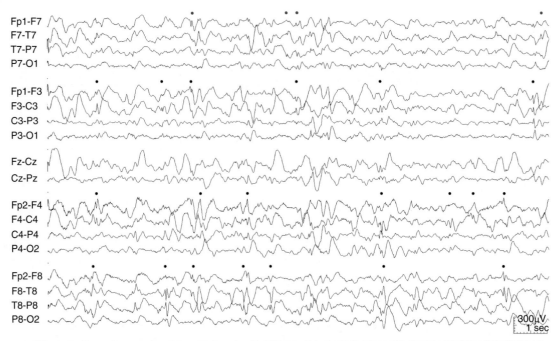

Figure 10.69 A pattern of multifocal spikes is seen (dots) during light sleep. Unless the different spike foci can be shown to belong to a single benign developmental epilepsy syndrome (on the basis of the patient's history and the location of the spikes), the multiplicity of spike locations seen here suggests the presence of a diffuse epileptic encephalopathy, usually associated with some degree of cognitive abnormality. Also note that, based on the calibration bar in the lower right corner of the figure, these spikes are of relatively higher voltage than they may appear at first glance.

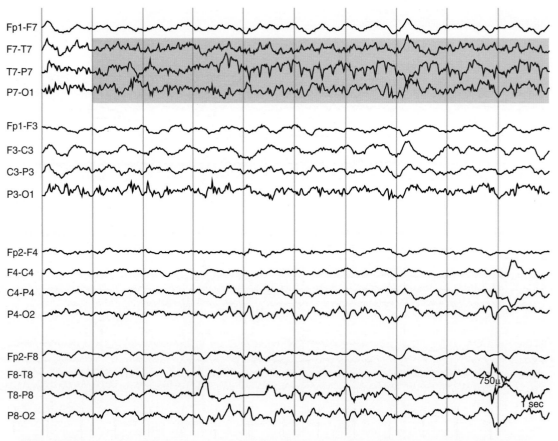

Figure 10.70 The seizure discharge seen in the left temporal chain seems, at first glance, to have a fairly constant firing frequency. When the spike frequency is formally measured at the beginning of the page and at the end of the page (see shaded rectangles), it can be seen that the discharge has slowed from 5 Hz to 4 Hz over these 8 seconds.

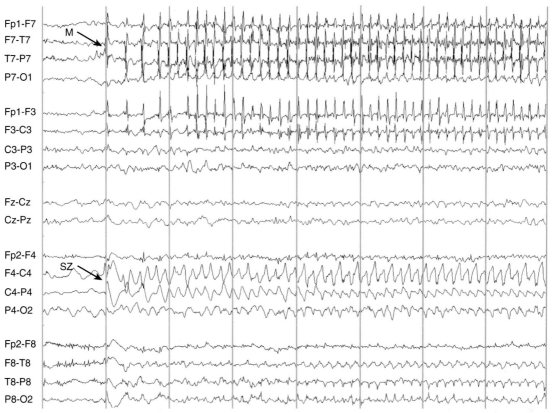

Figure 10.71 A seizure discharge (SZ) is seen beginning in the right central area in a teenage boy with Rasmussen encephalitis, a degenerative disorder that usually involves a single hemisphere. Because this discharge happens to involve the face area of the motor strip, the rhythmic left facial twitching caused by the seizure can be seen as repetitive muscle artifact related to the twitching (M) over the left frontotemporal area.

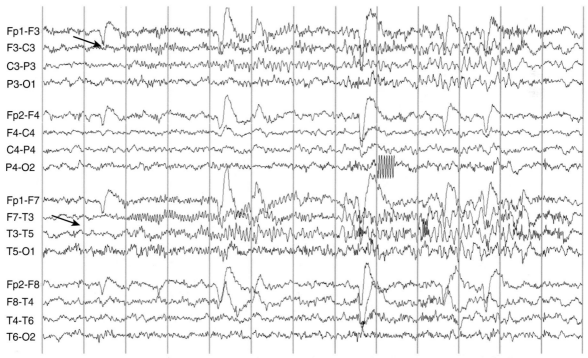

Figure 10.72 A fast seizure discharge is seen to begin in the left temporal area (arrows) quickly spreading to the left central area (montage setup: left parasagittal chain over right parasagittal chain, left temporal chain over right temporal chain). Throughout the course of the discharge, the firing frequency slows and the discharge terminates by the last second of the page. An event marker for this seizure, pressed by a caretaker, can be seen in the P4-O2 channel.

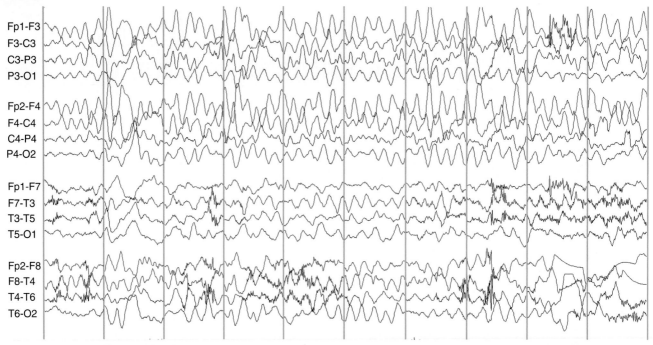

Figure 10.73 These high-voltage, hypersynchronous waves represent an arousal hypersynchrony rather than a seizure discharge. These waves happen to have maximal voltage over the parasagittal areas. The fact that the waves retain a steady frequency throughout helps distinguish between the two possibilities.

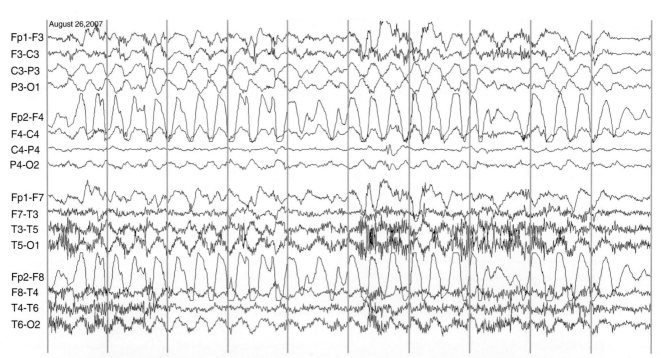

Figure 10.74 The repetitive and rhythmic waves seen on this page are caused by chest physical therapy artifact rather than a seizure discharge. Because the head movement caused by the rhythmic chest percussion jostles each electrode in an unpredictable way, high-voltage deflections are seen from some electrodes that are adjacent to electrodes that manifest little or no deflection, indicating that the apparent discharge has no plausible electric field and is the result of motion artifact.

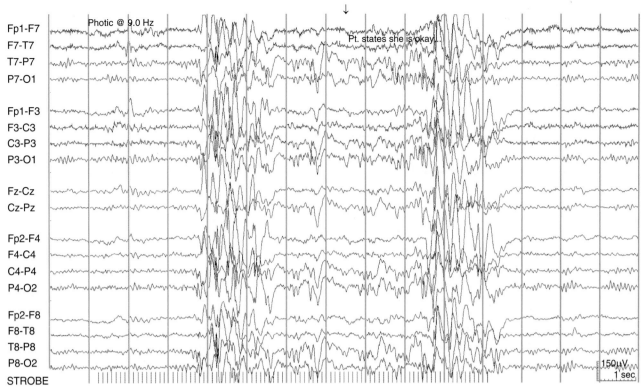

Figure 10.75 Two generalized spike-wave bursts are elicited by strobe stimulation. The generalized (rather than primarily posterior) distribution of the discharge and its high-voltage increase the chance that this represents a true photoparoxysmal response.

should have a plausible electric field. The process of distinguishing artifact from cerebral activity is discussed in Chapter 4, "Electroencephalographic Localization," and Chapter 6, "Electroencephalographic Artifacts."

A minority of seizure discharges do not match the patterns of the lengthier, evolving seizure discharges described earlier. As discussed earlier, myoclonic seizures are very quick seizures often associated with bursts of polyspikes that may be too short to show evolution or rhythmicity in the usual sense. The characteristic, brief electrographic pattern of infantile spasms was described earlier and occasionally consists of a single, diffuse slow wave with complex topography, sometimes with discernible superimposed fast activity. When carefully analyzed, that fast activity may also be seen to decrease in frequency over its brief duration; however the fast component of the discharge is not always visible. As already shown, some seizures may be associated with an electrodecremental pattern in the EEG as well.

REVIEW QUESTIONS

1. Regarding seizure types and seizure syndromes, which of the following is true?
   a. It is unwise to diagnose a seizure type without concurrent EEG.
   b. The most powerful tool in diagnosing a seizure type is to know its semiology.
   c. Seizure syndromes are best diagnosed with concurrent video/EEG.
   d. Most seizure syndromes can present at any age.

2. According to different definitions of epilepsy, a patient can be diagnosed with epilepsy if
   a. the MRI shows a focal cortical dysplasia (FCD) in the temporal lobe.
   b. the patient has experienced prolonged febrile seizures.
   c. the patient has had a single seizure but other testing suggests that the patient's recurrence risk is similar to a person who has experienced two or more seizures.
   d. the EEG is abnormal.

3. Considering current and past nomenclature systems,
   a. infantile spasms are a type of myoclonic seizures.
   b. dyscognitive seizures are usually generalized seizures.
   c. partial seizures are a milder type of generalized seizure.
   d. complex partial seizures are synonymous with focal seizures with impaired awareness.

4. Regarding automatisms, they
   a. are driven by seizure discharges in mesial temporal lobe structures.
   b. are expected to express contralateral to focal seizure discharges.
   c. represent loss of suppression of automatic cortical programs that are then allowed to "run," rather than the direct effect of a seizure discharge.
   d. may represent the aura of a seizure.

5. Regarding auras,
   a. when they begin to occur more frequently, it is more likely that the patient will experience an actual seizure.
   b. seizure medications rarely treat them effectively.
   c. they can give useful localizing value.
   d. they can be considered an annoyance, but beyond that have little clinical significance.

6. Regarding the proper approach to diagnosing seizures,
   a. a seizure type is most often confidently diagnosed based on observers' descriptions.
   b. in the absence of a successful seizure recording on EEG, the provider should not proceed to a diagnosis of seizures.
   c. staring seizures are synonymous with absence seizures.
   d. a negative EEG during a clinical episode excludes the diagnosis of epileptic seizure.

7. A myoclonic seizure is
   a. a clonic jerk that involves contraction of myocytes.
   b. a seizure type that can occur in multiple seizure syndromes.
   c. always an epileptic phenomenon.
   d. a sign of a severe epilepsy.

8. Which of the following must be seen to make the diagnosis of "classic 3 Hz generalized spike wave?"
   a. a 3 Hz discharge.
   b. a truly generalized discharge.
   c. discharges with clear spike-wave morphology.
   d. none of the above

9. All are true regarding atypical absence seizures EXCEPT which of the following?
   a. They are not expected in childhood absence epilepsy.
   b. They lack the abrupt onset and termination seen in typical absence seizures.
   c. They are usually encountered in persons with cognitive disability.
   d. They begin as typical absence seizures and evolve to atypical absence seizures.

10. The concept of developmental and epileptic encephalopathy is meant to capture the idea that
    a. the seizures themselves cause a deterioration in the patient's neurologic function.
    b. a patient's pre-existing encephalopathy predisposes them to the seizures.
    c. seizure medications can dull a patient's cognitive status.
    d. the patient's neurodevelopmental problems are more likely caused by the epilepsy rather than a genetic problem.

11. Febrile seizures in children represent
    a. a milder form of epilepsy.
    b. a disorder caused by mesial temporal sclerosis (MTS).
    c. a syndrome of provoked seizures, therefore not an example of epilepsy.
    d. not a form of epilepsy, but often followed by epilepsy.

12. Examples of the age-dependent encephalopathies include which of the following?
    a. Benign childhood epilepsy with centrotemporal spikes (BCECTS or SeLECTS).
    b. West syndrome.
    c. Temporal lobe epilepsy.
    d. All of the above.

13. The diagnosis of Benign Rolandic Epilepsy (or BCECTS or SeLECTS) is considerably less likely if the story includes
    a. grand mal seizures occurring out of wakefulness.
    b. discharges that consistently occur on only one side of the brain.
    c. an EEG in which the discharges fail to show a "tangential dipole".
    d. school problems related to attentional difficulties.

14. Classic EEG findings in JME (juvenile myoclonic epilepsy) include
    a. a high-frequency photic driving response.
    b. occipital sharp waves activated by sleep.
    c. polyspikes-wave discharges during patient startle.
    d. None of the above.

15. Medial temporal lobe epilepsy refers to seizures arising from
    a. the medial half of the temporal lobe.
    b. temporal neocortex.
    c. the hippocampal formation.
    d. the inferior, medial, and superior temporal lobe gyri.
16. EEG features that support the idea that a particular waveform represents an EEG seizure are
    a. abrupt onset and termination and variations in amplitude.
    b. abrupt onset and termination and variations in frequency.
    c. abrupt termination with arousal from sleep.
    d. activation of pattern on falling asleep.
17. Concurrent recordings with invasive electrode grids and scalp EEG have shown that seizure discharges confined to the hippocampus
    a. often cannot be recorded on the scalp.
    b. most often project to the anterior temporal electrodes.
    c. most often project to the parasagittal and vertex electrodes.
    d. often are recorded best over the contralateral temporal lobe.

ANSWERS

1. ANSWER: **B**. Although a concurrent EEG is very useful for the diagnosis of seizure type, with the exception of absence seizures it is uncommon that an actual EEG recording of the patient's seizure is available to the provider to aid in diagnosis. In the large majority of cases, the diagnosis of seizure type is based on the seizure's semiology and, secondarily, on specific clinical information (including interictal EEG and imaging). Seizure syndromes are best diagnosed knowing the constellation of clinical findings surrounding the patient, including taking into account the syndrome's characteristic age at onset, the patient's neurocognitive status, imaging results, etc.

2. ANSWER: **C**. The essence of giving a diagnosis of epilepsy is the idea that you have discerned that the person has a continuing tendency to unprovoked seizures. A patient who has experienced only a single seizure but has an abnormal EEG or other abnormal neurological status or testing may have a recurrence risk over 50%, or a risk similar to a person who has already experienced two unprovoked seizures (the earlier diagnostic criterion for epilepsy). An abnormal MRI finding of a temporal lobe FCD alone is not sufficient to diagnose epilepsy—the patient must also have experienced seizures. Not all patients with an FCD necessarily develop seizure disorders. Prolonged febrile seizures represent provoked seizures and, therefore, do not qualify as the unprovoked seizures necessary to diagnose epilepsy. Prolonged febrile seizures are, however, considered a risk factor for the development of later epilepsy. Many persons may have an abnormal EEG but never have seizures and, therefore, do not necessarily have epilepsy.

3. ANSWER: **D**. The newer term, focal seizures with impaired awareness, has been proposed as a replacement for the long-used term *complex partial seizure*, partly because the word *complex* was not clear as to its specific meaning (i.e., complex in what way?), and "impaired awareness" is very clear. Infantile spasms do not consist of a lightning-like jerk (the definition of myoclonic seizures), but rather resemble brief tonic seizures lasting approximately one second. *Dyscognitive seizure* is an obsolete term that originally replaced complex partial seizure but fell out of favor because the term was deemed awkward and not readily understandable by the lay public. Partial seizures are synonymous with *focal seizures*, the current preferred term, and are therefore not a type of generalized seizure.

4. ANSWER: **C**. Although automatisms may occur during temporal lobe seizures, they are not directly driven by mesial temporal lobe seizure discharges—they likely represent the release of pre-established cortical programs from suppression. Also, automatisms may occur in seizures arising from other cortical localizations, not just the mesial temporal lobe. When they lateralize, automatisms are often seen ipsilateral to the seizing hemisphere, suggesting that that an automatic motor program may be running from the non-seizing hemisphere. Auras are self-reported subjective phenomena at the beginning of a seizure, while automatisms are rarely reported by patients and occur later in the seizure's semiology.

5. ANSWER: **C**. The subjective nature of an aura can give useful localizing information as to where the seizure discharge is in its early stages. For instance, a seizure aura that consists of an unusual sound may be arising from auditory cortex. Because auras represent actual seizures, they are not a predictor of future seizures but rather an indicator that seizures are already occurring. Because auras are seizures, antiseizure medications have the potential to suppress auras. Some auras may spread to become more dramatic seizures. Their occurrence suggests that the patient's epilepsy is still active. It may occur, however, that antiseizure medications do not eradicate auras but successfully limit the spread of auras so that they do not evolve into bigger seizures.

6. ANSWER: **A**. Often the only information available to the clinician is the observer's description of the patient's behavior during and after a seizure event, and this is the most useful information in diagnosing seizure type. Interictal EEG and other testing may help confirm the diagnostic impression. Because it is often difficult to

record a patient's sporadic seizures on EEG, the diagnosis of seizure type usually has to be made without the benefit of an ictal recording. Although absence seizures are staring seizures, other seizure types can include staring, such as temporal lobe seizures. The term *absence* is reserved for the staring seizures that are accompanied by generalized spike-wave discharges, as may be seen in childhood or juvenile absence epilepsy—the term is not used for the staring behavior that may be seen in some focal seizures with impaired awareness. Although the EEG recording is usually positive during epileptic seizures, seizures arising from certain more distant cortical surfaces can be difficult to record on the scalp. Therefore, a negative EEG recording during a clinical spell cannot absolutely exclude the diagnosis of an epileptic seizure. However, the more involved the clinical spell (such as one that might resemble a GTC), the stronger negative EEG evidence is that the episode was non-epileptic.

7. ANSWER: **B**. Epileptic myoclonus can be seen in multiple epilepsy syndromes, both benign and severe. More benign examples include benign myoclonic epilepsy of infancy, and juvenile myoclonic epilepsy, while more severe syndromes include severe myoclonic epilepsy of infancy (Dravet syndrome), and the progressive myoclonic epilepsy syndromes. Although the term *myoclonus* seems to be a compound word suggesting any clonic jerk of the muscle, correct usage of the term is reserved for lightning-like muscle jerks that occur singly or in very brief clusters. Not all myoclonus is epileptic, with physiologic sleep myoclonus the most common example of non-epileptic myoclonus. Subcortical myoclonus and segmental myoclonus arising from the spinal cord are other examples of non-epileptic myoclonus.

8. ANSWER: **D**. What is referred to as "classic 3 Hz generalized spike-wave" often fires faster than 3 Hz at onset and can slow well below 3 Hz during its duration. The discharges are often not completely generalized and often show a clear bilateral superior frontal maximum (F3 and F4) with much lower voltage posteriorly. Finally, on close examination such discharges are often seen to show polyspike-wave morphology rather than simple spike-wave morphology.

9. ANSWER: **D**. Typical absence seizures (rather than atypical absence seizures) are the hallmark seizure type of childhood absence epilepsy. The two most distinctive characteristics of atypical absence seizures (compared to typical absence seizures) are poorly demarcated onset and termination and a slower firing frequency. Atypical absence seizures are most often seen in persons with intellectual disability. Atypical absence does not usually evolve from typical absence; usually the two seizure presentations are distinct.

10. ANSWER: **A**. Although with most epilepsies, the conceptualization is that a problem in the brain causes the seizures, the concept of developmental and epileptic encephalopathy implies that the seizures themselves are an important cause of functional impairment. Although overly aggressive use of epilepsy medications may dull cognitive function, epileptic encephalopathy implies that it is the seizures rather than the medications that are causing the dysfunction. Because most developmental and epileptic encephalopathies are thought to be genetic, both processes, the underlying genetic problem and the seizures, can be thought of as responsible for developmental problems.

11. ANSWER: **C**. Because they are considered provoked seizures, febrile seizures are not considered epileptic seizures and, therefore, not an epilepsy syndrome. MTS is not a cause of febrile seizures, but prolonged febrile seizures may be a cause of MTS later in life. Later epilepsy only appears in a small minority of children who experience febrile seizures in childhood.

12. ANSWER: **B**. The classic examples of the age-dependent epileptic encephalopathies include: EIEE (early infantile epileptic encephalopathy) which usually presents in the newborn period, West syndrome (infantile spasms) which typically presents later in the first year of life, and LGS (Lennox-Gastaut syndrome) which presents in early childhood or later. Temporal lobe epilepsy is not an age-dependent syndrome and can present at a wide variety of ages. Although BCECTS occurs during a specific age range, it is not considered an epileptic encephalopathy.

13. ANSWER: **A**. Grand mal seizures are not expected in BCECTS to occur out of wakefulness—they occur out of sleep. Although the centrotemporal spikes characteristic of this disorder are often seen over both hemispheres, the discharges may consistently occur only over one hemisphere in some patients. A tangential dipole is lacking in approximately half of children with rolandic epilepsy and is, therefore, not necessary for the diagnosis. Because attentional problems are a common comorbidity in rolandic epilepsy, their presence should not dissuade the clinician from the diagnosis.

14. ANSWER: **D**. Rather than the EEG findings listed above, the classic EEG findings in JME include fast spike-wave discharges, polyspikes-wave discharges (which is also the ictal correlate of the myoclonic jerks), and a photoparoxysmal response in some. The high frequency photic driving response (demonstration of photic driving at unusually high frequencies) is not considered an epileptiform abnormality. Occipital sharp waves may be seen in occipital epilepsy syndromes and lesional epilepsies, but are not an expected finding in JME. The polyspike-wave discharges of JME may drive episodes of epileptic myoclonus, but this is not related to startling the patient.

15. ANSWER: **C**. The term *medial temporal lobe epilepsy* is usually meant to describe seizures arising from the hippocampal formation and closely related structures, an evolutionarily and architecturally older part of the brain. Most of the temporal lobe, including much of the medial half, still consists of neocortex (including the parahippocampal gyrus and fusiform gyrus) which, although medially placed structures, are generally not included in

the formal definition of medial temporal lobe epilepsy. The inferior, medial, and superior temporal gyri form the lateral temporal lobe and are neocortical structures.

16. ANSWER: **B**. Abrupt onset and termination and variation in frequency are the most reliable signs of a seizure discharge. Abrupt onset and termination and variation in amplitude can be seen in a variety of rhythms, such as the posterior dominant rhythm with eye-closure and opening, and mu rhythms. A pattern that terminates on arousal from sleep likely represents a sleep rhythm as few epileptic seizures can be terminated by waking the patient. Although *interictal* discharges often accelerate on falling asleep, this is not a particular characteristic of epileptic seizure discharge patterns.

17. ANSWER: **A**. Seizure discharges wholly confined to the hippocampus often do not express on the scalp until they spread to adjacent (neocortical) structures. At that time, they may appear in the anterior temporal electrodes or vertex and parasagittal electrodes. Seizure discharges picked up contralateral to the seizing hippocampus suggest spread of the seizure to both temporal lobes.

SUGGESTED READINGS

Baram TZ, Shinnar S: *Febrile seizures.* San Diego, 2002, Academic Press.

Beaumanoir A, Bureau M, Deonna T, et al., editors: Continuous spikes and waves during slow sleep. Electrical status epilepticus during slow sleep. *Mariani Foundation paediatric neurology series:* 3, London, 1995, John Libbey Eurotext.

Bureau M, Genton P, Dravet C, Delgado-Escueta AV, Guerrini R, Tassinari CA, Thomas P, Wolf P, editors: *Epileptic syndromes in infancy, childhood and adolescence* 6th. Éditions, Montrouge, France, 2019, John Libbey Eurotext.

Commission on Classification and Terminology of the International League Against Epilepsy: proposal for revised clinical and electroencephalographic classification of epileptic seizures, *Epilepsia* 22:489–501, 1981.

De Negri M, Baglietto MG, Battaglia FM, et al.: Treatment of electrical status epilepticus by short diazepam (DZP) cycles after DZP rectal bolus test, *Brain Dev* 17:330–333, 1995.

Dehan M, Quillerou D, Navelet Y, et al.: [Convulsions in the fifth day of life: a new syndrome?], *Arch Fr Pediatr* 34:730–742, 1977.

Doose H, Gerken H, Leonhardt R, et al.: Centrencephalic myoclonic-astatic petit mal. Clinical and genetic investigation, *Neuropädiatrie* 2:59–78, 1970.

Fisher RS, Cross JH, French JA, Higurashi N, Hirsch E, Jansen FE, Lagae L, Moshé SL, Peltola J, Roulet Perez E, Scheffer IE, Zuberi SM: Operational classification of seizure types by the International League Against Epilepsy: Position Paper of the ILAE Commission for Classification and Terminology, *Epilepsia* 58(4):522–530, 2017 Apr. PMID: 28276060

Fisher RS, Acevedo C, Arzimanoglou A, Bogacz A, Cross JH, Elger CE, Engel J Jr, Forsgren L, French JA, Glynn M, Hesdorffer DC, Lee BI, Mathern GW, Moshé SL, Perucca E, Scheffer IE, Tomson T, Watanabe M, Wiebe S: ILAE official report: a practical clinical definition of epilepsy, *Epilepsia* 55(4):475–482, 2014 Apr. https://doi.org/10.1111/epi.12550. Epub 2014 Apr 14. PMID: 24730690

Hirsch E, French J, Scheffer IE, Bogacz A, Alsaadi T, Sperling MR, Abdulla F, Zuberi SM, Trinka E, Specchio N, Somerville E, Samia P, Riney K, Nabbout R, Jain S, Wilmshurst JM, Auvin S, Wiebe S, Perucca E, Moshé SL, Tinuper P, Wirrell EC: ILAE definition of the Idiopathic Generalized Epilepsy Syndromes: Position statement by the ILAE Task Force on Nosology and Definitions, *Epilepsia*, 2022 May 3. https://doi.org/10.1111/epi.17236. PMID: 35503716

Hirsch E, Velez A, Sellal F, et al: Electroclinical signs of benign neonatal familial convulsions, *Ann Neurol* 34:835–841, 1993.

Jeavons P, Bower B: The natural history of infantile spasms, *Arch Dis Childhood* 36:17–22, 1961.

Landau WM, Kleffner FR: Syndrome of acquired aphasia with convulsive disorder in children, *Neurology* 7:523–530, 1957.

Loiseau P, Duché B, Cordova S, et al.: Prognosis of benign childhood epilepsy with centrotemporal spikes: a followup study of 168 patients, *Epilepsia* 29:229–235, 1988.

Mizrahi E, Kellaway P: Characterization and classification of neonatal seizures, *Neurology* 37(12):1837–1844, 1987.

Pacia SV, Ebersole JS: Intracranial EEG substrates of scalp ictal patterns from temporal lobe foci, *Epilepsia* 38(6):642–654, 1997.

Panayiotopoulos CP: Benign childhood epilepsy with occipital paroxysms. In Anderman F, Beaumanoir A, Mira L, editors: *Occipital seizures and epilepsy in children*, London, 1993, John Libbey Eurotext.

Patry G, Lyagoubi S, Tassinari CA: Subclinical "electrical status epilepticus" induced by sleep in children. A clinical and electroencephalographic study of six cases, *Arch Neurol* 24:242–252, 1971.

Pearl PL, editor: *Inherited Metabolic Epilepsies,* 2nd edition, Demos Medical, 2018, Springer Publishing Company.

Picard F, Baulac S, Kahane P, et al: Dominant partial epilepsies: a clinical, electrophysiological and genetic study of 19 European families, *Brain* 123:1247–1262, 2000.

Scheffer IE, Berkovic S, Capovilla G, Connolly MB, French J, Guilhoto L, Hirsch E, Jain S, Mathern GW, Moshé SL, Nordli DR, Perucca E, Tomson T, Wiebe S, Zhang YH, Zuberi SM. ILAE classification of the epilepsies: Position paper of the ILAE Commission for Classification and Terminology. PMID: 28276062 PMCID: PMC5386840 https://doi.org/10.1111/epi.13709

Specchio N, Wirrell EC, Scheffer IE, Nabbout R, Riney K, Samia P, Guerreiro M, Gwer S, Zuberi SM, Wilmshurst JM, Yozawitz E, Pressler R, Hirsch E, Wiebe S, Cross HJ, Perucca E, Moshé SL, Tinuper P, Auvin S: International League Against Epilepsy classification and definition of epilepsy syndromes with onset in childhood: Position paper by the ILAE Task Force on Nosology and Definitions, *Epilepsia*, 2022 May 3. https://doi.org/10.1111/epi.17241. Online ahead of print. PMID: 35503717

Stafstrom CE, Velíšek L: *Developmental epilepsy: from clinical medicine to neurobiological mechanisms.* Singapore, 2019, World Scientific Publishing.

West WJ: On a peculiar form of infantile convulsions, *Lancet.* 1:724–725, 1841.

Wolf NI, Rahman S, Schmitt B, Taanman J-W, Duncan AJ, Harting I, Wohlrab G, Ebinger F, Rating D, Bast T: Status epilepticus in children with Alpers' disease caused by POLG1 mutations: EEG and MRI features, *Epilepsia* 50(6):1596–1607, 2009 Jun. https://doi.org/10.1111/j.1528-1167.2008.01877.x. Epub 2008 Nov 19

Wyllie E, Moosa ANV: Occipito-frontal sharp waves-An under-recognized electroencephalogram pattern in self-limited idiopathic childhood focal epilepsy, *J Clin Neurophysiol* 34(3):e9–e14, 2017 May.

11

Normal Variants in the Electroencephalogram

This section deals with a group of waveforms that may mimic abnormal waves but have now been recognized as normal variants. By definition, a normal variant is not associated with disease, be it epilepsy or another abnormal state. A few of the waveforms discussed in this chapter are of uncertain clinical significance: they are known to occur frequently in normal individuals but may be seen more often in people with epilepsy.

Many of the normal variant patterns described here bear some resemblance to epileptiform activity. The importance of developing proficiency in recognizing these patterns is to avoid mistaking them for epileptiform abnormalities. The basic features of these normal variants should be committed to memory so as to avoid the pitfall of reporting one of these variants as an epileptiform abnormality (Table 11.1).

NORMAL VARIANTS THAT MIMIC SINGLE EPILEPTIFORM WAVES

Positive Occipital Sharp Transients of Sleep

Positive occipital sharp transients of sleep (POSTS) are one of the most common normal variants seen in the EEG and can be considered one of the normal elements of sleep. The acronym POSTS tells the story of these distinctive waveforms: POSTS are of *Positive* polarity, they are seen in the *Occipital* areas; they have a *Sharp Transient* waveform, and they occur in *Sleep*. POSTS

TABLE 11.1 Summary Table of Selected Normal Variants	
Positive Occipital Sharp Transients of Sleep (POSTS)	Positive-polarity, low-voltage occipital sharp waves occurring in sleep, a normal sleep element
Lambda Waves	Triangular, low-voltage occipital sharps during wakefulness associated with searching eye movements
Small Sharp Spikes (SSS) or Benign Epileptiform Transients of Sleep (BETS)	Low-voltage spikes, synchronous or independent, unilateral or bilateral, with broad temporal field seen in adults during drowsiness and light sleep
Mu Rhythms	Arch-shaped rhythm in central areas during wakefulness, suppresses with contralateral hand movement
14 and 6 Hz Positive Bursts	Medium- to high-voltage, positive-polarity, arch-shaped bursts during drowsiness and light sleep in posterior temporal and occipital areas, mostly in children
Wicket Spikes/Wicket Rhythms	Arch-shaped rhythm of temporal areas during drowsiness and light sleep, mostly in adults
Breach Rhythms	Rhythm of regionally increased fast activity, sometimes with a spiky appearance, seen over areas of skull defects.
Rhythmic Temporal Theta Bursts of Drowsiness (RMTD) or Psychomotor Variant	Non-evolving, sharpened theta rhythm in temporal areas during drowsiness and light sleep
6 Hz Spike and Wave or Phantom Spike and Wave	Brief 6 Hz rhythms with inconsistent spike component seen in wakefulness and drowsiness, mostly in adults, following WHAM and FOLD patterns
Posterior Slow Waves of Youth	Theta and delta waves intermixed with posterior rhythm until mid-teenage years

FOLD = Female whose pattern has an Occipital emphasis, Low in amplitude, and seen in the Drowsy record; WHAM = Waking record, High in amplitude, Anterior in location, and especially in Males.

are "triangular" or V-shaped waves that are particularly prominent in light sleep (Figures 11.1 and 11.2). If not recognized as POSTS, these low-voltage discharges could potentially be mistaken for occipital sharp waves. Because POSTS are so common, the polarity of any low- to medium-voltage occipital sharp wave seen in sleep should be assessed before deciding that it is abnormal. Displaying POSTS in an appropriate referential montage should confirm their positive polarity and correctly identify them as POSTS rather than epileptiform discharges. POSTS

usually appear in a bilaterally synchronous fashion, although normal POSTS may manifest asymmetrical amplitudes. POSTS may occur in brief, semirhythmic runs. Although POSTS usually consist of low-voltage, V-shaped waves, they may occasionally assume a more spiky appearance (Figure 11.3).

Lambda Waves

Lambda waves are discussed with POSTS because their morphology and location are similar. The two are easily

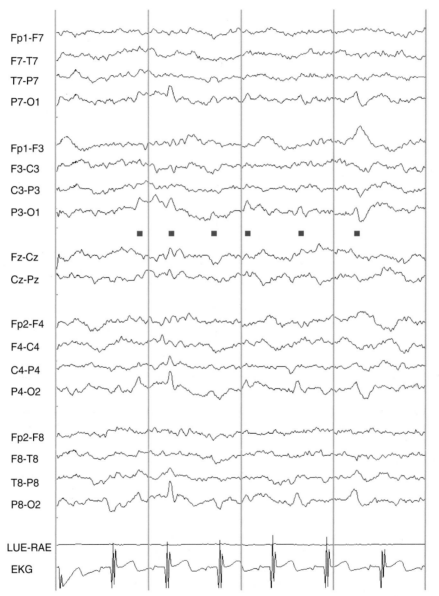

Figure 11.1 The distinctive triangular waves seen in the four occipital channels (P7-O1, P3-O1, P4-O2, and P8-O2) are examples of positive occipital sharp transients of sleep (POSTS; indicated by dots). The upgoing deflection of these waves in the occipital channels of this bipolar montage suggests two possible polarity/localization combinations. The first is that the upgoing wave implies that the parietal electrodes, P3 and P4, are "more negative" than O1 and O2 and that these waves could be caused by a negativity in the parietal areas. No clear phase reversal is seen anterior to the upgoing waves, however, raising the suspicion that a parietal negativity does not explain the waveform. The second possibility is the correct explanation: O1 and O2 should be considered "more positive" than P3 and P4, and a positivity in the occipital area is causing the deflection. The absolute polarity of the event—in this case, an occipital positivity—is most easily confirmed by displaying it in a referential montage (see Figure 11.2).

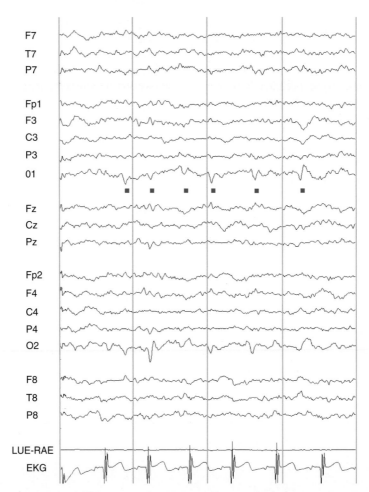

Figure 11.2 The same page of EEG shown in the previous figure is displayed in a referential montage. The clear downgoing deflections in the O1 and O2 channels (dots) clarify the positive polarity of these occipital discharges and confirm that they are an example of positive occipital sharp transients of sleep.

distinguished because lambda waves occur exclusively during wakefulness and POSTS are seen during sleep. Lambda waves also appear as low-voltage triangular waves in the occipital areas, reminiscent of the shape of the Greek letter λ, but they are distinctive in that they occur at the time of lateral searching eye movements. Confirmation that a low-voltage occipital sharp transient wave is a lambda wave is made easier by finding evidence of concurrent lateral eye movement artifact. Lambda waves may be either surface positive or surface negative in the occipital area (Figure 11.4). They are not as common as POSTS and are seen more frequently in children than in adults. Because they are related to searching eye movements, lambda waves are generally seen when the patient's eyes are open and the posterior rhythm is suppressed. Voltage asymmetry of lambda waves is not necessarily considered abnormal.

Small Sharp Spikes and Benign Epileptiform Transients of Sleep

The terms *small sharp spikes* (SSS) and *benign epileptiform transients of sleep* (BETS) are synonymous. These quick, low-voltage spikes are usually seen in the temporal areas with a broad gradient across the temporal chain. The upward and downward phases of the transients are usually of similar amplitude. They occur either unilaterally or bilaterally and, when bilateral, they may occur either synchronously or independently (Figure 11.5). SSS are seen in drowsiness and light sleep and tend to disappear with deepening sleep. SSS are considered by many to represent a normal variant but some authors still contend that the finding suggests an increased degree of epileptogenicity.

NORMAL VARIANTS THAT MIMIC REPETITIVE EPILEPTIFORM WAVES

Mu Rhythms

Mu rhythms are commonly encountered rhythms seen in the central areas during wakefulness, best recorded by the C3 and C4 electrodes. They are most often seen from later childhood into the adult years, although they are occasionally seen in very young subjects. The mu rhythm has a distinctive arciform (arch-like) or "comb-like" morphology (Figure 11.6). Because the mu rhythm is suppressed by voluntary motor activity in the opposite hand, the technologist can establish that a sharp central rhythm is a mu rhythm by requesting that

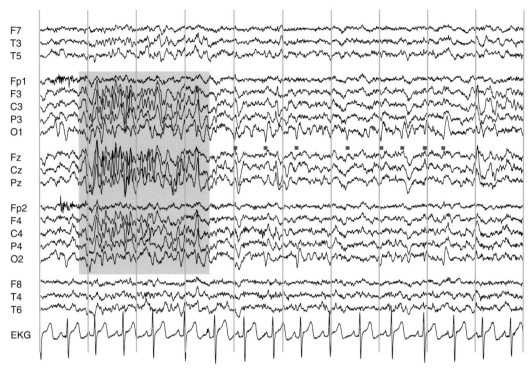

Figure 11.3 An example of Stage II sleep is shown in a referential montage (note the sleep spindles in the shaded area). Positive occipital sharp transients of sleep (POSTS) are seen in the O1 and O2 channels (dots). These POSTS have a more spike-like morphology than those seen in the previous example; the initial downgoing deflections indicate their positive polarity. These occipital waves are not synchronous with the electrocardiogram (EKG) complexes and therefore do not represent EKG artifact.

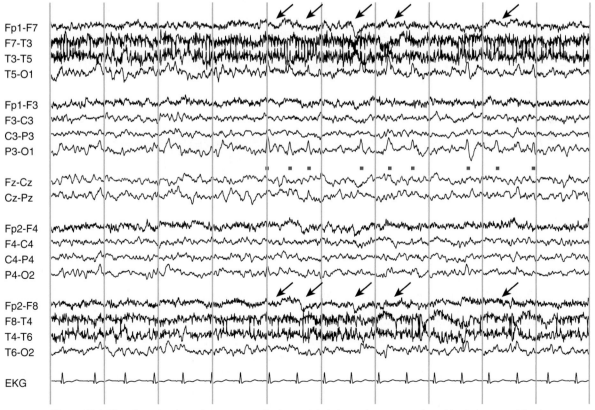

Figure 11.4 The triangular-shaped waves seen in the occipital channels are examples of lambda waves (dots). Lambda waves are associated with horizontal searching eye movements. Subtle lateral eye movement artifact (arrows) is seen in the frontal/anterior temporal channels with opposite polarity on each side (see Chapter 6, "Artifacts in the EEG" for further description of eye movement artifact).

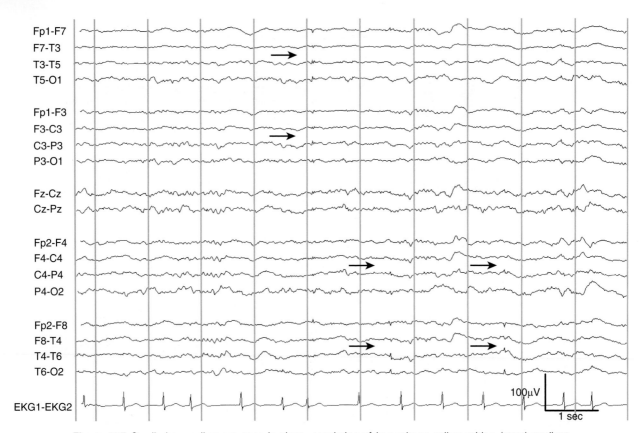

Figure 11.5 Small sharp spikes are seen in sleep, consisting of low-voltage spikes with a broad gradient across the temporal chains (arrows). In this typical example, the spikes are seen in both temporal areas independently.

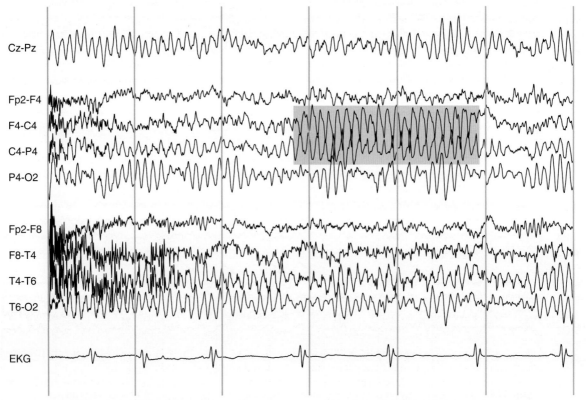

Figure 11.6 A mu rhythm is seen with maximum frequency in the right central (shaded) area, maximum in the C4 electrode. Note the typical morphology of the mu waveform, an arciform or comb-like rhythm, rounded on one side and sharpened on the other.

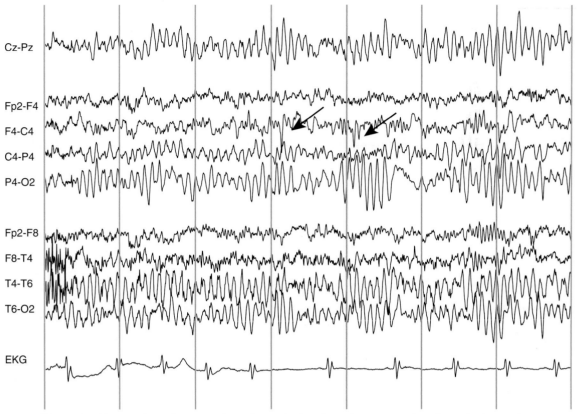

Figure 11.7 The two low-voltage transients (arrows) taken from the same tracing shown in the previous figure could be mistaken for low-voltage spikes. Comparing these transients to the mu rhythm shown in the previous figure, it becomes evident that these waveforms represent fragments of the patient's mu rhythm.

the patient move the contralateral hand and demonstrating that the rhythm disappears. Although classically suppressed by moving the contralateral hand, movement of the ipsilateral hand or planning to move the hand may also suppress the mu rhythm in some subjects.

Because this arciform rhythm is rounded on one side but sharpened on the other, there is some potential to mistake it for epileptiform activity. When mu rhythms occur in trains, it is not difficult to identify them correctly on the basis of their location, morphology, and suppression with movement, if necessary. Occasionally, fragments of a mu rhythm may resemble low-voltage spike activity (Figure 11.7). Apparent low-voltage central spikes can be confirmed to be a mu phenomenon by showing that the morphology of the spike fragment is similar to the mu waves when they occur in trains.

Mu rhythms may be seen either unilaterally or bilaterally. They may suppress independently. Asymmetrical expression of mu rhythms is not considered abnormal and is actually quite common. The mu rhythm tends to occur at a frequency similar to that of the patient's posterior rhythm and therefore varies with age. In some patients, the posterior rhythm's field blends into the field of the mu rhythm creating large zones of alpha activity in the posterior quadrants. Because of the similar frequencies and amplitudes of the two rhythms in such cases, it is not always clear where the posterior rhythm ends and the mu rhythm begins.

The mu rhythm and the posterior rhythm are the two main idling rhythms of the EEG: the mu rhythm is only seen during

contralateral motor inactivity and suppresses with movement. Similarly, the posterior rhythm is only present during visual inactivity and suppresses with eye opening or visual attention. A mu-shaped rhythm that does not necessarily suppress with movement is occasionally seen in the central midline (Cz) and is referred to as a "midline theta rhythm", also considered a normal variant.

Wicket Spikes and Wicket Rhythms

Because their morphology is quite similar to that of mu rhythms, wicket rhythms are discussed with mu rhythms. Wicket rhythms differ from mu rhythms in that they are seen in drowsiness and light sleep rather than wakefulness and have a predilection for the temporal rather than the central areas (Figure 11.8). Their arciform morphology is similar. Wicket rhythms range from 6 to 11 Hz with a voltage range of 60 to 200 μV (Reiher and Lebel, 1977). Similar to the situation seen with mu rhythms, it is possible to mistake a fragment of a wicket rhythm for epileptiform activity rather than a normal variant. Such fragments are called wicket spikes. Wicket spikes are distinct from temporal spike-wave discharges in that there is no aftercoming slow wave and they do not disrupt the underlying rhythm. The confirmation that a temporal spike is a wicket spike is best made by noting that the waveform is similar to that of the spikes when they occur in a train (as a continuous wicket rhythm) found elsewhere in the same tracing.

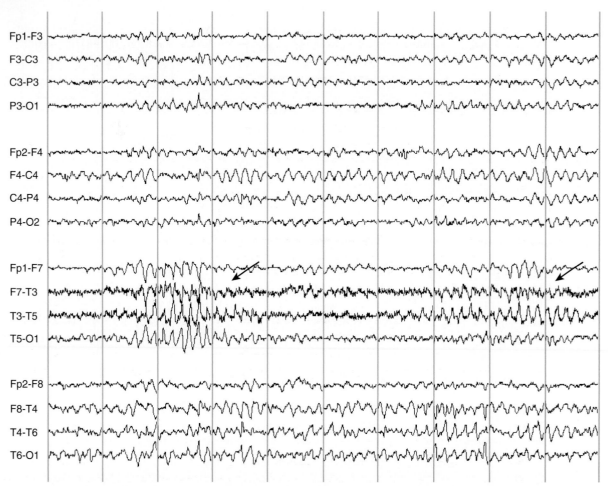

Figure 11.8 Brief trains of wicket spikes are seen in the left temporal area (arrows). Note the arciform morphology. A lower voltage wicket rhythm is present on the right (bottom four channels).

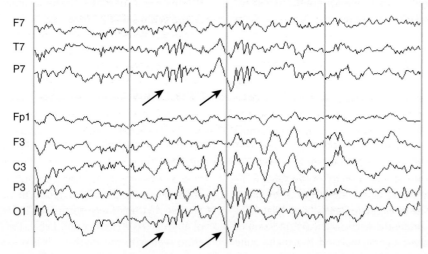

Figure 11.9 A close-up of 14 and 6 positive bursts is shown in a referential montage (arrows). Maximum positivity (indicated by downgoing deflections in a referential montage) of the 14 Hz bursts is seen in the left posterior quadrant (P7, T7, O1, and P3 electrodes).

14 and 6 Hz Positive Bursts

Often referred to simply as "14 and 6," 14 and 6 Hz positive bursts are seen most frequently in adolescence. The term *ctenoids* (a word that means "shaped like the teeth of a comb" or "like overlapping fish scales") has also been used for this phenomenon in the past but is no longer the preferred term. As the name implies, two versions of this variant are seen, one firing at a rate of 14 Hz and the other at 6 Hz. The 14 Hz form is more common (Figures 11.9 through 11.11). The discharges are most prominent in the posterior temporal and occipital

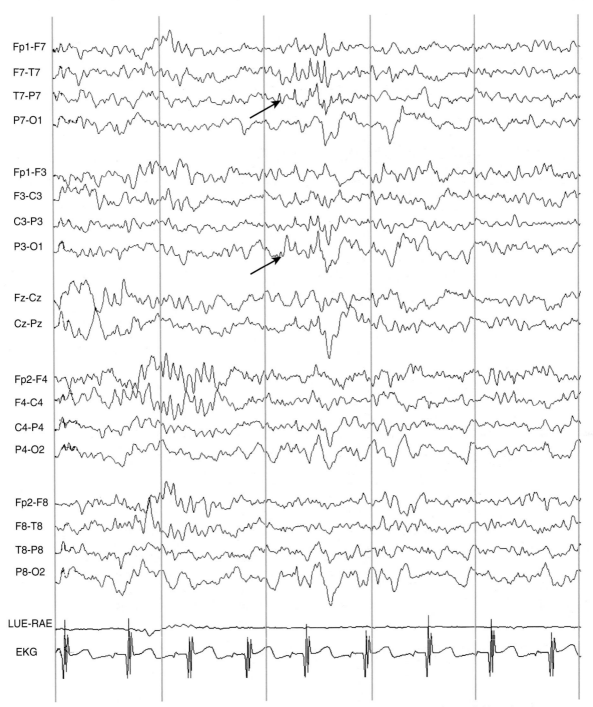

Figure 11.10 An example of 14 and 6 Hz positive bursts is shown in a bipolar montage (arrows). Note that the polarity and localization of the burst in this montage is somewhat ambiguous, appearing to be more anterior in the temporal chain than is actually the case. This appearance is caused by the positive polarity of the bursts, which is more easily understood when they are displayed in a referential montage (see Figure 11.11).

areas. The bursts consist of fast, arciform, or comb-shaped rhythmic discharges of low, medium, or high voltage in which the sharp phase has positive polarity and the rounded phase has negative polarity. It was initially asserted that 14 and 6 was associated with a variety of pathologic states, including epilepsy, but these bursts are now classified by most as a normal variant. The 6 Hz version of 14 and 6 is less commonly seen but felt to have the same significance; some patients manifest both forms in the same tracing.

Although 14 and 6 positive bursts may occur bilaterally, they usually do not fire synchronously. Asymmetrical occurrence of 14 and 6 positive bursts is not considered abnormal. Some authors believe that the 6 Hz component of 14 and 6 actually fires at 7 Hz and represents a subharmonic of the fundamental 14 Hz frequency, although true 6 Hz examples are seen. The bursts usually last 1 second or less, and there is no evolution in firing frequency during the burst. The distinctive wave morphology, frequency, and

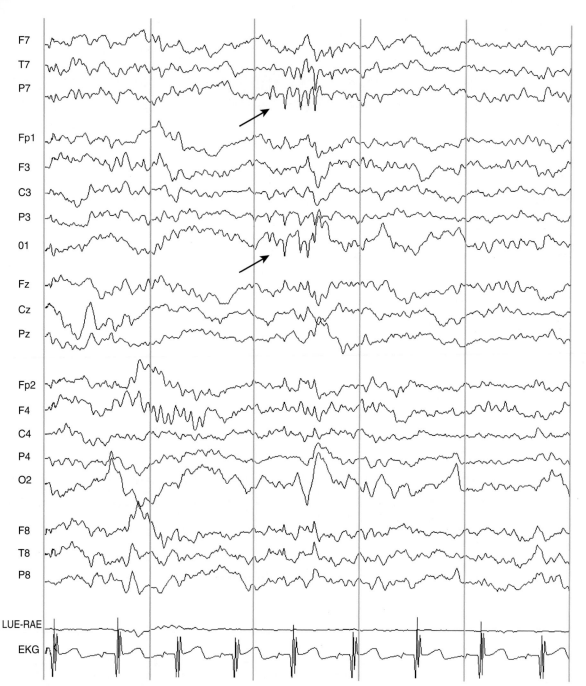

Figure 11.11 The same example of 14 and 6 Hz positive bursts from the previous figure is now displayed in a referential montage (arrows). The downgoing spikes in the posterior channels clarify the positive polarity of the bursts and the localization of their field to the left posterior quadrant.

positive polarity help to confirm examples of 14 and 6 Hz positive bursts.

Breach Rhythms

A breach rhythm results from a change in the transmission of EEG waves through the area of a skull defect, usually a postsurgical craniotomy site (Figures 11.12 through 11.14). For reasons that are not fully understood, faster activity is transmitted preferentially through the region of skull defects, causing breach rhythms to have a sharpened appearance. Because the voltage asymmetries caused by breach rhythms could be hard to interpret without knowledge of the patient's skull defect, EEG technologists are asked to include information about craniotomy scars along with the clinical history. There is still some question as to whether breach rhythms are simply caused by a reduction in the skull's insulation effect at sites where it has been surgically disrupted or are instead caused by some change in the underlying cortex caused by the previous surgical procedure. Breach rhythms sometimes bear a resemblance to mu rhythms or wicket rhythms, and some feel that they represent overexpression of these natural rhythms through the skull defect. It is important to identify breach rhythms so as

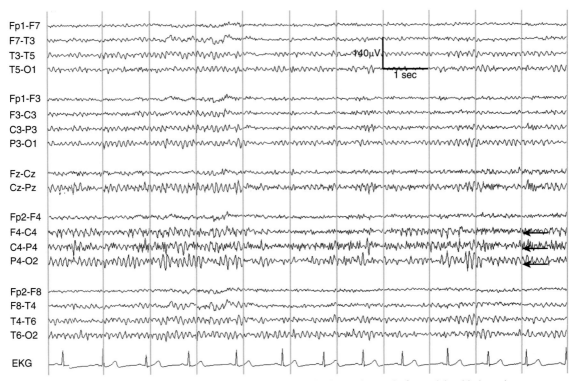

Figure 11.12 A breach rhythm is seen in the right parasagittal area (arrows) after a right-sided craniotomy. Note the higher voltage, sharpened rhythm in the F4-C4, C4-P4, and P4-O2 channels. (Image courtesy of Dr. Edward Bromfield and Dr. Barbara Dwortesky.)

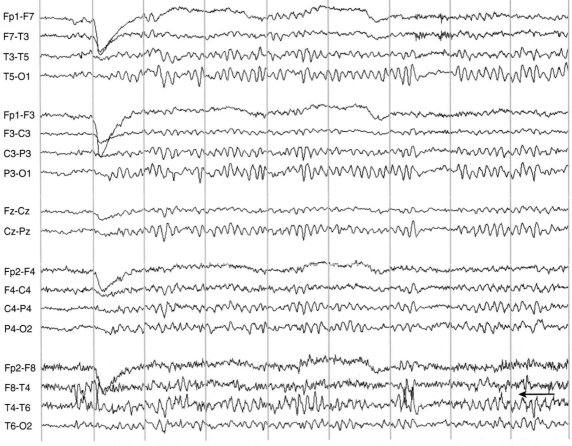

Figure 11.13 A breach rhythm is seen in the right midtemporal area (arrow) after a right temporal craniotomy. Note the arciform nature of the rhythm and compare with the homologous left-sided (T3) electrode. (Image courtesy of Dr. Jong Woo Lee.)

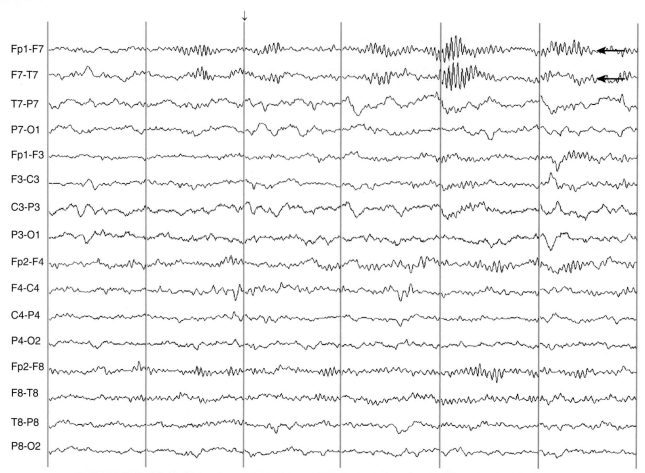

Figure 11.14 A breach rhythm is seen in the left anterior temporal area after a temporal lobectomy in a teenage boy (arrows). Compared with the previous examples, this rhythm has a more sinusoidal appearance.

not to misinterpret any observed voltage asymmetry and to avoid mistaking fragments of the breach rhythm for spikes.

Rhythmic Temporal Theta Bursts of Drowsiness or Psychomotor Variant

Originally also referred to as rhythmic midtemporal discharges (RMTD), rhythmic temporal theta bursts of drowsiness are also called *psychomotor variant* because of the discharges' resemblance to a temporal lobe seizure discharge. The use of the original term *RMTD* may persist because of the ease of using the abbreviation. Rhythmic temporal theta bursts can usually be easily distinguished from seizure discharges in that the frequency, amplitude, and morphology of the waveform do not vary throughout its course (Figure 11.15). These theta bursts are seen in both children and adults and may be seen in either or both hemispheres. The discharges have a distinctive morphology with trains of waves with rounded tops and sharpened bottoms as seen in the figure. This variant is seen in drowsiness and light sleep and is not felt to be associated with epilepsy.

Six per Second Spike-Wave Complexes or Phantom Spike and Wave

Six per second spike-wave complexes are also referred to as a *phantom spike wave* because of their short duration, usually

2 seconds or less. Phantom spike and wave is seen in wakefulness and mild drowsiness. The fact that it disappears with deeper sleep helps to distinguish it from epileptiform activity. These discharges are quick to appear and disappear, and the spike component of the spike and wave may only be intermittently evident.

In 1980, Hughes studied a large group of individuals with six per second spike-wave complexes. In this group, patients with certain characteristics, in particular those with high amplitude, frontal-maximum discharges, were more likely to have epilepsy. Individuals with lower voltage, posterior discharges were more likely to have been referred for "neurovegetative symptoms" such as headache, dizziness, and vertigo or other psychological complaints as opposed to seizures. He distinguished the two groups using the mnemonics WHAM (Waking record, High in amplitude, Anterior in location and especially in Males) and FOLD (Female whose pattern has an Occipital emphasis, Low in amplitude, and seen in the Drowsy record; Figure. 11.16).

Subclinical Rhythmic Electrographic Discharges in Adults (SREDA)

SREDA is a rare benign variant that, according to its name, is generally seen in adults, but very rare cases have been reported in younger subjects as well. SREDA may have a

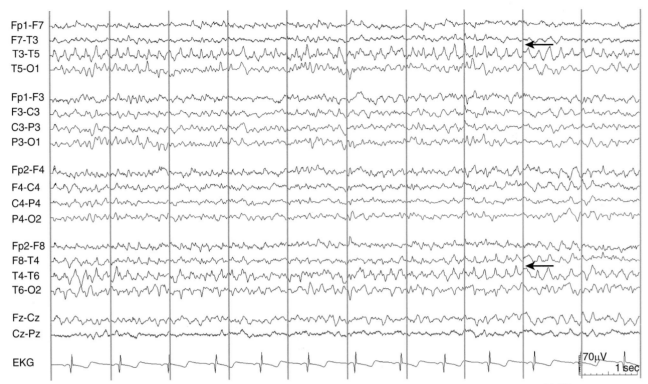

Figure 11.15 Rhythmic temporal theta bursts of drowsiness, also known as psychomotor variant or RMTD, are seen in each temporal area (arrows). The waves are sharp on one side and rounded or flat-topped on the other. The unchanging morphology and the constant frequency help to distinguish this from a seizure discharge—the "firing rate" is the same during the first second and the last second on the page.

diffuse distribution but is usually predominant in the posterior temporal and parietal areas. The pattern may begin abruptly as a theta rhythm or with monophasic sharply contoured waves that occur in a sputtering pattern that eventually coalesces into a sustained 4 to 7 Hz rhythmic pattern typically lasting 40 to 80 seconds (Figure 11.17). The pattern is not associated with any clinical change (Westmoreland and Klass, 1997). Like many of the variants discussed in this chapter, a possible association of SREDA with epilepsy or other disease states has not been definitely excluded.

GENERAL INDICATORS OF NORMAL VARIANTS

Especially for the beginning EEG reader, memorizing the various characteristics of the normal variants just described may seem a daunting task. Even if all of the normal variant patterns have not been committed to memory, certain features of apparent epileptiform discharges should prompt the reader to question the possibility of a normal variant.

High Frequencies

Many of the normal variants have fast firing rates. Whereas "classic" generalized spike wave discharges have a firing rate of 3 Hz and even "fast" spike-wave discharges have a firing rate of 4 to 5 Hz, many of the normal variants have firing rates of 6 Hz or above. Mu rhythms, wicket rhythms, 14 and 6 positive bursts, psychomotor variant, and phantom spike and wave all

have firing rates of 6 Hz or higher. Therefore, high-frequency spiking should cause the reader to consider whether the discharge may fit into the group of normal variants. True epileptiform spike-wave discharges occasionally have fast firing rates, but more moderate firing frequencies are the rule.

Monomorphic Rhythms

The normal variant discharges tend to consist of repetitive waves of similar shape and wavelength (breadth). Because wavelength is directly proportional to frequency, truly monomorphic waves do not vary in frequency. This feature of normal variants helps to distinguish them from seizure discharges and sometimes even from epileptiform activity. A run of the psychomotor variant pattern can be distinguished from seizure activity because it does not vary in frequency even during lengthy trains. In contrast, a hallmark feature of a seizure discharge is a speeding up or slowing down in firing frequency throughout its course. Even interictal polyspike discharges tend to slow down slightly in frequency over the course of a burst, whereas 14 and 6 Hz positive bursts do not. The reader can confirm this by showing that the width (wavelength) of the first wave of a 14 Hz positive burst is the same as the last.

Disappearance in Deeper Sleep

The normal variants described earlier appear in wakefulness or drowsiness and light sleep and tend to disappear with deepening sleep. In contrast, true epileptiform abnormalities often become activated by deeper sleep. Disappearance of a

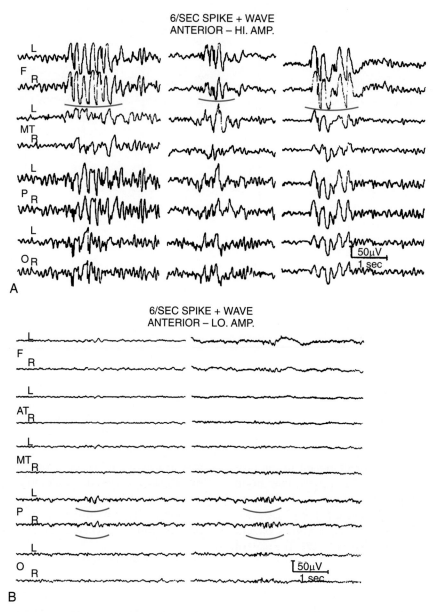

Figure 11.16 (A) Examples of frontal-maximum six per second spike and wave recorded from three separate patients (WHAM version) with higher amplitudes and anterior localization. (B) Examples of the occipital-maximum, lower voltage six per second spike and wave (FOLD version). (Adapted from Hughes JR: Two forms of the 6/sec spike and wave complex. *Electroencephalogr Clin Neurophysiol* 48:535–550, 1980.)

possible epileptiform discharge with deepening sleep should cause the reader to consider whether the discharge in question matches any of the normal variant patterns.

OTHER NORMAL VARIANTS

Posterior Slow Waves of Youth

Posterior slow waves of youth are theta and delta waves that intermix with the posterior rhythm in younger subjects (Figures 11.18 and 11.19). They are confined to the occipital areas and suppress with eye opening along with the posterior rhythm. Typically, these posterior slow waves briefly interrupt sustained runs of the posterior rhythm, sometimes making it

difficult to count. Posterior slow waves of youth appear after age 7 years and are commonly seen up to the middle of the second decade. They become distinctly less common during the late teenage years and are only rarely seen after age 20, by which time posterior slow waves may be abnormal. Posterior slow waves of youth usually occur singly and do not exceed the amplitude of the posterior rhythm by more than 50%. Amplitude asymmetries are not uncommon with these waves and are not necessarily abnormal.

K-Complexes and Related "Evoked Responses"

The k-complex is a normal element of sleep. K-complexes may occur either spontaneously or in response to an outside

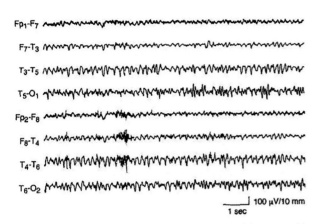

Figure 11.17 A typical SREDA pattern in a 52-year-old woman. Note the predominance of the pattern in the posterior quadrants and the intermittently sharpened features in the theta activity. Courtesy of Westmoreland and Klass.

stimulus such as a noise in the environment. Occasionally, the bursting characteristic of a k-complex could be mistaken for a generalized spike-wave discharge because of embedded sharpened features and their paroxysmal nature. Occasional intermittent increases in voltage during drowsiness or sleep caused by an environmental stimulus may represent a type of evoked response; these may, indeed, represent brief arousal rhythms. Figure 11.20 shows the EEG response of a 33-year-old woman to a noise in the environment during drowsiness. The EEG technologist should note the relationship of such bursts to environmental stimuli, as appropriate, to aid in interpretation.

Exaggerated Hyperventilation Response

Hyperventilation responses are typically more dramatic in children compared with adults. The hyperventilation response is also easier to elicit when blood sugar is lower. In the absence of dramatically asymmetrical findings or clear epileptiform discharges, there is no defined upper limit of voltage for a "normal" hyperventilation response (Figure 11.21), and hyperventilation hypersynchronies should not be considered abnormal based solely on voltage criteria at any age. The hyperventilation exercise we ask patients to perform during EEGs can be unpleasant and cause malaise or headache

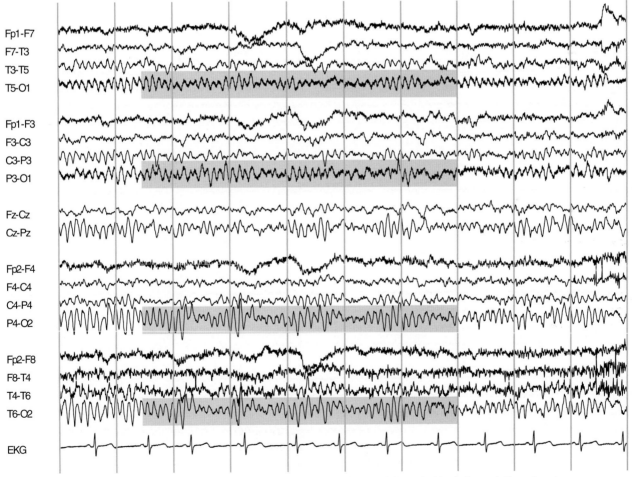

Figure 11.18 Posterior slow waves of youth are seen in the occipital channels (shaded areas). Note that the posterior rhythm does not have a flat baseline but instead rides up and down on low-voltage delta and theta waves. This degree of posterior slowing during wakefulness is commonplace from adolescence into the teenage years. Note that the posterior slow waves are well seen in the right occipital area (O2), but less prominent on the left (O1). An asymmetry of posterior slow waves of youth is not necessarily considered an abnormality.

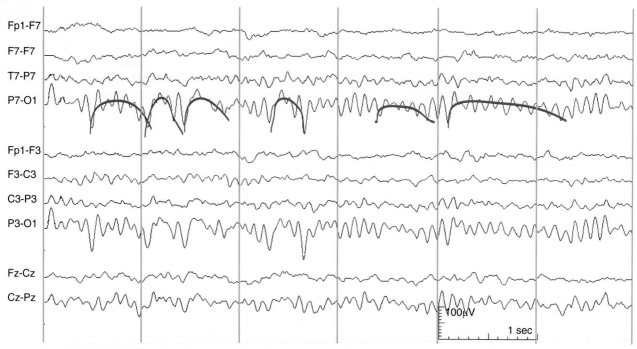

Figure 11.19 Posterior slow waves of youth are seen prominently in the P7-O1 and P3-O1 channels. Some of the intermixed delta and theta waves are marked with pencil in the P7-O1 channel to highlight the shifting baseline of the posterior rhythm caused by its superimposition on these posterior slow waves.

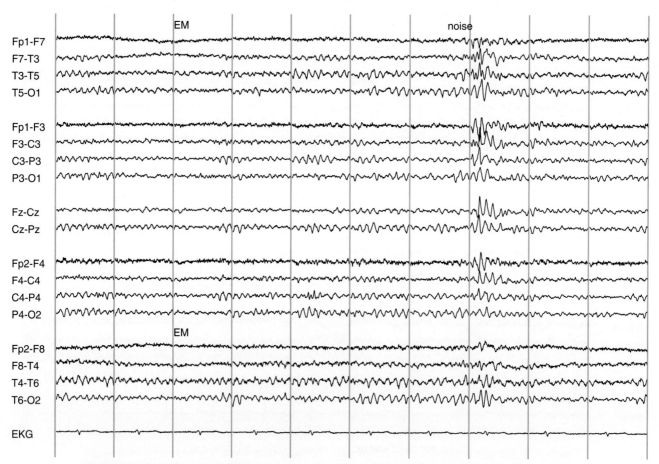

Figure 11.20 A brief increase in EEG voltage occurs in a 33-year-old woman in response to a noise in the EEG laboratory. Slow lateral eye movements (EM), indicated by a slight approximation of the Fp1-F7 and F7-T3 channels and a slight bowing apart of the Fp2-F8 and F8-T4 channels, and intermittent dropout of the posterior rhythm signal light drowsiness. Such brief increases in voltage from an outside stimulus may represent a brief arousal rhythm.

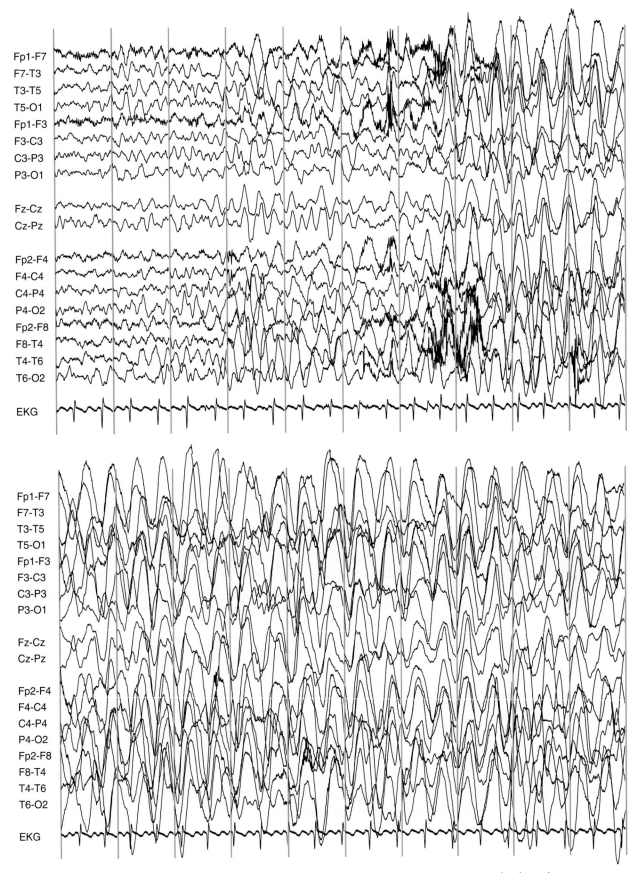

Figure 11.21 Even in patients who do not have epilepsy, the hyperventilation response can be dramatic, as it is in this young patient. In the absence of definite epileptiform features, very high-voltage hyperventilation responses should not be considered abnormal.

in some. Some patients, not feeling well during hyperventilation, may have a dreamy look and be slower to respond to questions. Hyperventilation works by driving down the blood CO_2 level, which causes cerebral vasoconstriction, decreasing blood flow to the brain and activating absence seizure activity if the patient is prone to them. From the clinical point of view, the dreamy appearance of hyperventilation-caused malaise and true absence seizure activity are usually not difficult to distinguish. With absence seizures, the patient almost always temporarily pauses the hyperventilation effort. Also, if asked to hold the arms outstretched in front during hyperventilation, this voluntary positioning will almost always droop during the event. Finally, high-voltage rhythmic slowing and true generalized spike-wave discharges should not be difficult to distinguish from one another on EEG.

Hypnogogic and Hypnopompic Hypersynchronies

Hypnogogic (on falling asleep) and hypnopompic (on arousal) hypersynchronies are highly rhythmic, medium- or high-voltage waves seen diffusely across the EEG either on transition into sleep or on arousal. At times, these hypersynchronies can be dramatic and may potentially be mistaken for epileptiform activity or seizure activity (Figure 11.22). Such hypersynchronies are usually easily distinguished from seizure activity on the basis of their occurrence at the time of sleep transitions and their monorhythmic nature: though the amplitude varies, the frequency of these rhythmic waves holds steady throughout their course, which helps distinguish them from seizure activity.

Photomyoclonic Response

The photomyoclonic response is the result of a reactive twitching of the facial muscles to strobe stimulation (Figure 11.23). This results in bursts of muscle artifact occurring in tandem with the strobe flash. In some instances, the muscle potential bursts could be mistaken for spike-wave discharges. When the muscle spikes and eyeblink artifacts are visually removed, no other abnormalities are seen. The photomyoclonic response is not associated with seizures and is therefore considered a normal variant.

Spiky Alpha

The posterior rhythm is usually a sinusoidal rhythm, but a variant morphology, "spiky alpha," may be seen in a minority of patients. Spiky alpha waves are rounded on one side and spiky on the other (Figure 11.24), similar to the arciform pattern seen with mu and similar rhythms. Spiky alpha variant is usually easy to recognize as such; the danger comes in finding fragments of spiky alpha and mistaking them for occipital spikes.

Slow Alpha Variant and Fast Alpha Variant

The slow alpha variant is a variant of the posterior rhythm in which a subharmonic frequency of the posterior rhythm (half the frequency) is either superimposed on or replaces the posterior rhythm itself. Figure 11.25 shows a patient with a 9 Hz posterior rhythm. Later in the page, a prominent 4.5 Hz rhythm is seen. Replacement of the posterior rhythm with a subharmonic frequency is considered a normal variant and should not be considered a slow-wave abnormality. More rarely, the posterior rhythm may be replaced with a higher harmonic frequency, typically a doubling of the fundamental posterior rhythm. This phenomenon is referred to as fast alpha variant (Figure 11.26). Note the resemblance of the fast alpha variant pattern seen in this figure to the example of a fundamental frequency superimposed on its harmonic (octave) frequency that was shown in Figure 3.11.

Cascading Vertex Waves

Vertex waves during Stage II sleep typically appear in a periodically repetitive fashion, often in conjunction with a spindle. In some patients, highly repetitive or "cascading" vertex waves may be seen for periods of time without pauses (Figure 11.27). Although their appearance may be dramatic, this pattern can be considered a normal variant of vertex wave expression.

Spindle Fragments and Posterior Rhythm Fragments

Sleep spindle rhythms typically appear in runs lasting from one to several seconds. Occasionally, a fragment of this normal waveform can appear, giving a misleading impression. Figure 11.28 shows two apparent sharp waves in the left central area. In fact, these are fragments of a sleep spindle, seen in a more typical form at the beginning of the page. Occasionally, fragments of the posterior rhythm may also appear singly, suggesting a single sharp wave (Figure 11.29). When the morphology of the suspected wave fragment can be seen to match perfectly with previous, easily recognizable examples of the posterior rhythm, the benign nature of the wave can be confirmed. Similar phenomena involving wave fragments of mu rhythms and wicket rhythms are discussed earlier in the chapter.

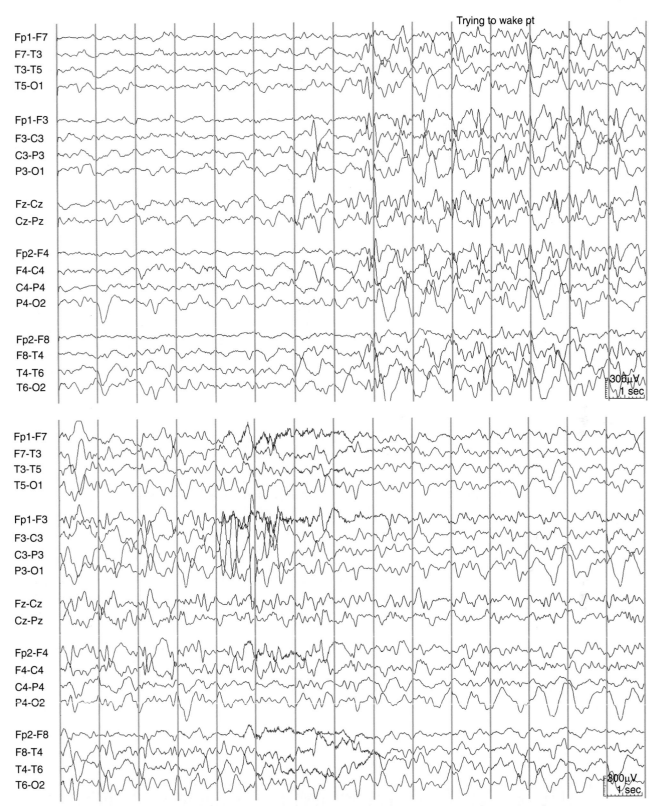

Figure 11.22 This example of a hypnopompic hypersynchrony (hypersynchrony occurring on arousal) occurs out of Stage II sleep when the technologist awakens the patient. This particular pattern consists of a mixture of rhythmic, high-voltage 1 Hz delta with a lower voltage 6 Hz theta rhythm. The fact that these frequencies do not evolve helps to exclude a seizure discharge. The hypersynchrony persists in the form of posterior high-voltage delta in the second half of the bottom page. The mild left-sided predilection of this hypersynchrony may still be within normal limits.

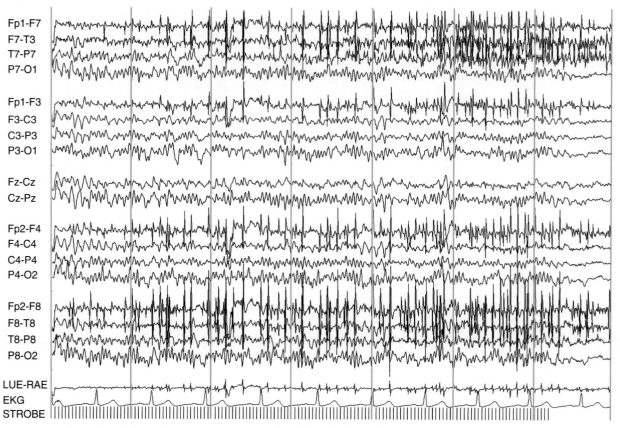

Figure 11.23 Repetitive muscle spikes are seen in the frontal areas during strobe stimulation. These artifactual spikes should not be mistaken for spike-wave discharges. The photomyoclonic response is seen more commonly in subjects with increased tension or anxiety. Visual observation of the patient shows that it is caused by rhythmic eye-twitching/blinking in time with the strobe. The timing of the strobe flashes is shown by the vertical lines in the bottom channel. A normal photic driving response is well seen in the occipital channels. Note that the occipital photic driving response terminates soon after the strobe stops flashing.

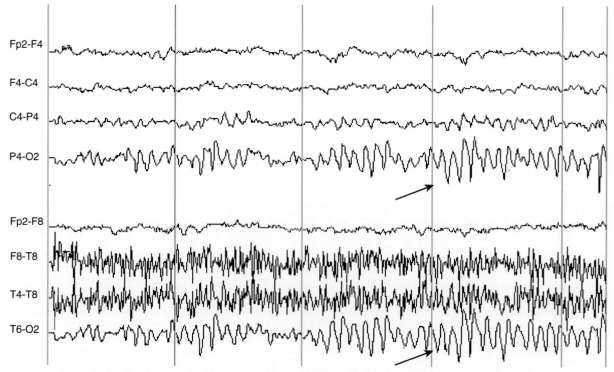

Figure 11.24 The posterior rhythm may become sharpened on one or both sides in some patients (arrows). This normal variant of the posterior rhythm is called spiky alpha variant.

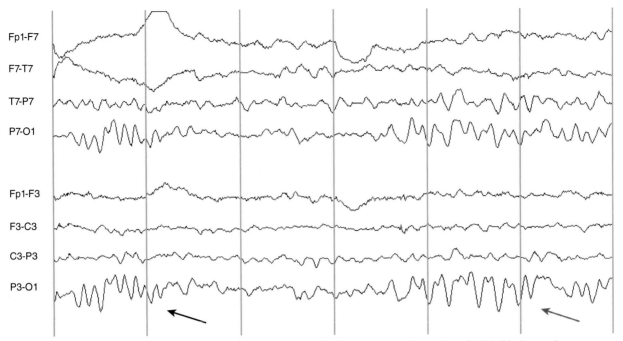

Figure 11.25 This patient with slow alpha variant has a fundamental posterior rhythm of 10 Hz (black arrow). At times a prominent and higher voltage 5 Hz rhythm is seen in the same region (gray arrow), representing a subharmonic of the fundamental 10 Hz rhythm. In this example, both the 5 Hz and the 10 Hz rhythm (in the form of notching of the 5 Hz rhythm) can be seen at the same time. In other patients, a pure subharmonic of the fundamental rhythm can be seen without notching by the fundamental frequency (e.g., a pure 5 Hz rhythm completely taking the place of the 10 Hz posterior rhythm). In such cases, the presence of slow alpha variant can be confirmed by finding the fundamental posterior rhythm frequency elsewhere in the record, which should be a higher multiple of the slower frequency.

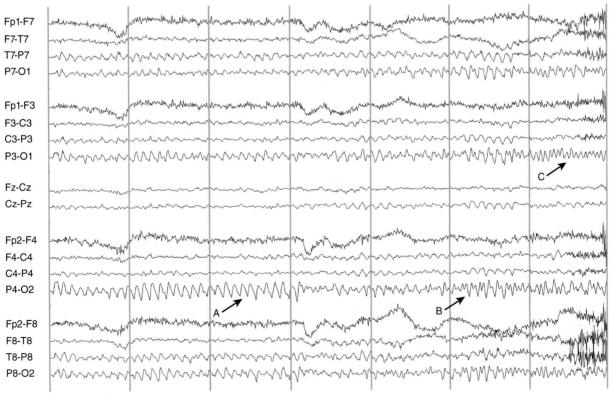

Figure 11.26 (A) This patient's fundamental posterior rhythm frequency is well seen. (B) A combination of the fundamental posterior rhythm and its first harmonic frequency (double the fundamental frequency) is seen in the form of a "notched" version of the posterior rhythm. (C) A pure version of the harmonic frequency, the "fast alpha variant."

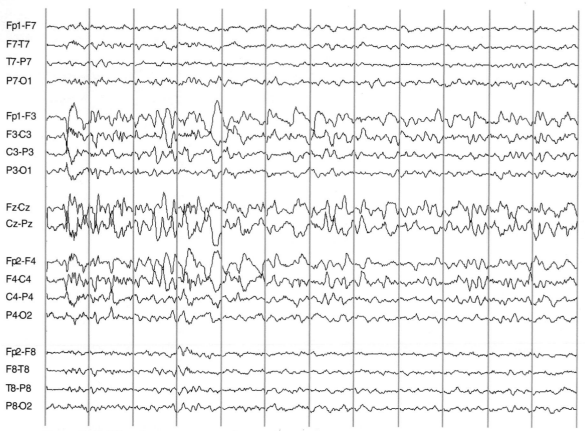

Figure 11.27 Although vertex waves usually occur in a repetitive, on-and-off pattern, less commonly they may be seen as relatively continuously appearing discharges. The maxima of these waves at Cz, C3, and C4 and the relative exclusion of the waves' field from the temporal areas help to identify them as vertex waves of sleep despite their repetitive nature.

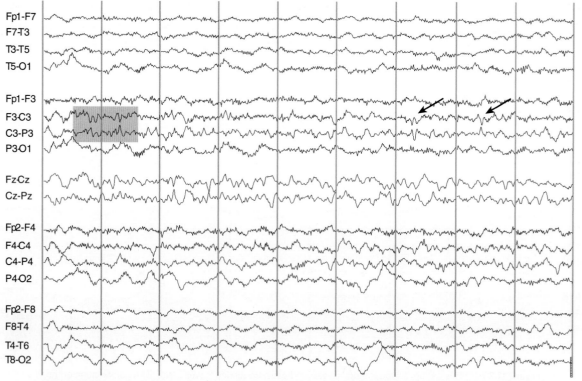

Figure 11.28 Two possible low-voltage spikes are noted in the left central region (arrows). The possibility that these represent low-voltage spikes can be excluded after it is recognized that they have the exact same morphology as the spindle wave seen at the beginning of the page (shaded area) and that they are examples of spindle fragments.

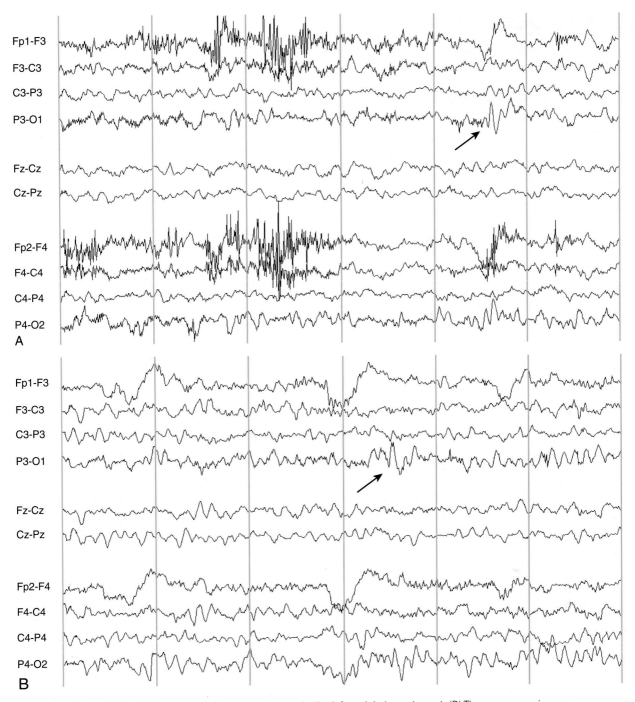

Figure 11.29 (A) An apparent sharp wave is seen in the left occipital area (arrow). (B) The same wave is now recognized in the context of the posterior rhythm (arrow), confirming that it is a posterior rhythm fragment rather than a sharp wave. The posterior rhythm fragment seen in Panel A was likely caused by rapid eye closure (note the eyeblink artifact in the frontal channels occurring at the same time as the wave fragment). The posterior rhythm wave indicated in Panel B can be distinguished from a spike since, even though it is of higher voltage than its neighbors, it neatly fits into the rhythm of the adjacent waves.

REVIEW QUESTIONS

1. Which is true of POSTS and lambda waves?
   a. Both have a triangular shape.
   b. Both have positive polarity.
   c. Both occur predominantly in sleep.
   d. Both are seen in a higher frequency in people with epilepsy.

2. Mu rhythms
   a. can be suppressed by having the patient move the contralateral hand.
   b. can be suppressed by having the patient move the ipsilateral hand.
   c. are considered an "idling rhythm" of motor cortex.
   d. All of the above.

3. Wicket rhythms can be distinguished from epileptiform activity or temporal lobe seizures because wicket rhythms
   a. don't evolve in frequency.
   b. don't evolve in wave morphology.
   c. fire at frequencies of 6 Hz and above, unlike interictal epileptiform activity.
   d. All of the above.

4. The positive polarity seen in 14 and 6 Hz positive bursts is best demonstrated by
   a. noting waves with downgoing sharp features.
   b. using transverse montages.
   c. using a referential montage with an indifferent reference electrode.
   d. using additional electrodes from the 10-10 system.

5. Posterior slow waves of youth
   a. are considered abnormal if of different amplitude on one side compared to the other.
   b. are abnormal if they occur asymmetrically.
   c. should disappear with eye closure.
   d. None of the above.

6. The photomyoclonic response
   a. is seen in the benign myoclonic epilepsies of childhood.
   b. is seen in the progressive myoclonic epilepsies.
   c. has no association with epilepsy.
   d. responds well to valproic acid.

ANSWERS

1. ANSWER: **A.** The triangular morphology of POSTS and lambda waves are similar. Although POSTS have consistently positive polarity, lambda waves may have either positive or negative polarity. Lambda waves are associated with searching eye movements and, therefore, are only seen during wakefulness. Neither POSTS nor lambda waves are believed to have any association with epilepsy and both are considered normal findings in the EEG.

2. ANSWER: **D.** The technologist can display suppression of a mu rhythm by asking the patient to move the hand (either hand in many patients). The mu rhythm can be considered an "idling rhythm" of the motor cortex, meaning that once the motor cortex becomes engaged in a task, the rhythm is suppressed.

3. ANSWER: **D.** The fact that wicket rhythms fire at such a high rate helps distinguish them from interictal spike-wave discharges, which tend to fire at slower rates. The individual waves of wicket rhythms tend to maintain a consistent wave morphology and frequency throughout their runs, unlike seizure discharges, which tend to evolve in amplitude, but especially in frequency.

4. ANSWER: **C.** Depending on the montage and location of the bursts, positive-polarity waveforms may manifest either downgoing or upgoing waves. A referential montage with a neutral reference is the best tool to show positive polarity of the sharp component of 14 and 6 Hz positive bursts. Transverse montages and additional electrodes from the 10-10 system may not help clarify the polarity.

5. ANSWER: **D.** Posterior slow waves of youth are not necessarily considered abnormal if they vary in amount or amplitude from side to side. Posterior slow waves of youth are characteristically seen superimposed on the posterior rhythm, indicating that are seen *during* eye closure.

6. ANSWER: **C.** Because it is not associated with epilepsy, the photomyoclonic response is not seen with increased frequency with any type of epilepsy, myoclonic or otherwise, and would not be expected to change with the use of valproic acid.

REFERENCES

Hughes JR: Two forms of the 6/sec spike and wave complex, *Electroencephalogr Clin Neurophysiol* 48:535–550, 1980.

Reiher J, Lebel M: Wicket spikes: clinical correlates of a previously undescribed EEG pattern, *Can J Neurol Sci* 4:39–47, 1977.

Westmoreland BF, Klass DW: Unusual variants of subclinical rhythmic electrographic discharge of adults (SREDA), *Electroencephalogr Clin Neurophysiol* 102(1):1–4, 1997 Jan. https://doi.org/10.1016/s0013-4694(96)96035-6. PMID: 9060848

SUGGESTED READING

Westmoreland BF: Benign electroencephalographic variants and patterns of uncertain clinical significance. In Ebersole JS, Pedley TA, editors: *Current practice of clinical electroencephalography*, ed 3, Philadelphia, 2003, Lippincott, Williams & Wilkins, pp. 235–245.

12

EEG Patterns in Stupor and Coma

Consciousness refers to a state in which one is fully aware of one's self and one's environment. The term *coma* refers to a state in which a person is unaware of self and surroundings, even if stimulated from the outside. Between consciousness and deep coma, there is a continuum of possible levels of responsiveness and awareness. Encephalopathy is a broad term that may be used to indicate a decrease in awareness; a patient who develops confusion and decreased awareness can be said to be "encephalopathic." Because many of the nuances of the neurologic examination are lost in the comatose patient, the EEG plays a special role in ascertaining the depth of coma and whether it may be improving or worsening. In addition, patients are often pharmacologically paralyzed in the ICU to assist with mechanical ventilation, a practice that severely limits the information gained from the neurologic examination. In such patients, the EEG may be the principle source of information regarding the patient's neurologic state.

Broadly speaking, the EEG may contribute information in the setting of coma in three ways. First, the pattern seen on a single EEG "snapshot" may suggest the depth and severity of the coma. Second, trends seen in repeat or serial EEGs can be a useful indicator of improvement or deterioration in a patient's status. Some of the specific EEG parameters used to follow such trends and their implications are discussed in this chapter. Third, in a minority of cases the EEG pattern seen in coma can give clues to the cause of the coma, such as the association of triphasic waves with hepatic and other metabolic encephalopathies or the unexpected discovery of continuous subclinical seizure activity. Focal findings or asymmetries in the EEG of a comatose patient may be the first indication of a structural brain abnormality, such as stroke.

INDIVIDUAL PARAMETERS OF THE EEG IN COMA

Voltage, Frequency, Reactivity, and the Presence of Normal Sleep Elements

There is a general correspondence between EEG coma patterns and the depth and severity of the coma. A variety of EEG attributes can be followed on serial testing to track a patient's progress in the comatose state. In patients who have a deteriorating neurological status, a parallel deterioration in the EEG is expected. Likewise, in patients with progressive neurologic improvement, a concomitant improvement in the EEG is expected. Thus, the EEG can serve as a useful adjunct to the clinical examination. The key parameters to follow in the EEG of the comatose patient are discussed below.

Slow-Wave Voltage

When low-voltage slow waves become intermixed with the patient's baseline background activity, this may be the first EEG sign of encephalopathic change (Figure 12.1). Increases in the amount and amplitude of slow-wave activity and decreases in the frequency of the slow-wave activity suggest an increasing severity of the encephalopathy. With deepening coma, slow-wave amplitude may continue to increase and high-voltage slow-wave patterns may be seen. Rather than intermixing with the faster background activity, the high-voltage slow-wave activity becomes the background and the faster rhythms disappear. As cerebral function is increasingly affected, however, slow-wave amplitude can only increase to a certain point. With yet more severe cortical dysfunction, neurons become less and less able to create higher voltages and slow waves may then begin to decrease in amplitude. With the most severe neurological processes, cortical function becomes depressed and the brain becomes less able to maintain slow-wave voltages, resulting in progressively diminished background activity and voltage. Thus, very low-voltage patterns in coma are considered more ominous than high-voltage slow-wave patterns. The EEG patterns associated with the most severe degrees of cortical dysfunction show marked suppression of voltages or even electrocerebral inactivity.

Given this described sequence of initially increasing, then decreasing slow-wave amplitude with increasingly severe encephalopathy, a linear relationship between slow-wave amplitude and severity of encephalopathy cannot be assumed. When amplitudes are seen to decrease, this could represent either a trend toward normalization or signal a trend toward voltage depression and increasing dysfunction. Usually these two circumstances are not difficult to distinguish as with improvement of the coma, diminishing slow-wave activity will be replaced by more normal, faster activity. In such cases, other EEG features (discussed below) such as frequency and reactivity of the background may help clarify the meaning of the change (Figures 12.2 and 12.3).

The evolution of slow-wave activity during the improvement phase of a neurologic process may be less tightly linked to the patient's neurologic status. The clearing of slow-wave activity often lags behind the patient's clinical improvement. In a patient who is recovering from a dramatic encephalopathy, EEG slow-wave activity may still be present even as the patient wakes up, sits up, and begins talking. The persistence

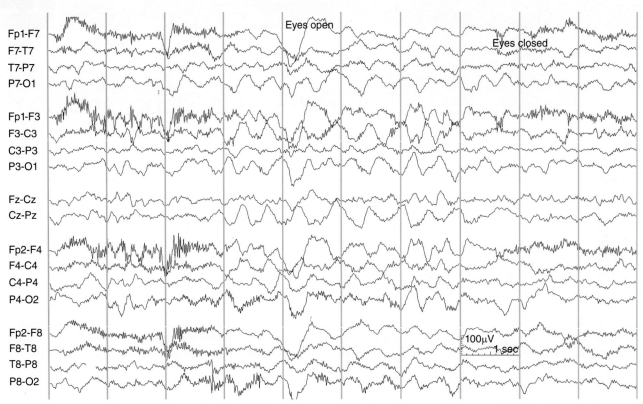

Figure 12.1 Medium- to high-voltage delta activity is seen superimposed on an otherwise unremarkable background in a stuporous 12-year-old boy with meningitis. In this case, the slow waves are intermixed with faster activity in the patient's background.

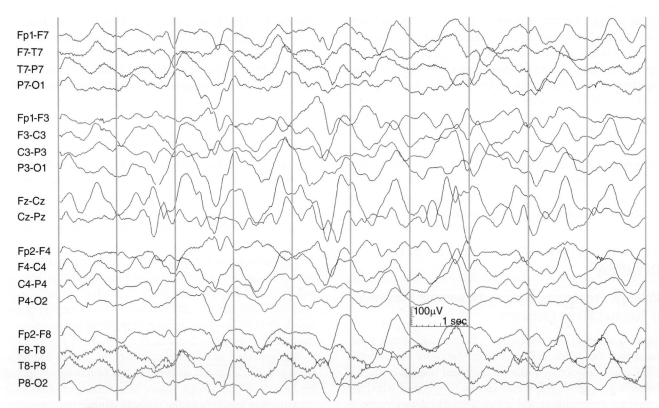

Figure 12.2 A typical slow-wave pattern in coma is shown with high-voltage semirhythmic delta waves. A small amount of intermixed theta activity is also seen, particularly near the vertex and in the occipital areas. Compare to Figure 12.3.

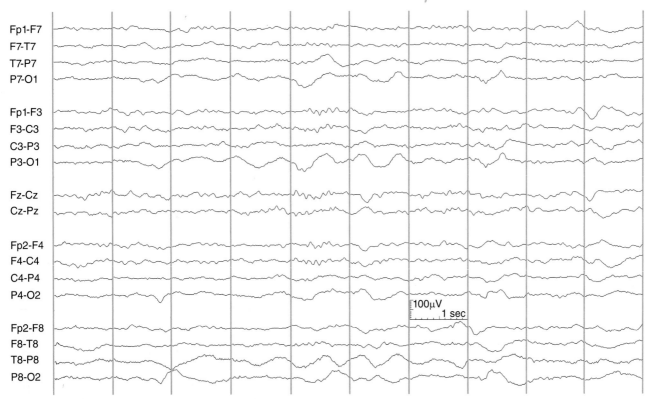

Figure 12.3 The EEG of the same patient seen in Figure 12.2 recorded 48 hours later. As discussed in the text, a decrease in slow-wave voltage in coma can signal either an improvement or a deterioration in the patient's state. In this tracing, the appearance of faster rhythms accompanies the decrease in amplitudes, clarifying that the drop in voltages represents a trend toward improvement.

of slow-wave activity in the face of an improving neurologic picture is not necessarily a negative neurologic sign as long as there is a trend toward EEG improvement. Likewise, the slow-wave activity that follows a seizure (postictal slowing) may persist well past the point that patients report feeling back to their pre-seizure baseline. Slow-wave activity may persist after a seizure for minutes, hours, commonly a few days, but occasionally for as long as 3 to 4 weeks depending on the type of seizure, the duration of the seizure, and the general neurologic health and age of the individual.

Slow-Wave Frequency

The relationship of slow-wave frequency to coma severity is more straightforward than it is for slow-wave amplitude. In general, decreasing slow-wave frequencies suggest increasing severity of encephalopathy. A decrease in slow-wave amplitude can be associated with either improvement or deterioration in neurologic status as described above. Counting wave frequency is a useful tool for distinguishing between the two possibilities. If background frequency is increasing, this is a good sign; slower slow waves suggest deterioration. A similar approach is taken when comparing two hemispheres with slow-wave activity, one with higher voltages than the other. Higher voltage slowing may mark the more affected (abnormal) hemisphere, but it also could be that the opposite hemisphere manifests lower voltages because it is the more abnormal side. In such cases, comparing the frequencies generated by each side may clarify which is the relatively "healthier" hemisphere, identified by its higher frequency.

Reactivity

EEG reactivity is an additional useful feature in assessing the depth of coma. The EEG is monitored for change when the patient is stimulated. The stimulus may be as simple as calling the patient's name or could include purposeful noxious tactile stimulation (examples include nailbed pressure, sternal rub, nasal tickle, trapezius squeeze, etc.). Intensive care unit procedures such as endotracheal tube suctioning or venipunctures also provide an opportunity to observe EEG reactivity. An unreactive EEG is one that shows no change in response to stimulation. Reactive EEGs show a change with stimulation, which may be seen in the form of an increase in amplitude and rhythmicity in low-voltage tracings or a relative flattening of the background in higher voltage tracings (the latter finding comparable to the voltage attenuation seen in noncomatose patients with arousal or alerting). The presence of reactivity in the EEG is considered a relatively good prognostic sign compared to when it is absent.

Presence of Normal Sleep Elements

The presence of identifiable sleep elements in the EEG in coma is associated with a relatively better neurologic prognosis. The presence of sleep features implies that there is enough functioning cerebral circuitry intact to generate these elements. Sleep spindles are the most commonly identified sleep feature in this setting. In rare cases, the higher centers that generate sleep elements are intact, but there has been a severe injury at lower levels of the central nervous system such as the brain stem, resulting in a poor outcome despite the persistence of sleep elements.

SPECIFIC EEG PATTERNS IN COMA AND NEUROLOGIC PROGNOSIS

The prognostic impact of the EEG patterns discussed here must always be interpreted in the context of the coma's underlying etiology. Although various EEG coma patterns have different reputations in terms of the severity of the encephalopathic state that they imply, even the most severe patterns can have a good final outcome if the etiology of the coma is inherently reversible. A good example of a reversible process is drug overdose. Patients with drug overdose may show, at least for a period of time, otherwise ominous EEG patterns such as burst-suppression, voltage depression, or even "flat" EEG patterns. After the drug effect has cleared, assuming there has been no permanent brain injury, the patient (and the EEG) may recover completely. This stands in contrast to the patient who shows a burst-suppression pattern or voltage depression after a prolonged cardiac arrest, a type of injury that is less likely to be reversible. In this group of patients, these EEG patterns have a more ominous significance.

Some of the most useful studies that have examined the prognostic impact of different EEG patterns in coma have limited the study group to patients with anoxic insults, such as those caused by cardiac arrest. This approach has the advantage of excluding the important variable of coma etiology from long-term outcome; however, the conclusions of these studies should only be extrapolated outside this etiologic group studied with caution. It is no surprise that two patients with the same EEG pattern in coma, such as a drug overdose patient and a patient with a malignant brain tumor, would have very different neurologic outcomes despite similar EEG findings. Because EEG patterns are dictated more by the function of the cerebrum than the brainstem, the minority of patients with devastating brainstem injuries but relative sparing of the cerebrum may have misleadingly benign EEG findings. The order that specific coma patterns are listed in the following subsections should not imply a strict ranking, although they are generally described in order of increasing severity.

Intermittent Rhythmic Delta Activity

Among EEG findings in encephalopathy, intermittent rhythmic delta activity (IRDA) lies at the mild end of the spectrum of encephalopathic EEG patterns. IRDA may appear in patients who are awake or who are mildly lethargic or stuporous. IRDA patterns are not associated with deeply comatose states and, in fact, are often seen in outpatients. IRDA tends to occur in the frontal regions in adults (frontal intermittent rhythmic delta activity, or FIRDA) and in the occipital regions in younger children (occipital intermittent rhythmic delta activity, or OIRDA; Figure 12.4). When encephalopathic states become more severe, IRDA patterns may be replaced by continuous slow-wave patterns. Various types of IRDA are discussed in more detail in Chapter 9, "The Abnormal EEG."

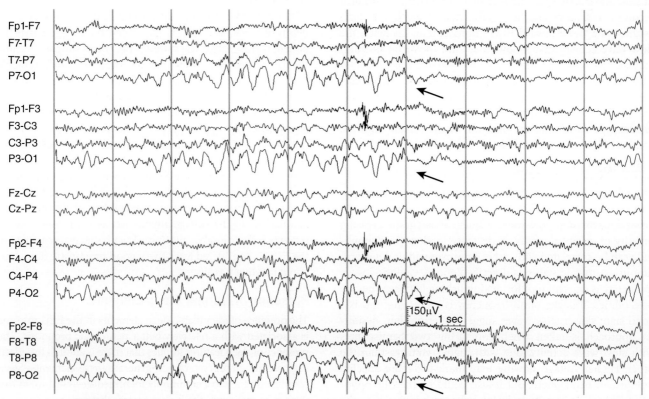

Figure 12.4 Occipital intermittent rhythmic delta activity (OIRDA) and excess fast activity are seen in a 9-year-old intensive care unit patient with postictal confusion (arrows). The increased fast activity is the result of treatment with lorazepam. Intermittent rhythmic delta activity is usually associated with mild encephalopathies.

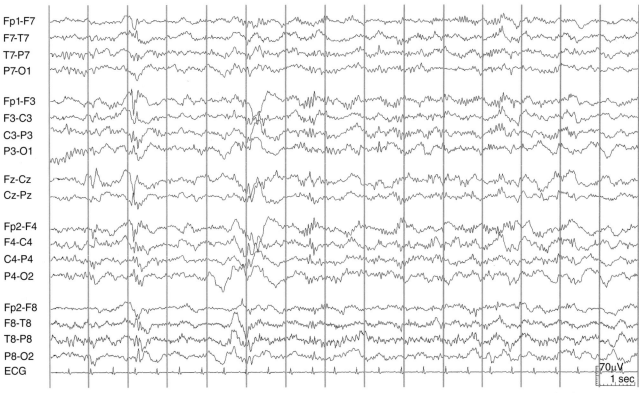

Figure 12.5 Exaggerated spindles are seen along with vertex waves in this comatose patient, representing an example of spindle coma.

Spindle Coma

Spindle coma may be indistinguishable from normal Stage II or III sleep (Figure 12.5). The term may be applied to generalized slow-wave patterns obtained in comatose patients in which sleep spindles can be identified, although in many examples of spindle coma the amount of spindle activity is exaggerated. Coma patterns that include normal sleep elements usually fall into better prognostic groups. This makes intuitive sense because the ability to generate normal sleep elements implies that the centers responsible for generating spindles, located in the diencephalon and above, are functionally intact. Some cases of spindle coma with poor outcome may be explained by patterns of damage that involve brainstem structures but have left higher cerebral structures relatively intact. Spindle coma can be distinguished from alpha coma (discussed later) in that, in spindle coma each spindle has a discrete duration and spindles should be maximally expressed in the frontocentral regions. Alpha patterns in alpha coma (discussed later) are more diffuse and continuous.

Continuous Slow-Wave Patterns

Diffuse slow-wave patterns are among the most frequently encountered EEG patterns in coma. Just as there is a continuum among alert, stuporous, and comatose states, so is there a continuum between the normal EEG and EEG patterns with various degrees of diffuse slowing. Diffuse slow-wave patterns are usually comprised of delta frequencies, but theta frequencies may be seen as well. Slow-wave patterns in coma are usually nonrhythmic. Rhythmic slow-wave patterns are more often seen in the setting of metabolic encephalopathies.

As described in the previous section on slow-wave voltage in coma, higher slow-wave voltages are generally considered "more healthy" than lower voltages, but the relationship between voltage and depth of coma is complex, because declines in slow-wave voltage may potentially be associated with either deterioration or improvement in clinical state. EEGs that show reactivity to noxious stimulation are generally associated with a better neurologic prognosis than those that are unreactive, and those with higher frequencies are generally prognostically better than those with lower frequencies.

As with other coma patterns, the underlying cause of the coma is a strong influence on outcome, often more important than the specific EEG pattern itself. Outcome after an anoxic event associated with delta slowing may be quite different from the outcome seen after a generalized seizure that is followed by similar delta slowing in the postictal period; there is the expectation that the latter pattern may be completely reversible.

Asymmetric voltages in slow-wave patterns suggest that an asymmetric process is at work. Diffuse processes, such as metabolic derangements, are usually associated with symmetrical patterns. The exception to this rule is the case of a symmetrical process acting on an asymmetrical brain. For instance, although most patients with hyperosmolar coma would be expected to show a symmetrical slow-wave pattern, a patient with hyperosmolar coma who has suffered a previous stroke may show an asymmetric pattern in reaction to the metabolic

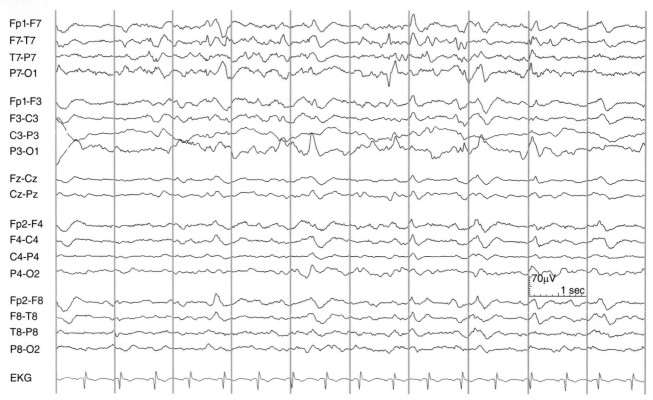

Figure 12.6 In this comatose patient, asymmetric slowing is seen with higher voltages over the left hemisphere compared with the right. Some sharp features are also evident over the left hemisphere. When slow-wave patterns are asymmetric, it is not always obvious which is the more severely affected side. In this example, fewer theta rhythms are seen over the lower voltage right hemisphere, suggesting that side may be more severely affected.

derangement; healthy brain regions may react differently to the metabolic abnormality compared to previously injured regions. As discussed earlier, it may not always be clear which side is more severely affected when slow-wave patterns are asymmetrical (Figure 12.6). Other findings superimposed on a slow-wave background such as periodic lateralized epileptiform discharges ("PLEDs or LPDs;" see Chapter 9) or epileptiform activity may suggest additional diagnoses.

Alpha Coma

The alpha coma pattern consists of diffuse alpha activity in the range of 8 to 13 Hz (Figure 12.7). Most reports have associated the alpha coma pattern after anoxic insult with a relatively pessimistic outcome, although with some exceptions. A similar pattern of diffuse alpha activity may be seen in toxic and metabolic encephalopathies, especially drug intoxications. In contrast to the post-anoxic state, when an alpha coma pattern is seen after drug intoxication it is expected to have a relatively more favorable prognosis.

Various theories have been put forward to explain the genesis of alpha rhythms in alpha coma. Some have suggested that the pattern is related to the spindle generator. Others have suggested that this alpha activity represents a paradoxically retained alpha-range activity related to the posterior rhythm. An additional possibility is that, because of diffuse cortical injury, the alpha activity of alpha coma represents a slowed version of the beta activity that is usually generated locally by the normal cortex. The dependence of neurological

outcome on the cause of coma after alpha coma is a reminder of the general importance of considering etiology in assessing prognosis in coma.

Triphasic Waves

The appearance and significance of triphasic waves is discussed in more detail in Chapter 9, "The Abnormal EEG," and an example is shown in Figure 9.39. The presence of triphasic waves is almost always associated with a state of depressed consciousness. Triphasic waves have been classically associated with metabolic derangement such as hepatic coma or renal failure but are occasionally seen after an anoxic insult and have also been observed in other disorders. The prognosis of patients with triphasic waves depends on the course of the underlying process.

Nonconvulsive Status Epilepticus

Among EEG coma patterns, prompt diagnosis of nonconvulsive status epilepticus (NCSE) is very important because it is a cause of coma that may be readily responsive to treatment with antiseizure medications. Both generalized convulsive status epilepticus (SE) and focal SE with impaired awareness (previously complex partial SE) often evolve into states that resemble coma.

It is important to be aware of the natural progression of convulsive SE. Patients with continuous generalized seizures destined to have SE often begin by having repetitive, outwardly observable generalized convulsions. However, as the

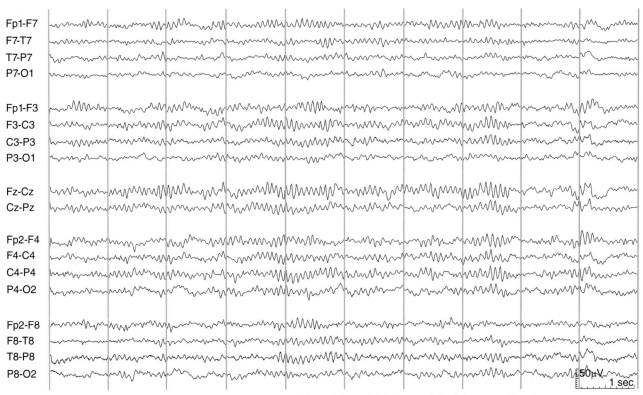

Figure 12.7 An alpha coma pattern is seen with diffuse alpha activity. Prognosis in alpha coma differs in cases caused by anoxia as opposed to those caused by drug effect.

generalized seizure discharges repeat the convulsive movements become less prominent, eventually culminating in a state in which the patient lies unresponsive and motionless even as the same generalized electrographic seizure discharges might continue in the EEG. Patients with initial convulsive SE may transition to this nonconvulsive state within 30 minutes or less of seizure onset. This progression from convulsive to nonconvulsive SE, along with the metabolic derangements that may accompany it, are illustrated in Figure 12.8. Similarly, prolonged focal seizure activity with impaired awareness will evolve to a stuporous or comatose state, sometimes with cyclical fluctuations in responsiveness (Figures 12.9 and 12.10). Careful observation of patients with either initial tonic-clonic SE or NCSE resulting from prolonged focal seizures with impaired awareness may reveal intermittent, subtle rhythmic movements in the face or limbs, but absence of this finding cannot be relied on to exclude the diagnosis of occult SE.

Different definitions of SE have used different time limits to define the entity. Some earlier definitions used this 30-minute time point as a cutoff for a definition of SE based on the transition that occurs at about this time toward both systemic decompensation and neuronal injury related to excess excitatory neurotransmitter release. Current definitions use shorter durations in order to encourage earlier treatment of seizures that do not terminate on their own. The strategy for how to set a duration limit for SE is philosophical. Although the idea behind setting a 30-minute limit as above based on the timing of when physiologic injury might begin seems sensible, much shorter durations are now used in order to trigger

SE treatment algorithms well before 30 minutes of seizure activity has occurred.

NCSE may have a variety of causes ranging from the patient with an idiopathic epilepsy who experiences a seizure that fails to terminate to the patient in whom NCSE occurs as a terminal event after severe anoxic, metabolic, or neoplastic processes. When NCSE is caused by a severe, irreversible injury the electrographic seizure pattern may evolve to a low-voltage pattern and eventually to a "flat" EEG. Specific EEG criteria for the diagnosis of NCSE have been proposed by a consensus committee and are referred to as the "Salzburg Criteria." These are discussed below in the section on the 2021 ACNS Terminology.

Absence status epilepticus (ASE) can present as a confusional state, although many patients retain the ability to walk and converse, albeit in a confused fashion, despite the presence of continuous generalized spike-wave discharges. Therefore, ASE is less likely to present with a true coma presentation.

Burst-Suppression Patterns

Burst-suppression patterns consist of periodic bursts of polymorphic activity, often containing sharp features, separated by periods of voltage suppression (Figure 12.12). Each burst looks different from the next. In a minority of patients, a myoclonic movement may accompany each burst. Burst-suppression patterns have been associated with anoxic injury and are generally associated with a poor prognosis for neurologic recovery. In infants and children, and especially in the minority of patients in whom the pattern improves promptly, outcome may be somewhat better. Burst-suppression patterns

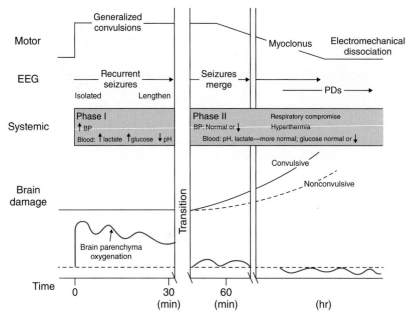

Figure 12.8 Summary of systemic alterations and brain metabolism in SE. Various events are aligned with respect to a time line. Note discontinuities in the time line and the designation of a critical transition period after 30 minutes of SE. (Adapted from Lothman E. The biochemical basis and pathophysiology of status epilepticus. I 1990 May;40(5 Suppl 2):13–23.)

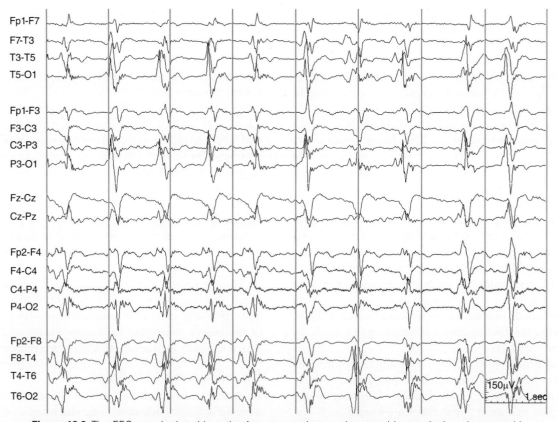

Figure 12.9 The EEG reveals that this patient's unresponsiveness is caused by continuing electrographic seizure activity or nonconvulsive status epilepticus. The pattern consists of repetitive periodic discharges.

can also be caused by drugs, either by drug overdose or the purposeful use of drugs, such as barbiturates, to induce coma. The post-anoxic and pharmacologic versions of burst suppression are usually easily distinguished by history and laboratory testing. Pharmacologic burst-suppression patterns

have the potential for complete reversibility and are therefore in a separate prognostic group.

The purest form of burst-suppression is an unrelenting pattern that does not cycle to other patterns, is present on every page of the EEG, and is unaffected by outside stimuli. Lower

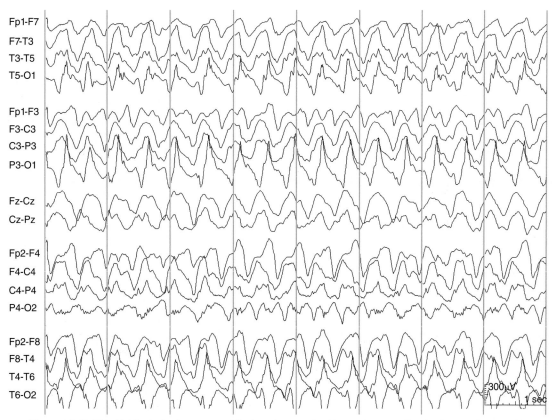

Figure 12.10 This highly rhythmic pattern with sharp features in this comatose patient is also consistent with nonconvulsive status epilepticus.

voltage bursts and longer and flatter interburst intervals correlate with increasing severity. Transitional versions of burst suppression that change, or even pause, with outside stimuli (so-called *reactive burst suppression*) are probably associated with a better prognosis than the pure form of the pattern.

Voltage Depression

Low-voltage records in coma (tracings in which voltages persistently do not exceed 20 µV in any head region) are considered severely abnormal. The pattern suggests a degree of injury so severe that the cerebrum cannot generate significant voltages. Voltage depression may be seen after continued deterioration of a burst-suppression pattern in which the bursts have disappeared leaving only the periods of suppression. It may also be seen near the end of a sequence of progressive voltage decline in a slow-wave pattern as described earlier. In addition to a *low-voltage* pattern being defined as showing most or all voltages below 20 µV, the newer American Clinical Neurophysiology (ACNS) 2021 terminology has introduced the term *suppressed* for a record with all voltages <10 µV (further described below).

Certain pitfalls in the diagnosis of voltage depression should be avoided (Figures 12.13 and 12.14). The term implies a persisting pattern, but some patients have a period of voltage depression after a seizure though this period should be short-lived. Voltage depression also may occur transiently after anoxia. Therefore, very short tracings are inadequate to establish a diagnosis of voltage depression. Standard instrument settings may hide some features of a low-voltage EEG and may even suggest electrocerebral inactivity unless appropriate adjustments to amplifier gains are made. Finally, a small percentage of normal adults may have a very low-voltage EEG pattern during wakefulness; the foregoing discussion of low-voltage patterns only applies to recordings obtained from patients in coma.

General Ranking of EEG Patterns from Alertness to Deepening Coma

Normal Background
Appearance of IRDA (intermittent rhythmic delta activity)
Loss of (faster) alpha and beta rhythms from the background, appearance of (slower) theta and delta rhythms
Pattern similar to Stage II sleep with presence of spindles, but without arousals
Predominant delta pattern with increasing voltage and diminishing frequency, sleep forms absent, loss of reactivity
Burst-suppression pattern, with progressively decreasing voltage of bursts and increasing duration of interburst intervals
Reduction and eventual suppression of all EEG voltages
"Flat" tracing

This table provides a general ranking of EEG patterns seen with increasing depth of coma. Few, if any, individual patients will pass through all of these patterns.

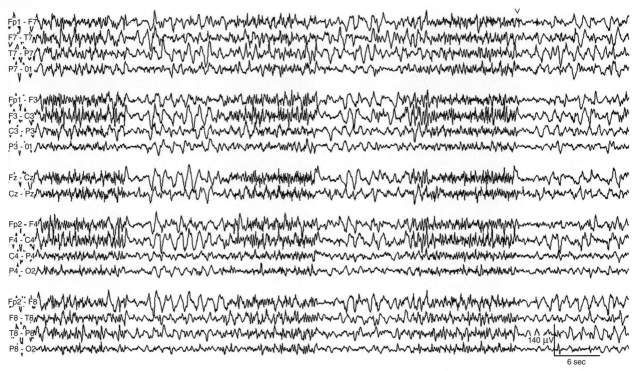

Figure 12.11 Cyclic Alternating Pattern of Encephalopathy (CAPE) is a very rare pattern believed to consist of alternating sleep states. Note that this page of EEG is highly compressed at 5 mm/sec in order to show multiple cycles of the alternating pattern (also note 6-second calibration bar). In this particular example, 6 Hz theta activity alternates with 1-Hz delta activity.

ACNS 2021 CRITICAL CARE EEG TERMINOLOGY

In an attempt to create a common vocabulary for classifying EEG patterns recorded in critical care settings (intensive care units or ICUs) "to aid in future research involving such patterns," the ACNS has published guidelines to standardize terminology, with the first set published in 2005, followed by 2012 guidelines, and most recently a 2021 version: *American Clinical Neurophysiology Society's Standardized Critical Care EEG Terminology: 2021 Version*. The current guidelines have the advantage of having undergone several iterations with comments solicited from the larger community of electroencephalographers. Interrater reliability was also assessed for several of the categories.

Exactly how this ACNS Terminology should be used for everyday EEG interpretation does not have a straightforward answer given the complexity of the system you will see summarized below. In proposing the terminology, the authors of the system did not propose that all ICU EEGs be scored by the system in clinical practice. The core publication describing the proposed terminology and definitions reviewed here is not short, running to 29 pages. The main publication is supplemented by a useful appendix consisting of 35 pages of sample illustrations of the different patterns defined in the ACNS Terminology. Recognizing that the primary publications are lengthy, condensed versions have also

been published. Just based on the length of the publication you may already have a sense that this terminology system is fairly complicated. Although this proposed terminology system boasts considerable precision, this precision comes at the price of considerable complexity, as the specifics of some of the definitions can be quite cumbersome to work through, much less to commit to memory. The varied opinions EEG readers may have of this terminology may depend on the purpose individual users might have for using the new system. When conducting research on a particular EEG pattern, excellent reliability is required in defining whether a specific EEG is or is not showing an example of the particular pattern being studied. If you are conducting a study on the meaning of a certain pattern and would like to compare your results to a study done at another center on the same pattern, if both research groups have used the same terminology system and definitions, then the studies can be compared with a good amount of confidence that they are likely discussing the same EEG phenomenon. Of course, most EEG interpretation is not done in the context of research studies, but to provide clinical care for patients. The question then comes up as to how much of this classification system should be used for reporting of EEGs in the context of clinical practice, which is the main focus of this text.

The pitfalls of implementing precise definitions are not always obvious. An example to consider is how defining even the simplest terms, such as *abundant, frequent,*

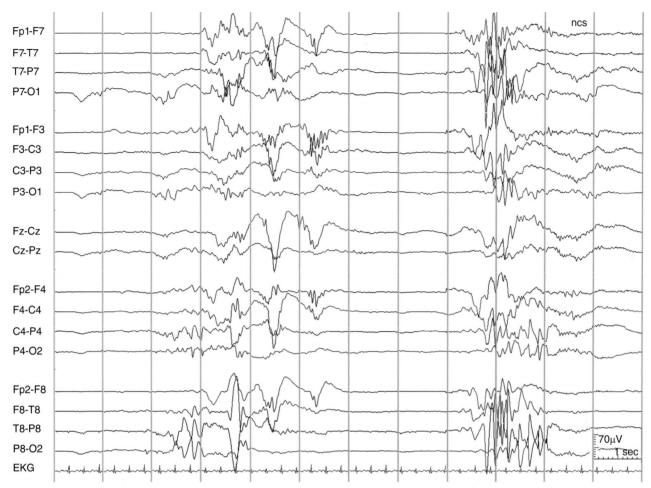

Figure 12.12 A burst-suppression pattern is seen with high-voltage polymorphic bursts separated by periods of suppression. NCS = no clinical signs.

occasional, and *rare* (e.g., in terms of prevalence of a spike discharge) might not be a good thing. After all, you may have read a report describing "rare spike-wave discharges" and wondered exactly how many were actually seen. The 2021 definitions of these terms for sporadic epileptiform discharges (*abundant*: ≥1 per 10 seconds, *frequent*: ≥1 per minute but less than 1 per 10 seconds, *occasional*: ≥1 per hour but less than 1 per minute, *rare*: <1 per hour) do seem to answer the question, especially if you have some confidence that the writer of the report you just read uses the 2021 system stringently. If you like the idea of using these precise new definitions, you have the option of either memorizing their quantitative definitions or keeping a listing of the definitions handy at all times when writing reports. This may take some effort, but you may be invested enough to do it. There is another side of the coin to this problem, though. When your report is received by the ordering provider, will they have the same definition list memorized or near at hand?—probably not! If not, to some extent much of your effort in using the strict definition of terms has gone to waste if the receiver of the report, who after all may be considered the "final customer" for your careful work, cannot understand it without going to a reference. Perhaps it would be simpler to write "approximately one spike-wave

discharge was seen per minute" or "two spike-wave discharges were seen in this recording" if you feel would like to reliably communicate the frequency of a finding to your reader. The simplicity of this approach is that neither you nor the ordering provider needs to seek out a terminology table to understand what you have to say. Ironically, in this example, converting the message from "two spikes were seen" to "rare spikes were seen" actually blurs the precision of the report, even though the word "rare" does have a precise definition in the guidelines. And for those of you who may feel brave enough to memorize the meanings of these terms, care should be taken that when used in different contexts, the same words may have different meanings in the ACNS Terminology. For instance, the same voltage descriptors (e.g., "high," "low") are defined differently when describing amplitude of background patterns as opposed to periodic or rhythmic patterns.

Therefore, each laboratory needs to decide what portion of this terminology system to adopt for the purpose of routine reporting of tracings recorded in its ICUs, balancing the time and effort required to codify each finding according to this system with the potential benefit such detail may or may not translate into in terms of clinical decision-making for the patient. In fact, few electroencephalographers will be able to

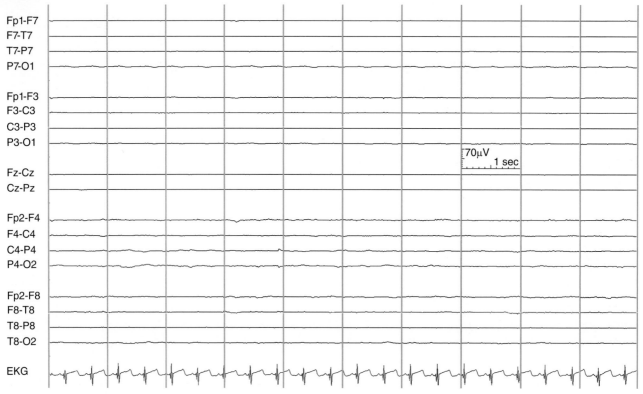

Figure 12.13 This EEG of a comatose patient is displayed at a sensitivity of 7 µV/mm and appears flat. Especially when electrocerebral inactivity is suspected, sensitivities of 2 µV/mm should be used (see Figure 12.13).

memorize all the parameters and specific coding definitions set forth in this new system, implying that full use of the terminology system would, indeed, require that a version of the system always be at hand. Most laboratories will likely adopt many of the terms from this new classification, but not necessarily decide to code every ICU EEG according to all the parameters set forth.

A summary of the 2021 ACNS Terminology is presented below in order to give the reader an idea of how it works. This description is included here recognizing that, while many laboratories will not wish to routinely use the complete system to code ICU EEGs, many of the terms introduced have already come into common use in the EEG community and, at a minimum, it will be useful to be familiar with them. A few of the more lengthy definitions have been simplified—the idea is to present here the essence of the definitions without some of the more complicated modifications set forth in the original report in favor of readability. Therefore, this summary is not all-inclusive but is designed to give the reader an idea of the general construct of the ACNS Terminology system. Those interested in additional detail are referred to the original publications, which are referenced at the end of this chapter.

GENERAL STRUCTURE OF THE ACNS 2021 TERMINOLOGY SYSTEM

The 2021 terminology publication includes six sections regarding the core description of the findings that might be found

and described in any ICU EEG, though almost all reports will require the use of fewer sections since not all of the patterns each of the sections deals with will likely be present in any given EEG recording. The six main sections include (A) background, (B) sporadic epileptiform discharges (C) rhythmic and periodic patterns (RPPs), (D) electrographic and electroclinical seizures, (E) brief potentially ictal rhythmic discharges (BIRDS), and (F) ictal-interictal continuum (IIC). The proposal publication also includes a G-section that gives recommendations for how often the EEG findings should be reported to the clinical team, and an H-section that is an optional section that suggests a standard way to quantify the burden (amount) of certain abnormal findings that may be present in the record.

Because some of the sections of the terminology system are actually subsets of larger categories, the general scheme of the system may be better understood by reviewing Figure 12.15. Looking at the top boxes of the figure, all reports would include a description of the background (the schema for description of the background is described below) followed by a list of any possible abnormalities that may be superimposed on that background. There are four main groupings of these abnormalities including (1) epileptiform discharges (this group includes two subgroups according to whether the discharges occur sporadically or rhythmically, which is then further broken down into more subgroups), (2) electrographic or electroclinical seizures (subdivided into briefer seizures versus the status epilepticus versions of these seizure types), (3) BIRDS, and (4) IIC. Each group and subgroup of these findings are described in more detail below.

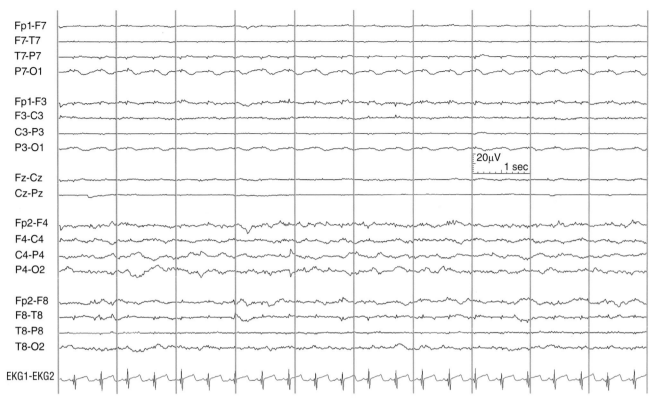

Figure 12.14 When the same page of EEG as was shown in Figure 12.12 is displayed at a sensitivity of 2 μV/mm, a small amount of definite electrocerebral activity is seen over the right hemisphere (bottom eight EEG channels). No electrocerebral activity is seen over the left hemisphere and midline, however. Pulsation artifact is seen in the channels that include O1.

BACKGROUND

Because all EEG tracings have a background, a background description should be given for all studies. This is in distinction to all of the following possible sections that describe findings (e.g., epileptiform patterns, etc.) that may or may not be present in any particular EEG recording and therefore may or may not require description. The 10 possible parameters to describe the background include symmetry, frequency, posterior dominant rhythm, continuity, reactivity, state changes, presence or absence of a cyclic alternating pattern of encephalopathy (CAPE), voltage, anterior-posterior gradient, and breach effect are expanded on below.

Symmetry: background asymmetries may be present in terms of *amplitude*, *frequency*, or both. **Frequency:** the background frequency is reported for the most aroused state (which usually results in reporting the highest background frequency). If present, the **posterior dominant rhythm** and its frequency are reported. The degree of background **continuity** is described as *continuous*, *nearly continuous*, or *discontinuous* (discontinuous if as much as 10 to 49% of the record consists of suppression). If over 50% of the background consists of suppression, then it is scored as *burst-suppression*. The terms *burst-suppression* and *suppression-burst* are considered synonymous. The term *suppression* is used when the suppressed periods are ≤10 μV and *attenuation* if the periods of lower voltage are

greater than 10 μV but less than 50% of the higher background voltage (in which case, the term *burst-attenuation* is used). If more than 99% of the record is below 20 μV it is scored as *low voltage* and if below 10 μV as *suppression*. If suppressions or attenuations are induced by stimulation, an *SI* (stimulus-induced) modifier is used.

EEG **reactivity** is scored as *reactive*, *unreactive*, *unclear*, or *unknown* (i.e., not tested). Reactivity implies a change in EEG pattern, usually frequency or amplitude; the appearance of muscle or eyeblink artifact with stimulation does not constitute reactivity. One less common form of reactivity is the appearance of *stimulus-induced rhythmic, periodic, or ictal-appearing discharges (SIRPIDs)*. **State changes** refers to alternation between a more aroused and less aroused state, with each state required to last at least 60 seconds, occurring either spontaneously or with stimulation, and are scored as either *present* or *absent*. If present, they are further described as present with K-complexes and spindles, present but with abnormal K-complexes and spindles (abnormality is then described), or present but without K-complexes and spindles. **Cyclic Alternating Pattern of Encephalopathy (CAPE)** is a rare EEG pattern in which the EEG alternates between a more aroused state and a less aroused state, with each pattern lasting at least 10 seconds and at least six cycles of the pattern are seen. It may represent an instability of the brain's control system of sleep state. CAPE is scored as either *present, absent*, or *unknown/unclear* (See Figure 12.11).

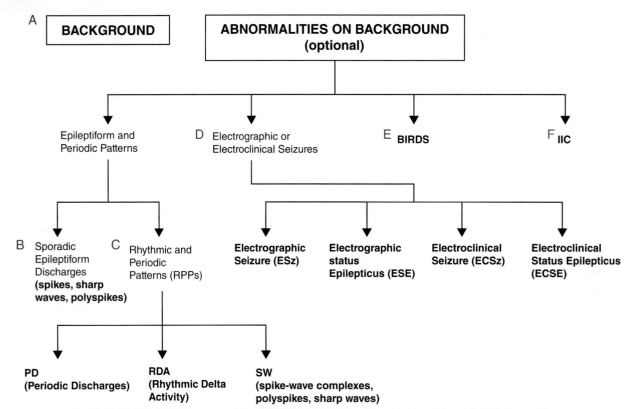

Figure 12.15 The overall structure of the ACNS Terminology consists of a description of the EEG background, which is described for all tracings, followed by a list of optional additional findings depending on whether or not they are present in the study. Each abnormality category is described further in the text. The red letter labels shown in the figure correspond to the sections A through F of the classification wherein the element is described.

Voltage of the background is measured from the peak to the trough of the background waves in a standard longitudinal bipolar montage. It is rated as *high*: ≥150 μV, *normal*, *low*: <20 μV, or *suppressed*: <10 μV. The **anterior-posterior (AP) gradient** (the presence of faster frequencies and lower voltages anteriorly and slower frequencies and higher voltages posteriorly) is scored as *present*, *absent*, or *reversed*. Finally, the *presence* or *absence* of a **breach effect** and its location (the preferential transmission of faster rhythms through the area of a skull defect, often related to a previous neurosurgical procedure and less often head trauma) is noted. Breach rhythms are discussed in more detail in Chapter 11, "Normal Variants in the Electroencephalogram."

ABNORMALITY LIST (OPTIONAL SECTIONS)

Now that the background pattern has been described, next comes what is essentially an abnormality list, the list of additional findings that might possibly be superimposed on the background described in the initial section. The first two major categories are for epileptiform and rhythmic patterns and for seizures. Two additional smaller categories are available to describe findings that do not easily fall into the ictal or interictal groups: brief potentially ictal rhythmic discharges or BIRDS (patterns that resemble electrographic seizures but are shorter than the definition allows for) and the ictal-interictal continuum or IIC (patterns that the electroencephalographer

cannot confidently classify as ictal or interictal). Each of these groups is described in more detail below.

Regarding epileptiform discharges (which, by definition, do not include seizures), this terminology system categorizes epileptiform abnormalities into two groups: those that occur in an unpredictable way against the background, like paint spattered on a canvas—*Sporadic Epileptiform Discharges*—and those that occur in a rhythmic or predictable pattern for some amount of time—*Rhythmic* and *Periodic* Patterns, or RPPs. There are three types of abnormalities that can be categorized as RPPs: periodic discharges (PD), rhythmic delta activity (RDA), and SW (spike-wave complexes, polyspikes, and sharp waves). Note that when any epileptiform discharge might occur sporadically, it would appear under the Sporadic Epileptiform Discharges group, but if it occurs rhythmically or periodically, it would be classified in the RPP group.

SPORADIC EPILEPTIFORM DISCHARGES

This section refers to the scoring of any **spikes**, **sharp waves**, or **polyspikes** that are not periodic or rhythmic, and therefore sporadic. The definition of these terms is standard and refers back to the 2017 glossary by Kane et al. and was also described in Chapter 3, "Commonly Used Terms in Electroencephalography." The standard distinction between a spike and sharp wave is used, with a spike defined as having a pointed apex and a base between 20 and 70 msec and a sharp wave with a base between 70 and 200 msec in duration. The prevalence of the discharges is scored as either *abundant*: ≥1 per 10 seconds, *frequent*: ≥1 per minute, *occasional*: ≥1 per hour, or *rare*: <1 per hour. In this terminology, sharply contoured slow waves are not considered epileptiform. Also, spike-wave complexes are not explicitly included here, but since these can occur sporadically, it would seem reasonable to include them in this group as well.

RHYTHMIC AND PERIODIC PATTERNS (RPPs)

This section describes any rhythmic or periodic pattern found in the tracing. These patterns have been split into three categories: **periodic discharges (PD), rhythmic delta activity (RDA), and spike-and-wave activity (SW)**. The SW group includes not just spike-and-wave activity, but also polyspike-and-wave or sharp-and-wave discharges as long as they occur in a rhythmic train. The key feature that distinguishes periodic discharges from rhythmic discharges is that each discharge in a series of periodic discharges is separated by some *intervening background activity* from the next periodic discharge, while rhythmic patterns such as RDA or SW in the context of this RPP section are not separated from each other by any intervening activity and occur in trains.

PD refers to any waveform of less than 0.5 seconds duration (or if longer than 0.5 seconds having no more than three phases) that repeats at nearly regular intervals and has relatively uniform morphology. Otherwise, discharges of >0.5 seconds and of more than three phases are defined as **bursts**. Note then that PD consists of repetitive, similar-appearing waveforms with some intervening background activity separating each example. The interval between individual PDs should be somewhat regular and not vary by more than 50%. To qualify as PD, the pattern must repeat for at least six cycles.

RDA refers to repetitive, similar-appearing waveforms occurring between 0.5 and 4 times per second with no intervening background activity between each waveform. Although the waveforms can be as simple as sinusoidal delta waves, they also may be more complex and include sharp features. To qualify as rhythmic, a pattern must repeat for at least six cycles.

SW refers to any runs of spike-, polyspikes-, or sharp-and-slow wave complexes that repeat regularly, also for at least six cycles. When the waveform of either PD or SW (but not RDA) shows a negative-positive-negative polarity, the modifier "with triphasic morphology" can be added.

Main Term 1 and Main Term 2

These three possible categories of rhythmic and periodic patterns, PD, RDA, and SW, are described using Main Term 1 and Main Term 2. The PD, RDA, and SW are considered *Main Term 2* in the classification and is preceded by a modifier, which is Main Term 1. *Main Term 1* specifies the distribution of the Main Term 2 pattern and is described below and serves as a prefix to Main Term 2. As an example, since the Main Term 1 modifier for generalized is "G," an example of RDA that occurs in a generalized distribution would be termed GRDA. There are five possible choices for Main Term 1: **G, L, BI, UI**, or **Mf**, as described below.

Generalized (G). At first glance, the term *generalized* would seem to describe a waveform that appears over all brain areas at once. In this terminology, however, the "G" term for generalized is actually used more broadly. It is used for any waveform that is bilaterally synchronous and symmetric. Thus, although the "G" term would still be used to describe waveforms that are commonly considered generalized (i.e., at least to some extent seen over all brain areas at once), this definition allows discharges that might occur quite focally but synchronously and symmetrically to be scored as generalized. For instance, purely bifrontal or purely bioccipital discharges whose field does not encompass all brain areas would still be termed generalized according to this terminology. G patterns may be further localized by the terms *frontally predominant, occipitally predominant, midline predominant*, or *generalized, not otherwise specified*.

Lateralized (L). This term is used for any waveform that is unilateral, be it focal, regional, or hemispheric in distribution. (This contrasts with the previous common use of the term *lateralized* that referred specifically to broader hemispheric patterns—see the description of periodic lateralized epileptiform discharges, or PLEDs, in Chapter 9, "The Abnormal EEG.") It may also be used for waveforms that have some bilaterality, as long as they are of consistently higher amplitude over one hemisphere or if the waveform shows a consistent lead-in on one side (i.e., its onset consistently precedes its pair in the opposite hemisphere). To further specify which of these circumstances is present, the additional modifiers unilateral, bilateral asymmetric, or bilateral asynchronous can be used.

Bilateral Independent (BI). This term refers to waveforms that occur independently (asynchronously) but simultaneously in opposite hemispheres.

Unilateral Independent (UI). This term is used to describe two or more discharges occurring in the *same* hemisphere during the same period but independently.

Multifocal (Mf). The Mf modifier is used for discharges that occur in three or more locations, with at least one in each hemisphere.

Main Term 1 and Main Term 2 to Describe all PD, RDA, and SW			
Main Term 1		**Main Term 2**	
G	Generalized	PD	Periodic Discharges
L	Lateralized	RDA	Rhythmic Delta Activity
BI	Bilateral Independent	SW	spikes, polyspikes, and sharp waves
UI	Unilateral Independent		
Mf	Multifocal (≥ 3 loci in 2 hemispheres)		

Main Modifiers

The quantitative definitions of the English-language main-modifier words are included here. The ACNS Terminology authors point out that, even though these terms are meant to refer specifically to the waveforms described in this version of the terminology, they could conceivably be used for all EEG waveforms.

Quantitative Definitions of Descriptors		
Prevalence (percent of record containing the pattern)	**Duration** (typical duration of pattern)	**Voltage** (of PD, SW, or RDA—not for use to describe background voltage, which has different definitions for its descriptors)
Continuous: ≥90%	Very long: ≥1 hour	Very Low: <20 μV
Abundant: 50% to 89%	Long: 10 to 59 minutes	Low: 20 to 4 μV
Frequent: 10% to 49%	Intermediate: 1 to 9.9 minutes	Medium: 50 to 149 μV
Occasional: 1% to 9%	Brief: 10 to 59 seconds	High: ≥150 μV
Rare: <1%	Very brief: <10 seconds	

Evolution. A waveform can evolve in terms of voltage, location, and/or morphology. Strict guidelines are set out in the original guidelines as to what type of changes do and do not qualify as evolution in each of these parameters. Patterns can be defined as evolving, fluctuating, or static.

The Plus (+) modifier may be added only to PDs and RDA but not SW. A "+" modifier means that a pattern looks more ictal than usual. All "+" cases must be further categorized as +F (superimposed fast activity—for PDs and RDA only, and only when those patterns are present and the fast activity is not part of the background), +R (superimposed rhythmic delta—for PD only), or +S (associated with sharp or spike-like activity—not for SW patterns). Combinations such as +FR or +FS are possible.

A surprisingly large part of the terminology is devoted to the classification of a relatively rare but interesting finding, **Extreme Delta Brushes** (EDB). These consist of fast activity superimposed directly on either PDs or RDA in a time-locked pattern (i.e., not a case where the fast activity involves all of the background, but rather it is only seen superimposed on the PD or RDA waveform), and would therefore be coded as either PDs +F or RDA +F. In this case the finding is termed either definite EDB or possible EDB. EDBs have a strong association with an autoimmune disorder, anti-NMDA receptor encephalitis, but have also been described in febrile infection-related epilepsy syndrome (FIRES), an explosive presentation of refractory seizures after fever, mostly described in children. The clinical setting of EDB is also discussed in Chapter 10, "The EEG in Epilepsy."

ELECTROGRAPHIC AND ELECTROCLINICAL SEIZURES

How to define what constitutes an electrographic seizure has been a longstanding challenge in EEG. Because, essentially by definition, the term *electrographic* implies that there is no clinical change caused by the discharge, the assessment must be made solely on the appearance and features of the waveform. In the ACNS Terminology, the definition of electrographic seizures is largely based on the Salzburg criteria for the diagnosis of *nonconvulsive status epilepticus*. Note that this is somewhat different from creating a definition for diagnosing single electrographic seizures, so this extension of the Salzburg criteria to the ACNS Terminology definition has a slightly different goal. For all of its possible imperfections, the Salzburg-based criteria have the advantage of simplicity. The ACNS Terminology defines **Electrographic Seizures** (ESz) as consisting of the following:

(1) "Epileptiform" discharges averaging over 2.5 Hz for ≥10 seconds (e.g., more than 25 discharges in a 10-second period). OR
(2) Any pattern with definite evolution and lasting ≥10 seconds.

This differs slightly from the original Salzburg criteria that allowed for discharges qualifying under part two of this definition if they showed evolution (as stated above), but also if they didn't necessarily show evolution but responded to antiseizure medications or if they were associated with subtle clinical signs. (Note here that an electrographic seizure would not have any clinical signs by definition, but since the Salzburg criteria dealt with *non-convulsive* SE, subtle signs were possible. Also, because the Salzburg criteria were defined with an SE state in mind rather than for single seizures, it would be more likely that there would be an opportunity to observe a response to antiseizure medication treatment.)

The choice of a "10-second rule" understandably created quite a lot of discussion and the authors admit that the cutoff used for these criteria was completely arbitrary. Indeed, it is easy to imagine scenarios that would appear to make any specific cutoff for duration internally contradictory. For instance, imagine a patient who has 50 examples of 11- to 12-second electrographic seizures that conform to the definition. The patient also has a few examples of a nearly identical discharge but these are only 9 seconds long. Stepping back, it would seem quite likely that, from the brain's point of view, whatever the 12-second discharge is, the 9-second discharge is just a slightly shorter version of the same phenomenon and that the 10-second boundary for the definition is artificial. Or consider a patient on a pharmacologic paralytic agent with 8-second discharges that look highly suspicious for electrographic seizures but do not fit the definition because of duration. After stating in your report that they are not electrographic seizures because of their inadequate duration, a colleague points out to you that the previous day, before having received paralytic agents, that patient had the same 8-second discharges and each was associated with tonic stiffening. If they were clearly seizures yesterday, why are they not seizures today?

Therefore, we must admit to ourselves that creating a perfect definition for electrographic seizures is currently impossible and we will have to live with the imperfections that would be associated with any definition. The important aspect of this realization is to keep the arbitrariness of this definition in mind and not be overly rigid about using the definition for clinical decision-making. To create a dramatic example of being too rigid about the definition, you would not want to be a neurologist who would aggressively treat a patient with numerous 11-second electrographic "seizure" discharges with antiseizure medications, but provide no additional therapy for the same patient if the discharges were only 9 seconds long, declaring that you knew they were not seizures based on the ACNS Terminology and, therefore, they did not require treatment!

The word *epileptiform* was placed in quotation marks in the above definition to call attention to the fact that its meaning in this definition is slightly at odds with the official definition given elsewhere in the terminology. The general definition of "epileptiform" in the ACNS Terminology specifically excludes any wave (even with a sharp component, such as a sharply contoured slow wave) that lasts longer than 200 msec. For the purposes of this electrographic seizure definition, such waves may be considered epileptiform. This makes sense since a discharge firing at 2.5 Hz that would qualify under this definition could have a duration of 400 msec. Therefore, the definition allows for any repetitive discharge with a sharp component firing at $\geq$2.5 Hz and lasting $\geq$10 seconds, or any pattern (with or without sharp features) with definite evolution that lasts $\geq$10 seconds.

Electrographic Status Epilepticus (ESE) is defined as an electrographic seizure lasting for $\geq$10 continuous minutes or for a total duration of $\geq$20% of any 60-minute period of recording.

Electroclinical Seizures (ECSz) are defined as any EEG pattern that is time-locked to a clinical manifestation or any pattern that shows both EEG and clinical improvement with antiseizure medications. (There is no minimum duration in the definition, which is sensible as certain well-known electroclinical seizures, such as epileptic myoclonus, may last even less than 1 second.)

The definition of **Electroclinical Status Epilepticus (ECSE)** is similar to the definition of ESE as regards time limits: $\geq$10 continuous minutes or for a total duration of $\geq$20% of any 60-minute period of recording. An exception to the 10-minute rule is made for a seizure with bilateral convulsive activity, which only needs to last $\geq$5 minutes to qualify as ECSE.

BRIEF POTENTIALLY ICTAL RHYTHMIC DISCHARGES (BIRDS)

The BIRDS definition is designed to capture some, but not all of the phenomena of discharges that look like possible electrographic seizure discharges but that last less than 10 seconds and therefore do not qualify as electrographic seizures according to the ESz definition above.

BIRDS are defined as:
Generalized or focal activity >4 Hz that lasts between 0.5 and 10 seconds (six full cycles required), but is
- not consistent with a known normal pattern or benign variant (to exclude spindles, mu-rhythms, etc.)
- not part of a burst-suppression or burst-attenuation pattern
- and does not have a clinical correlate

but has at least one of the following:
- (a) Evolution ("evolving BIRDS")
- (b) Similar morphology and location as epileptiform or seizure discharges seen in same patient
- Sharply contoured but without "a" or "b"

Once again, and similar to the issues with the definition of electrographic seizures discussed above, the 10-second limitation in the BIRDS definition must be acknowledged as arbitrary. It may or may not be appropriate to think of Ms. A., a patient with short electrographic seizures, and Ms. B., a patient with similar, but shorter discharges that qualify as BIRDS, as being in very different clinical categories.

ICTAL-INTERICTAL CONTINUUM (IIC)

The choice of the term *IIC* is considered unfortunate by many. First, the very use of the term implies that there is a continuum between interictal epileptiform activity and seizure activity. If you have spent years as an electroencephalographer working at distinguishing seizure from non-seizure activity, learning that there is a continuum (rather than a border) between the two may come as a shock, since the existence of a "continuum" implies that there is no such border at all. Electroencephalographers have for years recognized that patients may have spikes in the EEG that are interictal and that don't require administration of emergency antiseizure medication, but at other times may have very similar-appearing spikes in more rapidly evolving trains, often accompanied by clinical signs, which require prompt treatment (seizures). Implicit in these examples is the idea that 30 spikes that occur singly are qualitatively different from 30 spikes that occur in a seizure train, including the ability to generate a convulsion and perhaps even the risk for brain injury. In other sections, the ACNS Terminology itself takes great pains in defining a sharp boundary between electrographic seizures, electrographic status epilepticus, and interictal epileptiform discharges. The very terms *ictal* and *interictal* imply this separation. The authors of the ACNS Terminology also thought along these same lines and explicitly stated that the IIC as a concept does not represent a new or separate diagnosis on page 25 of the publication, though this disclaimer has been missed or misunderstood by many. The problem is that the words that make up the term *ictal-interictal continuum* may seem to imply a different meaning—that there is a continuum and that a patient may be shifting about on that continuum, implying the existence of a type of blurred state between seizure and interictal discharges. Whether or not such a blurred state actually exists, a neurophysiological question that has certainly not yet been worked out and is at odds with both traditional practice in EEG interpretation and seizure treatment in the ICU, the authors of the new terminology did not, indeed, appear to be trying to define a new entity. The ACNS Terminology makes clear that the IIC term is synonymous with "possible ESz" or "possible electrographic SE." Perhaps a more accurate term would be "I don't know if what I am looking at is a seizure or not," which would generate an unwieldy acronym, but be more explanatory of what the term means. Similar to its use in other areas of the ACNS Terminology, perhaps modifiers such as "unclear" or "uncertain" would have been more fortunate choices. There certainly are EEG patterns that defy easy classification as seizure discharges as opposed to interictal activity. When there is worry that such a pattern could indeed represent seizure discharges or be causing ongoing brain injury, a trial of antiseizure medications may be warranted.

The ACNS Terminology describes specific types of discharges that can qualify to be considered as being on the IIC. While according to the definition, an electrographic seizure should have a PD or SW pattern that fires more than 25 times over 10 seconds, a similar discharge that fires between 10 and <25 times over 10 seconds can be scored as being on the IIC. A similar discharge that fires from 5 to 10 times on average over 10 seconds but has a plus modifier (implying "looks more ictal") or which shows fluctuation can also be scored as being on the IIC. Finally, any lateralized rhythmic delta activity (e.g., LRDA, BIRDA, UIRDA, and MfRDA, but not GRDA) that fires >1 Hz and lasts >10 seconds and merits a plus modifier or shows fluctuation can be scored as IIC. Perhaps the term *IIC* should best be thought of as meaning "It Isn't Clear."

So what to make of this classification? Many of the definitions are exacting. Consider that one of the strictest and most longstanding definitions in electroencephalography is that a spike is less than 70 msec in duration and a sharp wave is of more than 70 msec duration. At the same time, it is also recognized that there is no clinical situation in which clarifying that a discharge is a spike versus a sharp wave changes the diagnosis. (Another way of putting it is that there is no practical situation where one might say, "If it's a spike then it's Disease 'A,' but if it's a sharp wave then it's Disease 'B.'") This suggests that the apparent precision of all these definitions really should be taken with a grain of salt and certain of the strict distinctions made by our classifications may not have *clinical* importance. On the other hand, this terminology system was created by a group of very knowledgeable individuals with a vast collective knowledge of EEG with the goal of creating a useful research tool, and there is a lot to be learned from their insights in how they created this classification system. The ACNS has published a reference chart to help understand the definitions without referring to the main publication (Figure 12.16).

EEG RECORDING IN SUSPECTED CEREBRAL DEATH

The role of the EEG in the patient with suspected brain death is not straightforward. The original definition of death as the cessation of all vital signs became impractical with the advent of modern intensive care and mechanical ventilation. In response, an ad hoc committee was convened at Harvard Medical School in 1968 to establish a definition of irreversible coma or brain death that could replace the older definitions that were based on breathing and presence of a heartbeat when necessary in intensive care settings when mechanical ventilation would be in use. The guidelines attempted to identify individuals with "no discernible central nervous system activity" (see "A definition of irreversible coma," 1968, cited below). The guidelines were designed to create a new legal definition of death such that when the criteria set forth for the diagnosis of brain death are met, the patient can be legally declared dead and removed from the ventilator. The specific guidelines for determination of brain death vary among countries, jurisdictions, and even among individual hospitals. Almost all official criteria require a complete lack of responsiveness, lack of CNS-driven patient movement, lack of respiratory effort when the patient is taken off the ventilator during a proscribed trial period, and absent brainstem function, with all assessments made according to strict guidelines.

The role of EEG in diagnosing brain death varies by location; an EEG showing electrocerebral inactivity (ECI) is usually *not* required to make the determination of brain death, though the test can serve as an adjunct to the diagnosis when necessary. Patients with true ECI recordings, especially when two such recordings are obtained 24 hours or more apart, rarely experience neurologic recovery. An ECI recording considered alone (i.e., apart from the context of the patient's history and the brain death neurologic examination) should not be considered synonymous with brain death. To make matters more complicated, a small fraction of patients who fulfill legal criteria for brain death may still have some deflections on the EEG of cerebral origin (a phenomenon more frequently seen in children than in adults) when the test is obtained.

EEG recordings performed in the setting of suspected cerebral death are almost always carried out in ICUs. The large amount of electrical equipment in most ICUs can make this setting an electrically hostile environment and increases the challenge of obtaining clean EEG recordings at the high amplifier gains necessary for determination of ECI (Figure 12.17). Nevertheless, with careful technique, satisfactory EEG tracings for this purpose are obtainable. As can be seen from the figure, describing the EEG as "flat" or "isoelectric" often is not technically accurate as EEGs that demonstrate true ECI often have deflections caused by a variety of artifacts (e.g., pulse, EKG, respiratory/ventilator, etc.) due to the high amplifier gains required for these recordings.

Because of the gravity of the question at hand, an EEG performed with the goal of establishing a complete lack of brain wave activity or ECI should meet certain minimal technical standards. The most recent guidelines from the American Clinical Neurophysiology Society were published in 2016 ("Guideline 6," 2016) and are summarized in the following list.

Electrocerebral inactivity is defined as the **absence** of nonartifactual electrical activity over 2 µV measured from peak to peak when the following appropriate recording techniques are used:

ACNS Standardized Critical Care EEG Terminology 2021:
Reference Chart

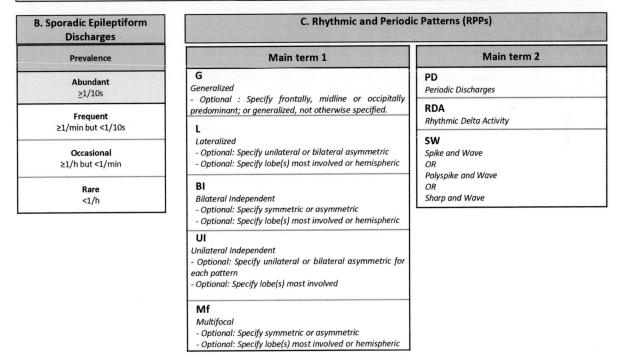

				A. EEG Background						
Symmetry	Background EEG frequency	PDR	Continuity	Reactivity	State Changes	Cyclic Alternating Pattern of Encephalopathy (CAPE)	Voltage	AP Gradient	Breach effect
Symmetric	Delta	Present Specify frequency	**Continuous:** <1% periods of suppression (<10 μV) or attenuation (≥10μV but <50% of background voltage)	Present	Present with normal stage N2 sleep transients	Present	Normal ≥20 μV	Present	Present
Mild asymmetry <50% Amp. 0.5-1/s Freq.	Theta	Absent	**Nearly continuous:** 1-9% periods of suppression attenuation	SIRPIDs only	Present but with abnormal stage N2 sleep transients	Absent	Low 10 to <20 μV	Absent	Absent
Marked asymmetry ≥50% Amp. >1/s Freq.	≥Alpha			Absent	Present but without stage N2 sleep transients	Unknown/unclear	Suppressed <10 μV	Reverse	Unclear
			Discontinuous: 10-49% periods of suppression or attenuation	Unclear	Absent				

Highly Epileptiform Bursts (Present or Absent)

If Burst-suppression or Burst-attenuation then specify if:

Identical Bursts (Present or Absent) ←

Burst-suppression or **Burst-attenuation:** 50-99% periods of suppression or attenuation

Suppression: >99% periods of suppression or attenuation

Epileptiform Findings (including Rhythmic and Periodic Patterns)

B. Sporadic Epileptiform Discharges

Prevalence
Abundant ≥1/10s
Frequent ≥1/min but <1/10s
Occasional ≥1/h but <1/min
Rare <1/h

C. Rhythmic and Periodic Patterns (RPPs)

Main term 1	Main term 2
G *Generalized* - Optional : Specify frontally, midline or occipitally predominant; or generalized, not otherwise specified.	**PD** *Periodic Discharges*
L *Lateralized* - Optional: Specify unilateral or bilateral asymmetric - Optional: Specify lobe(s) most involved or hemispheric	**RDA** *Rhythmic Delta Activity*
BI *Bilateral Independent* - Optional: Specify symmetric or asymmetric - Optional: Specify lobe(s) most involved or hemispheric	**SW** *Spike and Wave* *OR* *Polyspike and Wave* *OR* *Sharp and Wave*
UI *Unilateral Independent* - Optional: Specify unilateral or bilateral asymmetric for each pattern - Optional: Specify lobe(s) most involved	
Mf *Multifocal* - Optional: Specify symmetric or asymmetric - Optional: Specify lobe(s) most involved or hemispheric	

Figure 12.16 This reference chart is published alongside the main ACNS 2021 Terminology Publication.

Major modifiers

Prevalence	Duration	Frequency	Phases[1]	Sharpness[2]	Absolute Amplitude	Relative Amplitude[3]	Stimulus Induced or Stimulus Terminated	Evolution[4]
Continuous ≥90%	Very long ≥1 h	4/s	>3	Spiky <70 ms	High ≥150 µV	>2	SI *Stimulus Induced*	Evolving
		3.5/s	3			≤2	ST *Stimulus Terminated*	Fluctuating
Abundant 50-89%	Long 10-59 min	3/s		Sharp 70-200 ms	Medium 50-149 µV			
		2.5/s	2					Static
		2/s	1	Sharply contoured >200 ms	Low 20-49 µV		Spontaneous only	
Frequent 10-49%	Intermediate duration 1-9.9 min	1.5/s						
Occasional 1-9%	Brief 10-59 s	1/s			Very low <20 µV		Unknown	
		0.5/s		Blunt >200 ms				
Rare <1%	Very brief <10 s	<0.5/s						

Minor modifiers

Onset	Triphasic[5]	Lag	Polarity[2]
Sudden ≤3 s	Yes	A-P *Anterior-Posterior*	Negative
Gradual >3 s	No	P-A *Posterior-Anterior*	Positive
			Dipole
		No	Unclear

Plus (+) Modifiers

No +
+F *Superimposed fast activity – applies to PD or RDA only* **EDB** (*Extreme Delta Brush*): A specific subtype of +F
+R *Superimposed rhythmic activity – applies to PD only*
+S *Superimposed sharp waves or spikes, or sharply contoured - applies to RDA only*
+FR *If both subtypes apply – applies to PD only*
+FS *If both subtypes apply – applies to RDA only*

NOTE 1: Phases: Applies to PD and SW only, including the slow wave of the SW complex
NOTE 2: Sharpness and Polarity: Applies to the predominant phase of PD and the spike or sharp component of SW only
NOTE 3: Relative amplitude: Applies to PD only
NOTE 4: Evolution: Refers to frequency, location or morphology
NOTE 5: Triphasic: Applies to PD or SW only

D. Electrographic and Electroclinical Seizures

Electrographic Seizure (ESz)

Either:
A) Epileptiform discharges averaging >2.5 Hz for ≥10 s (>25 discharges in 10 s), OR
B) Any pattern with definite evolution and lasting ≥10 s

Electroclinical Seizure (ECSz)

Any EEG pattern with either
A) Definite clinical correlate time-locked to the pattern (of any duration), OR
B) EEG *and* clinical improvement with a parenteral anti-seizure medication

Electrographic Status Epilepticus (ESE)

An electrographic seizure for either
A) ≥10 continuous minutes, OR
B) A total duration of ≥20% of any 60-minute period of recording.

Electroclinical Status Epilepticus (ECSE)

An electroclinical seizure for either
A) ≥10 continuous minutes, OR
B) A total duration of ≥20% of any 60-minute period of recording, OR
C) ≥5 continuous minutes if the seizure is convulsive (i.e., with bilateral tonic-clonic motor activity).
Possible ECSE: An RPP that qualifies for the IIC (below) that is present for ≥10 continuous minutes or for a total duration of ≥20% of any 60-minute period of recording, which shows EEG improvement with a parenteral anti-seizure medication **BUT** without clinical improvement.

E. Brief Potentially Ictal Rhythmic Discharges (BIRDs)

Focal (including L, BI, UI or Mf) or generalized rhythmic activity >4 Hz (at least 6 waves at a regular rate) lasting ≥0.5 to <10 s, not consistent with a known normal pattern or benign variant, not part of burst-suppression or burst-attenuation, without definite clinical correlate, and that has at least one of A, B or C below:

Definite BIRDs feature either:
A. Evolution ("evolving BIRDs") OR
B. Similar morphology and location as interictal epileptiform discharges or seizures in the same patient

Possible BIRDs are
C. Sharply contoured but without (a) or (b) above

F. Ictal-Interictal Continuum (IIC)

1. Any PD or SW pattern that averages >1.0 Hz but ≤2.5 Hz over 10 s (>10 but ≤ 25 discharges in 10 s); OR
2. Any PD or SW pattern that averages ≥0.5 Hz and ≤1 Hz over 10 s (≥5 and ≤10 discharges in 10 s), and has a plus modifier or fluctuation; OR
3. Any lateralized RDA averaging >1 Hz for at least 10 s (at least 10 waves in 10 s) with a plus modifier or fluctuation;
AND
4. Does not qualify as an ESz or ESE.

Figure 12.16 Cont'd

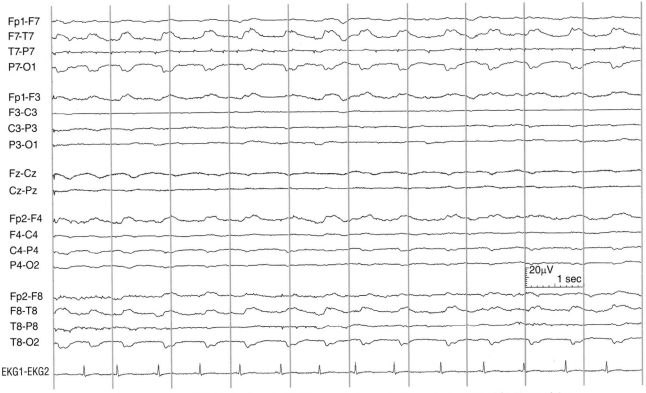

Figure 12.17 This page of EEG is displayed at 2 μV/mm and shows electrocerebral activity (ECI). None of the waves seen are of cerebral origin. Tracings displayed at the amplifier gains necessary for determination of ECI are prone to large amounts of artifact. On this page, several channels show pulsation artifact. Note how the various pulsation artifact waveforms in this EEG follow the EKG's QRS complex, as expected. Beyond the use of high amplifier gains, several other procedural requirements must be met as described in the text before the EEG diagnosis of ECI can be formally made.

1. A **full set of electrodes** should be used, including the midline electrodes, Fz, Cz, and Pz, with the exception of areas that may be inaccessible because of recent surgery or trauma. All major brain areas should be covered.
2. Interelectrode impedances should be **between 100 ohms and 10,000 ohms**. Impedance testing should be done during the study.
3. The integrity of the recording system should be verified to confirm that the apparent low-voltage tracing was not caused by a disconnection in the recording apparatus. This is done by **tapping the individual electrodes** and confirming the presence of the tapping artifact on the recording.
4. A **double-distance montage** with some interelectrode distances greater than 10 cm should be used during at least some portion of the recording. Greater interelectrode distances increase the chance of detecting low-voltage activity. An extracephalic electrode placed on a limb (e.g., the right hand) can help identify artifacts. An electrocardiogram (EKG) channel should also be applied to help identify EKG artifact.
5. The record should be recorded at a sensitivity of **2 μV/mm for at least 30 minutes** to minimize the possibility of missing a 2 μV signal. Calibration testing should be done with calibration pulses of low voltage (e.g., 2 or 5 μV, to mimic the low-voltage signals being sought).
6. Appropriate filter settings should be used with a **bandpass of 1 to 30 Hz** or wider (low-frequency filter set at 1 Hz or below and high-frequency filter set at 30 Hz or above). The 60 Hz notch filter may be used, but a segment of the EEG should then be recorded without the notch filter for comparison.
7. **Additional monitoring techniques** should be used to distinguish artifact from brain wave activity at the high amplifier gains used. This may include an EKG and a respiratory channel, if necessary, to monitor ventilator artifact which can also be confirmed by video.
8. There should be **no EEG reactivity** to intense tactile, auditory, or visual stimuli.
9. The recording should only be made by a **qualified EEG technologist**.
10. If the diagnosis of ECI is **uncertain, the recording should be repeated**.
11. **Notation of medications and physiologic variables**, including temperature, blood pressure, and blood oxygen saturation, should be made.

REVIEW QUESTIONS

1. In general, regarding slow wave amplitude,
   a. increasing amplitudes reliably mark a worsening of coma.
   b. increasing amplitudes reliably mark an improvement of coma.
   c. decreasing frequency marks a worsening of coma.
   d. increasing frequency marks a worsening of coma.

2. Regarding the EEG in coma,
   a. a "flat" EEG usually portends impending death.
   b. the presence of sleep spindles is a generally positive prognostic sign.
   c. testing EEG reactivity in coma by sternal rub is not useful because, by definition, a person in coma cannot feel external stimuli.
   d. a poor EEG pattern after drug overdose is more predictive of a negative prognosis than a poor EEG pattern after cardiac arrest.

3. Which is true?
   a. Triphasic waves are considered diagnostic of hepatic encephalopathy.
   b. IRDA can mark the deepening of coma.
   c. Alpha coma after cardiac arrest is associated with a relatively poor prognosis.
   d. Alpha coma should suppress when the patient's eyes passively or actively open.

4. Regarding status epilepticus (SE),
   a. the cessation of body jerking is a reliable sign that seizure medications have been effective.
   b. SE is diagnosed after 30 minutes of continuous seizure activity.
   c. focal seizures are not considered a cause of SE.
   d. if an individual is treated for generalized convulsive SE, the patient's ability to resume conversation can be considered a reliable sign that the SE has terminated.

5. In the case of a burst-suppression EEG,
   a. even in the absence of a known reversible cause, burst-suppression is generally associated with a favorable prognosis.
   b. it is expected that the bursts are of similar duration compared to the interbursts.
   c. in certain cases, doctors will purposely induce burst-suppression in order to treat seizures.
   d. medications that induce burst-suppression should be avoided as the bursts may damage nerve cells.

6. Which of these attributes is NOT true of both periodic patterns and rhythmic patterns?
   a. Both may have sharp forms.
   b. Both may fire under 2 Hz.
   c. Both may be of low voltage.
   d. Both may be separated by intervening background activity.

ANSWERS

1. ANSWER: **C.** Slow wave amplitude is not linearly associated with depth of coma because, as coma deepens, slow-wave amplitudes may increase, then decrease. Therefore, neither statement A or B is correct. A reduction in slow-wave frequency in a comatose EEG does suggest a worsening of coma, while an increase in frequency usually marks an improvement.

2. ANSWER: **B.** A flat EEG may be seen in a patient on the verge of death, but it is important to also take into consideration the cause of the coma, since certain drugs in high doses may also flatten the EEG but the flat tracing may be completely reversible. Even in coma, some patients will be able to show EEG reactivity to auditory or tactile stimuli, which is a relatively positive prognostic sign. The EEG pattern in coma is less predictive of outcome when the cause of the coma is reversible, such as drug overdose, as compared to a coma caused by a cardiac arrest.

3. ANSWER: **C.** Although triphasic waves are associated with hepatic encephalopathy, they are not diagnostic of that disorder and other causes need to be considered. IRDA is not a pattern of deep coma, but is rather seen in earlier stages of encephalopathy, often in ambulatory patients. Alpha coma may not be associated with a poor outcome when seen after a reversible process such as drug overdose, but when it occurs after cardiac arrest it is a much more worrisome pattern. Alpha coma patterns are not expected to change with patient eye-opening or closure.

4. ANSWER: **D.** The natural course of SE is that the outwardly evident convulsive movements will cease after a period of time, even though the EEG seizure discharge (and therefore the SE) is continuing. The 30-minute time limit for SE is based on an older definition of SE that is no longer in common use. Any type of seizure, if prolonged, can produce an example of SE, including focal seizures. If a patient who has experienced a prolonged generalized convulsion can begin to converse, this would be a reliable indication that the seizure has terminated.

5. ANSWER: **C.** In the absence of a reversible cause, burst-suppression EEGs are often associated with a poor neurological prognosis. There is no set rule regarding the relationship between burst and interburst duration in burst-suppression, but the interbursts are typically considerably

longer than the individual bursts. Pharmacologically-induced burst-suppression, as may be induced by medications such as pentobarbital, can be an effective treatment for otherwise refractory SE.

6. ANSWER: **D.** The key part of the definition of a periodic pattern is that the individual complexes must be separated by background activity. With rhythmic patterns (e.g., runs of spike-wave discharges), on the other hand, each waveform is not separated by intervening background activity. Both types of activity may have sharp forms. The 2 Hz firing rate and low-voltage parameters do not distinguish between periodic patterns and rhythmic patterns.

SUGGESTED READINGS

A definition of irreversible coma. Report of the Ad Hoc Committee of the Harvard Medical School to Examine the Definition of Brain Death. *JAMA* 205:337–340, 1968.

Bennett DR and the Collaborative Study of Cerebral Death: Atlas of electroencephalography in coma and cerebral death: EEG at the bedside or in the intensive care unit, New York, 1976, Raven Press.

American Clinical Neurophysiology Society Guideline 6: Minimum technical standards for EEG recording in suspected cerebral death, *J Clin Neurophysiol* 33:324–327, 2016.

Hirsch LJ, Fong MWK, Leitinger M, et al. American Clinical Neurophysiology Society's Standardized Critical Care EEG Terminology: 2021 Version, *J Clin Neurophysiol* 38:1–29, 2021.

Hirsch LJ, Fong MWK, Leitinger M, et al. American Clinical Neurophysiology Society's Standardized Critical Care EEG Terminology: 2021 Version. *J Clin Neurophysiol.* 2021; Supplemental Digital Content 1, http://links.lww.com/JCNP/A134.

Hirsch LJ, Fong MWK, Leitinger M, et al. American Clinical Neurophysiology Society's Standardized Critical Care EEG Terminology: 2021 Version. *J Clin Neurophysiol.* 2021; ACNS Standardized Critical Care EEG Terminology: Condensed Version. Supplemental Digital Content. http://links.lww.com/JCNP/A139.

Kane N, Acharya J, Benickzy S, et al: A revised glossary of terms most commonly used by clinical electroencephalographers and updated proposal for the report format of the EEG findings. Revision 2017, *Clin Neurophysiol Practice* 2:170–185, 2017.

Leitinger M, Beniczky S, Rohracher A, et al. Salzburg Consensus Criteria for Non-Convulsive Status Epilepticus—approach to clinical application, *Epilepsy Behav* 49:158–163, 2015 Aug. PMID: 26092326.

Lothman E: The biochemical basis and pathophysiology of status epilepticus, *Neurology* 40(5 Suppl 2):13–23, 1990 May. PMID: 2185436

Posner JB, Saper CB, Schiff ND, Plum F: *Plum and Posner's Diagnosis of Stupor and Coma* Oxford and New York, 2007, Oxford University Press.

13

The Electroencephalogram of the Newborn

Newborn EEG interpretation is considered a particularly challenging area. An understanding of the appearance of the normal newborn EEG was achieved considerably later than for EEGs of childhood and adulthood. In fact, before the 1960s, it was not generally accepted that there was scientific or clinical value to be found in the analysis of the EEGs of newborns.

The relatively slower progress in the field of neonatal electroencephalography has been related to several factors. In almost any laboratory, the number of newborn EEG studies performed is considerably smaller than the number of studies performed in older age groups. Thus, any given reader likely has less clinical experience reading tracings from the neonatal age group compared with older children and adults. Also, to establish the basic foundations of neonatal EEG interpretation one must know the appearance of the normal neonatal EEG, which, in turn, requires that we know which patients are neurologically normal. Neurologic normality is more difficult to ascertain in newborns because of the inherent limitations in our ability to assess newborns neurologically. For that reason, the question of whether certain findings in the newborn EEG may be normal has remained controversial. In general, newborns are considered neurologically "normal" when the history, examination, imaging, and other neurological studies are normal. This definition is more difficult to apply in practice because most babies who have had an EEG have had it for some clinical indication, and the presence of an indication immediately brings up the possibility that something is amiss. Finally, there was an early bias toward believing that typical premature tracings were abnormal because their discontinuous appearance resembled patterns such as burst-suppression that are known to be abnormal in older individuals.

THE CONCEPT OF POSTCONCEPTIONAL AGE

The EEG of newborns is strikingly different from that of older children and adults. In fact, the best-known elements of the mature EEG (posterior rhythm, sleep spindles, vertex waves) do not make their first appearance until 6 to 8 weeks after a term delivery. In the context of electroencephalography, a newborn's degree of prematurity is stated in terms of postconceptional age (CA). The CA at birth is equivalent to the gestational age and is usually established using the date of the mother's last menstrual period, but other information such as early fetal ultrasounds and the baby's physical examination can be used to modify the estimate. In this use, CA is being used as a shortcut expression for post-menstrual age

(date since last menstrual period) and, therefore, a bit of a misnomer. By definition, a full-term newborn born on its due date has a CA of 40 weeks. Newborns delivered before 37 weeks are considered premature. Note that a 3-week-old newborn who was delivered at 38 weeks gestational age is considered to have a CA of 41 weeks for the purposes of EEG interpretation. The current CA is derived by adding the gestational age at birth to the current age in weeks (time since birth or "legal age").

One of the underlying assumptions of neonatal electroencephalography is that the expected appearance of a healthy newborn's EEG is based on its CA. Whether it was born prematurely or not, the EEG of a healthy newborn is generally assumed to evolve at the same rate whether the baby is inside or outside the womb. Certain pathological processes may, however, interrupt this orderly maturation. Therefore, a normal baby born at 41 weeks CA is generally expected to have an EEG structure similar to that of a normal 5-week-old baby who was at born 36 weeks CA.

From extreme prematurity to term to the post-term period, the appearance of the neonatal EEG evolves dramatically. In fact, on the basis of the various EEG features described here, an experienced neonatal electroencephalographer should be able to estimate the CA of a newborn to within approximately 2 weeks based on the appearance of the EEG tracing. It has been claimed that when the CA estimate suggested by an otherwise normal neonatal EEG differs from the estimate based on the baby's dates or physical examination, the EEG-based assessment is more likely to be correct. Figures 13.1 and 13.2 show the striking changes in the appearance of the cortical surface between 31 weeks CA and 40 weeks CA (term). It should come as no surprise then that the appearance of the EEG evolves rapidly in premature babies.

Recording Technique

Opinion varies as to whether a full or reduced electrode set should be used for neonatal recordings. Some authors assert that the head is smaller, and therefore it is reasonable to apply fewer electrodes to the smaller head of the newborn. The opposing view holds that if the neonatal brain is conceptualized as a shrunken version of the adult brain, each lobe, gyrus, and cortical circuit is proportionally smaller, and the electric fields of discharges will be correspondingly smaller, requiring the usual (non-reduced) number of electrodes to achieve the same anatomic resolution of electric fields. Our laboratory uses a full complement of electrodes from the 10-20 system in newborns and even in most premature infants; reduced

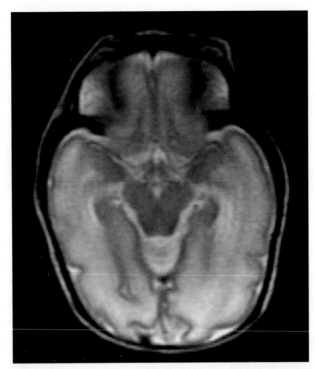

Figure 13.1 A T2-weighted magnetic resonance imaging scan of the brain of a normal baby at 31 weeks CA shows the relatively smooth appearance of the cortical surface and the rudimentary gyral pattern seen at this gestational age. In this sequence, cerebrospinal fluid appears white. Prematures between 24 and 30 weeks CA have an even less developed cortical folding pattern.

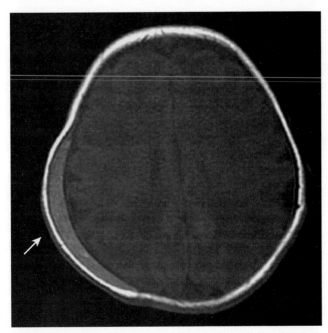

Figure 13.2 A T2-weighted magnetic resonance imaging scan of a term baby (40 weeks GA) shows that the complexity of the gyral pattern is now similar to that seen in adult patterns brains. Considering the dramatic evolution of the visual appearance of the brain between 24 and 40 weeks gestation, it is no surprise that EEG patterns during this time period evolve in a dramatic way as well.

electrode sets are only used for premature infants with the smallest head sizes. Although reduced (double-distance) electrode applications have been shown to record the majority of normal and abnormal EEG activity and may also be better tolerated by the premature infant whose scalp skin is more sensitive, occasionally a highly focal seizure discharge or other highly focal finding may be missed. In addition, difficulties with artifact identification represent a hidden pitfall of the use of sparser electrode arrays. When a deflection is seen in a single channel, denser electrode arrays help determine whether an electric field surrounds the event, increasing or decreasing the chances that it is of cerebral origin as opposed to an electrical artifact.

Additional leads are applied to help assess sleep state; to some extent, a neonatal EEG recording resembles a polysomnogram. The added leads may include a nasal thermistor to measure respirations, ocular leads (one placed just above the outer canthus of one eye and the other just below the outer canthus of the other eye), and a submental electrode to monitor chin muscle (electromyographic or EMG) activity. Additional leads may include a strain gauge placed on the abdomen to record respiratory muscle effort and limb leads to document movements. Notations made by the recording technologist on the EEG record should also carefully document the appearance of the baby. Notations such as "appears asleep," "has hiccups," "feeding," "eyes closed," or "moving" help the reader assess sleep state and evaluate artifacts especially when these features cannot be seen clearly in any simultaneous video recording (Figure 13.3).

Traditionally, newborn EEGs have been recorded at "half" paper speed (15 mm/sec). Although this practice may have originally been motivated in part by the urge to save paper on the longer recordings of newborns, the compression of the EEG resulting from slow paper speeds can make it easier to identify some discontinuous or bursting patterns, both normal and pathological. Certain delta patterns are easier to appreciate when displayed at slow paper speeds. For these reasons, slow paper speeds are still preferred by most readers for review of newborn EEG recordings. Ideally, a neonatal EEG record should include all stages of sleep—wakefulness, quiet sleep, and active sleep—which often requires recording times over 1 hour to allow assessment of sleep architecture.

A "QUICK TOUR" OF THE MAJOR NEONATAL EEG SLEEP STAGES

Similar to the "quick tour" of the adult EEG shown in Chapter 2, "Visual Analysis of the EEG," what follows is a brief overview or "tour" of the main sleep stages of the newborn EEG and also how the technique of neonatal EEG recording differs in a few ways from that of older patients. Because the appearance of the newborn EEG evolves considerably through prematurity and approaching term, no single tracing can demonstrate all of the key findings because they appear at different gestational ages.

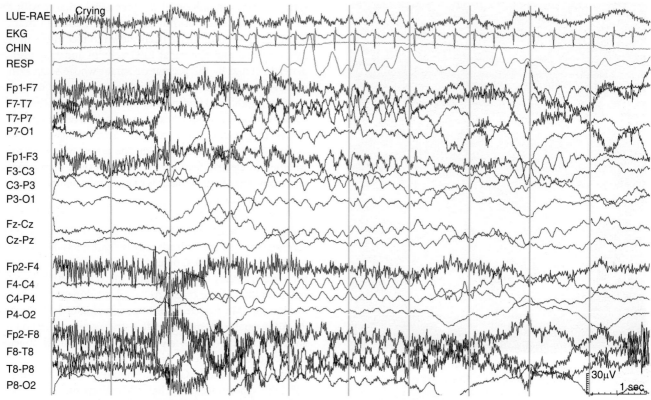

Figure 13.3 Rhythmic waves seen in the 4th to 7th seconds of this neonatal recording represent patting artifact. Because caretakers often attempt to soothe a crying baby by patting, patting artifact is a common finding in the newborn EEG. This type of rhythmic artifact may, in some cases, mimic an electrographic seizure. In general, however, caretakers tend to pat babies at a fairly steady frequency, while seizure discharges typically change in frequency throughout their duration.

In children and adults, the appearance of the EEG tracing itself more or less defines sleep state—but not so in newborns. In newborns, one EEG background may be associated with several sleep states, and individual sleep states are associated with a variety of EEG backgrounds. To make things even more interesting, the way that EEG background patterns mesh with the neonatal sleep states differs at different gestational ages. Information from polysomnographic channels and behavioral observations are often necessary to define the current sleep state. We start by reviewing the five main background patterns of the newborn EEG, followed by the three main newborn sleep stages, and how the described background patterns relate to the different sleep stages.

THE FIVE COMMON EEG BACKGROUND PATTERNS SEEN IN NEWBORNS

The features that we are most accustomed to seeing in the waking and sleep EEGs of older patients, such as the posterior rhythm, sleep spindles, and vertex waves, are not seen in newborns. Rather, specific types of EEG background patterns and elements are seen at different stages of maturity. These five principle EEG background patterns were originally described by the "French School" of neonatal electroencephalography. Although this system has not remained in common usage in all laboratories, it remains a useful construct for interpreting

and describing neonatal EEGs. Inherent to the categorization of EEG backgrounds into these five groups are both the benefits and disadvantages of simplification, trading off ease of use with the problem of loss of nuance, in addition to the inevitability of encountering patterns that may not easily fit into one of the proscribed categories. Nevertheless, this system works surprisingly well, especially for normal or near-normal newborn EEGs near term. Additional characteristic waveforms that appear at specific CAs and are superimposed on these patterns, referred to as EEG *graphoelements*, are described later.

Normal neonatal EEG background patterns may be either continuous or discontinuous. The first step in classifying a background pattern is assessment of the degree of continuity. A discontinuous pattern is a pattern in which EEG activity seems to alternately "turn on" and "turn off" for varying amounts of time. In a continuous pattern, there are no recognizable regional pauses in activity (Figure 13.4). The first three background patterns described here are continuous patterns, and the final two patterns are discontinuous patterns.

The Low-Voltage Irregular Pattern

As the name implies, this pattern consists of continuous low-voltage irregular (LVI), mixed frequencies, with delta and theta activity most prominent. Voltages generally range from

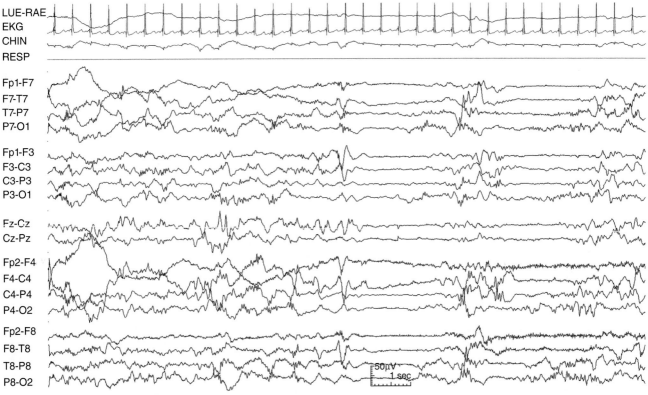

Figure 13.4 This page of EEG shows a transition from a continuous pattern, seen on the left half of the page, to a discontinuous pattern, seen on the right half of the page. The two periods of relative flattening (interburst intervals) seen on the right half of the page mark this portion of the tracing as discontinuous. LUE = left under eye, RAE = right above eye.

15 to 35 µV. An example is shown in Figure 13.5. As described later, the LVI pattern may be seen during both wakefulness and active sleep. The LVI pattern is not expected to be seen during quiet sleep.

The Mixed/Medium (M) Pattern

The M pattern is similar to the LVI pattern, but with somewhat higher voltages and a more prominent contribution of slow activity. It, too, is a continuous pattern with mixed frequencies and medium voltages (Figure 13.6). The "M" term is derived from the original French term for this pattern, *activité moyenne* (meaning medium or average activity), though the pattern is also sometimes translated as "mixed pattern." The M pattern can be seen during any sleep stage. During active sleep, the LVI pattern is most characteristic, but the somewhat higher voltages of the M pattern may also be seen, especially during the first period of active sleep that is seen just after the baby falls asleep. Similarly, during wakefulness, either the LVI or M pattern can be seen. In quiet sleep, the tracé alternant and high-voltage slow (HVS) patterns (described next) are most characteristic, but the M pattern may also be seen. It is evident that, because it is possible to see the M pattern in any stage of wakefulness or sleep, polysomnographic findings and observed behaviors are key to correct determination of sleep stage when the M pattern is present.

The High-Voltage Slow (HVS) Pattern

The HVS pattern is characteristic of quiet sleep; it only rarely makes an appearance in other sleep stages. Like the LVI and M patterns, the HVS pattern consists of continuous, irregular mixed frequencies, but with higher voltages (50–150 µV). Delta frequencies are more prominent (Figure 13.7).

As described below, the last two patterns are discontinuous patterns (tracé discontinu and tracé alternant) and are the primary patterns of quiet sleep from the earliest post-conceptional ages to 38 weeks CA. As the baby gets closer to term, the tracé alternant pattern is replaced by the HVS pattern.

It is not difficult to identify the three continuous background patterns in neonatal EEG. The LVI, M, and HVS patterns all consist of *continuous* irregular, mixed frequencies. The main distinguishing feature among these three continuous patterns is voltage.

The Tracé Discontinu Pattern

The tracé discontinu pattern (French for "discontinuous tracing") is a pattern of early prematurity, seen primarily at 30 weeks CA and before. As the name implies, tracé discontinu is a highly discontinuous pattern consisting of very high voltage polymorphic bursts, often containing large amounts of sharp features that may even resemble prolonged high voltage polyspikes (Figure 13.8). The dramatic bursts of tracé discontinu are

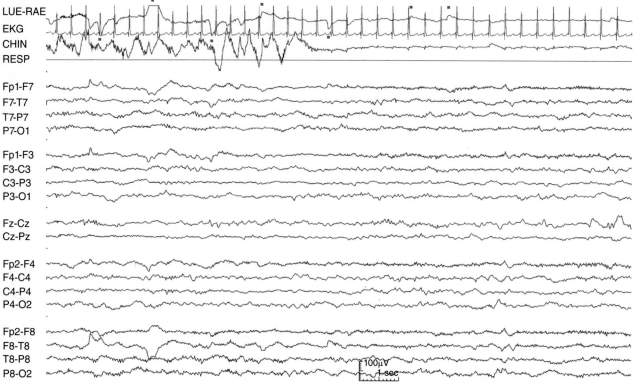

Figure 13.5 An example of a low-voltage intermixed (LVI) pattern is shown, with relatively nondescript mixed frequencies. The LVI EEG pattern is characteristic of both wakefulness and of active sleep. The triangular deflections seen in the top (ocular) channel represent rapid eye movements (dots) indicating that this is an example of active sleep. Although the LVI pattern can be seen in both active sleep and wakefulness, the lack of muscle and motion artifact in this tracing are strong indicators that the baby is asleep. LUE = left under eye, RAE = right above eye.

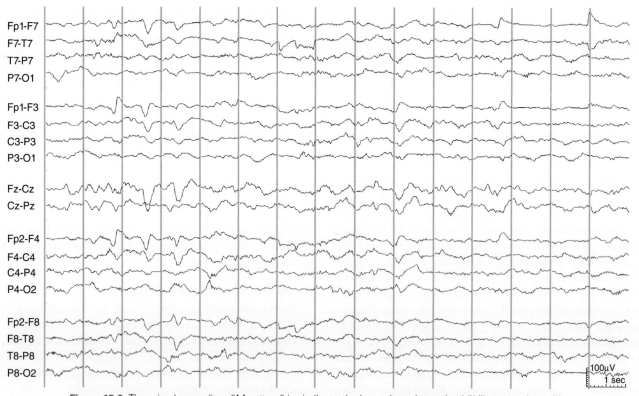

Figure 13.6 The mixed or medium "M pattern" is similar to the low-voltage intermixed (LVI) pattern, but with higher voltages. The M pattern may be seen in any of the sleep stages, including wakefulness, quiet sleep, and active sleep. Assignment of sleep state when the M pattern is present depends on other recording parameters such as technologist observations and information from the polysomnographic channels.

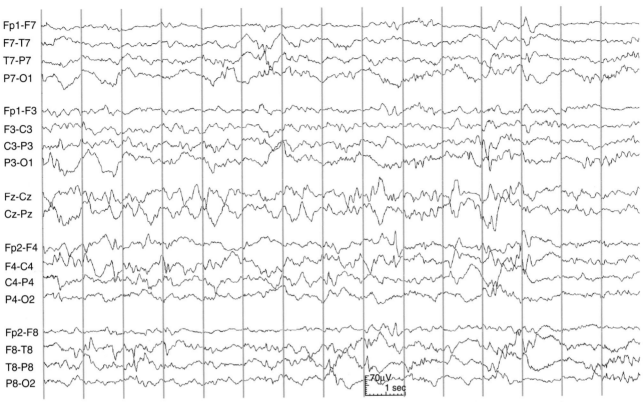

Figure 13.7 This segment of high-voltage slow (HVS) pattern was obtained during quiet sleep in a term newborn. Voltages are higher than were seen in the previous two patterns, but frequencies remain mixed and the waves are irregular. The HVS pattern is particularly associated with quiet sleep.

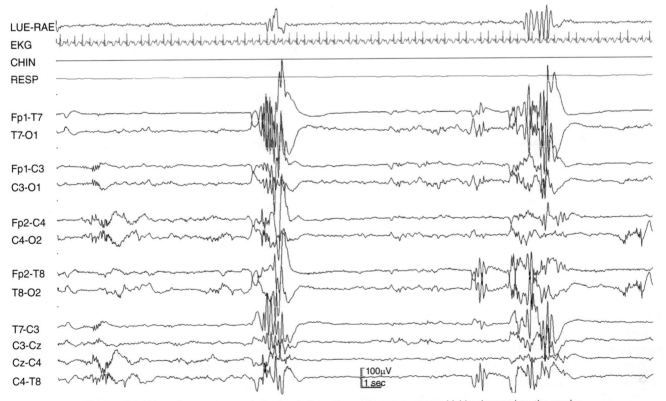

Figure 13.8 When first encountered, the tracé discontinu pattern may appear highly abnormal to the reader accustomed to interpreting adult EEGs. High-voltage bursts containing large amounts of polymorphic activity, often very sharp as in this example, are seen synchronously in both hemispheres. The bursts are separated by quiet periods of varying duration. Because the bursts are of high voltage, it is no surprise that they are picked up by the eye channel (LUE-RAE) as well, whose electrodes are close to the frontal lobes. LUE = left under eye, RAE = right above eye.

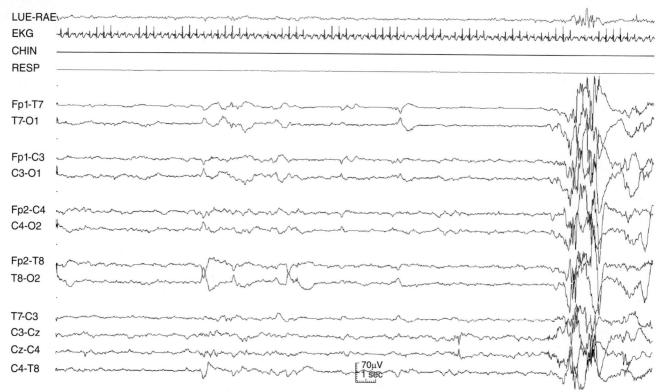

Figure 13.9 In this example of tracé discontinu, the interburst periods are particularly lengthy; note the time scale at the bottom of the figure. The plentiful spikes seen within the bisynchronous bursts are considered a normal feature of the tracé discontinu pattern. At the earliest CAs, the flat periods between bursts can be quite lengthy, sometimes exceeding 20 seconds. LUE = left under eye, RAE = right above eye.

separated by equally dramatic flat periods that may exceed 10 to 20 seconds in length in the most premature babies (Figure 13.9). Because of its resemblance to burst-suppression, a well-known pathologic pattern in adult EEG, it took some time for neonatal electroencephalographers to confirm that this was a normal pattern of early prematurity. The bursts of tracé discontinu are almost completely bisynchronous, which is to say that the bursts occur in both hemispheres at the same time. This bisynchrony is one of several characteristic features that can help distinguish the tracé discontinu pattern from the other discontinuous pattern, tracé alternant, described next.

The Tracé Alternant Pattern

Tracé alternant (French for "alternating tracing") is the hallmark pattern of quiet sleep in newborns. Tracé alternant is a discontinuous pattern consisting of bursts of mixed activity lasting 2 to 8 seconds with interspersed flatter periods referred to as "interbursts" lasting 4 to 8 seconds (Figure 13.10). Generally, the bursts and interbursts are of similar duration. The bursts normally contain a variety of activity, including sharp transient activity and also delta brush activity in more premature babies (described later).

When tracé alternant makes its first appearance after the 30 weeks CA, the quiet interburst periods are longer and flatter than at later CAs. Also, at earlier CAs, the bursts of tracé alternant show the least amount of synchrony between the two hemispheres—many of the bursts occur in one hemisphere at a time. As the baby approaches term, the tracé alternant pattern evolves in three ways. First, the bursts are not as widely separated

(the interburst intervals become shorter). Second, the interburst intervals evolve from being relatively flat, showing only small amounts of activity, to showing increasing amounts of activity, so much so that as term approaches it may become difficult to tell where a burst ends and a quiet period begins. Finally, the degree of interhemispheric synchrony of the tracé alternant bursts increases toward term, although it may never reach complete synchrony. The pattern shown in Figure 13.11 has, indeed, achieved complete synchrony, although this does not always occur. Even after term the degree of interhemispheric synchrony of tracé alternant is never required to exceed 75%, meaning that in normal babies, a small amount of asynchrony may always be seen. Also, note the increased amount of activity in the interbursts in Figure 13.10 compared to Figure 13.11. The tracé alternant pattern should only be seen during quiet sleep stages, which makes sleep staging considerably easier when this pattern is identified. Therefore, with increasing gestational age, the tracé alternant pattern manifests shorter interbursts, the interbursts have higher voltage activity, and there is increased interhemispheric synchrony to the bursts.

The differences between tracé alternant and tracé discontinu are both qualitative and quantitative. Quantitative differences in tracé discontinu compared with tracé alternant include longer interburst intervals, more sharp activity within bursts, and near complete synchrony. Qualitatively, in tracé discontinu the interburst intervals are expected to be essentially flat, whereas varying amounts of continuous activity are expected during the interburst intervals of tracé alternant, especially at later CAs. Between 30 and 34 weeks CA, the

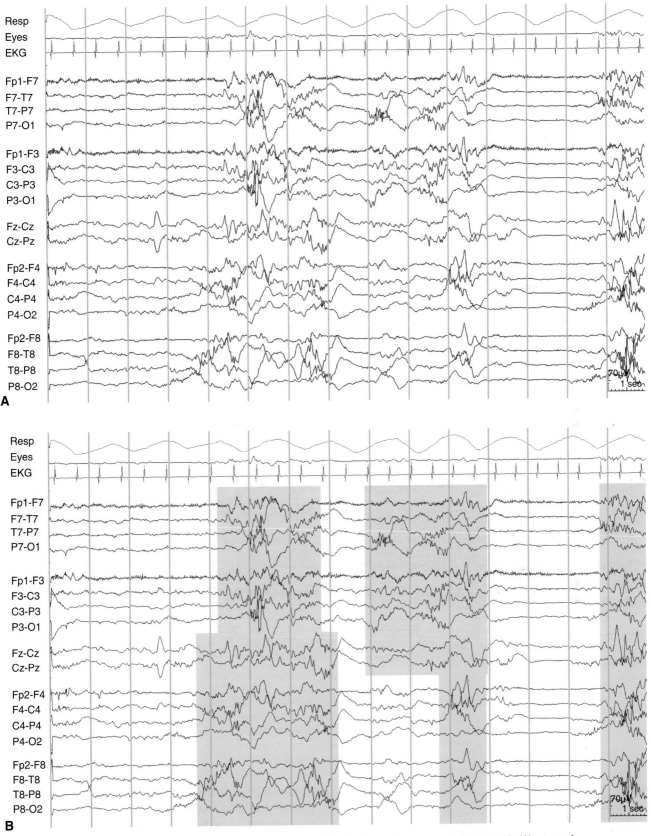

Figure 13.10 The distinctive, discontinuous pattern of tracé alternant is shown. In this example (A), most of the bursts are bisynchronous with bursting activity and suppressions occurring in each hemisphere more or less at the same time. Some amount of asynchrony is noted, however. The lower panel (B) shows the same page of EEG as was shown in Panel A, now with shading marking the approximate beginning and end of each burst. Note each burst contains a fair amount of sharp activity. The regular respirations and lack of eye movements confirm that this is an example of normal quiet sleep.

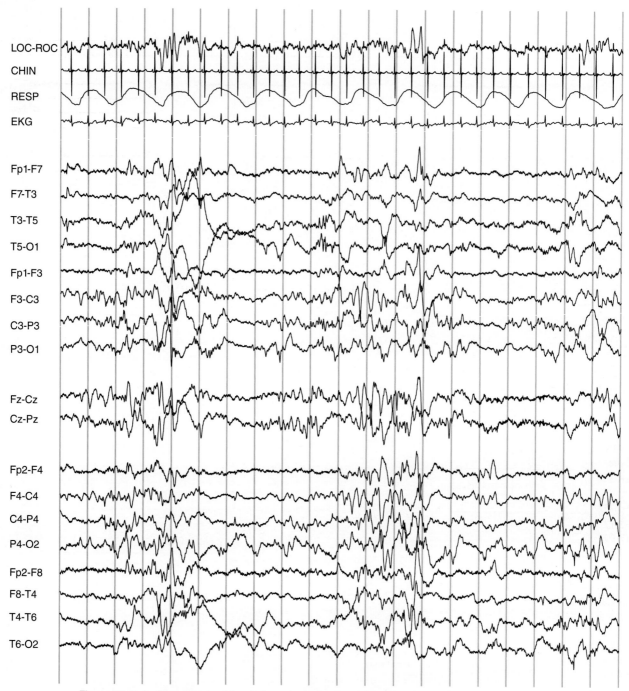

Figure 13.11 In this example of tracé alternant the bursts and suppressions are completely synchronous. The time scale has been compressed to make the discontinuous pattern easier to appreciate. Although clearly of lower voltage than the bursts, the periods between bursts contain a fair amount of activity. This and the high degree of synchrony suggest that the baby is near term. Also note the highly regular respirations, another hallmark of quiet sleep.

evolution of tracé discontinu to tracé alternant during quiet sleep occurs on a continuum.

The Evolution of Interhemispheric Synchrony

In contrast to tracé alternant, the tracé discontinu pattern is almost completely synchronous between the hemispheres. This leads to a distinctive sequence in the evolution of inter-hemispheric synchrony through the weeks of prematurity.

In the most premature babies (before about 30 weeks CA), there is nearly complete interhemispheric synchrony in the tracé discontinu pattern, which is seen in all clinical sleep/wake states. When the tracé alternant pattern first appears (at approximately 30 weeks CA), the pattern is initially significantly asynchronous. This is followed by a gradual return of interhemispheric synchrony as the tracé alternant matures and the baby approaches term. Therefore, the EEG is synchronous in extreme prematurity, becomes moderately asynchronous in "middle" prematurity, and becomes synchronous again near term.

SLEEP STAGES IN THE NEWBORN

The three main sleep stages of the newborn are active sleep, quiet sleep, and wakefulness. The French School, realizing that there was no other gold standard for defining when a baby was awake or asleep, defined the concept of "asleep" simply enough as a state during which the baby persistently held the eyes closed. These three newborn sleep stages correspond to and will evolve into the well-known stages of REM sleep, slow-wave sleep, and wakefulness seen in older subjects.

Active Sleep

During active sleep, the baby is seen to squirm, grimace, and have an agitated appearance, yet the eyes remain closed. In fact, these movements may lead an observer to think that the baby is on the verge of waking up. Respirations are irregular, and occasional respiratory pauses may be seen. Rapid eye movements of sleep are seen, both on the eye channels of the EEG and by casual observation of the baby's eyelids; darting movements of the corneal bulge can be seen under the baby's eyelids. The chin EMG lead picks up phasic bursts of muscle activity that correspond to facial muscle movements, such as

grimacing or other movements. However, in between facial movements, chin EMG activity is low. The EEG typically shows an LVI pattern that is similar to what is seen during wakefulness (Figure 13.12). Although most active sleep periods are associated with an LVI pattern, the initial period of active sleep that occurs as a baby first falls asleep may show a somewhat higher voltage EEG pattern, such as an M pattern, compared with later active sleep stages.

Active sleep in neonates is analogous to REM (dream) sleep in children and adults, although there are two interesting distinctions. First, although older subjects experience a form of paralysis during dream sleep, presumably so that dreams are not physically acted out, as the name implies, babies move actively during active sleep. Second, whereas the first REM sleep stages typically appear only after children or adults have been asleep for some time (as was described in Chapter 2, "Visual Analysis of the EEG"), newborns enter active sleep as their first sleep stage, as they transition from wakefulness to sleep. REM sleep at sleep onset is not expected in adults, except in patients with narcolepsy in whom this phenomenon is one of the hallmarks of the syndrome.

Quiet Sleep

The term *quiet sleep* derives from the quiet appearance of the baby during this sleep stage. Respirations are deeper and regular, and there are few, if any, limb movements. Outwardly,

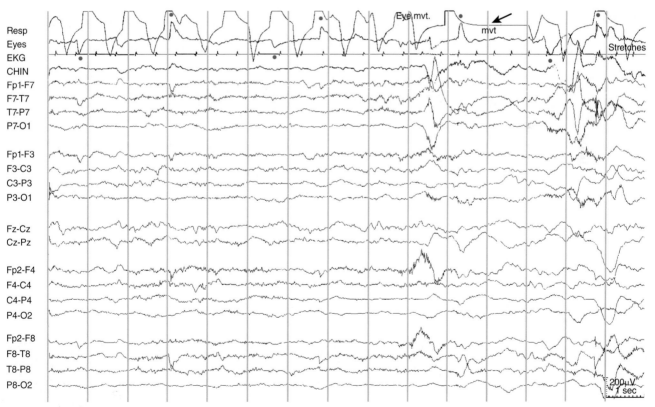

Figure 13.12 An example of active sleep is shown. Note the low-voltage irregular (LVI) pattern in which overall voltages are low save for examples of superimposed motion artifact. The respiratory (top) channel shows irregular respirations and a brief respiratory pause (arrow), consistent with active sleep. The oculogram (second channel) shows sharp deflections representing horizontal rapid eye movement of sleep (dots), the hallmark of active sleep.

the baby appears to be in a deep sleep state. REMS are not seen (see Figure 13.9). The chin EMG lead, perhaps surprisingly, shows a high level of tonic muscle activity, with comparatively more EMG activity than is seen during the periods between body movements in active sleep. After term as the baby gets older, quiet sleep patterns eventually meld into the more mature slow-wave sleep patterns.

The EEG pattern seen during quiet sleep before term is the distinctive tracé alternant pattern, a discontinuous pattern with periods of high-voltage mixed activity separated by periods of relative quiescence. As the baby approaches term, an HVS pattern gradually replaces the tracé alternant pattern during quiet sleep stages. During this transitional period, which occurs during the weeks just before and after term, some babies manifest an HVS pattern at the beginning of a quiet sleep epoch, which may then transition to a tracé alternant pattern with deepening quiet sleep.

Wakefulness

In wakefulness, the baby's eyes are open and the activity level may vary considerably, from relaxed wakefulness (often seen just after feeding) to states of considerable agitation and crying. Breathing can be mildly irregular when the baby is calm to very irregular when the baby is more active. Recorded eye movements are irregular and include voluntary tracking and searching movements. These searching movements during wakefulness are usually easy to differentiate from the REMS of active sleep, which are faster and are more prominent in the horizontal plane.

The EEG pattern during wakefulness usually consists of an LVI pattern that may include a large amount of superimposed motion artifact depending on the baby's level of activity (Figure 13.13). The somewhat higher voltage, M pattern may also be seen. The EEG patterns seen during wakefulness can be quite similar to those seen during active sleep and, at times, it can be difficult for the reader to determine whether a page of EEG represents active sleep or wakefulness. This distinction is usually not difficult to make for the EEG technologist who is directly observing the baby and knows whether the baby's eyes are open or closed, the key factor in making this distinction. This situation highlights the importance of the technologist making frequent observational notes while recording newborn EEGs, especially if good video of the baby is not available.

Transitional Sleep and Indeterminate Sleep

For the sake of completeness, two additional sleep states are defined. The term *transitional sleep* is used for periods when the EEG transitions from one sleep state to another, including elements of both states. Some babies spend a considerable amount of time in these transitional states. The term *indeterminate state* is used for stages that cannot be assigned clearly to any of the aforementioned groups.

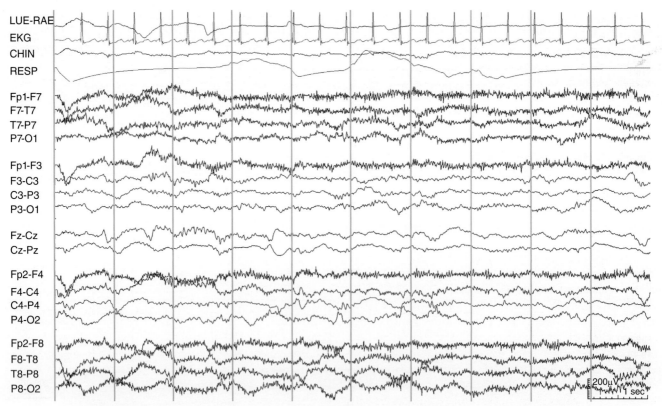

Figure 13.13 A page of wakefulness is shown with the EEG showing an M pattern. The technologist's observation that the baby's eyes are open and the moderate amount of muscle and motion artifact imply wakefulness. Eye movements are seen in the eye channel (labeled "LUE-RAE"); however, they do not clearly have the classic "sharp" or triangular morphology of horizontal rapid eye movement sleep and likely represent voluntary or searching eye movements.

TABLE 13.1	Summary of Most Common Features of the Major Neonatal Sleep States		
	Quiet Sleep	**Active Sleep**	**Wakefulness**
EEG Pattern	Tracé alternant or high voltage slow	Low voltage irregular	Low voltage irregular or medium
Breathing	Very regular, deeper, slower	Irregular, with some pauses	Irregular, variable
Body Movements	Few movements, peaceful appearance	Squirming, sucking, grimacing, but eyes closed	Calm, active, or crying, eyes open
Eye Movements	Little or none	Horizontal REMS	Searching, consistent with having eyes open
Chin EMG	High tonic activity	Low tonic activity (measured in between movements)	Usually phasic

REMS = rapid eye movements, EMG = electromyogram.

Table 13.1 summarizes the features of the three main sleep states of the newborn after they have become well differentiated.

TYPICAL EVOLUTION OF NEONATAL SLEEP STAGES NEAR TERM

Sleep State Cycling in the Newborn

Typical sleep state cycling is depicted thus (W = wakefulness, AS = active sleep, QS = quiet sleep):

$$W \rightarrow AS \rightarrow QS \rightarrow AS \rightarrow QS \rightarrow AS \rightarrow W \rightarrow W \rightarrow W \rightarrow AS \rightarrow QS$$
$$\rightarrow AS \rightarrow QS \rightarrow W \dots$$

Active sleep is usually the first sleep stage on falling asleep followed by quiet sleep. Periods of active sleep and quiet sleep then alternate until the next waking period. Periods of transitional sleep that may include the features of both sleep states may be interposed between well-defined active sleep and quiet sleep epochs. Newborns normally sleep for as many as 20 hours out of a 24-hour day. Each complete sleep cycle lasts approximately 60 minutes but with wide variation. Typically, newborns spend about half of their sleep time in active sleep and half in quiet sleep. The fraction of sleep time spent in dream sleep decreases with age; adults spend only about 20% of the night in REM sleep.

After remaining in active sleep for approximately 20 to 25 minutes, if the baby remains asleep, a transition to quiet sleep is expected. The changes associated with the transition from active sleep to quiet sleep are more dramatic than those associated with transition from wakefulness to active sleep. First, as the baby's sleep quiets, muscle and motion artifact disappear from the record. The breathing pattern noted in the respiratory channels becomes very regular, and eye movements are rare. A tracé alternant pattern then appears (or HVS in infants closer to term). The baby thereafter alternates between quiet sleep and active sleep until arousal. Between sleep stages, brief transitional states may be seen with elements of both types of sleep present at the same time (e.g., irregular breathing accompanying a tracé alternant pattern).

EEG Architecture in More Premature Infants

The orderly sleep structure described in the previous section characterizes infants nearing term. Very premature newborns, however, lack this sleep structure. The earliest EEGs in clinical practice are recorded in babies at 23 to 24 weeks gestational age, which is considered near the limit of viability. In fact, EEGs are only occasionally obtained in such premature infants, partly because of the extreme fragility of their skin but also because seizures are believed to be uncommon at these very early CAs. At these early gestations, the predominant EEG background is tracé discontinu, consisting of bilateral complex bursts separated by prolonged periods of electrical quiescence. The period of electrical quiet may last longer than 20 seconds. Between 24 and 30 weeks CA, there is a tendency for the flat portions of tracé discontinu to become shorter and the amount of activity during the interburst to increase. It may come as a surprise to learn that there is no reliable relationship between sleep state and EEG appearance before 30 weeks CA; the tracé discontinu pattern is seen during both wakefulness and sleep, even though periods of wakefulness and sleep are clinically distinguishable.

The Emergence of Continuity

The first state seen with continuous activity in the premature infant is active sleep, appearing at approximately 30 weeks CA. When active sleep periods finally appear, continuous LVI or M patterns (with REMs) make their first appearance. Continuous activity during wakefulness first becomes well established at approximately 34 weeks CA. The final sleep stage to manifest continuous activity is quiet sleep. As described earlier, the discontinuous tracé alternant pattern is typically seen during quiet sleep, but at approximately 38 weeks CA the continuous HVS pattern makes its first appearance. During this transition, both tracé alternant and HVS patterns may be seen during quiet sleep at different times in the same baby. Even though the HVS pattern predominates during quiet sleep after term, fragments of the discontinuity of the tracé alternant pattern may be seen during quiet sleep up to 46 to 48 weeks CA. After 48 weeks CA, any discontinuity in the EEG is considered abnormal. In summary, the EEG first becomes continuous at 30 weeks CA in active sleep, at 34 weeks CA in wakefulness, and at 38 weeks CA in quiet sleep.

AN ORDERLY APPROACH TO NEONATAL EEG INTERPRETATION

The first step in visual analysis of a page of newborn EEG is asking the question, what state is this? As the EEG is sequentially examined from beginning to end, the reader attempts to identify the various sleep states the baby may be cycling through as described in Table 13.1: wakefulness, active sleep, and quiet sleep. Do the sleep stages have the expected structure according to the baby's reported CA? For example, in a baby nearer to term, during wakefulness is there an LVI or M pattern? Often the presence of motion artifact in the tracing, video, and technologist comments confirm that the child is awake and active. As the baby falls asleep, the reader will expect to see a first sleep stage, most likely active sleep. Because wakefulness and active sleep are both associated with either an LVI or M pattern, the transition may not be obvious based on the EEG alone. Active sleep is marked by closed eyes, the appearance of REMs, and a relative reduction in body movements and crying. After a period of active sleep, does the EEG become discontinuous (tracé alternant)? Does the baby quiet, and do the respirations become regular with disappearance of REMS, marking the onset of quiet sleep? The presence of this type of normal sleep cycling is a positive clinical sign. Although the absence of expected sleep architecture may be related to CNS pathology, it is important to keep in mind that there are many other possible explanations for disrupted sleep architecture (noises, medications, cooling therapy, and other procedures), especially on hospital inpatient units. In the absence of other explanatory circumstances, the fewer features of normal sleep stage structure noted, the greater the worry of brain pathology.

EEG GRAPHOELEMENTS

During the late 1950s and early 1960s, in addition to describing neonatal sleep states, the "French school" of electroencephalography described certain specific waveforms in the normal newborn EEG that appeared and disappeared at specific CAs, calling these features *graphoéléments*. The concept of EEG graphoelements remains useful. Familiarity with the different neonatal EEG graphoelements and the CAs and sleep states during which they are expected to appear helps the reader "date" the EEG in terms of apparent CA. It also helps to avoid labeling normal elements as abnormal.

Temporal Sawtooth Waves

Temporal sawtooth waves are seen in the EEG most prominently between 26 and 32 weeks CA, declining thereafter. They are a hallmark finding of the EEG between 28 and 30 weeks in particular. Temporal sawtooth waves appear as 4 to 6 Hz sharply contoured theta waves of varying voltage seen in each midtemporal area (Figure 13.14). Because sleep states are not yet well defined at these CAs, they are not particularly associated with a specific state.

Delta Brushes

The delta brush is one of the most distinctive waves of prematurity. Delta brushes have also been called *beta-delta complexes* and *ripples of prematurity*. They consist of a delta wave

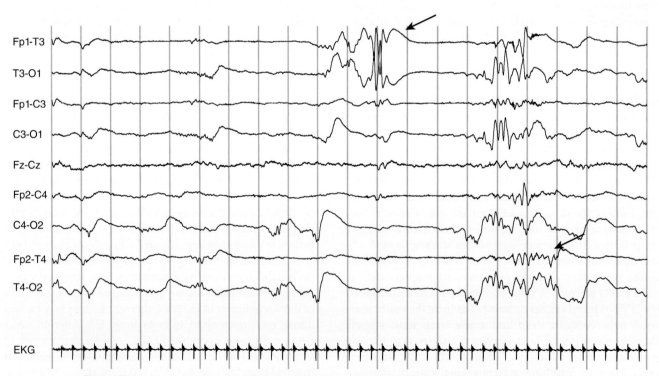

Figure 13.14 Temporal sawtooth waves are among the most characteristic waves seen in the EEG between 27 and 28 weeks CA. Sawtooth waves consist of brief runs of sharp theta activity seen over each temporal lobe (arrows).

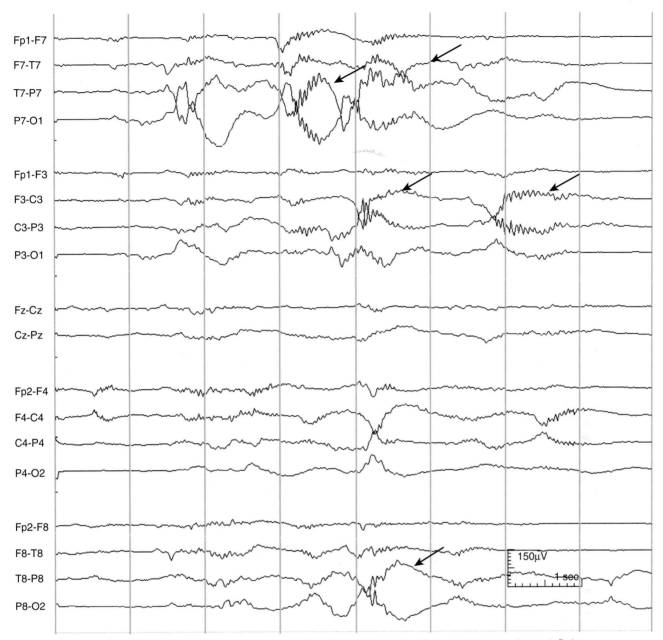

Figure 13.15 Delta brushes consists of a "brush" or "ripple" of activity riding on a delta wave (arrows). Delta brush activity peaks at 34 weeks CA. The amplitude of both the fast activity and the slow component vary in different examples. Delta brush activity tends to be most prominent in the posterior quadrants, as seen in this segment.

with superimposed fast activity that may have a wide range of frequencies, from 8 to 22 Hz (Figure 13.15). Delta brushes show a predilection for the posterior quadrants (central, temporal, parietal, and occipital areas) and are not often seen frontally.

Delta brushes make their first appearance at 26 to 28 weeks CA at a time when sleep stages are not well differentiated. They are initially seen in the central areas. They reach their peak density in the EEG at about 34 weeks CA, by which time they are also prominent in the occipital areas. When quiet sleep becomes a distinct sleep stage, delta brushes are particularly seen as a part of the tracé alternant pattern of quiet sleep; they are only rarely seen during well-established active

sleep or wakefulness. By 39 to 40 weeks, CA delta brushes have all but disappeared and should be absent by 44 weeks CA. Similarly, by this CA the tracé alternant pattern has been replaced by the HVS pattern during quiet sleep.

Sharp Transients

In the wider world of electroencephalography, spikes and sharp waves have the connotation of both being abnormal and associated with seizures. In neonatal electroencephalography, both of these biases must be reversed. First, not only may sharp activity in the EEG be normal, certain sharp discharges are actually expected in newborn EEGs as normal graphoelements. Second, when abnormal sharp activity is seen in newborns, such discharges may be associated with brain injury but not specifically with seizures as they are in older individuals. Therefore, even abnormal sharp waves in babies are not considered an epileptiform abnormality. To avoid the negative connotation of the terms *spike* and *sharp wave*, such discharges in the newborn EEG are referred to as sharp transients.

Frontal Sharp Transients (*Encoches Frontales*)

Frontal sharp transients, also referred to by the original French term *encoches frontales* (frontal notches—pronounced on-KOSH fron-TAL), consist of high-voltage, usually bilateral, frontal sharp waves (Figure 13.16). They may have a biphasic morphology, and the primary phase has negative more often than positive polarity. Occasionally unilateral examples are seen, but when one-sided, the number of discharges seen on each side should remain similar. Encoches frontales are seen most often in quiet sleep and are only rarely seen in active sleep or wakefulness; large numbers of frontal sharp transients during wakefulness or active sleep are considered abnormal. These transients first appear at about 34 weeks CA and become less common after term. They should not be seen at all after 48 weeks CA.

Temporal Sharp Transients

Temporal, central, or centrotemporal sharp transients with negative polarity are expected in normal newborn EEGs and may be seen during both the LVI and higher voltage M patterns, or during the tracé alternant, or HVS portions of the tracing (Figure 13.17). Such sharp activity is an *expected* feature of the discontinuous neonatal EEG patterns: tracé alternant and tracé discontinu. Sharp activity may be especially plentiful within the bursts themselves. The sharp transients described here are those that occur outside the context of the bursts, during continuous EEG states.

There is probably no lower CA limit of normal for temporal sharp transients. Temporal sharp transients are a particularly common feature of the newborn EEG between 35 and 42 weeks CA. After 44 weeks CA, they are uncommon, and they are considered abnormal after 48 weeks CA.

The Emergence of Vertex Waves and Spindles

Sleep spindles appear in the EEG between 6 and 8 weeks after term (46–48 weeks CA), and vertex waves of sleep follow soon after at 8 weeks or thereafter. During infancy and up to 18 to 24 months of age, there is a tendency for sleep spindles to occur asynchronously over each hemisphere. After 2 years of age, sleep spindles occur synchronously over both hemispheres. During the transitional stage between spindle asynchrony and synchrony during the second year of life, the spindles may be asynchronous in light sleep but become more synchronous as Stage II sleep deepens. Spindle duration tends to be longer in infants (several seconds) and shortens toward adulthood (approximately 2 seconds).

When Are Sharp Transients in the Temporal, Frontal, and Other Areas Considered Abnormal?

Establishing strict criteria of normality for neonatal sharp transients that occur outside of tracé alternant bursts has not been easy. It has already been stated that some amount of frontal and temporal sharp transient activity should not just be "passed" as normal but is actually an expected feature of the newborn EEG. However, it has been shown statistically that abnormal babies may manifest higher numbers of sharp transients than do normal babies. This pair of facts suggests that there may be some specific upper limit to the amount of sharp transient activity a baby may have beyond which a tracing should be considered abnormal. An exact limit, however, has been difficult to define. As readers of neonatal EEGs gain experience, they become accustomed to the wide range in the

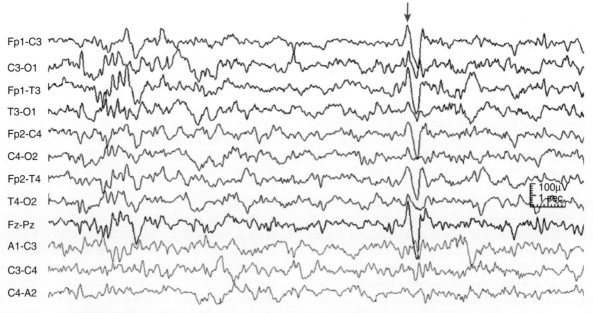

Figure 13.16 A single frontal sharp transient is seen (arrow) in this double-distance montage.

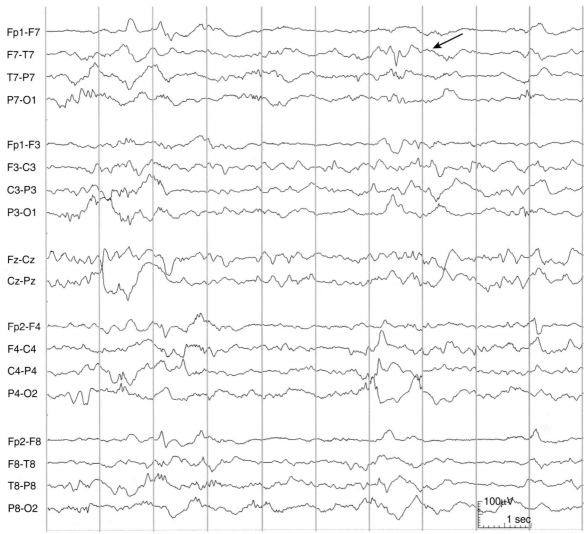

Figure 13.17 A temporal sharp transient is seen, maximum in the T7 electrode (arrow). Normal temporal sharp transients usually occur singly, are of low to moderate voltage, and should be seen to the same extent over each temporal lobe throughout the record. (Image courtesy of Dr. Sanjeev Kothare.)

number of sharp transients that are usually seen in a newborn record, giving a benchmark against which to decide how many is "too many." One sharp transient per minute has been considered to be within the normal range by some, though exceeding this frequency by some amount is not necessarily considered abnormal. When it is felt that a tracing clearly shows too much sharp transient activity, the abnormality is referred to as "excess neonatal sharp transients." The reader must take care not to be overly aggressive in calling neonatal EEG tracings abnormal solely on the basis of the abundance of these discharges, keeping in mind that a baseline number of these transients is considered completely normal. This is true especially if the observed sharp transients do not manifest any of the abnormalities described in the next section. Many babies whose *only* EEG abnormality is an excess of neonatal sharp transients have a favorable developmental outcome.

Normal neonatal sharp transients can probably be seen in any brain area, although there is a tendency for transients to be more widely distributed at earlier CAs and to concentrate in the central, temporal, and frontal areas nearer term. Transients seen in the midline electrodes are more often associated with abnormality, but still may be normal.

Other Features of Abnormal Sharp Transients

Apart from the frequency of their appearance, certain other features are felt to mark sharp transients as abnormal. These include very high voltage (>150 μV), asymmetrical appearance (considerably more on one side than the other), polyphasic rather than the usual monophasic or diphasic morphology, repetitive discharges in one location, and, sometimes, positive polarity (discussed later). Certain locations are felt to have a higher association with abnormality than others. Sharp transients occurring in the midline, such as at the Cz electrode, are more often seen in abnormal babies. Some authors feel occipital sharp transients are abnormal, but others do not. When a sharp transient is deemed abnormal, it is felt to mark a nonspecific brain injury rather than an epileptiform abnormality, which is to say that it is that it is not specifically associated with an increased risk of seizures.

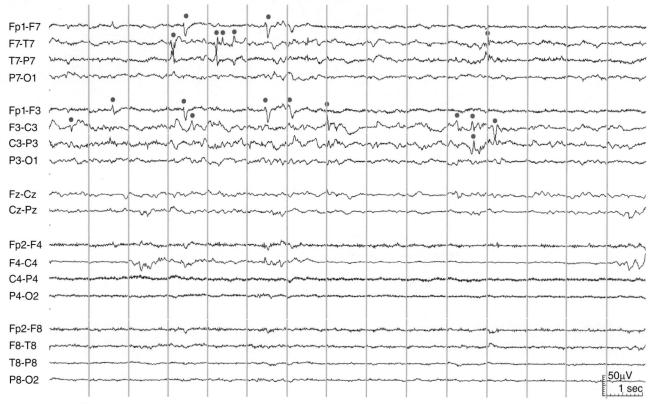

Fp1-F7
F7-T7
T7-P7
P7-O1

Fp1-F3
F3-C3
C3-P3
P3-O1

Fz-Cz
Cz-Pz

Fp2-F4
F4-C4
C4-P4
P4-O2

Fp2-F8
F8-T8
T8-P8
P8-O2

50μV
1 sec

Figure 13.18 Multiple sharp transients are seen over the left hemisphere (dots) but not over the right. Although not of particularly high voltage, the repetitive and asymmetric nature of these transients marks them as abnormal. This baby experienced a stroke in the left hemisphere.

Figure 13.18 shows excessively repetitive sharp transients in the left temporal area of a baby who experienced a stroke in that area.

Central and Temporal Positive Sharp Waves

When first described, central positive sharp waves in newborns were felt to be strongly associated with intraventricular hemorrhage (IVH). These central positive sharp waves are now understood to be associated with multiple disorders; however, they are particularly characteristic of injury to the deep white matter structures in premature infants, including IVH and periventricular leukomalacia. The positive polarity of such sharp waves is indicated by the distinctive phase reversal seen in bipolar montages in which the peaks of the sharp wave point away from (rather than toward) each other indicating positive polarity (Figure 13.19). Temporal positive sharp waves have also been associated with IVH and hypoxic-ischemic injury in the past; however, they have also been described in normal infants, possibly related to the sharp temporal theta discharges (sawtooth waves) that have already been described.

BACKGROUND ABNORMALITIES OF THE NEONATAL EEG

Of all the parameters that can be examined with regard to the neonatal EEG, the feature most predictive of a baby's final developmental outcome is the EEG background. The topic of neonatal EEG background was comprehensively reviewed by Holmes and Lombroso (1993). Various background abnormalities encountered in the neonatal EEG are described next, generally in order of decreasing severity.

Electrocerebral Inactivity and Voltage Depression

Electrocerebral inactivity (ECI) implies a complete lack of electrical activity recorded from the brain. The term should be reserved for recordings that have been performed with stringent technique. (The proper recording techniques for possible ECI tracings and the concept of brain death are discussed in more detail in Chapter 12, "EEG Patterns in Stupor and Coma," but are summarized here as they pertain to newborns.) The specific recording technique necessary to make a formal diagnosis of ECI includes the use of double-distance electrode montages, proper electrode impedances, confirmation that the EEG apparatus is connected properly by tapping the individual electrodes, and that noxious stimulation maneuvers have been performed on the baby to try to elicit EEG activity. The tracing must be of adequate duration and the cutoff frequency for the low filter should be set adequately low ($\leq 1\,Hz$). Recording sensitivities of $2\,\mu V/mm$ should be used, at least for a portion of the tracing. At such high amplifier gains, it can sometimes be difficult to distinguish true brain wave activity from electrical artifacts, which are magnified at these settings. Synonyms used for ECI include electrocerebral silence and "isoelectric" EEG (Figure 13.20).

Note that the presence of an ECI tracing is not equivalent to the diagnosis of brain death. The diagnosis of brain death must be backed up by multiple elements of the neurologic examination and sometimes by specific types of

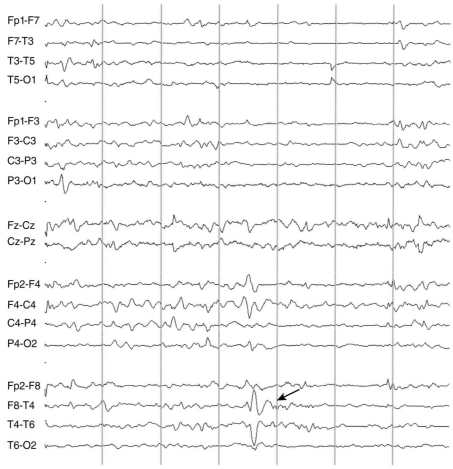

Figure 13.19 A positive sharp wave is noted in the right midtemporal area with a positive phase reversal seen in T4 (arrow). Neonatal positive sharp waves have been associated with deep white matter lesions.

neuroimaging; the specific legal definition used to declare brain death depends on the jurisdiction and is particularly difficult to apply in the case of newborns in whom a separate, specialized set of criteria is used. It should not be surprising that an EEG showing ECI is not equivalent to brain death. The scalp-recorded electroencephalogram records electrical activity from the cortical surface, but the diagnosis of brain death implies complete inactivity of both the brain surface and deeper brain structures, such as the brainstem (medulla, pons, and midbrain), structures that are distant from scalp EEG electrodes. In fact, in most settings, an EEG recording is not required to establish the diagnosis of brain death.

Not infrequently, the reader will encounter an EEG in which no definite electrocerebral activity can be identified but that has not been recorded with the strict technique described here and in Chapter 12, "EEG Patterns in Stupor and Coma". Such tracings may be described as showing "no definite electrocerebral activity" or colloquially as "flat" but in these cases, the more absolute designation of ECI should not be used. In such cases, the report should state that the strict technique necessary to make a diagnosis of ECI was not used for the recording.

Of course, when the EEG diagnosis of ECI is made, the lack of electrocerebral activity must persist throughout the whole tracing and the recording must be of sufficient duration. It is important to note that some babies experience a complete but transient

suppression of EEG voltages after a seizure. The EEG tracing may similarly flatten and recover after a transient hypoxic-ischemic insult. In cases of transient flattening after a seizure, however, the EEG only remains flat for several minutes, and activity should be seen to recover soon after. Occasionally, a seizure may have occurred by chance just before a recording was started, and the fact that observed voltage suppression is a postictal change is not obvious. In such cases, some electrical activity should return after several minutes. Rarely, high levels of sedative agents may also flatten the EEG.

The large majority of babies with an ECI pattern have a poor neurologic outcome, including death or severe disability. The longer the pattern persists, the more certain the poor prognosis.

Voltage depression in the form of low voltage, invariant patterns that lack sleep features are also associated with a poor neurologic prognosis, but the outcome is somewhat more variable. The specific limits for the definition of low voltage patterns has varied, with some using voltages persistently below 20 μV, and more recently 10 μV, for this cutoff (Figure 13.21). When serial EEG studies document improvement in the pattern, the prognosis may also be improved. When a second EEG tracing is obtained approximately one week after the initial study and it continues to show a severely abnormal background, this can confirm a poor prognosis, while an improvement in background can indicate a more positive prognosis.

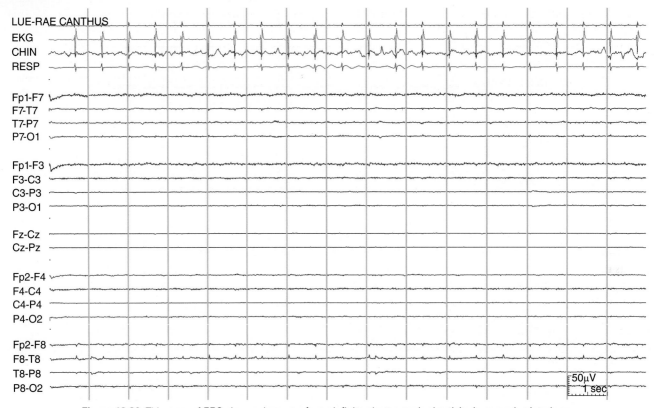

Figure 13.20 This page of EEG shows absence of any definite electrocerebral activity in an asphyxiated newborn. At the high amplifier gains used for such recordings, artifacts may become prominent in the tracing. In this example, the low-voltage electrocardiogram artifact noted in several channels would not be mistaken for brain waves because of its rhythmic, monomorphic nature.

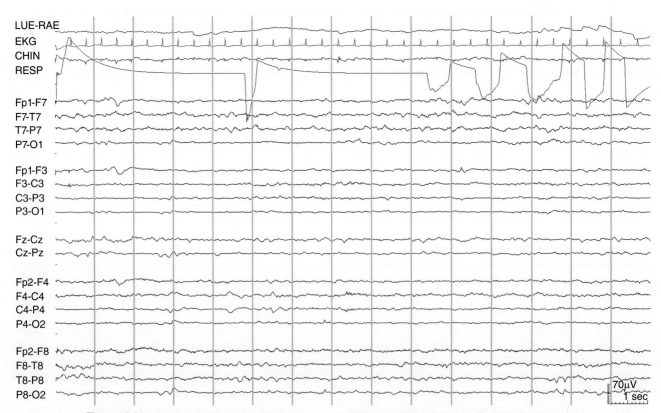

Figure 13.21 Although small amounts of electrocerebral activity are detected, nearly all activity in this tracing is below 20 μV and sleep features and cycling are lacking, signifying voltage depression. Note the high amplifier gains used as suggested by the scale in the lower right-hand corner. When persistent and if not explained by reversible causes, voltage depression is often associated with a poor neurologic prognosis.

Apart from suspecting widespread cortical damage as the explanation for low-voltage records, the electroencephalographer must consider other possible explanations. These include causes of diffuse scalp swelling, such as caput succedaneum or extensive subgaleal hematomas, or intracranial causes such as extra-axial fluid collections, such as subdural hematomas or hygromas or pus collections.

Burst-Suppression Patterns

Burst-suppression patterns consist of high-voltage bursts across the brain, in most patients bilaterally synchronous but in some interhemispherically asynchronous. The bursts are separated by flat periods (Figures 13.22 and 13.23). Burst-suppression patterns are persistent (i.e., they are not governed by a sleep-wake cycle), and they are usually not responsive to outside stimuli. When a burst-suppression pattern changes with outside stimulation, the prognosis is relatively improved. The diagnosis of burst-suppression in the neonate is somewhat more difficult because the normal discontinuous patterns in very premature newborns, tracé discontinu and tracé alternant, bear some resemblance to burst-suppression. It is usually not difficult to distinguish burst-suppression from tracé alternant, a pattern that has more interburst activity and that may include normal forms such as delta brushes. Tracé alternant should not be invariant, which is to say that it should appear and disappear during the recording as sleep cycling occurs. In fact, any pattern that cycles on and off should not be labeled burst-suppression, which is typically a monotonously persistent pattern. Tracé discontinu can be more difficult to distinguish from burst-suppression in very preterm infants. The diagnosis of burst-suppression in this post-conceptional age group should only be made with hesitation and should be confirmed by serial recordings. So-called *permanently discontinuous* patterns probably represent a variant of burst-suppression.

With some exceptions, burst-suppression is associated with a dismal neurologic outcome. Babies who show improvement on a 1-week follow-up EEG tend to do considerably better than those who do not. Aside from being associated with hypoxic-ischemic or hemorrhagic injury, a burst-suppression pattern is also the hallmark finding in several epileptic syndromes of infancy, including early myoclonic encephalopathy, early infantile epileptic encephalopathy, and pyridoxine-dependent seizures (these disorders are discussed in more detail in Chapter 10, "The EEG in Epilepsy"). High therapeutic levels of barbiturates may also contribute to the appearance of a burst-suppression pattern in newborns, but this effect is probably not common. Finally, monotonously discontinuous patterns seen in babies undergoing therapeutic hypothermia may not carry a dismal prognosis compared to true burst-suppression.

Electrographic Seizure Activity

The presence of electrographic seizure discharges in the EEG background is generally considered a poor prognostic sign; however, newborns who manifest seizure activity can be divided into different prognostic groups. The most distinctive of these groups is the newborn with repetitive seizures arising from the same location. Unilateral seizures are highly suggestive of a focal lesion, such as neonatal stroke or, less commonly, cerebral dysgenesis in that area. The prognosis in these babies depends on the nature of the underlying lesion.

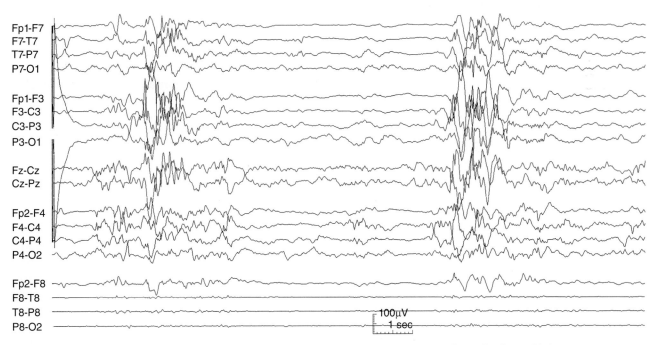

Figure 13.22 The burst-suppression pattern shown in this segment appears as "angry" polymorphic bursts of activity across both hemispheres separated by flatter periods. This pattern continued monotonously throughout the tracing. Note the lower voltages in the right temporal chain (bottom four channels) related to a subdural hematoma over the right temporal lobe.

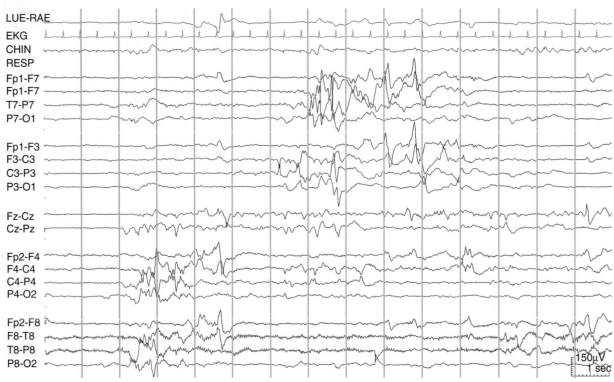

Figure 13.23 This unremitting burst-suppression pattern differs from the previous example in that the bursts occur asynchronously over each hemisphere. The lack of sleep cycling, either clinical or electrographic, during the rest of this recording confirms that this is a burst-suppression pattern rather than a normal sleep pattern.

Among those children with seizures arising from both hemispheres, children who only manifest sporadic seizure activity, as a group, have a better prognosis than those who have unremitting electrographic seizure activity (electrographic status epilepticus). In severely asphyxiated babies, continuous electrographic seizure activity may even progress to an ECI pattern, although some babies instead may show considerable improvement. Most babies with continuous seizures on EEG have sustained a significant neurologic injury.

Amplitude Asymmetries

When a persistent amplitude asymmetry is seen, the extra-axial causes of voltage asymmetry listed earlier (such as fluid collections in the various extra-axial spaces) should be excluded by the clinician. Asymmetries of 25% or more are generally considered significant. It is good practice to confirm a potential voltage asymmetry with a referential montage. Large voltage asymmetries may be caused by strokes, hemorrhages, or cerebral dysgenesis. Marked asymmetries may be associated with a poor prognosis, which is usually determined by the nature of the underlying lesion.

Generalized slowing and focal slowing are uncommon findings in newborn EEGs and are not considered standard abnormality types in the newborn EEG. The impression of focal slowing over one hemisphere may actually represent a voltage asymmetry, and the possibility that it is the opposite side that is abnormal because of low voltage should also be considered.

When amplitude asymmetries are transient, they may not be clinically significant. An unusual example of asymmetry is seen in prematures in whom one hemisphere may appear to "fall asleep" by attenuating before the other. This relatively uncommon phenomenon should only be seen once in a recording, in which case it is not considered abnormal.

Abnormal Sleep Architecture

It is difficult to appreciate sleep architecture abnormalities until 34 weeks CA. Sleep structure abnormalities range from a complete lack of sleep cycling to more subtle disruptions in expected sleep patterns. In many EEG records with abnormal sleep structure, the abnormal sleep architecture may be only one of many abnormalities present, and the coexisting abnormalities may have more prognostic significance. Abnormal sleep structure as a sole finding may have other possible explanations, such as sleep interruptions related to the intensive care unit environment, administered medications, and so forth. Furthermore, lack of normal sleep cycling as an isolated abnormal finding will often improve by the time of a follow-up tracing. Therefore, this is considered one of the milder background abnormalities, and many babies whose only EEG abnormality is abnormal sleep structure will eventually do well. Conversely, in a baby for whom there is worry of significant neurologic injury, the presence of normal sleep cycling can be considered a reassuring sign.

Immature Patterns and EEG Dysmaturity

Estimation of a baby's CA by EEG standards proceeds along two parallel pathways, summarized in Figure 13.24. The first step is depicted by the top three bars in the figure. These summarize the EEG pattern expected in each of the three sleep

POST-CONCEPTIONAL AGE IN WEEKS

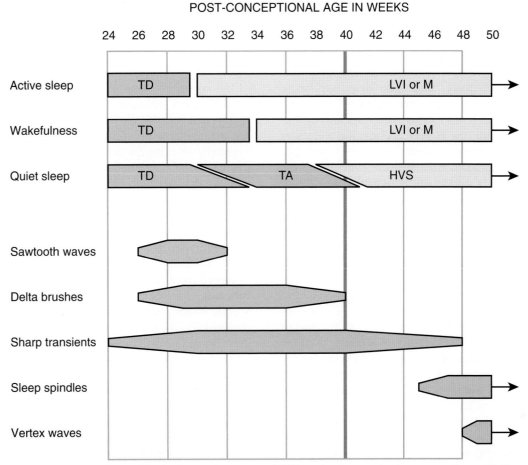

Figure 13.24 A summary of the background patterns and EEG graphoelements is shown according to CA. The group of three bars on the top of the figure refer to background patterns and the bottom five show the timing of the appearance of graphoelements. Note that the tracé discontinu pattern is seen in all sleep stages before 30 weeks CA, before which differentiation between wakefulness and sleep can only be made on the basis of the baby's clinical appearance and specific sleep stages are therefore hard to differentiate based on the EEG pattern alone. The continuous background patterns, LVI, M, and HVS, are highlighted in lighter red to emphasize the stages during which continuous activity is seen. The bottom five bars show the timing of the appearance and disappearance of different EEG graphoelements by CA. HVS = high voltage slow, LVI = low voltage irregular, M = mixed/medium pattern, TA = tracé alternant, TD = tracé discontinu.

stages: active sleep, wakefulness, and quiet sleep, according to CA. The bottom portion of the figure represents the second step: identification of graphoelements in the EEG and the CAs they are associated with. Each step of the analysis supplements the other. The top half of the figure shows that, before 30 weeks CA, the tracé discontinu pattern is generally expected in all sleep/wake states. For instance, if a baby has tracé discontinu in all states and temporal sawtooth waves are seen, the tracing would then be consistent with a CA of approximately 28 weeks. If a baby has well-established tracé alternant during quiet sleep and there are copious delta brushes, because delta brush activity is maximum at 34 weeks CA, the tracing would be suggestive 34 weeks CA.

The process is further fine-tuned by noting the quality of the tracé discontinu or tracé alternant pattern. As mentioned, in tracé alternant, interburst intervals become progressively shorter toward term, there is increasing activity seen during the interbursts, and interhemispheric synchrony increases. Although specific ranges for duration of interburst intervals have been suggested for different CAs, these figures

should not be handled too strictly, as abnormal developmental outcome for babies who have strayed outside these ranges has not been established. The voltage and amount of activity present during interbursts may also provide clues as to CA, with voltages <25 μV seen before 34 weeks, voltages of about 25 μV seen at 34 to 36 weeks, and voltages >25 μV after 37 weeks (Tsuchida et al., ACNS Guidelines, 2013). In that publication, the maximum duration for normal interbursts was set at 20 seconds for 30–33 weeks CA, 10 seconds for 34 to 36 weeks CA, and 6 seconds for 37 to 40 weeks CA. It was also acknowledged that a strict relationship between duration of interburst intervals and patient outcomes had not been settled. For that reason, and especially when it is the only abnormality, EEG records that show only small deviations from these stated normal values should only be considered mildly abnormal.

Taking all of these observations into account, this process may allow the reader to estimate the CA of a baby to within approximately 2 weeks. When the CA estimate based on the history and examination does not match the CA suggested by the EEG, it is worthwhile to reexamine the baby's clinical gestational age assessment. When the CA suggested by the EEG is more than 2 weeks earlier than the clinically derived CA, the EEG is said to have an immature or dysmature pattern. Such dysmature patterns should be considered a nonspecific abnormality and are considered to be among the mildest background abnormalities. The EEG should be more than 2 weeks "dysmature" before any clinical significance should be associated with the apparent developmental lag in EEG maturation. Examples of EEG dysmaturity could be a tracing of a 38-week CA baby that still shows copious delta brush activity (as might be seen at 34 weeks) or an excessively asynchronous tracé alternant pattern with flat interbursts near term (a stage by which the pattern should have become mostly synchronous and interburst activity should be richer). While babies whose only EEG abnormality is an immature pattern are presumed to have sustained a mild and possibly reversible neurologic insult, a large number of such babies are neurologically normal at follow-up.

ELECTROGRAPHIC SEIZURE DISCHARGES

Because many newborn EEGs are obtained with the goal of excluding or confirming the presence of seizures, the EEG reader is frequently called on to assess the EEG tracing for seizure activity. In contrast to the EEGs of older children and adults, the background of the normal newborn EEG contains little rhythmic activity. Familiar rhythmic forms such as the posterior rhythm and sleep spindles seen in the EEGs of older individuals have not yet appeared in the newborn EEG. The main continuous EEG background patterns of newborns, LVI, M, and HVS, consist of irregular activity; the discontinuous patterns of tracé discontinu and tracé alternant have even less of a tendency toward rhythmicity. Except in rare examples, as discussed subsequently, electrographic seizure activity in newborns consists of rhythmic activity. This fact makes identification of neonatal seizures considerably easier. *Any rhythmic activity of sufficient duration in the newborn EEG is suspicious for seizure activity.* Although historically the lower limit of discharge duration required by others to declare a rhythmic discharge an electrographic seizure has varied, a 10-second lower limit for ictal rhythmic discharges in neonates is reasonable, though admittedly arbitrary. Note that this limit is designed for electrographic-only seizures, which is to say it refers to EEG seizures without a clinical accompaniment. There is no declared minimum time limit for electro*clinical* seizures. EEG patterns that resemble seizures but last less than 10 seconds have been referred to as BRDS (i.e., brief rhythmic discharges, similar to the brief potentially ictal rhythmic discharges or BIRDS described in older patients and discussed in the previous chapter).

Typically, neonatal seizure discharges consist of rhythmic waves in a focal distribution, sometimes with sharp features and sometimes not. The morphology of the discharge can range from repetitive sharp waves, spikes, or even polyspikes, to a rhythmic sinusoidal pattern (Figure 13.25). In some cases the discharge can be so focal as to be confined to a single electrode (Figure 13.26) but even the most focal discharge will usually affect other nearby electrode contacts to some extent throughout its course, which can help distinguish such highly focal seizures from single-electrode artifact. During its evolution, a neonatal seizure discharge may migrate from one location to another in the involved hemisphere and may also appear to "spread" to the opposite hemisphere as in Figure 13.27, although an independent, simultaneous onset in the opposite hemisphere may also explain this appearance. Neonatal seizure discharges generally fire at a rate of 1 to 3 Hz and occasionally faster, although it is more common for seizure discharges to fire at the lower end of this range. Especially when the discharge is accompanied by clonic activity, the rate of the jerking is usually nearer one per second than the top end of this range.

It is said that newborns cannot have truly generalized seizures, and this is probably the case. For instance, generalized spike-wave discharges are not seen in the newborn. Presumably, the cortical circuitry of very young babies is not organized in a fashion capable of mounting generalized discharges. Mimics of generalized discharges can occur, however. In some cases, a baby may have a seizure discharge ongoing in both hemispheres at once. In many such cases, the discharges are not truly synchronous and the discharges are actually bilateral but independent (Figure 13.28). Clinically, a seizure is occasionally seen with bilateral extremity jerking, suggesting a generalized discharge. In some such cases, the EEG may show a unilateral discharge in which the seizure outflow causes bilateral synchronous limb movement. In such cases, close analysis may show that the movements may be of different intensity on each side. In other cases, close inspection reveals that the jerking movements are not synchronous but bilaterally independent.

Neonatal seizures that consist of nonrhythmic or non-repetitive discharges occur more rarely. For instance, high-voltage single generalized polyspikes may result in whole body myoclonic jerks. Tonic seizures and clonic seizures in newborns are usually associated with rhythmic seizure discharges. When a rhythmic discharge is identified in a newborn EEG, often the biggest challenge is distinguishing between a true seizure discharge and a rhythmic artifact related to breathing, the pulse, or equipment in the ICU setting.

CLASSIFICATION OF NEONATAL SEIZURES

Types of Possible Clinical Seizure Activity and Their Relationship to EEG Seizure Discharges

In 2020, a new classification scheme for neonatal seizures was proposed, distinct from the general ILAE seizure classification described earlier. Since the 1980s, the neonatal seizure classification in most common use has been Volpe's 1989 revision of his own previous classification. The seizure types included clonic, tonic, myoclonic (focal or generalized), and subtle seizures (Table 13.2). Even at the time (and based on the seminal work of Mizrahi and Kellaway), there was a clear understanding that certain of the seizure types listed in the 1989 revised classification, subtle seizures and generalized tonic seizures in particular, were usually not associated with a seizure discharge on EEG but they were included to keep the classification comprehensive as to the different types of movements newborns could manifest. Nevertheless, this distinction was often lost in summaries of the

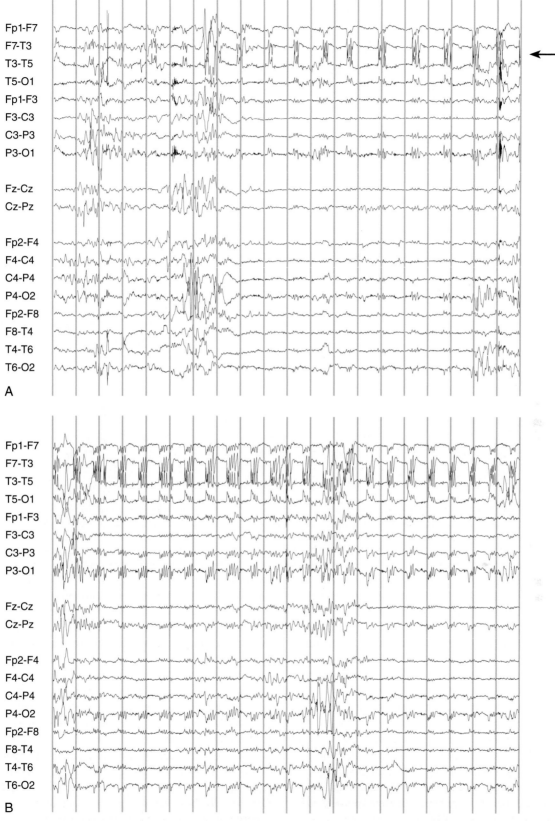

Figure 13.25 An electrographic seizure discharge is seen in the left temporal area, maximum in the left mid-temporal electrode, T3 (arrow). In this example, the discharge consists of a repetitive polyspike rather than a rhythmic sharp wave or slow wave. The discharge begins at the beginning of the first page (A) and increases in amplitude and complexity throughout its course, first spreading to the left occipital area (O1) and then to both occipital areas (O1 and O2) (B).

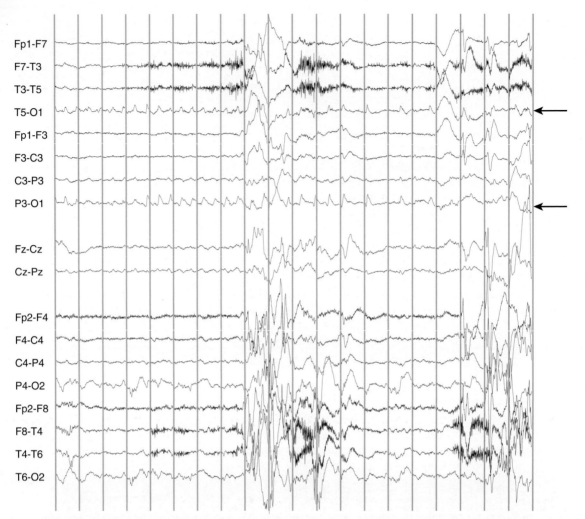

Figure 13.26 This seizure discharge begins as a run of rhythmic sharp waves recorded exclusively from the left occipital (O1) electrode (arrows). In some cases, a seizure discharge may start and stop remaining localized to a small area. For those worried that this deflection could represent a single-electrode artifact, note the small deflections in the C3-P3 channel that would not be present if the discharge were only related to a single electrode (O1). During the last 3 seconds of the page, however, the discharge can be seen to have rapidly spread to involve a broader area over the left hemisphere. The evolution of this discharge is shown in the next figure.

classification. This left many with the impression that, because they were present in the classification, these clinical behaviors were often believed to represent epileptic seizures in newborns. Historically, many unusual (and, indeed, abnormal) behaviors in newborns have been overdiagnosed as epileptic seizures by both neonatologists and neurologists alike.

In the original classification, subtle seizures described in neonates included movements such as "swimming," "boxing," or "hooking" movements of the upper extremities; "bicycling" movements of the lower extremities; orobuccolingual movements such as sucking or lip-smacking, eye opening, or complex eye movements; and pure apneas. Even at the time these classifications were introduced, these behaviors were controversial as to their cause as it was known that they were often not associated with a concurrent EEG seizure discharge. Indeed, rather than representing epileptic seizures, these behaviors may represent the unmasking of automatic reflex behaviors at times when the cerebral cortex is not functioning normally and is unable to suppress these reflex sequences. This question is of considerable importance because, if these behaviors are nonepileptic,

treatment with antiseizure medications would not be indicated. The story becomes even more complicated considering that, even if nonepileptic, these behaviors may be the result of cortical injury and may coexist with true EEG seizure discharges occurring at other times in the same baby. Finally, the fact that, for instance, persistent bicycling movements in a newborn may not, after all, represent seizure activity should not be perceived as all-together reassuring—the presence of the movements may still indicate a serious cerebral injury.

Among these subtle behaviors, apneas are perhaps the most difficult behavior to diagnose correctly. The great majority of apneas in newborns *are not related* to seizure activity. Occasionally, however, an epileptic seizure may manifest as a pure apnea in a newborn unaccompanied by clear motor or other behavioral change. Whether apneas in the newborn require EEG investigation depends heavily on the clinical context in which they occur.

The odds that an apparent clinical seizure event is associated with an EEG seizure discharge is strongly associated with the type of behavior observed. Not surprisingly,

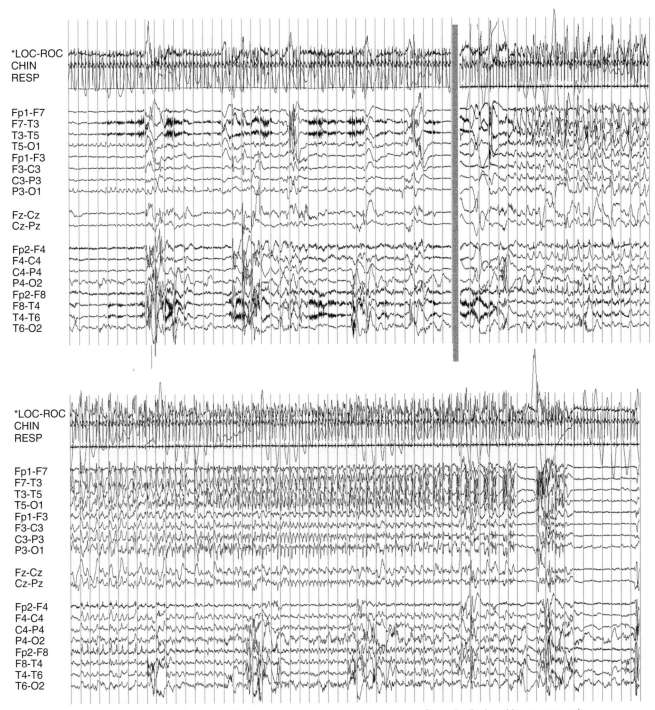

Figure 13.27 The seizure for which the onset is shown in the previous figure is displayed in compressed form to demonstrate its propagation. Each vertical division represents 1 second. The vertical gray bar denotes an area in which several seconds of the tracing have been removed to aid in the display. The seizure begins in the left occipital area and spreads more widely in the left hemisphere. Soon after the vertical gray bar, an independent discharge begins in the right hemisphere. Note that this pattern does not represent a generalized discharge as the seizure's firing frequency differs between the left and the right hemispheres. LOC = Left outer canthus, ROC = Right outer canthus.

simultaneous video/EEG recordings of babies at risk for seizures have shown that focal clonic activity is highly correlated to electrographic seizure activity. In contrast, whole body tonic stiffening, a dramatic clinical behavior that resembles the tonic phase of generalized tonic-clonic seizures in older subjects, does *not* have a strong association with EEG seizure discharges in newborns. In newborns, whole body stiffening may actually represent nonepileptic posturing in the setting of CNS dysfunction or perhaps a brainstem release phenomenon in a baby in whom cerebral cortex is not able to carry out its usual role in suppressing such behaviors. *Focal* tonic limb stiffening, however, is highly correlated with EEG seizure activity. Focal and multifocal myoclonic jerks are usually nonepileptic, but generalized myoclonic jerks have a higher

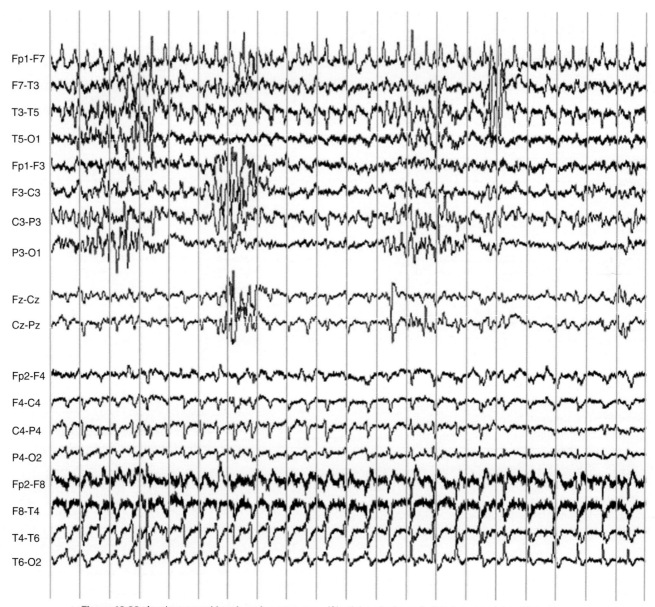

Figure 13.28 An electrographic seizure is seen to engulf both hemispheres in this term newborn. Close examination shows that the discharges in each hemisphere are bilateral but independent rather than synchronous.

TABLE 13.2	Volpe Neonatal Seizure Classification	
Clinical Seizure	Association With Electrographic Seizures
SUBTLE	Occasional
CLONIC	
Focal	Common
Multifocal	Common
TONIC	
Focal	Common
Generalized	Uncommon
MYOCLONIC	
Focal, Multifocal	Uncommon
Generalized	Common

Adapted from Volpe, 1989.

rate of association with seizure discharges on the EEG (see Mizrahi and Kellaway).

The new ILAE classification has made things somewhat clearer by discarding the old "subtle seizure" category, but it has been replaced by a category of "automatisms seizure," which may prolong the confusion. This most recent ILAE modification of seizure types and seizure syndromes for newborns had a goal of paralleling the general ILAE 2017 classification of seizure types for older patients (discussed in Chapter 10, "The EEG in Epilepsy"). Several differences in how neonatal seizure types should be classified, however, were immediately noted. First, almost all neonatal seizures are believed to be of focal onset. Because seizures with true generalized onsets in newborns are felt to be extremely rare, the usual first step of dividing seizures into those with focal versus generalized onsets was abandoned. Because assessment of awareness in newborns cannot be assessed ascertained in a practical way, the distinction of aware seizures versus those with impaired awareness was also not included. Likewise, because it is

TABLE 13.3 ILAE 2021 Classification of Electroclinical Neonatal Seizure Types

MOTOR
Automatisms
Clonic
Epileptic spasms
Myoclonic
Tonic
NON-MOTOR
Autonomic
Behavior arrest
SEQUENTIAL
UNCLASSIFIED

Adapted from Pressler et al. 2021.

essentially impractical to diagnose sensory, cognitive, and emotional phenomena in newborns, those seizure types are not part of the classification. Atonic seizures were not included because of the stated challenges of recognizing a sudden loss of tone in newborns who are often in the supine position.

At the same time, certain additions were made to the neonatal seizure classification. In recognition of the fact that a large fraction of newborn seizures are seen on EEG only and are not associated with clinical manifestations (especially in the setting of hypoxic-ischemic encephalopathy), electrographic-only seizures are now a part of the classification of newborn seizures. Finally, because it was felt that a distinctive seizure type occurs in newborns during which a sequence of seizure manifestations may occur sequentially in a particular order but without a single predominant feature, a sequential seizure type has been added. The classification of neonatal seizures with motor manifestations is shown in Table 13.3.

Again, the simple presentation of this list as above could seem to imply that all of these behavioral changes when observed in neonates may represent an epileptic seizure. In fact, the table that presents these seizure types in the actual classification publication annotates each seizure type with significant qualifying information, including that several of these manifestations are rarely epileptic, especially when they occur in isolation. This brings up a challenge in creating these classifications: balancing the goal of including all possible seizure types in the classification with the disadvantage of implying by their inclusion in the list that certain

specific behaviors that rarely represent seizure activity are, in fact, frequent clinical seizure manifestations in babies when they are not. A simple example of this would be an autonomic seizure manifesting by as an increase in heart rate. Although it is *possible* that an epileptic seizure may manifest solely by an increase in heart rate (and therefore merit inclusion in the classification), the percentage of episodes of isolated increased heart rate in newborns that are actually caused by epileptic seizures is vanishingly small. Automatism seizures are another good example of this problem. Most automatisms in newborns are oral, such as rhythmic or mechanical-appearing sucking movements on the endotracheal tube in an intubated infant. Such movements, especially in isolation, rarely represent epileptic seizure activity.

Clonic activity is the most reliably diagnosed seizure type in the newborn. Epileptic spasms are rare in the newborn, as the infantile spasms seen in West syndrome usually present after 3 months of age. Whole body tonic seizures/epileptic spasms are, however, the hallmark seizure type of the very rare early infantile developmental epileptic encephalopathy (previously early infantile epileptic encephalopathy or EIEE). Note that, outside of this syndrome, while focal tonic stiffening frequently represents epileptic seizure activity in the newborn, generalized tonic stiffening is very rarely an epileptic seizure manifestation in newborns, unless noticeably asymmetric. As mentioned above, autonomic signs such as changes in vital signs or apnea may occur alongside other seizure manifestations in newborns, but are only rarely the *sole* sign of epileptic seizures. Likewise, isolated behavioral arrest is very difficult to assess in newborns. Further descriptors for the five types of motor seizures—automatisms, clonic seizures, epileptic spasms, myoclonic seizures, and tonic seizures—are added, including unilateral, bilateral, bilateral symmetric or asymmetric, focal, or multifocal. Again, the completeness of this classification results in classified seizure types that are rarely thought to occur, such as bilateral clonic seizures (almost all such apparent examples show *asymmetrical* bilateral clonic activity when closely examined, driven either by a unilateral seizure discharge, or alternatively by bilateral independent discharges).

Table 13.2 serves as a reminder as to which types of clinical behaviors seen in newborns are most likely to represent true epileptic seizures. Focal and multifocal clonic activity often represent true seizure activity, as does focal tonic stiffening and generalized myoclonus. So-called subtle seizures, generalized tonic stiffening, and focal or multifocal myoclonus often do not represent epileptic seizures. Seizures that cause generalized, symmetric clonic activity, common in older patients (i.e., GTCs) are not expected in newborns.

REVIEW QUESTIONS

1. The concept of post-conceptional age (CA) is used because
   a. it is presumed that, in healthy babies, brain maturation proceeds at the same rate both inside and outside the womb, even when birth is premature.
   b. after premature birth, brain maturation proceeds at approximately half the rate compared to what it would have been in utero.
   c. it is easy to ascertain, even though the baby's body weight is a more reliable predictor of what EEG maturity should be than CA.
   d. a baby's CA is difficult to know with certainty, this parameter should not be relied upon in assessing neonatal EEGs.

2. In the case of premature babies,
   a. EEG electrodes should be applied by using a table of absolute measurements according to the baby's weight.
   b. the standard 10-20 method should be used determine electrode placement, just as it is used in adults.
   c. it is proper to apply electrodes at double-distance to compensate for the fact that the babies heads are smaller.
   d. electrode positions are usually visually estimated, because it is not practicable to measure an intubated premature baby's head.

3. The additional polysomnographic leads are applied for newborn EEGs because
   a. sleep disturbances are common in newborns.
   b. this is the best way to screen for apneas in newborns.
   c. the additional PSG measurements aid considerably in assessing sleep state.
   d. sleep state can be difficult to assess without information about chin EMG activity.

4. All of the listed neonatal EEG patterns are continuous except
   a. tracé alternant.
   b. LVI pattern.
   c. M pattern.
   d. HVS pattern.

5. Before 30 weeks CA, the only reliably continuous sleep state is
   a. wakefulness.
   b. active sleep.
   c. quiet sleep.
   d. None of the above.

6. In newborn EEG,
   a. tracé discontinu is considered the equivalent of burst-suppression.

b. tracé alternant is only seen during quiet sleep.
   c. active sleep in newborns evolves into slow-wave sleep in younger children.
   d. the mixed "M" pattern is a reliable sign of quiet sleep.

7. The tracé discontinu pattern
   a. is the hallmark pattern of extremely premature infants.
   b. consists of multifocal bursts.
   c. should not include periods of suppression longer than 10 seconds in otherwise normal prematures.
   d. is often seen as a precursor to seizure activity.

8. Regarding interhemispheric synchrony in the newborn EEG,
   a. it gradually increases with increasing CA.
   b. it gradually decreases with increasing CA.
   c. it starts out low, then reaches its peak just after 30 weeks CA, and then is lost by term.
   d. None of the above.

9. In quiet sleep,
   a. respirations are irregular.
   b. chin EMG activity is lower than in active sleep.
   c. the tracé alternant pattern predominates, then HVS.
   d. REMS can be seen under the baby's eyelids.

10. When considering the presence of EEG graphoelements in estimating CA,
   a. delta brushes peak at about 34 weeks CA.
   b. temporal sawtooths peak at about 28 weeks CA.
   c. temporal sharp transients are considered abnormal after 48 week CA.
   d. All of the above.

ANSWERS

1. ANSWER: **A.** If healthy, a baby's EEG is expected to evolve in the same fashion whether it is inside or outside the womb. Body weight is not used to assess GA as nutritional and many other factors can affect body weight. Even in premature babies, the GA can be established with certainty in most cases using data like the date of the mother's last menstrual period, dating from early fetal ultrasounds, and physical examination soon after delivery.

2. ANSWER: **B.** The advantage of the 10-20 measurement, which uses percentage measurements rather than absolute measurements, is that it can be used for all head sizes, from small prematures to adults. Only the very smallest premature babies require a reduced electrode set—the full 10-20 electrode set can be placed in most newborns. Electrodes are always placed based on tape measure measurements, not by visual estimation.

3. ANSWER: **C.** The main purpose for placing polysomnographic electrodes is as an aid to assessing sleep state rather than to diagnose sleep disorders in newborns. Although functioning respiratory channels on the EEG may aid in assessing sleep apneas, most hospitalized newborns are already on cardiorespiratory monitors that can alert the staff to apneas in real time. Of all the additional PSG electrodes, chin EMG activity may contribute the least in assessing sleep state.

4. ANSWER: **A.** The LVI, M, and HVS patterns are all continuous, mixed frequency patterns, differing mostly by their respective voltages. The tracé alternant pattern, however, is a discontinuous pattern.

5. ANSWER: **D.** Before 30 weeks CA, tracé discontinu, a discontinuous pattern, can be seen in all sleep states: wakefulness, active sleep, and quiet sleep. The first sleep state to become reliably continuous is active sleep, which occurs at 30 weeks CA or thereafter.

6. ANSWER: **B.** Although the tracé discontinu pattern does bear some resemblance to a burst-suppression pattern, its clinical significance is completely different from burst-suppression, which is a pathologic pattern. Instead, the tracé discontinu is a normal, physiologic pattern expected in very early prematurity. Tracé alternant is essentially seen in quiet sleep and perhaps in some transitional sleep states adjacent to quiet sleep. Active sleep evolves into REM sleep after the newborn period, not slow-wave sleep. The M pattern can be seen in any sleep state.

7. ANSWER: **A.** Tracé discontinu is the hallmark EEG pattern of extreme prematurity. The bursting pattern of tracé discontinu is a predominantly bisynchronous (rather than multifocal) bursting pattern. Periods of suppression in tracé discontinu may exceed 10 seconds, even in healthy premature infants, and the earliest prematures may have the longest periods of suppression. Although the bursts of tracé discontinu can contain angry-appearing

polymorphic activity, the pattern is not an indicator of impending seizure activity.

8. ANSWER: **D.** Interhemispheric synchrony does not steadily increase or decrease as very premature infants approach term. Rather, EEG synchrony follows a U-shaped curve. It is highly bilaterally synchronous in early prematurity (tracé discontinu), then becomes much less synchronous with the appearance of early tracé alternant, and then becomes increasingly synchronous near term with later tracé alternant.

9. ANSWER: **C.** In quiet sleep, respirations are highly regular. Chin EMG activity is higher in quiet sleep compared to active sleep. REMS seen under closed eyelids are a characteristic of active sleep rather than quiet sleep.

10. ANSWER: **D.** All of these listed benchmark CAs are characteristic of their respective graphoelements. For those who read neonatal EEGs, these figures are good to commit to memory.

SUGGESTED READINGS

Anders TF, Emde RN, Parmelee AH, editors: *A manual of standardized terminology, techniques and criteria for scoring of states of sleep and wakefullness in newborn infants*, Los Angeles, 1971, UCLA Brain Information Service.

Ellingson RJ: EEGs of premature and full-term newborns. In Klass DW, Daly DD, editors: *Current practice of clinical electroencephalography*, New York, 1979, Raven Press, pp 149–177.

Holmes GL, Lombroso CT: Prognostic value of background patterns in the neonatal EEG, *J Clin Neurophysiol* 10:323–352, 1993.

Hrachovy RA: Development of the normal electroencephalogram. In Levin KH, Lüders HO, editors: *Comprehensive clinical neurophysiology*, Philadelphia, 2000, WB Saunders, pp 387–413.

Dreyfus-Brisac C: Ontogenesis of sleep in human prematures after 32 weeks of conceptional age, *Dev Psychobiol* 3:91–121, 1970.

Lombroso CT: Neonatal polygraphy in full-term and premature infants: a review of normal and abnormal findings, *J Clin Neurophysiol* 2:105–155, 1985.

Mizrahi EM, Kellaway P: Characterization and classification of neonatal seizures, *Neurology* 37:1837–1844, 1987.

Monod N, Pajot N: Le sommeil du nouveau-né et du prématuré. I. Analyses des études polygraphiques (mouvements oculaires, respiration et E.E.G.) chez le nouveau-né à terme. [The sleep of the full-term newborn and premature infant. I. Analysis of the polygraphic study (rapid eye movements, respiration and EEG) in the full-term newborn], *Biol Neonat* 8:281–307, 1965.

Pressler RM, Cilio MR, Mizrahi EM, Moshé SL, Nunes ML, Plouin P, Vanhatalo S, Yozawitz E, de Vries LS, Vinayan KP, Triki CC, Wilmshurst JM, Yamamoto H, Zuberi SM: The ILAE classification of seizures and the epilepsies: Modification for seizures in the neonate. Position paper by the ILAE Task Force on Neonatal Seizures. Epilepsia. 62(3):615–628, 2021. https://doi.org/10.1111/epi.16815. Epub 2021 Feb 1.

Shewmon DA: What is a neonatal seizure? Problems in definition and quantification for investigative and clinical purposes, *J Clin Neurophysiol* 7:315–368, 1990.

Tharp BR: Electrophysiological brain maturation in premature infants: an historical perspective, *J Clin Neurophysiol* 7:302–314, 1990.

Torres F, Anderson C: The normal EEG of the human newborn, *J Clin Neurophysiol* 2:89–103, 1985.

Tsuchida TN, Wusthoff CJ, Shellhaas RA, Abend NS, Hahn CD, Sullivan JE, Nguyen S, Weinstein S, Scher MS, Riviello JJ, Clancy RR, American Clinical Neurophysiology Society Critical Care Monitoring Committee: American clinical neurophysiology society standardized EEG terminology and categorization for the description of continuous EEG monitoring in neonates: report of the American Clinical Neurophysiology Society critical care monitoring committee, *J Clinc Neurophysiol* 30:161–173, 2013.

Volpe JJ: Neonatal seizures: current concepts and revised classification, *Pediatrics* 84:422–428, 1989.

Zuberi SM, Wirrell E, Yozawitz E, Wilmshurst JM, Specchio N, Riney K, Pressler R, Auvin S, Samia P, Hirsch E, Galicchio S, Triki C, Snead OC, Wiebe S, Cross JH, Tinuper P, Scheffer IE, Perucca E, Moshé SL, Nabbout R: ILAE classification and definition of epilepsy syndromes with onset in neonates and infants: Position statement by the ILAE Task Force on Nosology and Definitions, *Epilepsia.*, 2022 May 3. https://doi.org/10.1111/epi.17239. PMID: 35503712

14

A Brief Introduction to Invasive EEG Monitoring for Epilepsy Surgery

Mark H Libenson, Aristides Hadjinicolaou, and Avantika Singh

INTRODUCTION

Thus far, the EEG studies we have been examining in this text have been recorded through the application of standard electrodes placed on the scalp or nearby. Of all EEG recordings done, the vast majority are, indeed, recorded via scalp electrodes. The purpose of this chapter is to serve as an introduction to EEG recordings obtained with invasive monitoring techniques, via electrodes placed either directly on the surface of the brain, or within the substance of the brain itself. This type of invasive EEG recording is performed in planning for epilepsy surgery, usually in specialized epilepsy surgery centers. Although the technique for electrode placement for invasive recordings differs greatly from that of applying scalp electrodes, the EEG patterns that are recorded from invasive electrodes are surprisingly similar to those of scalp recordings. This is to say that the large majority of the skills that you have learned while reading scalp-recorded EEGs will also be useful in the interpretation of invasive monitoring studies.

TYPES OF EPILEPSY SURGERY

In the broadest sense, there are multiple categories of surgical procedures used to help treat epilepsy and invasive monitoring techniques are not necessary for planning for all types. Epilepsy surgery can involve focal resections/ablations, disconnection procedures, or neuromodulation. For example, in corpus callosotomy, the corpus callosum, the massive bundle of axons that connects the two hemispheres, is severed to prevent propagation of focal seizures that arise in one hemisphere from spreading to involve both hemispheres. In some patients, a successful division of the corpus callosum can convert drop attacks that are the result of secondary generalization to more minor focal seizures since they can no longer spread to the opposite hemisphere. Neuromodulation may also be considered a subset of epilepsy surgery, including placement of a vagus nerve stimulator (VNS), a responsive neurostimulator (RNS), or a deep brain stimulator (DBS). Invasive monitoring is rarely necessary in preparation for VNS and DBS placement; RNS or DBS placement is sometimes chosen when a prior invasive monitoring study has shown that resective surgery is not safe or possible because of proximity of the seizure onset zone to eloquent cortex.

Rather, invasive monitoring is primarily done in the planning of *resective/ablative* epilepsy surgery, which is the broad category of epilepsy surgery described below and for which invasive monitoring plays a major role.

In the sense used here, resective/ablative surgery includes a few general types of surgical procedures whose purpose it is to disable the seizure onset zone. This includes actual resective procedures such as corticectomy (removal of an area of cortex), ablative procedures that use laser heating to destroy tissue, as well as focal disconnection procedures in which a defined area of brain is anatomically (and, therefore, electrophysiologically) isolated from the rest of the brain. In this form of disconnection procedure, instead of physically removing a larger region of cortex, that area of cortex is left in place along with its blood supply and drainage, but all neural connections from that area with the rest of the brain are severed. The practical result of a disconnection procedure is the same as would occur had that area been physically removed. Interestingly, seizures may continue to occur in disconnected cortex and even be recorded by later scalp EEGs, but they no longer have any impact on the rest of the brain or the patient's well-being as the abnormal activity is restricted to the isolated island of tissue and the activity is not transmitted elsewhere. In certain cases in which larger areas of cortex are involved, the disconnection technique is favored over resection because it has been found to be prone to fewer postoperative complications.

CANDIDACY FOR EPILEPSY SURGERY

Which patients are candidates for epilepsy surgery? Treatment with antiseizure medications leads to satisfactory control of seizures in approximately two thirds of patients with epilepsy. Patients are considered to have drug-resistant epilepsy if they have failed to achieve seizure control with two or more appropriately chosen antiseizure medications. This definition and the number of medications chosen for the definition are partly based on the statistical probability of a patient achieving seizure control once a first, second, third (and so on) medication has been tried and failed. In large groups of patients, it has been shown that, if seizure control has not been achieved after two appropriate medications have been tried, the chance that a third (or successive) medication will achieve control is well under 10%. It is a general policy that, to be considered a surgical candidate, the patient should have drug-resistant epilepsy. This guideline reflects the idea that, in most cases, if an individual can achieve excellent seizure control on medication without undue side effects, then the risks of a neurosurgical procedure should be avoided.

The ideal candidate for epilepsy surgery would be an individual in whom all of the seizures arise from one specific area in the brain, that part of the brain is not eloquent, and that part of the brain is accessible for surgery. All three of these concepts can benefit from additional discussion.

A Single Source of Seizures

If our goal is to cure a patient's seizures by resecting a particular area in the brain, it would be ideal if 100% of the seizures arose from the area of proposed operation. In certain selected cases, an exception is made to this rule. If approximately 90% of the seizures come from one area (and the exact cutoff percentage used is somewhat patient-dependent), a procedure may still be considered with the expectation that it will be "palliative." In such cases where it is known that the very large majority, but not all of the seizures, arise from the surgical target, the patient may be offered the procedure with the hope that, while complete seizure freedom will not be expected, the procedure may still allow the patient to benefit from a significant and meaningful reduction in seizure frequency.

Eloquent Cortex

In epilepsy surgery, injury to eloquent cortex is avoided. Although the term *eloquent* literally refers to speaking well, in the world of epilepsy surgery the term refers to any importantly functional area of cortex. This includes the language areas, both expressive and receptive (comprehension), but also includes principally the motor system, the sensory system, the visual system, and memory areas. A practical view of what it means to avoid eloquent cortex is that the resection will not result in undue or, ideally, any functional disability in the patient after the procedure. Significant effort is put into identifying areas of eloquent cortex and assessing their proximity to the proposed area of resection. The principal initial tool for identifying eloquent cortex is functional MRI (fMRI). However, with invasive electrodes in place, functional zones may be further defined through electrode stimulation ("cortical mapping"). By stimulating implanted electrodes, it is often possible to determine whether the electrode contact lies within a motor area (for example, the stimulus may cause the hand to contract or interrupt voluntary motor function), a sensory area (the stimulus may trigger a sensation), or a language area (the stimulus may interfere with the generation or comprehension of language). Alternatively, in patients who are old enough and cooperative, some amount of cortical mapping can be done during the resection procedure itself. In such cases, the patient is temporarily "woken up" from anesthesia with the cortex exposed and different areas are stimulated to identify function. For instance, awake intraoperative testing can help confirm that a particular area of cortex that was not previously recorded can be safely resected without damaging language function.

Surgical Accessibility

The concept of surgical accessibility has expanded in recent years. Certain areas of cortex are more difficult to access via open surgical techniques than others. For instance, operating on insular cortex (depicted in Figure 10.7 in Chapter 10, "The EEG in Epilepsy") via an open surgical procedure is considered a painstaking, lengthy, and risky procedure, mainly because this area lies behind the branches of the middle cerebral artery (MCA). Damage to even small branches of the MCA can lead to strokes in this highly functional area, making direct exposure of the insula challenging, and such procedures are often avoided for this reason. The more recent availability of laser interstitial thermal therapy (LITT) allows a minimally invasive approach to ablating epileptogenic tissue in the insula and other areas. With this technique, the target tissue is ablated by heating it with a laser that has been passed through the skull bone under stereotactic guidance. Other minimally invasive and non-invasive ablation techniques are in development and may become available in the near future.

ASSESSING PATIENTS AS CANDIDATES FOR EPILEPSY SURGERY

The assessment for candidacy for epilepsy surgery takes place in several steps and consists of the consideration of many different elements of the patient's story, including the patient's clinical information, a variety of formal testing and, of course, conventional EEG recording. The first step in attempting to localize a patient's seizure onset zone is analysis of the description of the seizure itself (the seizure's semiology). Patients with refractory epilepsy will likely already have a number of previous EEG recordings to analyze. This previous EEG data may already strongly point to a possible region of seizure onset via the location of interictal discharges and, in some cases, recordings of actual seizures from the scalp. Magnetoencephalography (MEG) studies may also furnish similar information.

The MRI is a pivotal test in the presurgical evaluation. The result of the MRI essentially divides patients into two groups: lesional and nonlesional. If an obvious MRI lesion has been identified as a likely source of the seizures, this can provide strong guidance for defining the proposed area of surgical resection and significantly increases the likelihood that any procedure will be successful. Persons who do not have a finding on MRI that points to the origin of their seizures are considered nonlesional cases. Nonlesional cases are considerably more challenging for surgical planning and, overall, have a lower success rate. In nonlesional cases, invasive monitoring is the principal technique used to identify the seizure onset zone.

PHASE I PRESURGICAL EVALUATION

A general schedule of evaluations called the *Phase 1 presurgical evaluation* is set up for individual patients to determine whether they are good candidates for epilepsy surgery. The

Phase 1 evaluation consists of an admission to an Epilepsy Monitoring Unit (EMU), which can last from a few days to a week or even longer. During this time, the patient is continuously recorded on conventional video EEG and seizures are recorded, if possible. Unless the patient is already having frequent spontaneous seizures at baseline, antiseizure medications may be reduced or discontinued in the EMU to facilitate the recording of seizures.

In addition to the MRI scan, a PET (positron emission tomography) scan may be performed. The PET scan creates a map of glucose utilization in the brain. Interestingly, *between* seizures, areas of cortex from which seizures arise tend to use *less* glucose than surrounding areas and, therefore, special attention is paid to darker areas on the scan. Some centers also use the technique of SPECT (single photon emission computed tomography) scanning, a technique that makes a map of cerebral blood flow at the time a radioisotope is injected. One SPECT scan is obtained in between seizures (the interictal SPECT scan) and another is obtained as soon after a seizure as possible, ideally only seconds after the seizure starts (the ictal SPECT scan). The interictal scan is then digitally subtracted from the ictal scan to show any zone of relative increased blood flow at the time of the seizure. This subtraction SPECT scan is then superimposed on the patient's MRI to aid in localization (this technique is also referred to as SISCOM: subtraction ictal SPECT coregistered to MRI). Finally, neuropsychological testing can also contribute to localization when there is a cognitive pattern suggestive of a lesion in a specific region.

LOCATING ELOQUENT CORTEX

The task of locating the region of brain from which the seizures originate is performed in parallel with the localization of different brain functions or "eloquent areas" and understanding their relationship to the seizure onset zone. For instance, if the patient's language resides in the left inferior frontal gyrus, whatever procedure is planned, it would be critical not to disturb that area in a way that might put the patient's language function at risk, as Broca's area typically resides in that area. Many eloquent areas are fairly consistently located in identifiable anatomical areas of the brain, such as visual cortex, which is nearly always located in the occipital lobes. As noted above, the primary technique for localizing functional areas of cortex is fMRI. Certain MEG techniques can also help localize certain functions. Additionally, transcranial magnetic stimulation (TMS) can be used to help identify the location of the motor cortex by delivering precise, brief magnetic pulses through the skull over different areas, looking for the locations that provoke a muscle twitch (usually in the hand). TMS may also be used to help identify expressive speech areas when a magnetic pulse over a specific location interrupts speech or generates a semantic error. The Wada test, a test during which one hemisphere of the brain is temporarily "put to sleep" by intracarotid injection of amobarbital was the original test used to help localize language and memory. The Wada test has been

substantially supplanted by fMRI, though it is still occasionally performed.

CONCORDANCE

The aim of collecting all these data through the tests mentioned above is to establish *concordance* of the data. Imagine a patient with refractory seizures whose seizure semiology strongly suggests an origin in the right temporal lobe, whose ictal and interictal EEGs show abnormalities in that area, and who has mesial temporal sclerosis in that temporal lobe on MRI. For such a patient with refractory seizures with that level of concordance of the clinical data, there would be considerable confidence that a right temporal lobectomy would be the appropriate operation. In such a case, intracranial monitoring may not even be necessary and the patient could conceivably go straight to surgery without the need for invasive monitoring. Of course, the clinical information gleaned from testing in real-world patients does not always line up as perfectly as it does in this example. In practice, it could be that the MRI finding is not as definite as suggested here, or that the EEG shows both some temporal discharges, but also discharges in other areas. In cases when concordance is not complete, additional information may be necessary to decide if a patient is a good candidate for epilepsy surgery and exactly what the best surgical procedure would be. In some cases, the findings may be so discordant as to indicate that the patient is not a viable candidate for resective/ablative surgery. In cases in which the Phase I information alone cannot adequately define the best surgical procedure for the patient, invasive monitoring may help define the target for resection.

PHASE II EVALUATION: INVASIVE EEG MONITORING

As mentioned, after the completion of a Phase I presurgical evaluation, certain patients with highly concordant data may be deemed appropriate for a single-stage resection. In such patients, the information gathered during the Phase I evaluation may be convincing enough as to the source of the seizures that the patient may go directly to surgical resection without invasive monitoring. The great majority of such cases are lesional cases. However, even in some lesional cases, it still may not be entirely clear whether the MRI abnormality is definitely the cause of the seizures, or the borders of the radiologic abnormality may not be clear. In others, there may be more than one MRI lesion and the identification of the causative lesion is not definite. In some, the MRI abnormality may partly overlie or be in close proximity to eloquent cortex. In such patients, invasive EEG monitoring may be necessary to best identify the borders of the epileptogenic zone. Likewise, in nonlesional cases, invasive monitoring may be the only way to define the epileptogenic zone.

THE CORTICAL ZONES

Although the concept of the epileptogenic zone has been around for many years, several different types of cortical zones involved in the generation of seizures were described and formalized by Rosenow and Luders. These zones are described here as they form a useful construct for thinking about how to plan and interpret invasive EEG monitoring studies.

The Epileptogenic Zone

The key cortical zone is the *epileptogenic zone.* The epileptogenic zone is defined as "the area of cortex indispensable for the generation of clinical seizures." Another way of thinking about the epileptogenic zone is that it is the smallest area of the brain which, if resected or disconnected, would result in the cessation of seizures. Therefore, the epileptogenic zone is the triggering area for seizures and without it, seizures, by definition, would not occur.

The Symptomatogenic Zone

The *symptomatogenic zone* is the area that, when involved with a seizure, produces the seizure's signs and symptoms (semiology). It is important to consider that the relationship between the epileptogenic zone and the symptomatogenic zone can vary. It is possible that the epileptogenic zone resides completely within the symptomatogenic zone, or alternatively it may be completely separate from it. If a patient happens to have a focal cortical dysplasia (FCD) precisely within the motor strip, that FCD may serve as the epileptogenic zone and when a seizure arises from it, cause immediate motor symptoms. Alternatively, a patient could have an epileptogenic zone in a silent area in the anterior frontal lobe. That patient's seizures may start in an anterior frontal area (anterior to the motor areas) and then spread posteriorly into the motor area where it causes the seizure's first (motor) symptoms. An outside observer may have the urge to believe that the seizure's triggering point was in the motor cortex because the seizure seemed to begin with motor symptoms; however, that would not be the case. Thus, in this example, the epileptogenic zone and the symptomatogenic zone are completely separate.

The Irritative Zone

The irritative zone is the area of brain that manifests interictal epileptiform discharges. These are usually detected by scalp EEG, MEG, or by invasive EEG studies. Although the irritative zone often overlaps with the epileptogenic zone, this need not always be the case. In some patients the irritative zone may be considerably larger than the epileptogenic zone.

The Seizure Onset Zone

The seizure onset zone is the area where the seizure actually starts. Although the definitions sound similar, the seizure onset zone may be larger than the epileptogenic zone, as only a subset of the area where the seizure is seen to start may be absolutely necessary to initiate a seizure. More rarely, the epileptogenic zone may be larger than the seizure onset zone. In such cases, if the seizure onset zone is completely resected, there may be remaining epileptogenic zone that did not participate in the patient's initially recorded seizures, but this area could still take over the seizure-triggering function after resection of the apparent seizure onset zone. In such

cases, which are fortunately less common, it is presumed that only the more frequent, low-threshold seizures were recorded during an invasive monitoring session, but higher-threshold areas of the epileptogenic zone that only trigger seizures more rarely are still capable of initiating seizures later. The seizure onset zone is often underestimated by invasive monitoring because the limited number of electrode positions in the brain may only be recording from a subset of the complete seizure onset zone.

The Epileptogenic Lesion

The epileptogenic lesion zone is usually defined by the high-resolution MRI, and less-so by PET scans. A patient may, however, have multiple potentially epileptogenic lesions and further EEG monitoring (scalp or invasive) may be necessary to sort out which is the causative lesion. When an epileptogenic lesion is present on MRI, an attempt to resect the entire lesion may be considered, but not possible. The comparative extent of the epileptogenic zone and epileptogenic lesion zone can vary in both directions. Especially with large lesions (e.g., tumors or strokes), there may be only one surface of the lesion that is actually triggering the seizures. In this case the epileptogenic zone may be considerably smaller than the lesional area. In some types of lesions (e.g., tubers, tumors, or cortical dysplasias), the seizures do not arise directly from within the lesions but from the cortex immediately adjacent to the lesion. In such cases, the lesion is felt to cause some type of irritative phenomenon in adjacent (perilesional) cortex. Alternatively, because of the limits of MRI resolution, MR images may somewhat underestimate the size of certain lesions, giving the impression that the seizure is arising from outside the strict confines of the radiologic lesion. Invasive monitoring with the placement of perilesional electrodes can help clarify these issues.

PLANNING AN INVASIVE IMPLANTATION

Surgical planning for electrode placement begins with a *hypothesis* that is formulated based on the presurgical evaluation described above. If it were possible to implant an unlimited number of electrodes and have contacts recording from every location in the brain at once, we could simply sit back and watch a hypothetical whole-brain recording of how and where the seizures start and spread out like a motion picture. In such a fantastical world, electrode placement would not require a lot of pre-planning or thought because every conceivable cortical location would be covered. Of course, in actual practice there are significant constraints to the number of contacts that can be safely placed in the brain as each additional electrode array or depth electrode confers a small but incremental risk to the patient, so this hypothetical "whole-brain implantation" is not practicable.

Implicit to the strategy of forming the pre-implantation hypothesis is the process of significantly narrowing down the list of possible epileptogenic zones that need to be demonstrated or excluded by the invasive monitoring study. The surgical implantation is designed to prove or disprove the main hypothesis, or to prove or disprove one of the alternative hypotheses, and also to clarify practical surgical questions such as the specific boundaries of the resection. For instance, a patient may have seizures that appear to arise from the temporal lobe but, before performing a temporal lobe resection, the possibility that the seizures may be coming from the insula or cingulate gyrus must also be tested. Thus, an implantation would be designed to establish from which of these regions the seizures are coming. Implantation plans without a coherent hypothesis often become "fishing expeditions" and are characterized by high numbers of electrodes that are trying to cast too wide a net because the areas of interest have not been sufficiently narrowed.

GENERAL IMPLANTATION STRATEGIES AND THE KEYHOLE PROBLEM

Imagine that you are implanting a patient in whom you strongly suspect that seizures are starting in the anterior temporal lobe. Based on your suspicion, you decide to place three electrodes in the suspicious anterior temporal lobe. You start the recording session and are pleased to see that the seizures are, indeed, present on those three electrodes, as expected. Believing you have chosen the right spot, you decide to resect the temporal lobe—but that decision, of course, would be premature. Although it is quite possible that you have, in fact, recorded the onset of the seizure successfully in the temporal lobe, it is also quite possible that the seizure started elsewhere (for instance the posterior temporal lobe, which you have not implanted), and subsequently spread to your three anterior temporal electrodes after onset. In this scenario, the true seizure onset zone is in the posterior temporal lobe and your planned anterior temporal lobectomy would not eradicate the patient's seizures. This illustrates the "keyhole" problem. If you are peering into a room through a keyhole, you can only see people and objects directly in front of the keyhole, but you would have no knowledge of people and activities in other parts of the room. Similarly, during an implantation, we can only see the area recorded by our implanted electrodes and we do not get information about what is happening in surrounding areas. Imagine four contiguous areas of brain: A, B, C, and D, and, in this case, the patient's seizures start in A and subsequently spread to B, to C, and then to D. If our implantation is designed only to record from positions C and D, we will observe during our recording that the seizure appears to start in C and then spreads to D. Such a recording could lead us to believe that C triggered the seizures, which then spread to D. We would be unaware that the true sequence of seizure spread was A to B to C to D and that A is the actual triggering epileptogenic zone. In theory, a well-planned implantation would help us to avoid this problem.

Ideally, our implantation would be planned in such a way that we have a *negative margin*. If we had designed our anterior temporal lobe implantation example such that, just posterior to the three active electrodes in the anterior temporal lobe, there was a row of EEG-negative electrodes, then our recording would be more convincing that the seizure did, indeed, start in the anterior temporal lobe rather than flow into the

anterior temporal lobe from some other location. Another clue to the possibility that the keyhole effect is at work might be if the patient's seizure symptoms start before the seizure onset is seen on the invasive electrodes. This would suggest that the seizure may have already started in some unrecorded area before appearing on our electrodes. Clearly, the optimal placement of invasive EEG electrodes is both an art and a science. It should be based on a well-thought out hypothesis and ideally establish negative margins for the resection as well.

INVASIVE ELECTRODE TYPES: GRIDS AND STRIPS VERSUS STEREO EEG ELECTRODES

Grids and Strips

There are two main types of procedures for invasive surgical monitoring based on the type of electrode hardware used. The first type is called *subdural grids and strips*. Grids and strips refers to electrode arrays that can be placed directly on the surface of the brain for the purpose of recording the cortical surface EEG. Many different sizes of grids are manufactured, such as 4 x 8 or 8 x 8 grids or arrays. Narrower arrays, such as 2 x 8 or 1 x 6 configurations, can be referred to as "strips" (Figure 14.1). For example, a combination of grids and strips could be placed over the parietal convexity, wrapped around the temporal lobe, or slipped between the hemispheres in the interhemispheric fissure. In certain cases, both grids and strips and depth electrode techniques can be combined—with the cortical surface exposed, depth electrodes can be manually placed alongside the grids and strips under direct visualization, perhaps with ultrasound guidance to aid in avoiding vessels. To place grids and strips, a window of skull bone must be removed (craniotomy) to expose the cortical surface. The

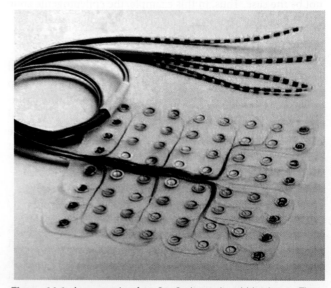

Figure 14.1 An example of an 8 x 8 electrode grid is shown. These electrode arrays are designed to record directly from the surface of the brain. Because of its relatively large size, this type of grid is often placed over the frontoparietal convexity. The four tails at the top of the image are color-coded and placed in a coupling device so that the position of each contact is preserved.

"tails" of the electrodes are tunneled out through the skull bone to allow for recording and the bone window is replaced. The patient's EEG is then monitored from these invasive electrode arrays for a period of time in the hospital, typically for about a week, though the duration can vary widely depending on how quickly seizure and other information is gathered. After this recording period, the patient returns to the operating room for removal of the grids and strips, and any cortical resection is done at the same time.

Subdural grids and strips have the additional advantage of allowing for orderly mapping of the cortical surface for the purpose of locating the motor areas, language areas, and so forth. This mapping can be done at the bedside after the patient has returned from the operating room and feels well enough to cooperate with the mapping. The geometry of an electrode array can be easier to understand compared to the relative positions of multiple stereo EEG electrodes recording from different structures at different angles.

Of course, the main disadvantage of subdural grids is that they can only record from the surface of the brain. Additionally, the positions in which they can be placed are limited by the location of the craniotomy. Certain placements, such as the interhemispheric fissure, can be challenging or even impossible in certain patients based on the anatomy of bridging vessels in that area. Patients who have had prior intracranial surgery can develop scarring and adhesion of the brain to the dura that can require painstaking and potentially injurious surgical dissection of the dura off the brain to permit grid placement. Areas of potential interest in deeper areas, such as insular cortex, are not accessible to recording with grids and strips. Finally, compared to the sEEG technique described below, the placement of grids and strips requires a craniotomy for placement and patient comfort is much more variable with this procedure, partly because of the additional volume of the "hardware" placed on the surface of the brain and possible fluid collections that may accumulate around the grids after placement.

Stereo EEG Electrodes

The second technique is stereo EEG (sEEG), in which depth electrodes are placed through small burr holes in the skull under precise stereotactic guidance in their desired locations. These long, thin electrodes, which can be under a millimeter in diameter, are typically available in a variety of lengths and contact spacing, ranging from approximately 4 to 18 contacts per electrode (Figure 14.2). A sEEG electrode has the potential to record from multiple disparate brain regions, such as the middle frontal gyrus at its entry point and the orbitofrontal gyri at its distal end. Subdural scarring does not limit sEEG electrode placement, but deficient skull, large cortical vessels, and cosmetic considerations can limit options for electrode trajectories. After placement of sEEG electrodes, the patient is similarly recorded for varying lengths of time. Again, one week is typical, though longer recording times are more feasible with this technique as patients with implanted sEEG electrodes tend to be more

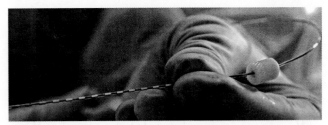

Figure 14.2 Before insertion, the stereo EEG electrode has a stylet (upper right of image) that stiffens the electrode and allows the neurosurgeon to maintain a straight insertion path for the electrode. The stylet is removed after electrode insertion. The electrode pictured has a diameter of 0.8 mm.

comfortable than those with grids and strips and the risk of infection may be lower, too. The electrodes are removed at the end of the recording period and some epilepsy surgery centers complete any cortical resection/disconnection or laser ablation at a later time, while others complete whatever procedure has been decided upon under the same anesthesia that is used for electrode removal.

The comparative advantages and disadvantages of the grids and strips versus the sEEG techniques have been debated through the years. Interestingly, in North America, between the two approaches, the grids and strips technique was historically the standard, especially before approximately 2015. At the same time, in Europe, and in particular, in France and Italy where the technique was pioneered, placement of stereo EEG electrodes has been the dominant technique for years. However, since approximately 2015, there has been a steady shift toward the use of stereo EEG implantations in North America and other parts of the world as well, and this is becoming the dominant technique in both North America and Europe.

Evolution of the Stereotactic Technique

Although others performed the very first stereotactic electrode implantations, the technique of placing multiple depth electrodes into the brain under stereotactic guidance for the study of epilepsy was predominantly pioneered and advanced by Bancaud and Talairach in Paris in the 1950s. To facilitate precise targeting of different brain structures, they created a detailed anatomical atlas of the human brain based on a three-dimensional coordinate system. This system was based on a line that joined the superior aspect of the anterior commissure and the inferior aspect of the posterior commissure when viewed from the side, which they called the *CA-CP line*. In addition, they defined vertical lines through the midpoint of each commissure, VCA and VCP. The anterior and posterior commissures were chosen because these structures were visible on pneumoencephalograms, the main brain imaging technique at the time. Bounding lines consisting of the most anterior, posterior, lateral, and inferior surfaces of the different lobes of the brain were then used to frame a three-dimensional grid whose subdivisions were proportional rather than absolute to accommodate brains of different sizes (Figures 14.3 and 14.4). Through post-mortem brain studies, they determined the anatomical location of different brain

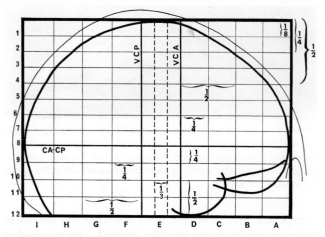

Figure 14.3 The Talairach proportional grid system is based on a lateral view of the brain using the anterior commissure and posterior commissure to define the "basal brain" or CA-CP line (CA = commissure antérieure, CP = commissure postérieure), which lies in the "interhemispheric medial plane" (midsagittal plane). Further anatomical lines were defined as VCA and VCP passing vertically through the anterior and posterior commissures, respectively. From there, a proportional grid was constructed using columns equal to the spacing between the VCA and VCP lines. The grid was then further subdivided in eighths, thirds, and quarters as shown. (Talairach J, Tournoux P: *Co-planar stereotaxic atlas of the human brain. 3-dimensional proportional system: An approach to cerebral imaging. Translated by Mark Rayport.* New York, 1988, Thieme Medical Publishers).

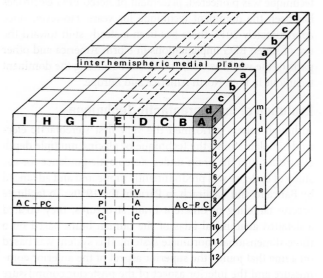

Figure 14.4 The interhemispheric medial plane grid shown in the preceding figure was then expanded laterally in the leftward and rightward directions to create orthogonal parallelograms as shown. Capital letters were used to denote columns in the antero-posterior direction, lowercase letters to denote columns in the transverse direction, and numbers for the various axial slabs, as shown. In this way, any specific parallelogram could be referenced with the combination of an upper case letter, a lowercase letter and a number, such as the shaded example of Ad1. An anatomical atlas was then created based on post-mortem brain studies that matched key brain structures to the various parallelogram coordinates of this system. Using this coordinate system and the known locations of various anatomical structures within this system, electrodes could then be passed through a special frame to specific depths in such a manner that specific brain structures could be accurately targeted and recorded. (Talairach J, Tournoux P: *Co-planar stereotaxic atlas of the human brain. 3-dimensional proportional system: An approach to cerebral imaging. Translated by Mark Rayport.* New York, 1988, Thieme Medical Publishers).

structures in this x-y-z coordinate system. Different anatomical structures could then be targeted by passing depth electrodes through the specific small slots of a metal grid (a "Talairach frame") stabilized rigidly adjacent to the patient's skull. Lateral angiography was performed to confirm that proposed trajectories would not damage blood vessels. This impressive work was done before the CT and MR imaging era. The great majority of the electrodes they placed were, therefore, orthogonal (i.e., parallel to the coronal, sagittal, or transverse planes), with occasional exceptions.

The placement of stereotactic EEG leads is now done using targeting computer software that uses the patient's own MRI on which the patient's vascular imaging (such as CT angiography) is superimposed by careful co-registration onto the MRI to confirm the safety of each trajectory. Stereo EEG electrodes can be placed using a stereotactic head frame, though specialized stereotactic robots are now available that can significantly speed up the procedure and minimize the risk of calculation error. These robots provide an accurately positioned entry guide for each pre-planned trajectory through which the neurosurgeon passes each electrode based on parameters from the electrode implantation plan. Thus, a nearly limitless variety of both orthogonal and oblique trajectories is possible, though entry points need to be reasonably perpendicular to the patient's skull to assure accurate implantation and good fixation. Also, certain entry points, such as the forehead, are not preferred so as to avoid a poor cosmetic result.

Whether by grids and strips or sEEG electrodes, intracranial EEG studies can provide beautiful, effectively artifact-free and informative recordings of seizure onsets and the networks by which they spread. The success of any particular implantation is highly dependent on the process for planning exactly where the electrodes will be placed and whether the recordings they generate are able to clearly support or refute the pre-implantation hypotheses. Stereo EEG electrodes have the impressive ability to describe a seizures onset and spread in three-dimensional space. An important advantage of sEEG electrodes over grids and strips is the ability to record from and resolve seizure activity in deep structures (such as the insula) that are effectively not accessible to recording on grids. Grid implantations have the advantage of allowing an orderly and dense interrogation of a cortical surface for cortical functions such as the sensory, motor, and language areas compared to sEEG electrodes. What follows are descriptions of implantations and recordings of two different patients with intractable seizures, one by the subdural grids and strips technique and one by implantation of sEEG electrodes.

EXAMPLES OF INVASIVE RECORDINGS

Subdural Grid Placement for Temporal Lobe Epilepsy

The strategy behind performing a grids and strips procedure for an 8-year-old boy with a 3-year history of refractory seizures is shown. The seizures consisted of staring, lip-smacking, and picking at his shirt, followed by bilateral motor activity. His MRI was normal. His scalp EEG showed both interictal discharges and actual seizures arising from the left temporal lobe. His language was found to be on the left side by fMRI. Based on these findings, the boy was presumed to have left temporal lobe epilepsy and the plan was to further delineate the seizure onset zone using grids and strips.

The planning for the placement of subdural grids started with drawing a cartoon of the proposed grid placement (Figure 14.5). Note the challenges of depicting the position of the 2 x 8 grids, which are flat when taken out of the package but are flexible enough to be wrapped around convex cortical surfaces. The strategy for this case was to wrap four 2 x 8 grids around the lateral temporal lobe going from front to back, with the distal contacts of these grids (the contacts farthest away from the electrode tails) recording from the floor of the temporal lobe. The fifth, left-most grid depicted in the figure records from the frontal lobe just above the Sylvian fissure and extends to record the subfrontal area as well. A 1 x 8 strip was slipped along the mesial temporal surface. The goal of this placement strategy is to record from extensive areas of the lateral temporal lobe, the base of the temporal lobe, and the mesial temporal lobe surface to design the best resection

that would identify the seizure onset zone and also allow for functional testing at the bedside. The subfrontal grid was placed to exclude the unexpected possibility that the seizures were actually of frontal origin.

The planning cartoon represents a pre-operative vision of where the grids will go; however, the patient's own anatomy, including the location of larger blood vessels, can require variations from the proposed pre-operative plan that will be decided in the operating room at the time of grid placement. The operative photograph shown in Figure 14.6 shows the relationship of the grids to one another when they are actually placed, and also documents the positions of each grid's "tail" (the wire that carries the electrical information from the contact to the recording apparatus). Tail position is important because the tail is always adjacent to the highest electrode numbers on the grid (e.g., 8 and 16 in the case of a 2 x 8 grid) and also helps confirm the grid's orientation on x-rays and scans. Tail position aids in confirming the orientation of the grid and helps avoid serious errors such as misinterpreting information from the tracings incorrectly thinking that the strip's position is rotated 180° from its true position. Note that, in the operating room picture, only a portion of the grids is visible as the neurosurgeon has slipped each grid under the

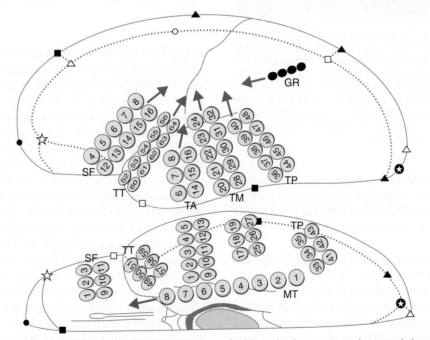

Figure 14.5 As part of the planning for the placement of grids and strips, a cartoon is created showing the proposed positions of the various grids and strips to achieve the desired coverage. Note that the top half of the cartoon shows the left hemisphere as viewed from the side, and the bottom of the image shows the basal view of the left hemisphere. Proceeding from left to right, a subfrontal grid (SF) is proposed for the lateral frontal lobe with the distal contacts continuing to the floor of the frontal lobe. A series of four 2 x 8 temporal strips, TT, TA, TM, and TP (abbreviated to denote the temporal tip, and the anterior, medial, and posterior portions of the temporal lobe), is then wrapped around the lateral surface of the temporal lobe with the distal contacts of the strips continuing to the floor of the temporal lobe. A 1 x 8 strip, MT (mesial temporal), is threaded around the temporal lobe tip to the mesial surface of the temporal lobe. Four grounding electrodes are seen in the upper right. Note that, for every grid and strip, the position of its tail, denoted by the arrows, is always adjacent to the highest contact numbers in each row on the array (e.g., contacts 8 and 16 are nearest the tail for the SF grid and contacts 1 and 9 are most distal). Once in the operating room, it may not always be possible to place the grids and strips exactly as was planned before the procedure. GR = ground; SF = subfrontal; TT = temporal tip; TA = anterior temporal; TM = medial temporal; TP = posterior temporal; and MT = mesial temporal.

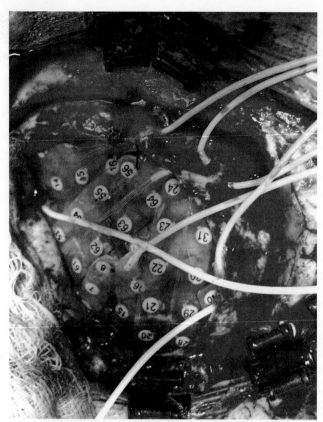

Figure 14.6 Photographs of the grid placement are taken in the OR to confirm the positioning of the arrays. The placement of the TT, TA, and TM grids are easy to match to the cartoon. Comparing the cartoon to this photograph, only contacts 14 and 15 are easily visible from the SF grid. Only contact 40 (the corner contact) is visible from the posterior temporal grid, TP. Only the tail of the MT grid is visible as the 1 x 8 strip has been slipped around the temporal lobe tip to run along the mesial temporal surface. Some of the electrode tails have already been tunneled through the dura.

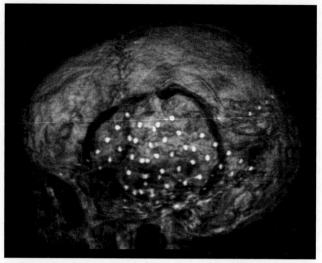

Figure 14.7 After the grids and strips have been placed, a CT-scan reconstruction is created with a special technique that changes the color of the electrode contacts based on their radiodensity to make their identification easier. A single image is shown from this postoperative CT, but the image can be "tumbled" in multiple planes to better understand the relative position of each contact. Note the hook-shaped lucency created by the bone window. The bone window was temporarily replaced immediately after placement of the subdural electrodes but will be removed and replaced again when the grids are removed at the end of the recording period and any resection is performed.

edge of the opening of the dural and bone window to reach its desired location. In practice, the final position of the grids as placed is usually similar to, but always differs to some extent from, the pre-operative proposed placement as drawn in the cartoon.

It may come as a surprise to learn that, even though the grids are placed under direct vision, it is not always completely clear where the exact positions of all the contacts are once they have been placed. This is explained both by the fact that parts of the grid are hidden under the skull bone, but also because, even under direct visualization, the identity of each of the exposed gyri is not always obvious. Figure 14.7 shows just one of many images that would be reviewed to confirm the location of all of the contacts in this case. This image is one of a series of images that can be "tumbled" in multiple directions to better understand the location of each contact in multiple planes. For instance, it will not be certain where the distal contacts of the TA grid seen in Figure 14.6 have reached until the post-operative scans have been reviewed.

Figure 14.8 shows the interictal recording obtained from a subset of the recording grids and strips placed in this patient. Note that the main discharges are seen in contacts TA 1 and

2, and TA 9 and 10. Post-operative scans confirmed that the positioning of these contacts is similar to what is depicted on the pre-operative cartoon of the grids shown in Figure 14.5. These four contacts are located on the base of the temporal lobe. Lower voltage discharges are also seen synchronously on the mesial temporal electrode contacts MT 5, 6, 7, and 8. This finding is harmonious with the placements indicated on the cartoon since contacts MT 5 through 8 are predicted to be very close to contacts TA 1, 2, 9, and 10. The precise relationship among all of these electrodes can best be determined by the various scans obtained after the grid placement.

Figure 14.9 shows that, in this patient's case, the patient's spontaneous seizure discharges do arise from the exact same location as the interictal discharges that were seen in the previous figure (though this is not always the case). Because the contacts on the TM grid that is situated just posterior to TA were not active with the discharges, this provided a good negative margin for planning the resection. After functional mapping confirmed that the patient did not rely on this region for language function, an anterior temporal lobectomy was done as shown in Figure 14.10. The patient had an excellent result from the procedure, achieving seizure freedom.

Stereo EEG Electrode Placement for Temporal Lobe Epilepsy

This 13-year-old right-handed girl had a 6-year history of weekly seizures that failed to respond to four antiseizure medications. She described that, during her seizures, she heard a repetitive banging sound and echoing in her ears during which she

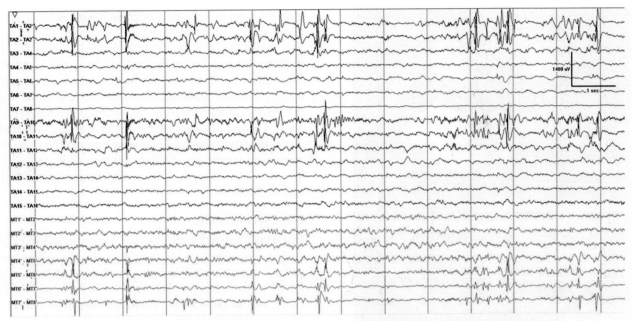

Figure 14.8 Only the tracings from the TA grid and MT strip are shown here for the sake of clarity. Discharges are seen on the most distal contacts of the TA grid: TA 1 and 2, and TA 9 and 10. Note the location of these contacts on the cartoon drawing. At the bottom of the tracing, synchronous interictal discharges are seen on the MT strip: MT contacts 5, 6, 7, and 8. The OR cartoon suggests that these contacts are adjacent to the active TA contacts and that all of these contacts are grouped together on the basal and mesial surfaces of the temporal lobe.

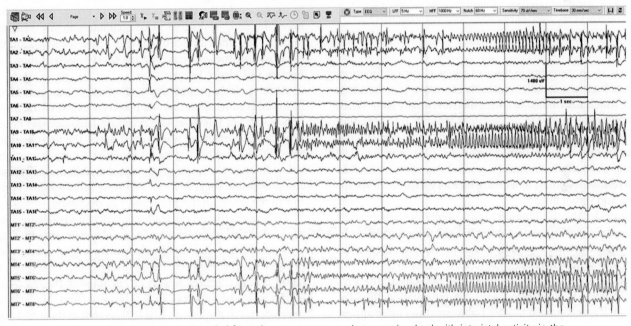

Figure 14.9 A seizure is recorded from the same contacts that were involved with interictal activity in the previous figure. In this patient, the seizures arose from the same location as the interictal activity, though that is not always the case.

was unable to understand the speech of those around her. The episodes often progressed to whole body jerking movements. Several of her typical seizures were captured on scalp EEG and showed left midtemporal to posterior temporal (T7/P7) onsets. Her MRI revealed an area suspicious for focal cortical dysplasia in the left temporal area, primarily in the middle temporal gyrus (Figure 14.11). Her PET scan showed a definite area of left

temporal glucose hypometabolism in a similar but somewhat larger region of the left temporal lobe (Figure 14.12).

Functional MRI (fMRI) showed left-sided language lateralization, though there was atypical additional contribution from the left frontal and temporal areas suggesting that her language area had undergone a degree of reorganization. This kind of functional rearrangement is not uncommon; when

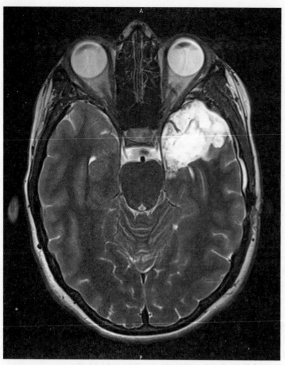

Figure 14.10 The patient returned to the operating room for removal of the grids and strips and, during the same procedure, a left anterior temporal lobe resection was performed as shown in this T2-weighted MRI scan in which the cerebrospinal fluid appears white. During the procedure, the exact positions of the active electrodes (TA 1, 2, 9, and 10 and MT 5, 6, 7, and 8) could be confirmed under direct vision.

there is an abnormality in the area where a cortical function, such as language, usually resides, that function often becomes more widely distributed in cortex than is typically seen. When such rearrangements occur, functions typically transfer either to areas adjacent to their usual location, or to homologous areas in the opposite hemisphere. Her neuropsychological testing showed above-average general cognitive ability but with relative weakness in working memory, expressive vocabulary, and verbal fluency.

Consider the thinking up to this point. The patient's seizure semiology suggests a potential seizure onset in auditory cortex, which is usually found in the lateral temporal lobe. The scalp EEG data with seizure onsets in T7/P7 also suggest a mid- to posterior temporal lobe onset. The PET scan finding is concordant with the information thus far, though it is recognized that PET abnormalities often appear to encompass a region somewhat larger than the true area of electrical abnormality. Finally, the MRI also localizes the lesion to lateral temporal cortex, albeit with indistinct margins.

A stereotactic EEG placement was planned in a collaborative fashion between the epilepsy neurologists and neurosurgeon with the goal of defining the boundaries of the patient's seizure onset zone, especially considering that the MRI lesion did not have sharp boundaries. Electrodes were placed even more posteriorly than the presumed area of seizure onset to facilitate mapping of her receptive language area, and also

with the hope of defining a negative margin for a safe, language-sparing resection. A schematic cartoon of the lateral and medial views of the patient's planned stereotactic EEG implantation is shown in Figure 14.13. Note that the goal of the implantation is to establish that the seizures are, indeed, coming from the radiologic lesion, but also to establish negative margins around the lesion and also to aid in mapping language. Figure 14.14 shows the appearance of sEEG electrodes in the operating room when placed through the scalp. The convention for naming sEEG electrodes used in this text follows the SENSA system, which is described at the end of this chapter, though other naming systems are also in use.

Interictal Recordings

Interictal discharges were observed soon after the recording started. Frequent spikes were seen from the superior temporal gyrus in the superficial contacts (T1bIb 6 and 7). In this case, the electrodes directly within the lesion in the middle temporal gyrus (T2a and T2b) did not happen to manifest interictal discharges (Figure 14.15).

Ictal Recordings

Thereafter, numerous typical seizures were captured (Figure 14.16). The earliest evidence of seizure onset was seen simultaneously in T2b (within the suspected lesion in the middle temporal gyrus) and T1bIb (in the cortex adjacent to the lesion in the superior temporal gyrus). This was followed by early spread to nearby contacts in the superior, middle, and inferior temporal gyri. The locations of the electrodes in the apparent seizure onset zone are shown in Figures 14.17 to 14.19.

At this point, a proposed area of resection came into focus; however, confirmation that the posterior extent of the resection would not interfere with receptive language was necessary. Cortical mapping was carried out at the bedside using the sEEG electrodes. Testing for receptive language by stimulating different electrode positions and simultaneously testing comprehension suggested that Wernicke's area was just posterior to the lesion, in the T1cIc and T2c electrodes.

To confirm that an electrode contact is in the seizure onset zone, electrical stimulation of the contact in question can provide additional confirmatory evidence if the stimulation provokes the patient's seizure. In this patient, cortical stimulation testing triggered seizures from some of the electrodes within the visible lesion (T2b 1-2) but also from the electrode just superior to the lesion (T1b 1-2), as well as those just posterior to the lesion (T2c). Based on this information, it was decided to perform a left subtotal temporal lobectomy.

The initial cortical exposure from the craniotomy is shown in Figure 14.20. As an adjunct to the surgical plan, electrocorticography (ECoG) was performed (Figure 14.21). ECoG consists of placing electrode grids directly on the brain, usually immediately before the actual resection is performed, and analyzing the position of any interictal surface discharges. ECoG can be useful because, after the sEEG data has been analyzed, limitations in the density of the electrode placement can at times result in a situation where not all resection

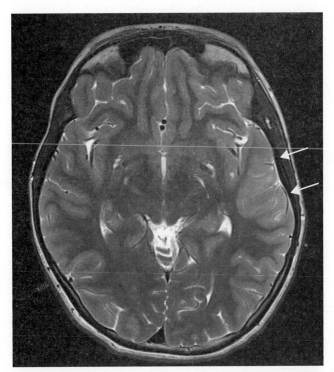

Figure 14.11 The patient's MRI showed a possible left temporal focal cortical dysplasia (arrows). Note that the overall signal is slightly brighter in this area. Even more importantly, the branching pattern of the white matter, which appears darker than the gray matter in this T2-weighted scan, is considerably reduced in this portion of the temporal lobe (compare to the opposite side).

borders have been definitely defined. ECoG data can sometimes provide supplemental information as to which areas of cortex are or are not active with epileptiform activity. This type of pre-resection ECoG recording has the advantage that the recording grid(s) can easily be moved to multiple different positions to make exploratory recordings in different areas, if necessary. It should be remembered, though, that ECoG data only represent interictal information as actual seizures are rarely observed on ECoG recordings. After the resection is completed, a second ECoG is often performed to document the extent to which the interictal discharges have been ablated, especially if they were observed on the pre-resection ECoG. ECoG is not always useful because even areas that are interictally active at other times may happen to be quiet during the snapshot of time that the ECoG is recorded. Depth of anesthesia may also play a role in suppressing interictal activity recorded on ECoG.

This patient underwent a lateral anterior temporal lobectomy. The post-resection photograph taken in the operating room is shown in Figure 14.22. A sagittal MRI scan shows the extent of the resection and is oriented similarly to the operating room photographs (Figure 14.23). Additional post-operative MRI scans showing the extent of the resection are shown in Figure 14.24. The patient remained seizure-free after her procedure, and there was no detrimental impact on her language. Pathology showed that the epileptic lesion was, in fact, a low-grade neuroepithelial tumor rather than the focal cortical dysplasia initially suspected.

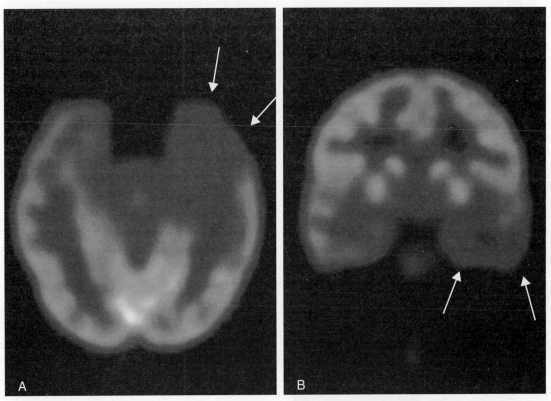

A   B

Figure 14.12 PET scans create a map of glucose utilization in the brain using the radiotracer ^{18}F-fluorode-oxyglucose. Brighter areas correspond to regions of increased glucose utilization. The image on the left shows a scan in the axial plane and the image on the right a scan in the coronal plane. The darker areas (arrows) in the left temporal lobe suggest a region of abnormally decreased glucose metabolism in that area.

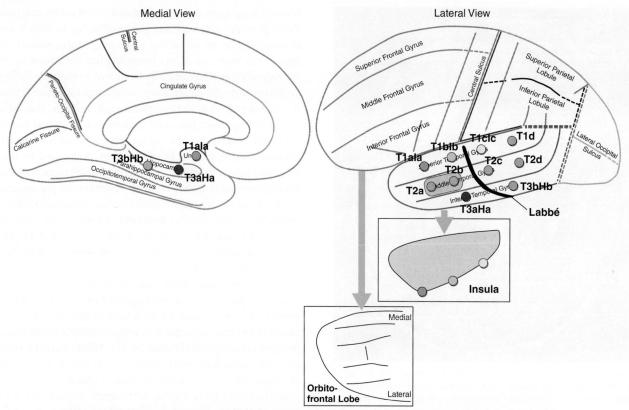

Figure 14.13 The drawing on the right side of the figure shows the proposed sEEG implantation entry points and includes two electrodes, T2a and T2b, that directly target the MRI lesion that is shown as a gray-shaded oval area in the temporal lobe. Additional electrodes are placed to surround the lesion and establish negative margins, and the more posterior electrode placements are designed to allow for testing of receptive language and identification of Wernicke's area. The drawing on the left side of the figure shows the medial surface of the left hemisphere and shows the electrodes that reach the medial surface (these are not additional electrodes but the same electrodes whose entry points are shown on the right). The insets on the right side of the figure show the targets of electrodes that reach the insula (three electrodes) and the orbitofrontal surface (no electrodes in this case). The location of the vein of Labbé, a useful anatomical landmark on the lateral temporal lobe convexity, is shown with a heavy black line. Note that, according to the rules of SENSA nomenclature, electrodes whose entry point is in the superior temporal gyrus have label prefixes of T1a, T1b, T1c, etc., from front to back. Electrodes that terminate in the insula have label names that terminate in Ia, Ib, and Ic, also from front to back, hence: T1aIa, T1bIb, etc. Electrodes that enter the middle temporal gyrus begin with T2 and those that enter the inferior temporal gyrus begin with T3. For a more complete explanation of the SENSA nomenclature, see the end of this chapter.

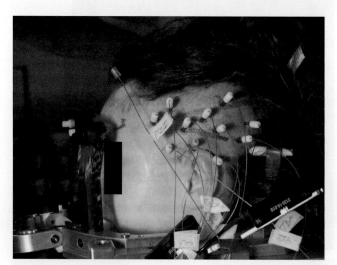

Figure 14.14 The anchor bolts for the sEEG electrodes are seen for this left temporal sEEG implantation. The patient's head is held by a rigid frame so that final entry points correspond exactly to the planned trajectories for each electrode.

UNIQUE ASPECTS TO CONSIDER WHILE READING INTRACRANIAL EEG

The basic skills acquired in reading scalp EEG also apply to intracranial recordings. Certain differences in the appearance of physiological rhythms, artifacts, ictal patterns, and the machine settings used for interpreting these studies are worth reviewing.

Sensitivity Settings

Because the electrodes used in invasive recordings lie directly in contact with the brain with no intervening insulators, it should not come as a surprise that the voltages recorded with these contacts require amplifier gains that are much lower than those used for scalp recordings. Although typical sensitivities used for scalp-EEG recordings might be between 7 and 10 µV/mm, those used for intracranial recordings are often in the vicinity of 50 µV/ mm (remembering that higher sensitivities correspond to

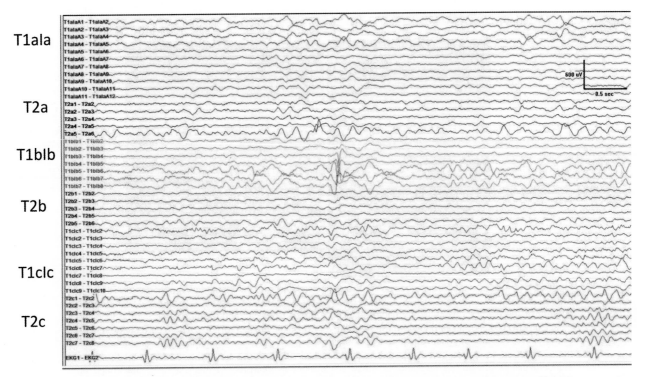

Figure 14.15 A single interictal discharge is seen in the middle of this page in the superior temporal gyrus in the superficial contacts of T1blb (maximum in contacts 6 and 7). Interestingly, in this case, the electrodes directly within the lesion in the middle temporal gyrus (T2a and T2b) did not happen to manifest interictal discharges in this or other pages of the recording.

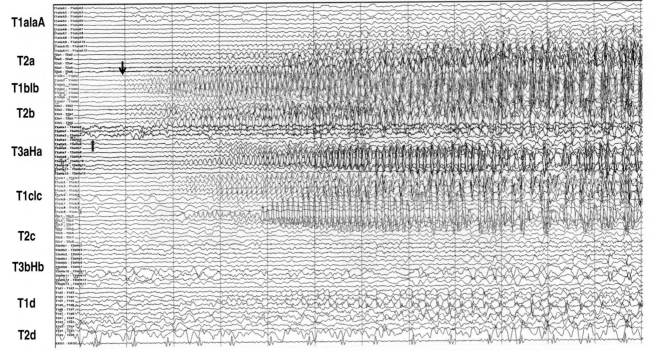

Figure 14.16 This page of stereo EEG shows how the patient's seizure spreads across various sEEG contacts. The dark black arrow shows the very earliest part of the seizure discharge, which occurred simultaneously in T2b (within the suspected lesion in the middle temporal gyrus), and T1blb (in the cortex adjacent to the lesion in the superior temporal gyrus). Spread to T1clc (in the superior temporal gyrus just posterior to the lesion) and other electrodes is seen soon after. The specific anatomical location of this seizure onset zone is easiest to appreciate in the following figures. Thereafter, the seizure spreads to nearby contacts in the superior, middle, and inferior temporal gyri. The seizure begins just under the black arrow as a very low-voltage 10 Hz sinusoidal discharge that increases in voltage over the next several seconds. Careful review of this page is necessary to appreciate the hippocampal rhythm (a phenomenon discussed in more detail later in this chapter) in contacts T3aHa 1 to 4 (gray arrow). The low-voltage fast activity superimposed on some sharpened theta rhythms seen in these contacts represents a physiologic hippocampal rhythm that was already ongoing before the ictal onset and is not a part of the seizure.

T1bIb

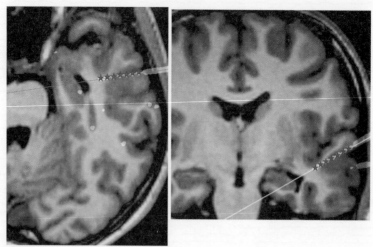

Figure 14.17 Two in-plane MRI images of the T1blb electrode are shown. Instead of showing the MRI image of a chosen electrode in one of the standard planes (axial, coronal, or sagittal), a plane that includes the entirety of the electrode is chosen. Imagine holding a pencil in the air and rotating a flat card around the pencil, always keeping the card flush to the pencil. Every possible position of the rotating card suggests one of the infinite number of possible planes that contains the pencil. In choosing in-plane MRI scans, although there would be an infinite number of possible choices, planes that most closely match one of the three standard planes are usually selected as these are easiest to interpret. In this example, the image on the left most closely matches the axial plane and the image on the right is a close match to the coronal plane. The T1blb electrode can be seen to enter the left superior temporal gyrus, most easily identified in the image on the right. The large sulcus seen just above the electrode is the Sylvian fissure leading down toward the insula. The red stars denote the contacts on the electrode where the seizure onset was seen.

T2b

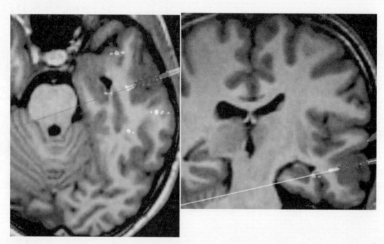

Figure 14.18 In-plane images of the T2b electrode show its entry into the middle temporal gyrus. Again, the image on the left is a close match to the axial plane and the image on the right is a close match to the coronal plane. The red stars denote the four contacts on the electrode where the seizure onset was seen.

lower amplifier gains). Recalling the basic principle discussed in Chapter 5, "Electroencephalographic Electrodes, Channels, and Montages and How They Are Chosen," that the closer any two contacts are to each other, all things being equal, the lower the voltage signal between the two is expected to be, all the more remarkable the high absolute voltages recorded from grid and sEEG electrodes are. The individual contacts on grid and strip electrodes are placed

fairly close together, typically 10 mm between contacts. Stereo EEG electrode contacts are often only separated by a few millimeters. Thus, the high voltages recorded from these intracranial contacts are all the more impressive compared to scalp recordings, but still expected. Sensitivities are adjusted for interpretation just as they are for conventional EEG recordings. Amplifier gains are set high enough so that detail in the signal is visible, but not so high that

T1cIc

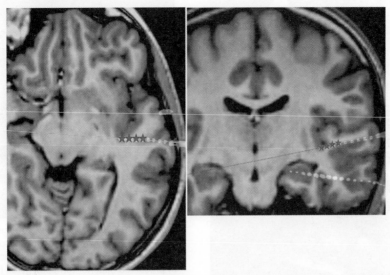

Figure 14.19 These in-plane images of the T1cIc electrode show the entry point of the electrode in the superior temporal gyrus, but posterior to the entry points of the T1bIb and T2b electrodes that were shown in the previous figures. The red stars show the locations of the deep contacts to which the seizure first propagates. By chance, the T3bHb electrode targeting the hippocampus is also captured in the image on the right and is seen passing below T1cIc.

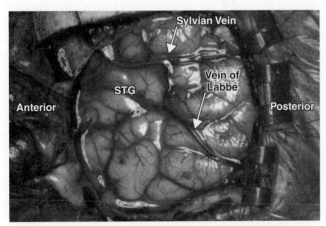

Figure 14.20 This photograph shows the appearance of the cortical exposure with the bone window removed. The patient's nose is toward the left side of the image (anterior) and the back of the head is toward the right side of the image (posterior). The Sylvian vein, which runs in the Sylvian fissure, can be seen to course horizontally and separates the frontal lobe (above the vein) from the temporal lobe (below the vein). The vein of Labbé can be seen coursing from the Sylvian vein down and to the right, eventually to anastomose with the transverse sinus (not visible). The vein of Labbé is frequently used as an anatomical landmark when planning temporal lobe resections. The superior temporal gyrus is labeled (STG). The previous entry point of one of the sEEG electrodes can be seen toward the bottom of the picture in the middle temporal gyrus.

adjacent channels cross each other and obscure features of the recording.

Filter Settings

We have already discussed the general strategies for choosing filter settings for conventional EEG recording in Chapter 7,

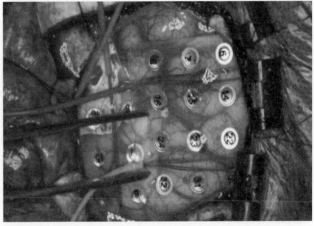

Figure 14.21 Electrode arrays (grids) are placed over the temporal lobe to obtain intraoperative electrocorticography (ECoG) recordings of interictal discharges. These recordings may help further define the exact boundaries of the resection.

"Filters in the EEG". The strategy for setting the high- and low-filter values (or "bandpass") for any recording are based on the goal of attenuating frequencies that are likely to contain unwanted activity, including artifact, and preserving and highlighting the EEG signals of interest as much as possible. Because both the types of unwanted activity and artifact and the frequency ranges of greatest interest to us differ between conventional and invasive EEG recording, filter setups for invasive recordings may differ from those used for conventional EEG.

Low Frequency Filters (LFFs)

One of the main advantages of the LFF in conventional EEG recording is its ability to filter out the large, slow deflections

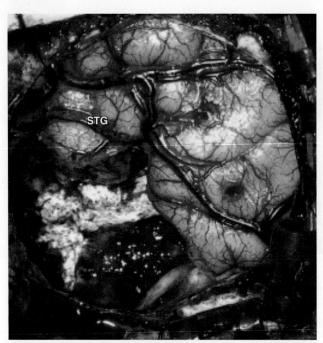

Figure 14.22 The anterior temporal lobe, which was located mostly to the left of the edge of the bone window visible in the left lower portion of this image and whose position is, therefore, not visible in this photograph, was substantially resected, with the exception of a portion of the superior temporal gyrus. To preserve receptive language, a portion of the superior temporal gyrus (labeled STG) was preserved. It can be seen that the remainder of the temporal lobe was resected almost back to the vein of Labbé (labeled in Figure 14.20. Compare to the post-operative MRI scans shown in the following figures.

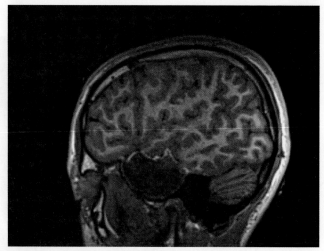

Figure 14.23 This post-operative sagittal MPRAGE MRI image has an orientation similar to the OR photographs shown in the previous figures. The anterior temporal lobe has been resected, but the island of preserved superior temporal gyrus (STG) that was seen in the previous figure is also evident on this MRI image and its relation to the entire temporal lobe resection (dark gray cavity) is now more clearly seen.

that are often caused by patient movements. Because of their protected position, intracranial contacts are not generally subject to this same type of motion artifact, but the LFF is still useful for other reasons. Although the identification of slow-wave activity is a key element of conventional EEG interpretation (such as identifying regions of abnormal slowing), the identification of regions of slow-wave activity is much less important in invasive studies. Instead, the emphasis in invasive studies is on the identification of epileptiform activity and seizure patterns, types of activity that lie in the higher frequency ranges.

With so many more channels displayed per page on invasive studies, vertical space is at a premium. Using stricter (higher) LFF cutoff frequencies helps keep each channel baseline within a more restricted horizontal area which, in turn, allows for the use of higher amplifier gains (lower sensitivities) without having adjacent channel crossings. Using aggressive LFF settings allows us to turn up the amplifier gain and create a larger display of the EEG signal, especially the lower-voltage, faster activity that is often of specific interest, though at the possible expense of losing the low-frequency component. LFF cutoff frequencies settings of 3 Hz, 5 Hz, and even 10 Hz can be used to advantage to interpret certain recordings. Figure 14.25 shows an example of using a "stricter" LFF setting of 10 Hz, a reading strategy that can help bring out the fast activity at the onset of a seizure. Note that with the LFF set at 10 Hz each channel's baseline is quite flat, which allows for use of higher amplifier gains. If using a stricter LFF setting

while scanning a stereo EEG study, it is advisable to go back and check the appearance of the recording from time to time without the use of the strict setting to see if any important activity may have been missed. This brings up the question of what type of important information might be lost if reading a stereo EEG study with a very strict LFF setting such as 10 Hz.

One important exception to our reduced interest in slower activity in invasive recordings is the identification of the so-called *DC shift*. The *DC shift* or *ictal baseline shift* is an interesting pattern that can be recognized on conventional EEG recordings at times, though it is considerably easier to identify on invasive recordings. A DC shift consists of a persistent shift of the EEG baseline up or down immediately preceding a seizure. Pinpointing The cortical areas that manifest such shifts may help identify the seizure onset zone. Although most signals in the EEG represent oscillating currents, such shifts that move the channel readout off the baseline, up or down, for a period of time represent examples of direct (DC) currents that are not typically a focus of interpretation of routine EEGs. The movement of the signal off the baseline without an immediate return to baseline represents a current flow in only one direction, different from an oscillating current with continued repeating baseline crossings (an alternating or AC current). In fact, even the standard LFF setting of 1 Hz that is used to suppress motion artifact in conventional EEG recordings can substantially impede the ability to recognize DC shifts. One of the main purposes of the LFF is to return a channel that has wandered away from the baseline back to its baseline (this property of the LFF is discussed in further detail in Chapter 7, "Filters in the EEG"). The display of the seizure in Figure 14.25 was chosen expressly to demonstrate this effect. Figure 14.26 shows the same seizure, but now with an LFF setting of 1 Hz. We now see that this seizure was associated with a dramatic DC shift that would have been missed if the reader had not also reviewed the seizure with a lower LFF setting.

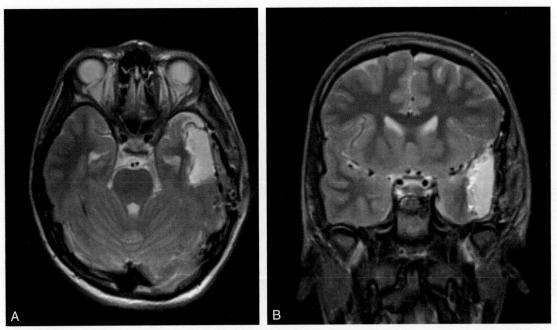

Figure 14.24 Axial (A) and coronal (B) T2-weighted images show the result of the left temporal lobe resection that was performed. The cerebrospinal fluid that fills the resection cavity appears white in these images.

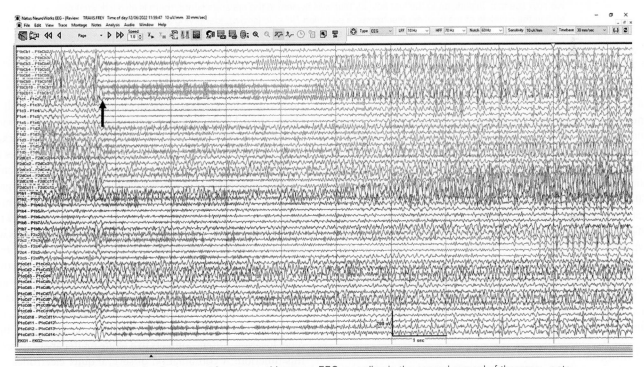

Figure 14.25 A seizure onset is seen on this stereo EEG recording in the second second of the page—note the sudden onset of fast activity in the F1bCb electrode (arrow). This page was displayed and interpreted using an aggressive LFF setting of 10 Hz to remove the slow component of the EEG signal. Note that this causes each channel baseline to be very flat, a desirable effect of the 10 Hz LFF setting. This allows the amplifier gains to be increased, making it easier to appreciate the fast activity at the beginning of the seizure. It is still important to analyze this seizure without the strict LFF setting of 10 Hz, as we shall see in the following figure.

High-Frequency Filters (HFFs)

Artifacts in the high-frequency range that are commonly seen in conventional EEG recording are much less of a problem with invasive recordings. In particular, muscle artifact and artifacts from jostling electrode contacts are usefully attenuated with the HFF in conventional EEG, but these types of artifacts are only rarely encountered in intracranial recordings. Because of the relative lack of worry for artifacts in the high-frequency bands in invasive EEG recordings, the use

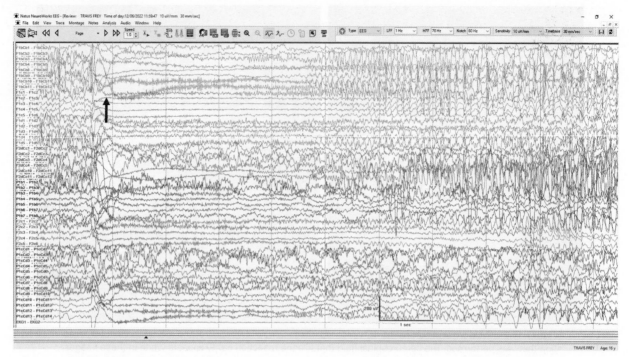

Figure 14.26 Displaying the same page of EEG as the previous figure but returning the LFF setting to 1 Hz, we now see that, in addition to the fast activity that was evident in the previous figure, there is also a dramatic shift in the baseline of the involved electrodes, a so-called *DC shift* (arrow). Identifying a DC shift may provide supplementary information helpful in localizing a seizure onset.

of restrictive settings for the high-frequency filter (HFF) is much less important. In studies in which there is a particular interest in recording very high-frequency activity (e.g., high-frequency oscillations or HFOs), the reader may choose to eliminate use of the HFF altogether. HFOs are low-amplitude, short-duration oscillations that occur at frequencies between 80 and 500 Hz. HFOs may be described as ripples (80–250 Hz) or fast ripples (250–500 Hz). Although some types of HFOs may represent normal physiological activity, certain types have been shown to be markers of epileptogenic cortex (though a detailed discussion of HFOs is beyond the scope of this text). When analysis of this high-frequency phenomenon is of particular interest, a correspondingly high sampling rate for recording the study will be necessary (see discussion of the Nyquist frequency in Chapter 7, "Filters in the EEG").

Montages

Although most laboratories use a standard set of montages for the interpretation of conventional EEG studies, because invasive implantation setups vary from patient to patient, invasive recording montages must be individualized for each patient's study, according to reader preference. Of course, the long sequences of contacts on a grid or sEEG electrode automatically suggest straightforward bipolar chain "montages," that compare adjacent electrode pairs of contacts (e.g., E1-E2, E2-E3…, etc), just as we have already seen in typical bipolar chains used in conventional EEG studies. The order in which these chains are displayed on the page depends on the reader's

preference. The ordering of the electrodes should usually follow some internal logic, such as ordering from front to back or top to bottom, to make the study most easily interpretable. When a large number of channels requires that two separate pages be used to display all channels, it can be efficient to place active electrodes, once these have been identified, on Page 1 and inactive channels on Page 2. This can make it easier to determine whether one contact fires first followed by another contact for both interictal and ictal activity. When certain electrodes are relegated to an "inactive" page, it is reasonable to check that page from time to time to confirm that it is remaining inactive.

Ideally, two sets of montages should be created for any study: a set of bipolar montages and a corresponding set of referential montages. Just as is done in conventional EEG, the electrode contact(s) chosen for the reference should be in a quiet location. Often, contacts in a white matter area can serve this function. A combination of several quiet electrodes can be averaged together to serve as a virtual reference electrode, or an average of all the electrodes used in the study may also be tried, much as is done when an average reference electrode is created in conventional EEG. Referential montages can make localization of any event more straightforward because, if the event is seen in that contact's channel, then it is present in that contact. In bipolar montages, it can be more difficult to sort out precise localization since each channel includes two electrode contacts, one of which may, in reality, be inactive. This is a particular issue when a deflection is seen at the beginning or end of a bipolar chain (e.g., E1-E2, E2-E3…,

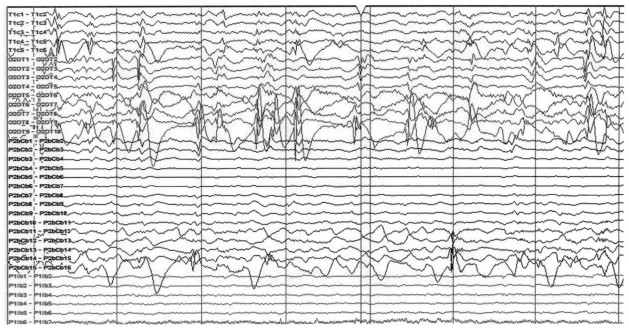

Figure 14.27 Note that several of the contacts in the P2bCb electrode appear quiet, specifically contacts 4 through 9. Usually a group of quiet channels like this suggests that they are traversing an area of white matter. This can be confirmed by reviewing the location of these contacts on MRI (see the following figure). Quiet channels are also noted in the P1lb electrode at the bottom of the page.

etc.). If a deflection is seen, for instance, in E1-E2, are both electrodes active, or is the deflection in E1-E2 solely caused by activity in E2? A referential montage setup such as E1-ref, E2-ref…, etc. makes this determination straightforward.

As already noted, the large number of channels in many invasive studies puts space on the display page at a premium. For this reason, the reader may choose to delete inactive channels from the reading montages with the goal of saving space on the page. With most sEEG implantation schemes, it is unavoidable that some number of the contacts will lie in the white matter, and white matter contacts are often low-voltage channels that do not convey useful information (Figure 14.27). For that reason, white matter contacts and other electrode positions that happen to be inactive because of their location (e.g., contacts that have not entered the substance of the brain and lie in the fixation bolt of the sEEG electrode) can be eliminated from montages. Before eliminating any white matter contacts from the reading montage, it should be confirmed that they are of low voltage both during background recording and during any interictal and ictal discharges. At the same time, the location of the electrode contacts in question should be reviewed on the patient's post-implantation imaging to confirm that the contacts proposed for elimination from the reading montages are, indeed, located in the white matter (Figures 14.28 and 14.29).

Interictal and Ictal Patterns

The appearance of interictal epileptiform discharges on intracranial EEG is fairly similar to that of conventional EEG and can include spikes, polyspikes, and low-voltage fast activity. The morphologies encountered may differ as a result of the proximity of the contacts to the origin of the recorded activity. Similarly, ictal patterns seen on invasive studies are usually similar to what is seen on scalp EEG though, again, the morphology can be more striking. Like scalp-recorded EEG, ictal patterns recorded on invasive studies are variable and include discharges that resemble rhythmic spikes or polyspikes, low-voltage fast activity, or rhythmic activity of abrupt onset that shows evolution.

Physiological Patterns on Intracranial EEG

It should come as no surprise that the various physiological patterns we see on conventional EEG recordings, such as the posterior rhythm, sleep spindles, mu rhythms, and so forth, may also be seen on intracranial recordings. Even readers adept at recognizing these patterns on conventional EEG may initially mistake these phenomena for abnormal activity when first encountered on invasive recordings. This occurs, in part, because a large part of the pattern recognition we use to identify these rhythms in conventional recordings is based on knowing where they are typically seen on the EEG page. When reading invasive EEG recordings, the relationship between location on the page and brain location is upended, and it is easier to be taken by surprise. Examples of a mu rhythm, the posterior dominant rhythm, and sleep spindles as they may appear on invasive recordings are shown in Figures 14.30 to 14.32.

Distinctive hippocampal rhythms, inaccessible to scalp EEG, can also be seen on sEEG electrodes implanted in the hippocampus. Compared to neocortex, the normal hippocampus can show a characteristic mixture of delta and theta rhythms in addition to increased beta activity (see Figure 14.33). Sometimes, the slower rhythms seen in the normal

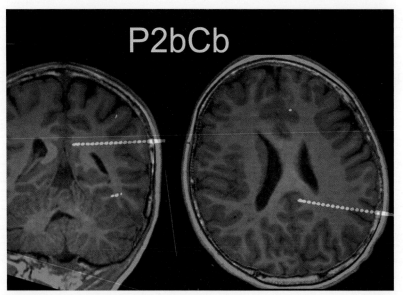

Figure 14.28 The in-plane MRI of the electrode P2bCb confirms that contacts 4 through 9 are, indeed, in the white matter (recall that the contacts are numbered so that the highest numbers are near the electrode's tail and the deepest contact is labeled contact #1). Confirmation that these contacts are located in the white matter and that the corresponding channels are of low voltage imply that they can safely be removed from the scanning montage.

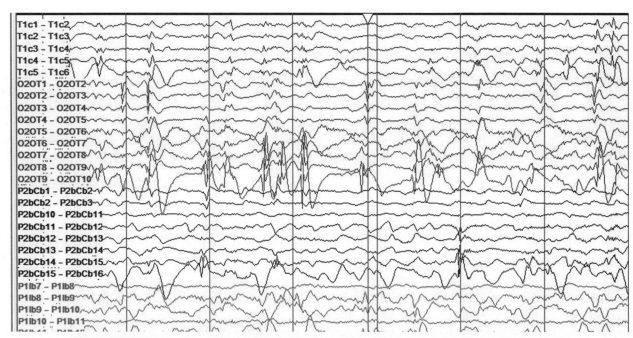

Figure 14.29 After removal of channels lying in the white matter, there is more space on the page for display of the active channels. In addition to the quiet P2bCb contacts identified in the previous figure, some of the quiet P1lb contacts (1 through 6) have also been eliminated from the montage. There is now considerably more "vertical space" on the page available to demonstrate the interictal discharges.

hippocampus may manifest sharpened contours that are somewhat suggestive of epileptiform activity, though they may represent normal physiologic rhythms.

Artifacts

Because of the protected location of the contacts, intracranial EEG studies are not subject to as many artifacts as we see on traditional scalp recordings. Muscle artifact, because of its high voltage, is occasionally transmitted through the skull and picked up at lower voltage by intracranial electrodes. Pulse artifact may be seen if a contact is near a pulsating vessel. With grid electrodes, occasionally an individual contact will not be in contact with the surface of the brain due to the conformation of the grid, creating an artifact. When voltages

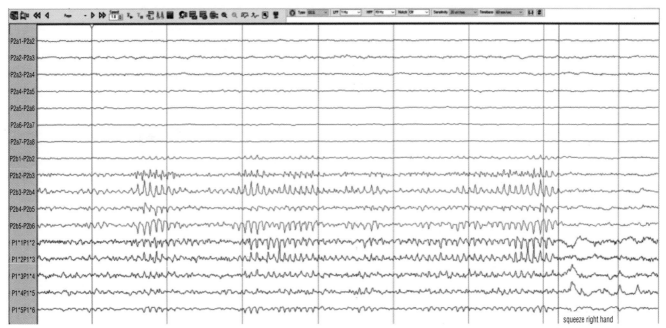

Figure 14.30 Similar to scalp EEG recordings, mu rhythms may initially catch the eye because of the sharp phase of this arciform rhythm, possibly suggesting epileptiform activity. This mu rhythm recorded on invasive EEG does, in fact, strongly resemble the mu rhythms we are accustomed to seeing on conventional recordings. If in question, the nature of this physiologic rhythm can be confirmed by demonstrating disappearance of the pattern when the patient is asked to move the contralateral hand, as was done here at the end of the page.

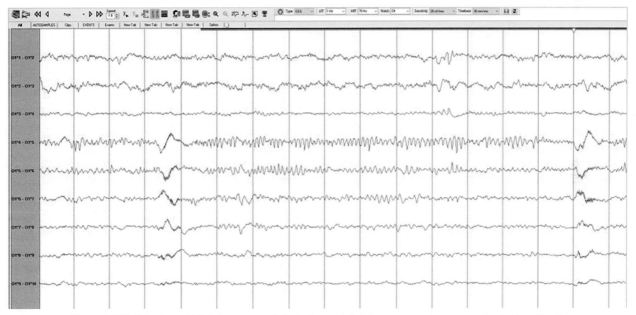

Figure 14.31 This sinusoidal alpha-range activity in the occipital area represents an example of this patient's posterior dominant rhythm. As expected, the rhythm was seen to suppress with eye opening.

are seen to progressively decrease from a grid electrode, the possibility that a fluid collection is forming under the grid, such as a hematoma, hygroma, or otherwise, should be considered. Artifacts caused by motion and electrical interference of the equipment connections running between the patient's head and the recording apparatus are not dissimilar to those seen on conventional EEG recordings.

SENSA NAMING SYSTEM FOR SEEG ELECTRODES

Thus far, there is no single standard for the naming of stereo EEG electrodes. Stone et al. at Boston Children's Hospital have proposed an efficient and easy-to-understand electrode-naming system that is presented here for those laboratories

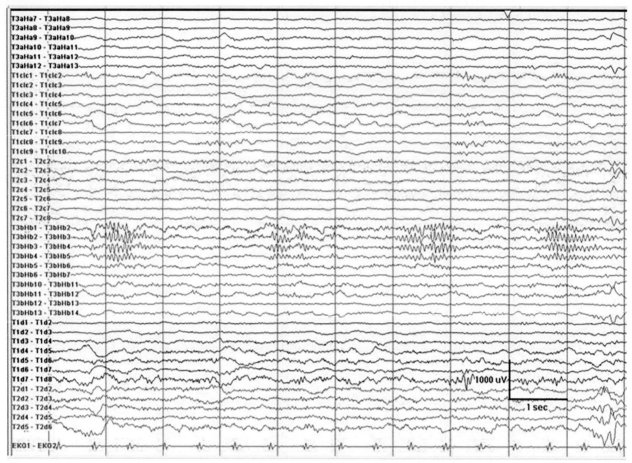

Figure 14.32 Sleep spindles are seen on this patient's invasive recording in the T3bHb electrode. The repetitive, non-evolving pattern of this 14 Hz activity confirms that it represents sleep spindles.

that may choose to adopt it. The system has the advantage that the name of the electrode suggests the electrode's basic positioning and trajectory. Currently, other naming systems are in use, but these naming conventions require that the reader memorize their standard electrode names, which may not be intuitive.

The SENSA (Standardized Electrode Nomenclature for Stereo electroencephalography Applications) names electrodes according to their entry point and their target.

Entry Point	Target	Contact #
T1b	OFa	3

The first component of the example electrode contact name above, T1bOFa3, is the abbreviation for the gyrus of entry. For instance, the superior, middle, and inferior temporal gyri are abbreviated T1, T2, and T3, respectively. Likewise, the superior, middle, and inferior frontal gyri are abbreviated F1, F2, and F3. When more than one electrode enters a particular gyrus, the gyrus abbreviation is suffixed with a lower case letter (e.g., 'a,' 'b,' or 'c') from front to back. For instance, if there are multiple entry points in the superior temporal gyrus, these would be denoted, from anterior to posterior, as T1a, T1b, T1c, etc. The prefix P1 is used for entry points in the superior parietal lobule and P2 for entry points in the inferior parietal lobule. O1 is used for entry points above the lateral occipital sulcus and O2 for entry points below the sulcus.

The second component of the electrode name represents the target of the electrode or where the electrode terminates, and is abbreviated in a similar fashion. For instance, electrode target abbreviations may include 'I' for insula, 'H' for hippocampus, 'A' for amygdala, 'OF' for orbitofrontal, 'PH' for parahippocampal gyrus, and so forth. Similar to the system for the first component, if there are two electrodes that happen to target the insula, then the most anterior target would be named 'Ia' the next most anterior target 'Ib' and so forth. Therefore, an electrode name such as T1aIb can be quickly coded and understood to be an electrode that enters the superior temporal gyrus more anterior than some other electrode(s), and arrives in the insula at a position posterior to one other electrode that has targeted the insula more anteriorly (and whose name would end in 'Ia'). The sixth contact of this T1aIb electrode would then be called *T1aIb6*. If there were only one electrode entering the superior temporal gyrus, the 'a' would not be required and the electrode would simply be named T1Ib. Likewise, if there were only one electrode targeting the insula, the 'b' would not be required and the electrode would be called *T1aI*. Based on the name of the T1bOFa3 electrode contact used in the example above, we can surmise that the electrode is the second most anterior to enter

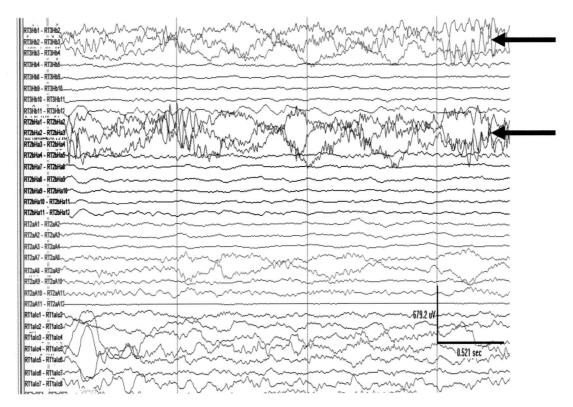

Figure 14.33 A normal hippocampal rhythm can be seen in contacts 1, 2, and 3, the deepest contacts of both the RT3Hb and RT2bHa electrodes (arrows). The remainder of the channels in this image are recording from neocortex and provide a good comparison to the hippocampal rhythm. Note the increase in delta and theta range activity seen in the hippocampus, in addition to the increased fast (beta) activity. Some of the slow wave contours appear sharpened, but they do not interrupt the underlying rhythm. (LFF = 1 Hz and HFF = 70 Hz).

the superior temporal gyrus, and that it terminates in the most anterior position in the orbitofrontal cortex compared to other electrode(s) that terminate there. When an electrode happens to end in a numeral because a target suffix has not been added, such as O1, an asterisk can be placed between the electrode name and the contact number to avoid confusion (e.g., O1*1, O1*2, etc.).

SUGGESTED READINGS

Bancaud J, Talairach J, Bonis A, et al: *La stéréo-électroencéphalographie dans l'épilepsie: informations neurophysiopathologiques apportées par l'investigation fonctionnelle stéréotaxique,* Paris, 1965, Masson and Cie.

Cardinale F, Cossu M, Castana L, Casaceli G, Schiariti M.P, Miserocchi A, Fuschillo D, Moscato A, Caborni C, Arnulfo G, Lo Russo G: Stereoelectroencephalography: Surgical methodology, safety, and stereotactic application accuracy in 500 procedures, *Neurosurgery* 72:353–366, 2013.

Lagarde S , Bonini F, McGonigal A, Chauvel P, Gavaret M, Scavarda D, Carron R, Régis J, Aubert S, Villeneuve N, Giusiano B, Figarella-Branger D, Trebuchon A, Bartolomei F: Seizure-onset patterns in focal cortical dysplasia and neurodevelopmental tumors: Relationship with surgical prognosis and neuropathologic subtypes, *Epilepsia* 57(9):1426–1435, 2016.

Lhatoo SD, Kahane P, Lüders HO, editors: *Invasive studies of the human epileptic brain. principles and practice,* Oxford, UK, 2019, Oxford University Press.

Stone S, Madsen J.R, Bolton J, Pearl P.L, Chavakula V, Day E: A Standardized Electrode nomenclature for stereoelectroencephalography applications, *J Clin Neurophysiol* 38(6):509–515, 2021.

Talairach J, Tournoux P: *Co-planar stereotaxic atlas of the human brain. 3-dimensional proportional system: An approach to cerebral imaging. Translated by Mark Rayport.* New York, 1988, Thieme Medical Publishers.

WHERE DO EEG WAVES COME FROM?

A final word on a central EEG physiology question: *what is the generator of the EEG waveform?* What follows here is a very brief review of the basic neurophysiology of how nerve cells fire and the electrical basis of EEG waves. Although this appendix may be of interest to readers who would like an introduction to the underlying physiology of brain waves, familiarity with these concepts is not obligatory for learning EEG interpretation and, like any good appendix, it can be removed from your initial introduction to EEG reading without ill effect. If your priority is to get to the nuts and bolts of reading EEGs immediately, you may decide to defer reading this section to a later time.

The Action Potential

Nerve cells "fire" via a physiologic mechanism called the *action potential.* It should be said at the outset that EEG waves are *not* actually formed from action potentials, nor are they the summation of action potentials, which may come as a surprise to some readers. Action potentials do play an indirect role in the production of EEG waves that is important enough that we will review the action potential concept here.

In the resting state, the voltage across the nerve cell membrane is not neutral—the charge on the surface of the membrane facing the inside of the cell is different from the charge on the outward-facing membrane: the inside of the membrane is negative and the outside of the membrane is positive. Note that this does not mean that the whole of the inside of the neuron is negatively-charged compared to the extracellular space. Rather, both the intracellular and extracellular spaces as a whole have a net neutral charge, but specifically in the region of the cell membrane there is a net negative charge clinging to the inside of the membrane and a net positive charge clinging to the outside (Figure A.1). Thus, the membrane is said to be *polarized.* At rest, this voltage difference across the membrane is approximately −70 mV (voltages are stated comparing the inside to the outside). Saying that the membrane is polarized is essentially synonymous with saying that there is a voltage drop or charge difference across the membrane.

When events lead to this resting negative-inside/positive-outside polarization being disturbed in a region of the membrane such that this charge difference might temporarily disappear, the cell membrane is said to be *depolarized* in that area. An action potential consists of a ripple of electrical depolarization that flows down the axon mediated by the quick opening and closing of specific ion channels, which is how a nerve cell fires. At the location where the ripple is passing down the axon membrane, that negative-inside/positive-outside polarization is actually briefly reversed, so that the inside of the membrane is very briefly positive (Figure A.2). Once the action potential passes a specific point on the membrane, the resting polarized state is restored.

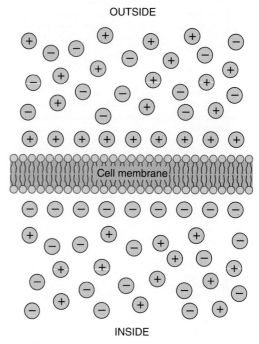

OUTSIDE

Cell membrane

INSIDE

Figure A.1 As a result of the work of the Na⁺/K⁺-ATPase pump as described in the text, the inside of the nerve cell membrane is more negatively charged than the outside of the cell membrane. Note that, overall, the intracellular and extracellular spaces carry a net neutral charge, both within the spaces and with respect to each other. The charge gradient is a local effect seen across the membrane itself.

When the action potential reaches the end of the axon and arrives at the synapse, it causes a neurotransmitter to be released into the synaptic cleft (whichever neurotransmitter that neuron "specializes" in). That neurotransmitter, in turn, will stimulate the next nerve cell on the other side of the synapse (referred to as the "postsynaptic" neuron). Therefore, nerve cell transmission runs by an *electrical* mechanism down the body of the cell and the axon, then by a *chemical* mechanism at the junction between cells (the synapse) where the action potential's arrival causes a chemical neurotransmitter to be released into the synapse.

The Effect of EPSPs and IPSPs

The released neurotransmitter binds to the postsynaptic cell and can effect a variety of voltage changes in that next cell's membrane (so-called *postsynaptic potentials*) depending on the particular neurotransmitter that was produced by the presynaptic neuron. Some neurotransmitters will cause the postsynaptic cell's membrane to become even more polarized (more negative-inside), and because this type of change makes the membrane even more stable (i.e., farther away from triggering an action potential), those neurotransmitters are said to be *inhibitory*. The electrical "blip" inhibitory neurotransmitters cause in the postsynaptic membrane that make it even more polarized are termed *inhibitory*

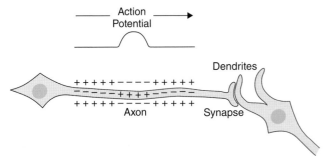

Figure A.2 This is a simplified depiction of an action potential flowing down an axon, from left to right. The cell body is on the left and its axon terminates in a synapse, allowing it to communicate with the dendrite of the next neuron in the chain (the postsynaptic neuron). Note that there is a resting potential across the membrane with a negative charge inside and a positive charge outside, except in the region of the action potential itself where the charge relationship is reversed. The action potential is a small region of charge reversal that propagates down the axon mediated by brief openings and closings of Na^+- and K^+-channels, as described in the text. The action potential travels down the membrane because the leading edge of this region of voltage reversal trips the nearby voltage-gated Na^+-channels to open in turn. This ripple of reversed charge flows down the axon toward the synapse, where its arrival causes the release of a packet of neurotransmitter into the synapse. Depending on the type of neurotransmitter the neuron in question releases, the arrival of the neurotransmitter on the postsynaptic neuron, shown on the right side of the figure, could either excite or inhibit the next nerve cell in line.

postsynaptic potentials (IPSPs). If the neurotransmitter produced by the presynaptic neuron has the effect of making the postsynaptic membrane less negative-inside, or more depolarized (i.e., closer to triggering an action potential), then it is said to be *excitatory*. The electrical "blip" excitatory neurotransmitters cause are termed *excitatory postsynaptic potentials* (EPSPs). As you may already know, the best-known excitatory neurotransmitter is glutamate and the best-known inhibitory neurotransmitter is gamma-amino butyric acid (GABA), but there are several others in each group. Note that, if excitatory, the neurotransmitter arriving on the postsynaptic nerve cell's membrane will generate an EPSP that may or may not be enough to evoke a new action potential in that postsynaptic neuron, depending on the quantity of that neurotransmitter released (Figure A.3). Even if there are a good number of EPSPs created in the postsynaptic cell's membrane causing some depolarization, it could be that IPSPs from other neurons are arriving at the same time counterbalancing the EPSPs, in essence protecting it from depolarizing. You can see that EPSPs and IPSPs can summate on the postsynaptic membrane determining whether or not that neuron will fire.

Setting Up the Transmembrane Potential

As mentioned, at rest the nerve cell has a charge or voltage difference set up across its membrane: inside-negative/outside-positive. How is this transmembrane charge set up and maintained by the cell? For a charge to be successfully maintained across a membrane a first, necessary property is

that the membrane be generally impermeable to the anions (negatively-charged ions) and cations (positively-charged ions) in solution surrounding it. If the membrane were very leaky, any charge across it would quickly dissipate. Because the cell membrane is generally impermeable to ions, the only way ions can traverse the membrane is when specific ion "pores" or channels briefly open to allow them to cross. There are many types of ion channels, each specializing in different ions and each having different properties in terms of what causes them to open and close and their influence on the cell.

The cell's machinery expends considerable energy to maintain this transmembrane potential. The key tool the cell uses to maintain this voltage difference is specialized proteins that float in the cell membranes called Na^+/K^+-(sodium-potassium) pumps. For these pumps to do their work, they consume energy in the form of ATP, and for that reason they are also called Na^+/K^+-ATPases (the term *ATPase* denoting that the pump breaks down ATP as an energy source in order to run). The trick of this pump is that it pumps three sodium ions (Na^+) out of the cell for every two potassium ions (K^+) it pumps into the cell. Note that if this ratio were just 2:2, you would expect to see higher Na^+ concentrations outside the cell and higher K^+ concentrations inside the cell as a result of the pump's work, but there would be no net impact on the distribution of charge inside and outside the cell—two cations would go in for every two cations going out. However, this pump works with a 3:2 ratio: there are 3 "+'s" being pumped out for every 2 "+'s" being pumped in. So, in addition to creating a difference in the concentrations of Na^+ and K^+ across the membrane, this uneven exchange in positively-charged ions also sets up a net negative charge on the inside of the membrane (where positive charges have been relatively depleted by the pump) as was shown in Figure A.1. Note that this pump sets up a negative charge on the inside membrane wall without directly moving negative charges—it does so by depleting positive charge from the intracellular side of the membrane. These pumps are constantly running in order to maintain these ionic and charge gradients, both to counteract the slow leakage of ions back across the membrane and also the effect of ion exchanges from the ongoing opening and closing of ion channels.

A "Party" Analogy to Illustrate Electrical and Chemical Gradients across the Neuronal Membrane

If this setup is hard to follow, consider the following analogy that is designed to mimic the transmembrane situation, but with people instead of ions. Two parties of equal size are taking place, but separated by a wall. One party is on the left side of the wall and the other is on the right. At the outset, each of the two parties has an equal number of boys and girls in attendance and the total number of people (boys and girls) on either side of the wall is the same at both parties. As long as the wall between the parties remains intact, the number of people on each side of the wall is equal and fixed, and the

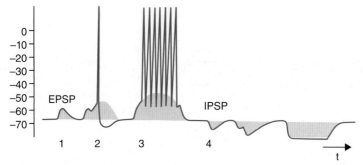

Figure A.3 This graph shows the voltage across the cell membrane and the impact of both EPSPs and IPSPs. At the very beginning of the voltage trace, the membrane is at its resting (negative-inside) voltage. Soon after, a first packet of an excitatory neurotransmitter arrives, opening a channel that allows a small amount of cations to flow into the cell, causing the inside to become briefly less negative ("EPSP"), but not so much that it crosses threshold voltage (1). This is the "small 'blip' of decreased negativity" described in the text. Immediately following this small EPSP, a small *group* of excitatory neurotransmitter packets arrives which effectively sum together and brings the membrane voltage below threshold, leading to the firing of a single action potential, the first sharp spike in the recording (2). A more prolonged train of EPSPs then causes a group of seven action potentials to fire (3). This is followed by a group of IPSPs that serve to hyperpolarize the cell membrane (4). In this way, it can be seen that the cell membrane integrates incoming EPSPs and IPSPs which, depending on their timing and preponderance, may or may not trigger an action potential.(Adapted from Speckmann E-J. Experimentelle Epilepsieforschung. Darmstadt: Wissenschaftliche Buchgesellschaft; 1986.)

boy/girl ratio and total number of partygoers in each room does not change. Now imagine that a turnstile is installed in the wall that separates the two parties. The turnstile operates in such a way that, every time it turns, it causes three girls to cross from left to right for every two boys it allows to cross from right to left. Running this turnstile for a period of time would result in two specific quantitative changes. First, the concentration of girls will rise in the room on the left and will fall in the room on the right. Similarly, the concentration of boys will rise in the room on the right and go down in the room on the left. The second change is that the total number of people (total of girls and boys) will increase in the party on the left but will decrease in the party on the right (Figure A.4A–C).

To add an additional twist, imagine that for some reason the partygoers' behavior is such that boys don't want to be near too many boys and girls don't want to be near too many girls–both boys and girls have a tendency to want to "spread themselves out" with respect to their gender. If boys or girls are highly concentrated in one area, they have an urge to want to migrate to areas where their concentration is lower. Finally, we will examine what the movement would be of girls and boys if girls-only and boys-only doors are installed in the wall under these conditions, with each type of door opening only briefly allowing only girls or only boys to switch rooms according to the preferences implied by these rules.

You may have already guessed how this analogy is working. The girls are Na^+-ions and the boys are K^+-ions. The turnstile is concentrating girls (or Na^+-ions) on the left side of the wall (the extracellular space) and boys (K^+-ions) on the right side of the wall (the intracellular space). Also, the excess of *people* (remember, both girls and boys have "positive charges" in this analogy) in the party on the left causes a net positive charge on the left side of the wall (or the outside of the cell) because

of the oversupply of both boys and girls on that side (both are "cations") and a net negative charge in the party on the right, or the inside of the cell, due to the relative absence of cations there.

Before we try a momentary opening of the girls-only or boys-only doors in the wall that separates the parties, we will add one more motivating factor. Imagine that there is a hot dog stand in the room on the right. Both boys and girls like hot dogs equally well and are similarly attracted, at least to some extent, to the idea of visiting the hot dog stand. The hot dog stand in this analogy represents an area of negative charge. Because both girls and boys have positive charges, they both feel a similar attraction to the idea of visiting the hot dog stand.

Now we will examine the behavior of girls if we open the girls-only door (Na^+-channels) or boys if we open the boys-only door (K^+-channels) in the separating wall, imagining that each is only opened for a few seconds. As we have set up the analogy, there are two forces in action: first, girls want to stay apart from girls and boys want to stay apart from boys no matter which side of the wall they are on and, second, both girls and boy have an interest in visiting the hot dog stand.

What happens when the girls-only door opens? It is pretty clear that the girls will immediately want to flow through their door from left to right because they have two good reasons to do so. First, there are too many girls present in the party on the left because of the operation of the turnstile, so going through the door will get them to a space where the concentration of girls is lower. This is the equivalent of flowing down a *concentration gradient*. Second, as hungry (positively-charged) people, they have an interest in visiting the (negatively-charged) hot dog stand. This is the equivalent of flowing down an *electrical gradient*. Therefore, in the case of the girls, both the concentration factor and the electrical factor work together to motivate them to go through the door from left to right.

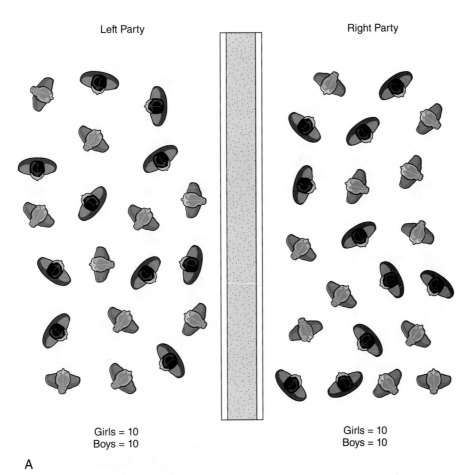

A

Figure A.4 This figure models the neuronal cell membrane by imagining two parties separated by a wall. At the start, each party has ten girls (red) and ten boys (gray) as shown in Figure A.4A. In Figure A.4B, a turnstile has been installed in the wall. It operates such that, for every revolution of the turnstile, three girls are transferred across the wall from left to right and two boys are simultaneously transferred from right to left. The figure shows the results of two revolutions of the turnstile. Now there are 16 girls and 6 boys in the party on the left, and 4 girls and 14 boys in the party on the right. In this party analogy, the girls represent Na^+-ions and the boys represent K^+-ions. Now that the turnstile has operated twice, two observations can be made: first, girls are more concentrated in the party on the left and boys are more concentrated in the party on the right; and second, there are more people in the party on the left (22) and fewer people in the party on the right (18). This corresponds to higher concentration of Na^+ outside the cell and the higher concentration of K^+ inside the cell. Regarding the new imbalance of the total number of partygoers at each party, because all of the "people" carry a positive charge in this example, the operation of the turnstile also creates a net positive charge outside the cell (the party on the left) compared to inside the cell (the party on the right).

In Figure A.4C, two additional changes have been made: there is a new hot dog stand installed in the party on the right—all partygoers are attracted to the hot dog stand to buy hot dogs. The hot dog stand represents negative charge, which will attract all of the ions in this example, Na^+ and K^+ alike, because both are positively charged. The other change is that two doors have been installed in the wall, a boys-only door and a girls-only door which, if opened briefly, will allow either just boys or just girls to flow through the doors in either direction according to their preferences.

There are two forces acting on each partygoer. First, if there is an area of high concentration of girls or boys, each will want to shift position from an area of higher concentration to an area of lower concentration in order to spread themselves out. The second force is that all partygoers have an urge to go toward the hot dog stand.

In this figure, it is clear that girls have two good reasons to cross from left to right if the girls-only door is opened: there are too many girls in the party on the left and the hot dog vendor also attracts them to the party on the right. This is analogous to the two forces, concentration gradient and electrical gradient, acting on Na^+-ions causing them to want to enter the cell when its channel is opened. However, in this example boys have conflicting incentives, wanting to flow from right to left because there are too many boys in the party on the right, but wanting to stay put in the party on the right because they, too, are attracted to the hot dogs there. Similarly, the K^+-ion is subjected to two forces, an urge to flow out of the cell because there is a lower K^+ concentration outside the cell, but also an attraction to stay inside the cell because of the negative charge there. For the case of actual nerve cells, the concentration effect happens to be stronger for K^+ than the electrical effect, which results in K^+ exiting the cell if a K^+-channel is opened.

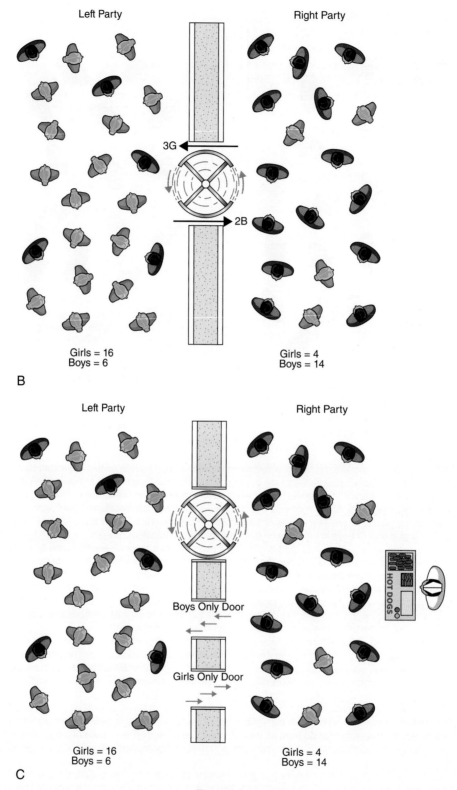

Figure A.4 (cont'd)

As for opening a boys-only door, the situation is more complicated as the boys will have mixed feelings about which direction to go. Because there are many more boys on the right side of the wall, they will have an urge to switch parties from right to left, toward the party where the concentration of boys is lower. On the other hand, there is a hot dog stand in their right-sided party, so they will also feel an urge to stay put on the right side of the wall because of their attraction to hot dogs. In fact, there is no way to predict in this example what the boys will do without a key piece of information: which is stronger for the boys, the urge to spread out or the urge to be near a hot dog stand? Returning to the cell membrane, K⁺-ions are highly concentrated inside the cell and sparser outside the cell, so if a K⁺-channel were opened, they should want to flow out of the cell along their concentration gradient. However, because they are positively charged and the intracellular environment has a negative charge, they should want to remain inside the cell. You cannot figure out the answer to this question unless you know which is greater, the force acting on K⁺-ions to flow out along their concentration gradient or the force urging them to flow inward along their electrical gradient to stay in the negatively charged intracellular space. As it happens, for the neuron the answer is that concentration gradient is a bigger factor for K⁺-ions than the electrical gradient, so when a K⁺-channel opens, K⁺-ions flow out of the cell *along* their concentration gradient but *against* their electrical gradient. Or put another way, for the boys, the hot dog loses.

When a channel specializing in Na⁺ opens in the cell membrane, sodium readily flows into the cell, driven both by its concentration gradient and its electrical gradient. These dual effects on the Na⁺-ion are so strong that, when a Na⁺-channel briefly opens as the first step in an action potential, the inflow of Na⁺-ions is so rapid that the transmembrane voltage shifts toward zero and actually overshoots so that it momentarily becomes positive inside and negative outside. It is only the quick opening of the K⁺-channel that immediately follows, discussed next, that brings the cell membrane back to its baseline, negative-inside polarized state. Figure A.5 summarizes the intracellular and extracellular environments and the forces acting on them for different ions.

Consider what might happen when a K⁺-channel opens. The concentration gradient force would attract K⁺-ions to flow from the inside to the outside of the cell, toward the space where the K⁺ concentration is very low. As discussed above, electrical forces would simultaneously provide an attraction for them to stay inside the cell, but the electrical effect is overwhelmed by the concentration effect resulting in a net outflow of K⁺-ions. Thus, when the K⁺-channel opens, there is a shift of positivity toward the outside of the cell, and the membrane repolarizes with the inner membrane regaining its negative charge. The opening of K⁺-channels can be thought of as restabilizing the cell membrane, allowing it to regain its resting polarized state. The quick depolarization and repolarization of the cell membrane seen with the action potential is therefore mediated by the quick opening and closing of Na⁺-channels followed immediately by the quick opening and closing of K⁺-channels. The ionic currents that cause an action potential to be seen as rippling past a specific location on the cell membrane are summarized in Figure A.6.

Chloride (Cl⁻) Ions

Although they were not part of the partygoer analogy above and are not directly involved in the firing of the action potential, chloride ions (Cl⁻) also play an important part in changes in membrane voltage. Cl⁻ happens to be far more abundant outside the cell compared to inside. Because of this steep

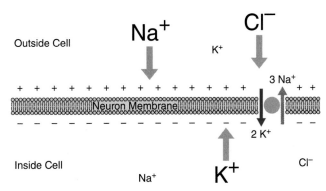

Figure A.5 A reminder of the net ionic forces that are acting across the membrane. First, the Na⁺/K⁺ pump works to concentrate Na⁺ ions outside the cell and K⁺ ions inside the cell. Because of the uneven 3:2 ratio of the Na⁺/K⁺ exchange, a net negativity develops inside the cell membrane and a corresponding positivity develops on the outside. Because of the action of the pump, if given the opportunity, the sodium ions outside the cell would want to rush inside the cell. Likewise, highly concentrated potassium ions inside the cell, if able, would exit the cell (the "concentration effect" that draws them out of the cell is greater than the "electrical effect" that tries to hold them in). Finally, chloride ions are considerably more abundant outside the cell and, if a chloride channel opens, those ions would flow into the cell making the membrane charge yet more negative and stabilized.

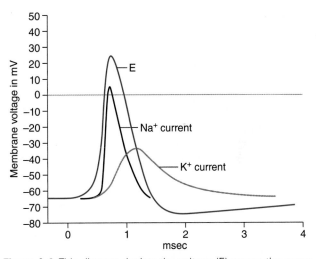

Figure A.6 This diagram depicts the voltage (E) across the neuronal cell membrane during an action potential (the red curve) and how Na⁺ and K⁺ currents contribute to its shape (black and gray curves). The red curve shows the voltage as it would be measured by a voltmeter placed across the membrane. The Na⁺ currents and K⁺-currents created by the opening of their respective channels are shown in black and gray, respectively. The initial rapid upswing of the voltage curve is initiated by the opening of Na⁺-channels which allows sodium ions to flow into the cell, depolarizing the membrane so rapidly that the transmembrane voltage briefly enters positive territory (voltages are measured relative to the inside of the cell). Soon after, potassium channels open, allowing K⁺-ions to flow out of the cell, repolarizing and even hyperpolarizing the cell membrane for a period of time before it returns to its resting negative potential. Note that the complete duration of the action potential is less than 2 milliseconds.

concentration gradient, opening a chloride channel causes Cl^- ions to rush into the cell (along its large concentration gradient but against its smaller electrical gradient), hyperpolarizing the membrane. Thus, opening a Cl^- channel has a stabilizing, *inhibitory* effect on the nerve cell membrane. The segregation of the different ions, Na^+, K^+, and Cl^- is made easier to remember by recalling the typical levels for these ions in serum, which can be seen to represent the extracellular space. Na^+ levels hover around 140, K^+ around 5, and Cl^- around 100 mEq/L, a good reminder of the distribution of these ions.

VOLTAGE-GATED CHANNELS PROPAGATE THE ACTION POTENTIAL

The quick opening of Na^+-channels followed by the quick opening of K^+-channels causes a momentary depolarization and repolarization at one spot on the cell surface, but the next question is, what causes this spot depolarization (the action potential) to move down the axon? Also, what makes the Na^+-channel open in the first place? The answer to both of these questions is explained by the fact that the Na^+-channel in question is *voltage-gated*. As its name implies, the voltage-gated Na^+-channel is triggered to open by anything that causes a significant dip in the membrane voltage (usually about –70 mV at rest) in its vicinity to fall under a certain *threshold voltage* level (usually around –50 mV or less). Any factor that causes the resting membrane voltage to depolarize below threshold voltage will trip open the voltage-gated Na^+-channels in the area of that depolarization. Of course, opening a Na^+-channel in an area of the membrane will cause a dramatic depolarization in that area, well below the threshold voltage (much bigger than, for instance, a single EPSP might cause). This causes the adjacent voltage-gated Na^+-channels to open in turn, a phenomenon that occurs in a repeated fashion down the cell membrane like a domino effect. Thus, voltage-gating is the key to how action potentials propagate down nerve cell membranes. If there is an initial opening of Na^+-channels at a certain location on the cell membrane, a large depolarization will occur in that area. This local depolarization is then sensed by adjacent Na^+-channels, which are then also triggered to open, causing Na^+-channels adjacent to them in turn to open, and so on, creating the ripple of depolarization that travels down the cell membrane that is the action potential.

Recapping the situation, for voltage-gated channels, if the membrane voltage is nudged just a little bit downward, say from –70 mV to –60 mV, nothing more happens—the channel remains in its closed, resting state. But if the nudge is big enough to bring the membrane voltage below the threshold voltage, this is the signal for the Na^+-channel to open, resulting in a torrent of sodium ions entering the cell, depolarizing the cell membrane completely in that area so much so that it is momentarily positive on the inside. In the action potential sequence, the K^+-channel opens close on its heels, which returns the membrane voltage to its resting, negative-inside state at that location. Adjacent voltage-gated Na^+-channels sense this nearby dramatic depolarization and

are triggered to open, too, causing a cascade of sequential Na^+-channel openings down the axon. This wave of depolarization propagates down the axon, comprising the action potential (as was depicted in Figure A.2).

It is important to keep in mind that this whole process of depolarization (mediated by the Na^+-channels) and repolarization (mediated by the K^+-channels) occurs very quickly, taking about 1 millisecond. The fact that the electrical "blip" of an action potential as might be measured by a stationary electrode over a point in an axon would only last about 1 ms will be important to consider later when asking whether EEG waves, or even spikes in the EEG, could represent action potentials. Note that in the EEG images shown in this text, one vertical division on the EEG page represents 1 second, implying that action potential spikes, if they were visible in the EEG, would have a width of one thousandth of the width of one of those vertical divisions. In fact, the action potential is much quicker and shorter than the fastest epileptic spikes we see in patients' recordings (not to mention the abundant slower waves). In the end, the action potential is not the answer to the question of what generates the EEG.

THE ANSWER: EPSPS AND IPSPS

The EEG signal we record on our EEG machines represents a summation of excitatory postsynaptic potentials (EPSPs) and inhibitory postsynaptic potentials (IPSPs), in particular as they impact the cell bodies and apical dendrites of pyramidal neurons that are near the scalp (Figure A.7) as explained below. Part of the explanation for why EEG waves recorded at the scalp look the way they do is related to the microscopic anatomical arrangement of how these pyramidal neurons are oriented in the cortex. Many large pyramidal cells are situated near the cortical surface, their axons travelling generally perpendicular to but away from the scalp. These pyramidal neurons accept many inputs, some excitatory and some inhibitory, in the form of large numbers of axons from other neurons that synapse on their cell bodies and dendrites. Each of these axons produces just one type of neurotransmitter, and that neurotransmitter may be either excitatory or inhibitory, as described below.

EPSPs are produced when the axon synapsing on the pyramidal cell uses a neurotransmitter that opens channels that *depolarize* the pyramidal cell membrane, generally by allowing the flow of positively charged ions into the cell. Glutamate is the best-known excitatory neurotransmitter and there are many classes of glutamate receptors on the neuronal membrane that specialize in binding glutamate. When a glutamate receptor on the pyramidal cell (which is the "postsynaptic" membrane in this case) binds glutamate, cations (such as Ca^{++} or Na^+) are briefly allowed to flow into the cell, partially depolarizing the membrane, bringing it closer to the threshold potential. This small "blip" of decreased negativity that the delivery of a packet of glutamate produces inside the cell membrane is an EPSP (see Figure A.3). If enough of these small "blips" (EPSPs) arrive at the same time, the membrane can be depolarized past the threshold voltage causing the voltage-gated Na^+-channels to open triggering an action potential to fire.

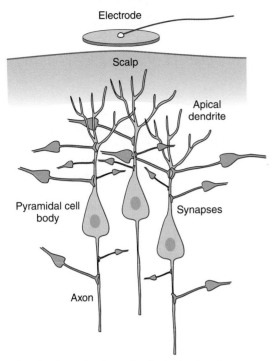

Figure A.7 A schematic of a scalp electrode placed over a group of pyramidal cell neurons. Note that, in general, pyramidal cell neurons are oriented in a parallel fashion and perpendicular to the scalp surface, with the apical dendrites of these neurons nearest the scalp. A large number of axons arriving from other neurons (e.g., interneurons) impinge on these pyramidal cell neurons, (shown with darker red cell bodies)and especially on their apical dendrites. The overlying scalp electrode summates the electrical activity that it detects below it. When, for example, a large amount of excitatory activity is occurring (i.e., EPSPs), Na+-channels are opened which causes a net shift of positive charge into the cells which is detected by the overlying scalp electrode as new net negativity in the extracellular space.

Conversely, other axons synapsing on the pyramidal cell release inhibitory neurotransmitters (e.g., GABA) which open Cl⁻ (chloride) channels. When Cl⁻ channels open (at least after the newborn period), because of chloride's concentration gradient (plentiful outside the cell and scarcer inside the cell), Cl⁻ tends to flow into the cell, making the inside voltage yet more negative, drawing it farther away from the threshold voltage and making it less likely that an action potential will fire. Many of the drugs used in the treatment of patients with epilepsy such as barbiturates (e.g., phenobarbital, pentobarbital) or benzodiazepines (e.g., diazepam, lorazepam, midazolam, clobazam) also work by opening chloride channels. Opening potassium channels will also increase the inside negativity of the nerve cell, as discussed above. Because these inhibitory neurotransmitters cause potentials that *hyperpolarize* the membrane bringing the voltage farther away from the threshold voltage that would trigger an action potential, these potentials are called inhibitory postsynaptic potentials

or IPSPs—they have the effect of making it less likely that the membrane voltage will fall below threshold causing an action potential to fire, even if there are some EPSPs occurring nearby.

Now, imagine a recording scalp electrode and the example of a number of EPSPs occurring on pyramidal cells and their dendrites just under its location on the scalp surface. As described above, the EPSP is associated with positive charge flowing into the cell (Ca⁺⁺ or Na⁺-channels open allowing these cations to disappear into the cell). The cell membrane effectively acts as an insulator, so scalp electrodes are only recording electrical activity from the extracellular space. From the scalp electrode's point of view, this net disappearance of positive charges into the cell looks like the appearance of a new net negativity. For that reason, EPSPs occurring near the scalp surface are most often seen as negative events by scalp recording electrodes. This is why the large majority of epileptic spikes, which can be considered an example of over-excitation, have negative polarity when measured from the scalp.

At this point you may wondering how it is that negative-polarity epileptic spikes might be recorded at the scalp without seeing their counterbalancing positivities. It is indeed the case that, if positive ions are entering the cell in one location (e.g., near the scalp surface), they must be exiting the cell somewhere else. As it happens, this counterbalancing efflux of positive charge occurs farther down the cell's axis, creating a complete current loop that balances charge, but at a location farther from the recording EEG electrode. Thus, the recording electrode does not "see" this part of the story because it occurs, on average, deeper to the scalp. Therefore, when recording the negativities associated with EPSPs from the scalp, we often do not see the deeper counterbalancing positivity. This is an example of the so-called *radially-oriented dipole* seen with most epileptic spikes—negativity on the scalp and positivity deep and distant and unmeasured by the recording electrode (radial and other dipoles are discussed further in Chapter 10, "The EEG in Epilepsy").

Of course, a single EPSP or IPSP, whatever its location, will not make a big difference in the EEG recording. However, when excitatory (or inhibitory) influences are synchronized, the recording electrode effectively summates the positivities and negativities going on below it, especially those nearest the scalp surface, displaying these voltage changes for us as an EEG wave. Thus, the EEG waves we interpret represent, for the most part, the summation of all of the EPSPs and IPSPs occurring on the cell bodies and especially the apical dendrites of the superficial pyramidal cell layer below the recording electrode. This electrical summation is facilitated by the fact that the pyramidal cells are oriented so that their apical dendrites are perpendicular to the cortical surface, as we saw in Figure A.7.

INDEX

Note: Page numbers followed by "*b*" indicate boxes, "*f*" indicate figures, "*t*" indicate tables.